INTRODUCTION.

It is not always, in the present state of our knowledge, that we can give absolute, characteristic contrasts.

It is easy to differentiate where remedies diverge ; but difficult to nicely discriminate where similar remedies converge, until their symptoms are almost identical ; and yet, just here individualization is most needed.

Failures arise first from defective judgment ; secondly from imperfect provings , thirdly from imperfect clinical reports ; fourthly from an imperfect comprehension of what symptoms should be compared.

Symptoms of minor import in the study of a drug in an individual may become quite characteristic when employed in comparison. Thus, *Belladonna* causes tonsilitis tending towards suppuration. This is certainly of less moment than the color, side and difficulty in swallowing water. But when compared with a medicine like *Apis*, which seldom causes suppuration of the tonsils, the contrast proves serviceable.

But with all their errors and imperfections, the comparisons have one use to perform—the main purpose for which they were transferred from private papers, intended for personal discipline, into printed papers. This use is to stimulate the study of Comparative Materia Medica.

We must determine which remedies agree, and which disagree ; we must know why some remedies, though similar in symptoms, are inimical in relation. We must distinguish between medicines, which are antidotes, and others which are complementary. Then we may be better prepared to systematize Materia Medica ; to abridge it without violence and to place it where it belongs, as the crown of science.

E. A. FARRINGTON.

CONTENTS

I. Differentiations of Remedies.—

COMPARISONS IN MATERIA MEDICA
WITH
THERAPEUTIC HINTS

DIFFERENTIATIONS OF SIMILAR REMEDIES

ABSCESSES AND BOILS

[**Remedies.**—*Arn. Ars. Bell. Calc-S. Carb-S. Carb-Veg. Cinch. Hep. Lach. Mag-C. Merc. Phos. Pic-Ac. Sil. Psor. Stram. Sul.*]

Arnica	&	**Silicea**
Crops of boils all over body—begin with soreness and go on to suppuration and are followed by another crop.		Furuncles, or boils which occur in crops and which do not heal readily, but continue to discharge a rather thin, watery (less commonly thick) and even ichorous pus, usually having a foul odor.
Arnica	&	**Kali Iodatum**
See above.		Crops of boils (in summer), which appear on head, chest or back.
Arnica	&	**Picric Acid**
See above.		Crops of pustules on face, which turn into small boils.
Arsenicum	&	**Carbo Vegetabilis**
When abscesses and boils become gangrenous with cutting, lancinating pains and extreme restlessness.		With burning pain like *Ars.* but without restlessness.
Belladonna	&	**Hepar**
Sudden violent symptoms : radiating redness, throbbing and tendency to suppuration—pus develops with lightning-like rapidity.		Indicated after *Bell.* when it fails to reduce the inflammation before suppuration commences, with sharp, throbbing, sticking pains and chills.
Hepar	&	**Mercurius**
See above.		Indicated after *Hep.* when pus has already been formed.

ABSCESSES AND BOILS *(contd.)*—

Mercurius & **Silicea**

See above.

Indicated after *Merc.* when the abscess has discharged and refuses to heal; pus keeps on forming and grows dark and fetid.

Phosphorus & **Silicea**

Abscesses with fistulous openings. Patients with irritable weakness.

Abscesses with fistulous openings. Patients with nutritive disturbances.

Silicea & **Sulphur**

See above.

When the benefit under *Sil.* ceases, an interpolation of a dose or two is necessary to rejuvenate the action of *Sil.*

APOPLEXY

[**Remedies.**—*Ap. Arn. Bar-C. Bell. Brom. Caust. Glon. Hell. Hyos. Lach. Op. Rhus-T. Stront-C. Tab. Verat-Vir.*]

Belladonna & **Lachesis**

In the initial stage, before the Paralysis sets in. The patient often starts from his heavy sleep, cries out, grinds his teeth, awakens frightened. Pulse is usually strong.

Indicated after *Bell.* when the pulse becomes quicker and more feeble and Paralysis is impending; head is hot, the face red, feet cold and the surface heat is irregularly distributed.

Belladonna & **Opium**

See above.

Indicated after *Bell.* Deep-red face. Stertorous breathing, convulsions. Tetanic rigidity of the body.

Hyoscyamus & **Lachesis**

Apoplexy, associated with convulsions.

See above.

Hyoscyamus & **Opium**

See above.

See above.

Lachesis & **Baryta Carb.**

Apoplexy in drunkards. See also above.

Apoplexy in drunkards with trembling of the limbs and well-marked Paralysis of the tongue.

Lachesis & **Opium**

Apoplexy in drunkards. See also above.

Apoplexy in drunkards. See above.

APOPLEXY *(contd.)*—

Lachesis	&	**Arnica**
Apoplexy followed by Paralysis. See also above.		Apoplexy associated with Hemiplegia or Paralysis, < left side. Pulse full and strong. Stertorous breathing. Aching soreness all over body.
Lachesis	&	**Baryta Carb.**
Apoplexy followed by Paralysis. See also above.		Followed by more or less severe Paralysis, *esp.* in old people. The patient is childish and has loss of memory. See also above.
Opium	&	**Apis**
See above.		Indicated after *Op.* Complete stupor or coma.

ASTHMA

[**Remedies.**—*Apis. Aral-R. Arg-Nit. Ars. Aur. Bar-C. Brom. Cact. Cad-Sul. Calad. Cap. Carbo-Veg. Cup. Dro. Ferr. Grp. Grin. Ipec. Kali-Bi. Kali-Chl. Lach. Lob. Lyc. Meph. Nat-Hypochlor. Nat-S. Nux-V. Plat. Pothos. Pulma-V. Rumex. Sep. Stict. Stram. Tereb. Yarba-S. Zinc. Zing.*]

Arsenicum	&	**Kali Bich.**
Expectoration is not tenacious.		Expectoration of stringy mucus.
Arsenicum	&	**Ipecacuanha**
The patient is besides himself with anguish.		A sensation, as of constriction of the chest, worse from least motion.
Cuprum	&	**Ipecacuanha**
Constriction of the throat; spasmodic symptoms predominate.		See above.
Drosera	&	**Mephites**
Asthma of the consumptives.		Indicated when *Drosera* fails.
Drosera	&	**Rumex**
Asthma of the consumptives.		Aggravation at 2 A.M.
Drosera	&	**Sticta**
Asthma of the consumptives.		Associated with splitting headache.
Ipecacuanha	&	**Lobelia**
See above.		A weak sensation in the epigastrium, which spreads up in the chest.

ASTHMA *(contd.)*—

Nux Vomica & **Zingiber**

Nux Vomica: Asthma of gastric origin; worse after a meal, after 12 o'clock at night, in the morning and always increased by cold air or any exertion, particularly when ascending a height; belching relieves.

Zingiber: Asthma of gastric origin; worse in the night towards morning. The patient has to sit up to breathe, but despite the severity of the paroxysms, there seems to be no anxiety.

BRONCHITIS

[**Remedies.**—*Amm-C. Amm-M. Balsam of Peru. Bry. Calc-P. Cap Carb-An. Carb-V. Dra. Kali-Bi. Kali-C. Lach. Lyc. Nat-A. Phos. Pix-L. Puls. Sang. Sul. Tereb. Yarb-S.*]

Ammonium Carb. & **Ammonium Mur.**

Ammonium Carb.: Heaviness in the chest, associated with *burning*. Coughs continually, but raises either not at all or with difficulty. Suited to fat, lazy and of indolent disposition.

Ammonium Mur.: Fat and sluggish—the legs disproportionately thin. Coldness between the shoulder-blades. Heaviness in the chest—as of a feeling of a lump in the chest, but without burning. Cough violent, during which the mouth is filled with saliva.

Carbo Animalis & **Carbo Vegetabilis**

Carbo Animalis: Suffocating hoarse cough producing shaking of the brain, as though the brain were loose in the head.

A cold feeling in the chest.

Expectoration is green, purulent and horribly offensive.

When the patient closes his eyes, he feels, as if he were smothering.

Carbo Vegetabilis: Spasmodic cough, with deep rough voice or aphonia.

Burning in the chest, with a great deal of rattling.

Expectoration, profuse; yellow and more fœtid than *Carb-An.*

Dyspnœa, worse on turning over in bed and dropping off to sleep.

Draconitum & **Balsam of Peru**

Draconitum: Yellowish purulent discharge—at first watery and burning; afterwards, of pus or muco-pus.

Balsam of Peru: The discharge is thick, creamy and yellowish-white muco-pus. *Loud rāles in the chest.*

Draconitum & **Pix Liquida**

Draconitum: See above.

Pix Liquida: Purulent expectoration, offensive in odor and taste. *Pain in the left bronchus.*

BRONCHO-PNEUMONIA

[**Remedies.**—*Acon. Ant-T. Bar-C. Chel. Hep. Ipec. Jab. Kali-C. Lyc. Phos. Sul. Tereb.*]

Aconite & **Antimonium Tartaricum**

Aconite: In the initial stage. High fever, with anxiety and restlessness, till the exudation has began.

Antimonium Tartaricum: Indicated after *Acon.* when the case begins in the right side, with great oppression and sharp, stitching pains in the chest and high fever. Mucous rāles are heard distinctly in the chest. Loose rattling mucus.

Aconite & **Ipecacuanha**

Aconite: See above.

Ipecacuanha: Indicated after *Acon.* Mucous rāles all through chest, both anteriorly and posteriorly. Spasmodic cough, usually attended with vomiting of mucus. There may be fever and the child may have difficulty in breathing.

Broncho-pneumonia or the capillary Bronchitis of infants caused by a warm, moist atmosphere. In such cases it often precedes *Ant-T.*

Antimonium Tartaricum & **Lycopodium**

Antimonium Tartaricum: See above.

Lycopodium: Loud rāles are heard all through the affected parts. The expectoration is thick and yellowish and there is fan-like motion of alæ-nasi.

Antimonium Tartaricum & **Sulphur**

Antimonium Tartaricum: See above.

Sulphur: When *Ant-T.* apparently well-indicated fails to control the symptoms. Loud rāles are heard all through the chest, *esp.* in the left lung. Atelectasis.

Ipecacuanha & **Antimonium Tartaricum**

Ipecacuanha: See above.

Antimonium Tartaricum: Indicated after *Ipec.* The cough grows less and less frequent—the chest is so filled with mucus, that the child cannot cough. He grows more and more drowsy.

Ipecacuanha & **Phosphorus**

Ipecacuanha: See above.

Phosphorus: Indicated after *Ipec.* when the inflammatory symptoms increase and Pneumonia supervenes.

CARBUNCLE

[**Remedies.**—*Anthrac. Ap. Ars., Canth. Carb-V. Hyos. Kali-Bi. Lach. Naja. Nit-Ac. Phyt. Rhus-T. Sec. Sil. Tar-C.*]

Arsenicum & **Anthracinum**

Pepper-box-like openings and dipping deeply into the cellular tissues. Cutting, lancinating, burning pains with *agg.* after midnight ; > by heat.

It has precisely the same symptoms as *Ars.* but to a more intense degree.

Arsenicum & **Carbo Vegetabilis**

See above.

The affected parts are bluish or livid and the discharges are offensive, with burning pains, but without restlessness.

Arsenicum & **Lachesis**

See above.

The surrounding area is swollen and purplish or blackish. Pus forms very slowly. Carbuncle near spine.

Arsenicum & **Phytolacca**

See above.

Lancinating jerking pains.

Arsenicum & **Secale**

See above.

> by cold.

Carbo Vegetabilis & **Arsenicum**

Without restlessness.

Most extreme restlessness.

Carbo Vegetabilis & **Silicea**

See above.

Non-malignant. Carbuncles between the shoulder and nape of neck.

Lachesis & **Hyoscyamus**

See above.

The patient is extremely nervous. Coma vigil, etc.

Lachesis & **Nitric Acid**

See above.

Hæmorrhagic tendency. Hæmorrhage, on slightest touch or without any touch.

Rhus Tox. & **Arsenicum**

Indicated in the beginning. The affected parts are dark-red. Red streaks or black.

Follows *Rhus-Tox.* See also above.

Rhus Tox. & **Carbo Vegetabilis**

See above.

Follows *Rhus-Tox.* See also above.

CARBUNCLE *(contd.)*—

Tarantula Cubensis &	**Arsenic**
Atrocious pains associated with great prostration and diarrhœa. Intermitting fever of evening exacerbation.	See above.
Tarantula Cubensis &	**Lachesis**
See above.	See above.
Tarantula Cubensis &	**Silicea**
See above.	See above.

CHOLERA

[**Remedies.**—*Arg-N. Ars. Cam. Carb-V. Colch. Cup. Eup-C. Hydr-Ac. Iris. Jat. Lach. Pod. Sec. Sul. Tab. Verat-A.*]

Arsenicum &	**Secale**
Restlessness prominent ; irritability of fibre. The patient wants to be warmly wrapped up. Rice-water stool.	*Tingling* or *formication all over the body.* The patient though cold, cannot bear to be covered ; wants to be cool. Stool copious—comes in spurt.
Camphor &	**Carbo Vegetabilis**
Intense prostration before any vomiting and purging. Indicated in the initial stage.	Prostration as the result of the drain on the system, by alvine discharge. Indicated in the later stage.
Carbo Vegetabilis &	**Secale**
The patient lies quiet—too weak to move, with passive hæmorrhage from the nose and bowels. The pulse is rapid, almost thread-like and intermittent.	Spasmodic twitching of the muscles of the various parts of the body ; the spreading asunder of the fingers. Almost pulseless. See also above.
Euphorbia Corrollata &	**Jatropha Curcas**
The patient wants to die ; cold sweat all over the body.	The vomited matters look like rice-water or the white of an egg. Purging like water from a hydrant. Cramps in the calves and coldness of the body.
Hydrocyanic Acid &	**Camphor**
Marked collapse, with sudden cessation of all discharges, as purging and vomiting.	Collapse before the purging and vomiting begin or with scanty discharges. See also above.

CHOLERA *(contd.)*—

Veratrum Album	&	**Arsenicum**
Cold sweat on the forehead—more marked. Restlessness—less marked. Stool—copious.		Cold sweat on the forehead—less marked. Restlessness—more marked. Stool—lesser in quantity than the other. See also above.
Veratrum Album	&	**Iris Versicolor**
Coldness of the body; collapse. See also above.		Absence of coldness and symptoms of collapse. Comes preferably at 2 or 3 o'clock in the morning.
Veratrum Album	&	**Podophyllum**
Sharp cutting pains in the abdomen. See also above.		Absence of pain. Stools liable to vary in color; come out with a gush and a splutter, like water from a hydrant.
Veratrum Album	&	**Secale**
Cold sweat on the forehead.		See above.
Veratrum Album	&	**Tabacum**
See above.		Nausea, accompanied by burning heat about the abdomen, the rest of the body being cold. The patient persists in uncovering the abdomen.

COLIC

[**Remedies.**— *Acon. Æth-C. Alumina. Bell. Bor. Bov. Caust. Cham. Cin. Cist. Coloc. Crot-T. Cup. Cycl. Dulc. Ipec. Lyc. Mag-C. Nux-V. Op. Plat. Plum. Rhus-T. Staph. Verat-A. Zinc.*]

Belladonna	&	**Colocynth**
Sharp pains, suddenly screaming out and bending *backward.*		Bending forward.
Chamomilla	&	**Colocynth**
In emotional colic—Hot face, red cheeks and hot perspiration.		In emotional colic—The severe pains cause the patient to double up for relief.
Colocynth	&	**Aconite**
The pains are atrocious; griping, cutting, etc. Force him to bend double or to press firmly against the abdomen, which gives him relief.		Inflammatory colic, which forces the patient to bend double, without any relief.

COLIC *(contd.)*—

Colocynth	&	**Bovista**
See above.		Finds relief from bending double and after eating. Red urine.
Colocynth	&	**Castoreum**
Nervous colic—griping. See also above.		Relief from pressure. Nervous colic with pallor, cold sweat and sudden loss of strength.
Colocynth	&	**Croton Tiglium**
See above.		Better from warm drinks.
Colocynth	&	**Magnesia Carb.**
See above.		Draws the limbs up to relieve the colic, frequently relieved by motion.
Colocynth	&	**Staphisagria**
In emotional colic. See also above.		In emotional colic— Crampy pains in the abdomen. Also complementary to *Colocynth,* stepping in to complete the cure when *Colocynth* is insufficient.
Colocynth	&	**Veratrum Album**
See above.		Forces the patient to bend double, but he must walk about for relief. Cold sweat on the forehead.
Cuprum	&	**Aconite**
Inflammatory colic, with a combination of neurotic with inflammatory symptoms.		See above.
Cyclamen	&	**Veratrum Album**
Flatulent colic arising from wind in the bowels, coming on at night, and relieved only by getting up and walking about.		See above.
Opium	&	**China**
Great deal of belching without relief.		Belching gives but temporary relief. Debility.
Opium	&	**Lycopodium**
Pressure downward on the rectum and bladder.		Sour taste with its belching. The flatulence tends upwards rather than downwards.

COLIC *(contd.)*—

Opium & **Nux Vomica**

Opium: See above.

Nux Vomica: Pressure *either* upward towards the chest, producing inconvenience in breathing, or downward towards the rectum and bladder, developing both urging to stool and desire to urinate.

Opium & **Veratrum Album**

Opium: See above.

Veratrum Album: Colic, as if the bowels were twisted ; abdomen tense. The longer delayed is the emission of flatus, the more difficult is it to pass.

Rhus Tox. & **Colocynth**

Rhus Tox.: The pain is relieved by bending double and *moving about.* Pains tearing down the thighs during stool.

Colocynth: The pain is relieved by bending double, but not from motion, although the severity of the pain may drive the patient to move about.

DIARRHŒA

[**Remedies.**—*Acon. Aloes. Als-S. Ant-C. Apis. Apoc. Aran. Arg-N. Arn. Ars. Bell. Bor. Bry. Calc-O. Calc-P. Cast. Cham. Cin. Cof. Colch. Crot. Dio. Dulc. Elaps. Elat. Eup-C. Ferr. Ferr-Ph. Gam. Gel. Ger. Grp. Grat. Hep. Iod. Ipec. Iris. Kali-Bi. Kali-Br. Lach. Lep. Lil-T. Lith-C. Mag-C. Merc. Nat-C. Nat-M. Nat-S. Nit-Ac. Nuph. Nux-V. Œno. Oln. Op. Opun. Paul. Pet. Phos. Phos-Ac. Pic-Ac. Pod. Psor. Puls. Rheum. Rhus-T. Rumex. Sil. Staph. Stram. Stront-C. Sul. Sul-Ac. Thuj. Verat-A.*]

Apis & **Bryonia**

Apis: Morning diarrhœa ; at every motion of the body the bowels move, as though the sphincter ani had no power.

Bryonia: Morning diarrhœa ; comes on as soon as the patient begins to move about.

Apocynum & **Aloes**

Apocynum: Stools, copious, yellow, watery and brownish ; contain undigested food and discharge with an expulsive force, like a cork from a bottle.

Aloes: Stools contain a jelly-like mucus, apt to be worse in the morning ; great prostration after stool. Colic—relieved by bending double.

DIARRHŒA *(contd.)*—

Apocynum & **Gamboge**

See above.

The stool is expelled all at once, after considerable urging and is followed by great relief; is preceded by excessive cutting about the navel.

Argentum Nitricum & **Cinchona**

The bowels move as soon as the patient drinks.

Diarrhœa after eating.

Argentum Nitricum & **Ferrum**

See above.

Diarrhœa as soon as the patient attempts to drink.

Argentum Nitricum & **Gelsemium**

Diarrhœa from great excitement, especially when the imagination has been played upon.
Diarrhœa from anticipation.

Diarrhœa appearing *suddenly* from excitement or the anticipation of some trying ordeals.

Arsenicum & **Cinchona**

Lienteric Diarrhœa—profuse; comes on during or after eating (more after than during); worse after midnight. Intense thirst.

Lienteric Diarrhœa—worse at night or after eating. Debilitating.

Arsenicum & **Ferrum**

Burning pain. See also above.

Lienteric Diarrhœa—without pain; apt to occur during meals.

Borax & **Mercurius**

Diarrhœa preceded by colic; associated with aphthous sore-mouth; mucous membrane around these aphthœ bleeds easily.

Diarrhœa accompanied by well-marked tenesmus; attended with sore-mouth with profuse salivation; water dribbles from the mouth.

Borax & **Staphisagria**

See above.

Diarrhœa associated with stomacace; cutting pains before and after stool, with a great deal of tenesmus of the rectum during stool and escape of flatus.

Bryonia & **Natrum Sulph.**

Morning Diarrhœa—comes on as soon as the patient begins to move about. Aggravated by hot weather. Less flatus.

Associated with a great deal of flatus.

DIARRHŒA *(contd.)*—

Bryonia	&	**Sulphur**
See above.		Morning Diarrhœa, hurrying the patient out of the bed.
Calcarea Ostrearum	&	**Castoreum**
Stools—greenish, more or less watery and sour.		Watery or greenish mucous stcols, with burning in the anus ; cutting colic before stool, better from pressure or bending double ; cutting about the navel.
Castoreum	&	**Gamboge**
See above.		Stools expel all at once, after considerable urging. See also above.
Chamomilla	&	**Bryonia**
Diarrhœa after anger. The symptoms are associated with *heat*. The face is pale with one cheek red. Tongue yellow.		Diarrhœa after anger. The symptoms are associated with chilliness. Tongue white.
Chamomilla	&	**Colocynth**
Soreness of the stomach, with soreness of the anus.		Colic relieved by bending double or from firm pressure.
Chamomilla	&	**Mercurius**
See above.		Much tenesmus.
Chamomilla	&	**Podophyllum**
See above.		Diarrhœa worse in the morning ; comes with a gush.
Cinchona	&	**Ferrum**
Worse at night or after eating ; attended with rapid exhaustion and emaciation.		Apt to occur during the meal.
Cinchona	&	**Iris Versicolor**
See above.		Lienteric Diarrhœa—associated with vomiting. The patient is worse at about 2 or 3 o'clock in the morning.
Cinchona	&	**Lachesis**
See above.		The abdomen is bloated ; very sensitive to touch about the waist.
Cinchona	&	**Oleander**
See above.		Lienteric diarrhœa ; the patient passes in his stools the food which he had eaten the day before.

DIARRHŒA *(contd.)*—

Cinchona & **Phosphoric Acid**

See above.

The stools are copious and frequent, but not attended with much debility.

Cinchona & **Podophyllum**

See above.

Gushing diarrhœa, comes in the morning, more during the day than at night.

Cinchona & **Strontiana Carb.**

See above.

Worse at night—the patient is scarcely off the vessel before he has to return. Better towards morning at 3 or 4 o'clock.

Colocynth & **Croton Tiglium**

Diarrhœa with griping, cutting, colicky pains, *relieved by bending over* or *from firm pressure.*

Movements are profuse and watery and gushing like water from a hydrant.

Colocynth & **Dioscorea**

See above.

Diarrhœa with griping colicky pains, *relieved by bending backwards.* The pains are apt to fly off to other parts of the body.

Croton Tiglium & **Euphorbia Corollata**

Colic better from warm drinks. See also above.

Mental state: the patient wants to die—is more marked.

Croton Tiglium & **Jatropha Curcas**

Nausea of a very aggravating character; attended by faintness and loss of sight.

Vomited matters look like rice-water, or the white of an egg.

Elaterium & **Croton Tiglium**

Olive-green stools.

Brownish-green stools.

Gelsemium & **Opium**

Diarrhœa from fright—the stools are copious, yellow and papescent. The tongue is coated white or yellowish.

Diarrhœa from fright—the image of the thing which caused the fright constantly appears before the mind.

Gelsemium & **Pulsatilla**

See above.

Diarrhœa from fright—the stools are greenish-yellow and slimy, or very changeable in color and worse at night; trembling; weeping.

DIARRHŒA *(contd.)*—

Gelsemium & **Veratrum Album**

See above.

Diarrhœa from fright—*cold sweat on the forehead.*

Geranium & **Œnothera**

Constant desire to go to stool, with inability for sometime to pass any faecal matter—then the bowels move without pain or effort ; mouth dry ; tip of the tongue burning.

Exhausting watery Diarrhœa —the evacuations are without effort and are accompanied by nervous exhaustion.

Hepar & **Calcarea Ostrearum**

Diarrhœa with sour stools ; worse during the day and after eating. The whole patient smells sour.

See above.

Hepar & **Magnesia Carb.**

See above.

Diarrhœa with characteristically sour stools—green and slimy ; preceded by much griping and rumbling in the bowels ; stools—like scum on a frog pond ; milk disagrees, causes pain in the stomach or passes undigested ; colic relieved by drawing the limbs or by motion.

Hepar & **Rheum**

See above.

Diarrhœa with sour stools—frequent, brown and frothy ; attended with a great deal of straining and violent pains.

Ipecacuanha & **Paullinia**

Diarrhœa with green stools.

Diarrhœa with profuse green stools, but odorless.

Leptandra & **Mercurius**

Urging to stool, griping colicky pains continue after stool.

Tenesmus continue after stool.

Magnesia Carb. & **Calcarea Ostrearum**

See above.

Sweat on the head, face and scalp ; damp and cold feet ; and enlargement of the abdomen.

Magnesia Carb. & **Colocynth**

Green, slimy stools.

See above.

Magnesia Carb. & **Chamomilla**

More deeper-acting than the other. See also above.

Yellowish-green stools, looking like chopped eggs.

DIARRHŒA *(contd.)*—

Magnesia Carb. & **Rheum**

See above.

Griping colic and twitching of the muscles of the face and fingers during sleep.

Nux Vomica & **Colocynth**

Stools scanty and there is frequent ineffectual urging.

See above.

Sulphur & **Dioscorea**

Morning Diarrhœa driving the patient out of the bed; stools change frequently in colour; may be slimy or watery. Soreness at the anus.

Morning Diarrhœa. See also above.

Sulphur & **Kali Bich.**

See above.

Morning Diarrhœa; the stools are watery and is followed by much tenesmus.

Sulphur & **Lilium Tigrinum**

See above.

Morning Diarrhœa, hurrying the patient out of the bed; stools papescent; causes an excoriating feeling at the anus.

Sulphur & **Natrum Sulph.**

See above.

See above.

Sulphur & **Phosphorus**

See above.

Morning Diarrhœa—*painless; green stools.*

Sulphur & **Podophyllum**

See above.

Morning Diarrhœa, driving the patient out of the bed; worse at noon; continues throughout the day.

Sulphur & **Rumex Crispus**

See above.

Morning Diarrhœa hurrying the patient out of the bed; associated with the characteristic cough of *Rumex*.

Veratrum Album & **Iris Versicolor**

Profuse watery stools—greenish, always associated with sharp cutting pains and often with cramps in the legs.

Absence of coldness; the patient is worse at about 2 or 3 o'clock in the night. See also above.

Veratrum Album & **Podophyllum**

See above.

Absence of pain. See above.

DIPHTHERIA

[**Remedies.**—*Ail. Alcohol. Amm-C. Amy. Ant-C. Apis. Ars. Ars-Iod. Arum. Bapt. Bell. Brom. Cam. Cap. Carb-Ac. Carb-V. Crot. Hydr-Ac. Ign. Iod. Kali-Per. Lac-C. Lach. Lyc. Merc-Bin. Merc-Cyan. Merc-Prot. Mur-Ac. Naja. Nat-A. Nit-Ac. Phyt. Ran-S. Rhus-T. Sul-Ac.*]

Apis & Arsenicum

Apis: Insidious advance. The throat has a varnished appearance as though the tonsils and fauces were coated with a glossy varnish. Early prostration. Feverish and drowsy at 3 P.M. Very high fever; pulse ranges from 130 to 140, and is very weak. Membranes form on either tonsil, oftener on the right than on the left and is thick like wash-leather. Often thirstless, in spite of fever. Stinging pain.

Arsenicum: The membrane has a dark hue and is gangrenous and there is fœtor. Thin, excoriating discharge from the nose. Adynamic fever and great somnolence, broken by starts, crying out in sleep and jerking of the limbs. Restlessness, especially after midnight; the urine is scanty and the bowels are either constipated or else there is an offensive Diarrhœa.

Apis & Kali Permanganatum

Apis: See above.

Kali Permanganatum: *Extreme fœtor.* The membrane is horribly offensive.

Apis & Natrum Arsenicosum

Apis: See above.

Natrum Arsenicosum: Despite the dark purplish hue of the throat, marked swelling and great prostration, there is not much pain.

Arsenicum & Arsenicum Iodatum

Arsenicum: See above.

Arsenicum Iodatum: Marked enlargement of the lymphatic glands.

Arum Triphyllum & Ailanthus

Arum Triphyllum: The throat is extremely sore and is covered with membrane, either, dark and offensive, or else, yellowish-white. The mouth is studded with ulcers, which appear principally on the inside of the cheeks, on the lips, and on the borders of the tongue. This ulceration is accompanied by salivation which is watery and very acrid. Great prostration. Restless tossing about.

Ailanthus: Torpidity—the patient becomes drowsy and lies in a profound stupor. Well-marked, excoriating, watery discharge from the nose, making the upper lip sore. Typhoid condition.

DIPHTHERIA *(contd.)*—

Arum Triphyllum	&	**Ammonium Causticum**
See above.		Diphtheria appearing in the nasal cavities, with a burning, excoriating discharge from the nose and great prostration.
Arum Triphyllum	&	**Amygdala Amara**
See above.		Sharp, lancinating pains in the swollen tonsils; the palate and fauces have a dark-red hue.
Arum Triphyllum	&	**Apis**
See above.		See above.
Arum Triphyllum	&	**Arsenicum**
See above.		See above. Indicated in severe cases.
Arum Triphyllum	&	**Baptisia Tinctoria**
See above.		The patient is very much prostrated and lies in a half-stupid state, almost like one intoxicated; the face is dark red and has a besotted look and the discharges from the mouth and nose are horribly offensive. Typhoid condition. Gangrenous tendency of the membrane. Sometimes the patient can swallow only liquids, but ejects solid food at once.
Arum Triphyllum	&	**Belladonna**
See above.		Congestion of the head, before the membrane has formed; violence of the initial symptoms.
Arum Triphyllum	&	**Kali Bichromicum**
See above.		The discharges are decidedly stringy. Pain in the throat extending to the neck and shoulder.
Arum Triphyllum	&	**Kali Permanganatum**
See above.		See above.

DIPHTHERIA *(contd.)*—

Arum Triphyllum & Lachesis

See above.

The membrane forms first on the left tonsil and spreads thence to the right and the *symptoms are worse from empty swallowing* and are often relieved by eating or swallowing solid food ; constant feeling, as of a lump on the left side, which descends with each act of deglutition but returns again. Aggravation after sleep and the throat is sensitive to the touch.

Arum Triphyllum & Lycopodium

See above.

Diphtheritic deposit travels from the right to the left side. The patient is always worse after sleep, even after a short nap. He is cross and irritable. Constant desire to swallow with violent stinging pains. Worse from swallowing drinks, especially cold drinks. Impending paralysis of the brain.

Arum Triphyllum & Mercurius Bin-iodatus

See above.

Inflammation of the left tonsil and formation of yellowish-grey membrane there. The symptoms are worse from empty swallowing, so that the simple attempt to swallow saliva, excites more pain than the swallowing of the food.

Arum Triphyllum & Mercurius Cyanatus

See above.

Membrane at first white ; becomes dark, threatening even to grow gangrenous. *Great weakness ;* blueness of the surface, coldness of the extremities, and weak pulse. The tongue is coated brown or in severe cases, even black. Nose-bleed.

DIPHTHERIA *(contd.)*—

Arum Triphyllum	&	**Mercurius Proto-iodide**
See above.		Deposit forms on the right side of the throat with accumulation of tenacious mucus in the throat. Thick yellow, dirty coating in the base and posterior part of the tongue, the tip and sides being red.
Arum Triphyllum	&	**Muriatic Acid**
See above.		Malignancy, most intense prostration—the patient seems to have scarcely life enough to move. Worse at 10 or 11 o'clock in the morning. The mouth is studded with deep ulcers having dark or black bases. *Involuntary stool and urine.*
Arum Triphyllum	&	**Naja Tripudians**
See above.		Impending paralysis of the heart. The patient is blue—awakes from sleep gasping. Thirst. Intermittent pulse.
Arum Triphyllum	&	**Natrum Arsenicosum**
See above.		Throat dark and purplish, with great swelling and prostration, but without much pain.
Arum Triphyllum	&	**Nitric Acid**
See above.		Great prostration and membranes in the throat and nose; there is distress and uneasiness in the stomach, with total rejection of food.
Arum Triphyllum	&	**Phytolacca**
See above.		Creepy chill and backache in the beginning. The throat dark-red, almost purple. Great burning in the throat, with aggravation from hot drinks. The patient is weak, and feels faint, when he sits up in bed.

DIPHTHERIA *(contd.)*—

Arum Triphyllum & **Rhus Tox.**

Arum Triphyllum: See above.

Rhus Tox.: The membrane is dark in color and bloody saliva runs out of the mouth during sleep. Inflammation of the glands of the neck, of a dark erysipelatous hue.

Cantharis & **Apis**

Cantharis: Severe burning and raw feeling in the throat; great constriction of the throat and larynx, amounting almost to suffocation, on any attempt to swallow water. Dysuria. *Marked debility*—as a sequel.

Apis: Early debility. See also above.

Cantharis & **Capsicum**

Cantharis: See above.

Capsicum: Burning blisters in the roof of the mouth. An odor from the mouth like that of carrion. The patient is worse when not swallowing.

Carbolic Acid & **Kali Permanganatum**

Carbolic Acid: Putridity associated with burning pains in the mouth, to the stomach. Dusky red face, pale about the mouth and nose. Rapid sinking of the vital force.

Kali Permanganatum: Painful throat; soreness of the muscles of the neck.

Carbo Vegetabilis & **Mercurius Cyanatus**

Carbo Vegetabilis: Nose-bleed. The face is pale and sunken and almost hippocratic. The blood flows persistently for hours, even for days; and is dark and rather fluid.

Mercurius Cyanatus: See also above.

Lachesis & **Apis**

Lachesis: See above.

Apis: Œdema of the throat; stinging pains and blisters on the borders of mouth.
See also above.

Lachesis & **Crotalus**

Lachesis: See above.

Crotalus: Persistent epistaxis—the blood oozes from the mouth.

DIPHTHERIA *(contd.)*—

Lachesis & **Lac Caninum**

See above.

Peculiar habit of alternating sides ; starting on one side, frequently the left, the soreness and swelling, and even the membrane, suddenly shift to the opposite side, only to return, in a few hours, to the starting point. The membrane is grayish-yellow and curdy, and if ulcers form they shine like silver-gloss.

Lachesis & **Lycopodium**

See above.

The right side mostly affected, and deposits travel to the left. Aggravation from 4 to 8 P.M. ; invades the nose—the patient cannot breathe through the nose. The child awakes from sleep, frightened or cross and angry. See also above.

Lachesis & **Naja**

See above.

Laryngeal Diphtheria ; the patient gasps at the throat, with a sensation of choking ; the fauces are dark-red ; fœtid breath ; short and hoarse cough with raw feeling in the larynx and upper part of the trachea.

Lachesis & **Nitric Acid**

See above.

A sensation, as of a fishbone, splinter or piece of glass sticking into the throat. Intermittent pulse. The nose is also invaded ; the discharge from the nose is watery and very offensive, excoriating every part it touches ; frequent epistaxis.

See also above.

Lycopodium & **Phytolacca**

See above.

Dark-red throat, worse on the right side. Inability to swallow hot drinks.

DIPHTHERIA *(contd.)*—

Muriatic Acid & **Nitric Acid**

Muriatic Acid

Yellowish-gray deposit. Very fœtid breath. Œdematous uvula. Intermittent pulse, associated with *involuntary stools* and *urine*.

See also above.

Nitric Acid

See above.

DYSENTERY

[**Remedies.**— *Acon. Aloes. Arn. Ars. Bap. Bell. Can. Cap. Carb-V. Cin. Colch. Coloc. Ferr-P. Kali-Bi. Lach. Merc. Nux-V. Rhus-T. Sul. Zinc-S.*]

Aconite & **Mercurius**

Aconite

The stools are scanty, bloody and slimy, with much tenesmus.

Autumnal Dysentery, when warm days are followed by cold nights.

Mercurius

Complementary. Tenesmus continues even after stool.

Cantharis & **Colocynth**

Cantharis

The stools, bloody and slimy and are *mixed with flakes that look like scrapings of the intestine*. The tenesmus is marked and is associated with dysuria.

Colicky pains, doubling the patient up ; they are of cutting, burning, griping, wandering character, which continue even after stools.

Colocynth

The stools may be fluid, copious, fæcal, flatulent, papescent, or slimy and bloody and preceded by severe tenesmus. The evacuations are provoked by the slightest food or drink as also the pain.

The griping colicky pains, relieved by bending double and by pressing firmly against the abdomen ; they are sometimes relieved by the emission of flatus or by stool ; the griping more often precedes the stool and is relieved afterwards, although sometimes it continues even after stool.

DYSENTERY *(contd.)*—

Cantharis & **Capsicum**

See above.

The stools are frequent but small ; bloody and slimy, and contain shaggy pieces ; attended with violent tenesmus and burning in both the rectum and bladder. There is thirst, and yet drinking causes shuddering and increases the pain. The pains and other symptoms are increased by the slightest draft of either warm or cold air.

Suited to flabby and stout persons.

Cantharis & **Colchicum**

See above.

Tympanitic distension of the abdomen. Stools—jelly-like white lumps, followed by violent tenesmus and constriction of the anus, tormenting the patient more than the urging

Cantharis & **Kali Bichromicum**

See above.

Follows *Cantharis ;* though the scrapings continue, the discharges become more jelly-like.

Cantharis & **Sulphur**

See above.

Complementary to *Cantharis,* when bleeding and tenesmus have abated but the stools are slimy with frequent sudden urgings ; or, when tenesmus has ceased but mucus and blood are still discharged.

Tenesmus continues from one evacuation to other.

Cantharis & **Zincum Sulphuricum**

See above.

The pains are referred to the sides of the abdomen.

Carbo Vegetabilis & **Arsenicum**

The abdomen is greatly distended and tympanitic. Burning pains situated deep in the abdomen, usually in one or the other of the bends of the colon. Stools are horribly offensive

Less tympanitic distension of the abdomen. Restlessness ; burning thirst—yet intolerance of water.

DYSENTERY *(contd.)*—

Carbo Vegetabilis & Cinchona

Carbo Vegetabilis: See above.

Cinchona: Discharges from the bowels are of a chocolate color ; horribly offensive ; coldness and great debility. Hectic symptoms. Anæmic symptoms.

Movements from the bowels are provoked by every attempt to eat and drink. Belching gives but temporary relief. The flatus is not so offensive and burning pains also are less marked.

Lachesis & Cinchona

Lachesis: General torpor, with hyperæsthesia of the cutaneous nerves.

Cinchona: Increased general sensibility. Hectic symptoms. Anæmic symptoms.

Lachesis & Kali Bichromicum

Lachesis: Blackish stools. Red, cracked, smooth tongue. The odor of the discharges are horribly offensive.

Kali Bichromicum: The discharges are jelly-like, sometimes mucous.

Nux Vomica & Aloes

Nux Vomica: The stools are bloody, slimy, watery and scanty. Frequent ineffectual urging to stool, ceasing as soon as the bowels move. Aggravation in the morning.

Aloes: The stool consists of blood and mucus (extraordinary quantity). The griping may or may not cease after stool.

Nux Vomica & Mercurius

Nux Vomica: See above.

Mercurius: The urging to stool does not cease with evacuation.

ECZEMA

[**Remedies.**—*Ant.-Cr. Ap. Ars. Bor. Cal-O. Clem. Cur. Grp. Hep. Nit-Ac. Nux-J. Petr. Psor. Ran-B. Rhus-T. Sel. Sep. Staph. Sul. Vio-T.*]

Arsenicum & Clematis

Arsenicum: Vesicles, which turn into pustules and form scabs, with copious scaling and much burning. A dry scaly desquamation.

Clematis: More rawness, *agg.* from washing. Moist, alternating with dry scabs.

Arsenicum & Graphites

Arsenicum: See above.

Graphites: Rough skin. Oozing of a gluous fluid.

ECZEMA *(contd.)*—

Arsenicum See above.	&	**Hydrocotyle Asiatica** Thick and scaly skin. but less burning.
Arsenicum See above.	&	**Kreosotum** Scales pile up into large masses.
Arsenicum See above.	&	**Rhus Toxicodendron** Vesicles on a red erysipelatous surface, chiefly about the genitals and on hairy parts, with itching, *agg.* at night, after scratching and in cold rainy weather.
Arsenicum See above.	&	**Sepia** Peeling follows vesicles, which were not surrounded by very red skin or it follows fine rash, worse about the joints or a circular eruption like harpes circinatus.
Calcarea Ostrearum On the scalp, with a tendency to spread downward, and over the face, forming thick crusts, which are often white, chalk-like deposits.	&	**Arsenicum** Bran-colored scabs on the head, coming down over the forehead. See also above.
Calcarea Ostrearum See above.	&	**Curare** Eczema of infants, worse about the face and behind the ears.
Kreostum Scaly eruption on the extensor surfaces of the limbs.	&	**Natrum Muriaticum** Scaly eruption on flexor surfaces and bends of joints.
Mezereum *Esp.* in scrofulous cases—hard thick, chalky crusts form, which crack and ooze copiously of pus. Itching is more intense at night when the patient is warmly wrapped up. Sometimes pimples surround the seat of the disease.	&	**Rhus-Toxicodendron** See above.

ECZEMA *(contd.)*—

Natrum Muriaticum & Sepia

Natrum Muriaticum

Has a particular affinity for the dorsa of the hand—the skin there becomes rough, dry and chapped.

See also above.

Sepia

With little ulcers about the joints of the hands.

See also above.

Rananculus Bulbosus & Antimonium Crudum

Rananculus Bulbosus

Eczema attended with thickening of the skin and formation of hard horny crusts.

Antimonium Crudum

Horny excrescences or callosities on the soles of feet.

Rhus Tox. & Apis Mellifica

Rhus Tox.

With burning, itching and tingling.

The cutaneous surface about the eruption is red and angry-looking.

If the face is attacked there is swelling of the eye-lids.

See above.

Apis Mellifica

With burning and stinging pains.

A red line marks the spread of the disease.

The eruption is moist, offensive and suppurating, at times impetiginous.

Selenium & Sulphur

Selenium

Tingling in spots.

Itching in the folds of skin and about the joints.

Sulphur

Harsh, rough skin, which very readily breaks out with eruption.

ENURESIS

[**Remedies.**— *Ant-C. Ap. Bell. Benz-Ac. Calc-O. Canth. Caust. Chlorum. Cina. Equi. Eup. Ferr-P. Gels. Grp. Hep. Hyos. Kre. Lina. Lyc. Mur-Ac. Nat-Hyp. Nat-M Op. Phos. Phos-Ac. Plant-M. Puls. Rhus-T. Scil. Sep. Sil. Sul. Zinc.*]

Antimonium Crudum & Lycopodium

Antimonium Crudum

Involuntary with cough day and night.

Enuresis in children who will be neither touched or looked at.

Lycopodium

Involuntary with cough at night ; during typhoid state.

Enuresis in children, who suddenly becomes obstinate.

Apis & Belladonna

Apis

With great irritation of parts, < at night and when coughing.

Urine clear, straw-colored.

Belladonna

Night and day, in girls and scrofulous children.

Urine contains white epithelia.

ENURESIS *(contd.)*—

Apis See above.	&	**Cantharis** After long retention.
Apis See above.	&	**Natrum Muriaticum** Night and day, when coughing, walking or laughing.
Causticum Involuntary, when coughing. Nocturnal enuresis in children during their first sleep. Children weak, weak-minded, totter when walking.	&	**Belladonna** Nocturnal enuresis in nervous children. See also above.
Causticum See above.	&	**Calcarea Ostrearum** Nocturnal enuresis in fat children. Also follows *Bell.*
Causticum See above.	&	**Chloral** Nocturnal enuresis, during the latter part of night.
Causticum See above.	&	**Equisetum** During the latter part of night, *esp.* in women, with urine containing blood and albumen.
Causticum See above.	&	**Ferrum Phos.** During day.
Causticum See above.	&	**Graphites** During the latter part of night.
Causticum See above.	&	**Kreosotum** During the first sleep. The patient urinates, while dreaming of the act. Profuse pale urine.
Causticum See above.	&	**Hepar** Wetting of the bed at night, when the urine voided passes very slowly.
Causticum See above.	&	**Hyoscyamus** In patients with great prostration.

ENURESIS *(contd.)*—

Causticum	&	**Phosphorus**
See above.		At night, in children who correspond to the *Phosphorus*-build ; in children who grow too rapidly.
Causticum	&	**Plantago Major**
See above.		During the latter part of the night. Profuse pale urine.
Causticum	&	**Pulsatilla**
See above.		During the latter part of the night.
Causticum	&	**Scilla**
See above.		Involuntary spurting of urine in old people.
Causticum	&	**Sepia**
See above.		At night, in little girls, during their first sleep.
Causticum	&	**Silicea**
See above.		During the latter part of the night. Also follows *Bell.*
Causticum	&	**Sulphur**
See above.		During the latter part of the night. Also follows *Bell.*
Cina	&	**Benzoic Acid**
Usually during the first sleep at night. The urine is pale and turbid ; sometimes has a very strong odor.		During the first sleep at night. The urine smells strong, like that of a horse.
Cina	&	**Kreosotum**
See above.		See above.
Cina	&	**Phosphoric Acid**
See above.		Enuresis during the forepart of the night. Urine with a very strong odor.
Cina	&	**Sepia**
See above.		See above.
Equisetum	&	**Linaria**
See above.		Enuresis, with frequent urging to urinate, causing the patient to rise at night.
Plantago Major	&	**Kreosotum**
Of children, in the latter part of the night. Also see above.		During the first sleep at night, See also above.

ERYSIPELAS

[**Remedies.**—*Anac. Apis. Bell. Bor. Cam. Can. Com. Crot.* ***Cupr.*** *Euph. Grp. Hep. Lach. Rhus-T. Sil. Stram. Sul.*]

Anacardium & **Rhus Tox.**

Erysipelatous eruptions on the face.

Erysipelas going from left to right.

Apis & **Belladonna**

The affected part exhibits a tendency to become œdematous; assumes a rosy-pinkish hue, which may turn to dark-purplish. *Nervous irritation*—a fidgety nervous state, a fretted feeling, which deprives the patient of sleep, although he feels sleepy. High fever, with dry skin and usually thirstless.

face is involved, the eye-lids protrude like sacs of water.

There is not much tendency to œdema or to the formation of vesicles. The pains are always acute, with throbbing in the affected parts. *Cerebral irritation*—the brain almost always sympathises markedly causing throbbing in the head and visions as soon as the patient closes his eyes; jerking in sleep. Full and hard pulse. Cerebral metastasis.

Apis & **Borax**

See above.

Erysipelas of the face, particularly of the cheeks. *A feeling as though a cobweb is on the face.*

Apis & **Cantharis**

See above.

The nose is involved, with larger blisters and more burning. Spreads to one or the other cheek, with the formation of vesicles which break and discharge an excoriating fluid.

Apis & **Rhus Tox.**

See above.

Special affinity for the scalp, the skin of the face and the genital organs. Travels from left to right, usually when attacking the face. The face is dusky-red. Formation of little blisters, which burn and sting, with preponderance of itching. The patient is restless, and drowsy. Aching of the limbs.

Belladonna & **Ailanthus**

See above.

The face is livid and mottled; profound stupor.

ERYSIPELAS *(contd.)*—

Belladonna & **Cuprum**

See above.

Convulsions; vigorous contraction of the flexor muscles.

Belladonna & **Crotalus** or **Lachesis**

See above

The face is purplish or of dark-bluish hue. The patient is weaker; the pulse more rapid and lacking in force. More drowsiness with muttering delirium.

Belladonna & **Sulphur**

See above.

Complementary.

Cantharis & **Graphites**

See above.

Chronic cases of Erysipelas commencing on the nose.

Lachesis & **Apis**

See above.

See above.

Lachesis & **Rhus tox.**

See above.

See above.

Lachesis & **Euphorbium**

See above.

Gangrene with Erysipelas of the face. The right cheek is of a livid or of dark-red hue. Vesicles form.

Rhus Tox. & **Stramonium**

See above.

Violent cerebral symptoms—congestion with more sensorial excitement; more restlessness and screaming out, as if terrified. There is *little or no fever.*

FEVER

[**Remedies.**— *Acon. Apis. Ars. Ars-I. Bap. Bell. Bry. Calc-O. Carb-V. Cupr. Ferr-P. Gels. Hyos. Ipec. Lyc. Merc. Myg. Nat-M. Ol-J. Op. Phos-Ac. Phos. Pod. Puls. Ran-B. Stram. Sul. Verat-V. Yar-S.*]

Aconite & **Apis**

Synochal fever—sthenic; decided chill, followed by dry hot skin; full, hard, bounding pulse; followed later by a warm, profuse, critical sweat with relief. Anxiety, restlessness and fear of death.

Symptomatology is opposed in every respect to typhoid state.

Chill followed by burning heat all over or heat in some parts and coolness in others; the skin is hot and dry or alternately dry and moist. Sweat is absent or breaks out only in spells soon drying off. Cri encephalique with cerebral irritation; dyspnœa.

FEVER *(contd.)*—

Aconite	&	Arsenicum
It never develops typhoid symptoms. See also above.		Fever running to typhoid state with putrid discharges. Intense, burning thirst, but intolerance of water or drinks little, but too often. The brain may remain perfectly clear. Aggravation after midnight.
Aconite	&	**Belladonna**
Indicated in the initial stages. See also above.		Fevers begin with symptoms of brain and spinal cord or which commence with the *Aconite-type* but have by extension involved the brain. Jerking in sleep; hallucinations; visions; and counting of death, rather than fear of it.
Aconite	&	**Bryonia**
It suits the hyperæmia, the congestion, or, even the chill, which precedes an inflammatory fever. The mind is excited and the patient is restless, tossing about the bed, full of fears.		Indicated when *Aconite* fails. The patient is perfectly quiet, because *motion aggravates his symptoms.*
Aconite	&	**Ferrum**
See above.		Inflammatory fevers—the discharges are blood-streaked. The pulse is full, but, rather soft.
Aconite	&	**Gelsemium**
See above.		Partial chill, beginning in the hands or running up and down the spine, followed by general heat—most decided about the face and head. Sweat is gradual and moderate, but always gives relief. The pulse is full and flowing, but not hard—the so-called water-hammer pulse. Associated with the above there is languor, muscular weakness, desire for absolute rest and drowsiness. It has never the violent tossing about.

FEVER *(contd.)*—

Aconite	&	**Sulphur**
See above.		The fever is remittent or continued, follows *Aconite*. The dry hot skin remains, even after the administration of *Aconite*, and there is no reaction or critical sweat; exacerbation each evening and a slight fall towards the morning, the fever never leaves entirely—the patient at first sleepless and restless, becomes drowsy and responds to questions very sluggishly, or slowly, as if not fully comprehending. The tongue is dry and red at the edges and tips, and speech a little thick.
Aconite	&	**Veratrum Viride**
See above.		A high degree of arterial excitement—the pulse is full and bounding and rapid. Laboured and difficult breathing.
Belladonna	&	**Mercurius**
Rheumatic fever—profuse, sour sweat, which gives no relief; the patient seems to soak everything about him with the sweat, and the more he sweats the less sign is there of improvement. See also above.		Rheumatic fever—follows *Belladonna*; when the fever has subsided somewhat but the sweat still continues.
Opium	&	**Gelsemium**
More drowsiness; the body is burning hot, even when covered with a copious sweat; desires to uncover.		See above.
Podophyllum	&	**Gelsemium**
During the fever the patient is sleepy and sometimes delirious.		See above.

FEVER *(contd.)*—

Pulsatilla & **Gelsemium**

The head is hot and the lips are dry; the patient constantly licks his lips to moisten them, yet he does not wish to drink. Sometimes one hand is cold, the other hot.

See above.

Sulphur & **Arsenicum**

See above.

Great restlessness and burning.

GANGRENE

[**Remedies.**—*Ant-C. Ap. Ars. Bell. Brom. Calc-O. Canth. Carb An. Carb-V. Cinch. Euph. Lach. Merc-Cor. Merc-Cyan. Plb. Ran-B. Rhus-T. Saly-Ac. Sec. Sil.*]

Apis & **Belladonna**

Gangrene, with stinging pain.

With throbbing pain.

Apis & **Cantharis**

See above.

With extreme irritation and inflammation with fever.
With vesicles.
With urinary complications.

Apis & **Rhus Toxicodendron**

See above.

Gangrene of exanthema; black.

Arsenicum & **Carbo Vegetabilis**

Burning pains, with extreme restlessness, agg. from cold, *amel.* by warmth.
Dry gangrene of old people.

With burning pains, but without restlessness.

Arsenicum & **Cinchona**

See above.

With hæmorrhage or after great loss of blood.

GANGRENE *(contd.)*—

Arsenicum	&	**Lachesis**
See above.		Gangrene of an ashy-grey color. Tingling, with heat and numbness. Marked blueness. With bluish-black vesicles. Inflammation which degenerates into gangrene. Tendency to gangrenous ulceration. Traumatic gangrene, when the edges of a lacerated wound turn black.
Arsenicum	&	**Rananculus Bulbosus**
See above.		Gangrene associated with fever and delirium.
Arsenicum	&	**Secale Cornutum**
See above.		With burning and numbness. With symptoms, *amel.* from cold. Dry gangrene, *esp.* of toes of the old people.
Calcarea Ostrearum	&	**Silicea**
Gangrene following canker-sores or stomatitis.		Gangrenous inflammation and ulcers.
Lachesis	&	**Euphorbium**
See above.		Gangrene, with erysipelas. The pains are boring, gnawing and digging in character, with itching and crawling when the pains are relieved.
Lachesis	&	**Secale Cornutum**
Gangrene of the toes. See also above.		Dry gangrene, *esp.* of the toes of the old people. See also above.

GOUT

[**Remedies.**—*Amm-P. Ant-C. Arn. Benz-Ac. Ber. Calc-O. Caust. Colch. Coloc. Guai. Kal. Led. Lith-C. Lyc. Nat-M. Puls. Rhod. Sab. Staph.*]

Berberis & **Benzoic Acid**

Berberis: Yellow, turbid and flocculent urine.

Benzoic Acid: The urine smells strong, like that of the horse.

Berberis & **Calcarea Ostrearum**

Berberis: See above.

Calcarea Ostrearum: Very offensive urine, with a white deposit. Gouty nodosities about the fingers.

Berberis & **Lycopodium**

Berberis: See above.

Lycopodium: The urine contains a lithic acid deposit.

Colchicum & **Pulsatilla**

Colchicum: The urine is dark-red and scanty. The great toe is involved and the paroxysms occur at night. Metastasis of Gout to the chest—a sensation, as if the chest were being squeezed by a tight bandage.

Pulsatilla: Gout—especially brought on by indigestion. Gouty synovitis. Feeling of soreness or of subcutaneous ulceration about the affected joints. Sharp, stinging pains—usually erratic ; pressure relieves ; worse from warmth and in the evening.

Followed by *Colchium.*

Ledum & **Colchicum**

Ledum: Characteristically travels upward. Gouty inflammation of the great toe ; the effusion is scanty, and tends to harden into nodosities ; acute tearing pains worse from the warmth of the bed and ameliorated by cold applications ; œdematous condition of the feet.

Colchicum: See above.

HÆMOPTYSIS

[**Remedies.**—*Acal--I. Acon. Bry. Cac. Calc-O. Carb-V. Elaps. Ferr. Ferr-P. Iod. Ipec. Laur. Led. Merc. Millef. Nit-Ac. Nux-V. Op. Phos. Puls. Rhus-T. Senec. Sul. Zinc.*]

Acalypha Indica & **Carbo Vegetabilis**

Hæmoptysis after dry coughing.

Burning pain in the chest. Great anxiety, but without any particular restlessness.

Aconite & **Cactus Grandiflorus**

The blood is bright-red ; anxiety and fever—invariably present.

Associated with strong throbbing of the heart and a sensation of constriction, as of a band about the chest. It has less anxiety and less fever.

Aconite & **Ledum**

See above.

Hæmoptysis of the drunkards or persons of rheumatic diathesis. The blood is dark-red but *foamy*.

Aconite & **Millefolium**

See above.

Profuse flow of bright-red blood but *without fever*.

Elaps & **Ferrum**

The blood discharged is dark in color.

Dark-red but coagulated blood. Associated with Phthisis.

Ledum & **Nux Vomica**

See above.

Hæmoptysis after a drunken spree or debauchery or violent emotion or suppressed hæmorrhoids.

Ledum & **Opium**

See above.

In drunkards : violent cough with expectoration of frothy mucus and blood ; the patient is drowsy with the cough. The chest is hot, but the limbs are cold.

Opium & **Senecio**

See above.

Bloody expectoration with the cough.

HÆMOPTYSIS *(contd.)*—

Phosphorus & **Pulsatilla**

Phosphorus: Associated with vicarious menstruation—the menstrual blood being too pale.

In chronic catarrh—with green mucus, blood-streaked.

Pulsatilla: Associated with vicarious menstruation—the menstrual blood being dark and clotted or colourless and watery.

Of incipient Consumption—with soreness in the chest, worse under the clavicles; burning pain especially in the region of the heart; stitches in the sides of the chest.

Rhus Tox. & **Sulphur**

Rhus Tox.: Hæmoptysis from over-exertion.

Sulphur: Hæmoptysis from congestion of the chest. Great difficulty in breathing. Violent palpitation of the heart.

HÆMORRHOIDS

[**Remedies.**—*Æsc-H. Aloes. Alum. Amm-C. Anac. Ant-C. Apoc. Ars. Arte-A. Bor. Cap. Carb-An. Carb-V. Coll. Goss. Grp. Ham. Ign. Lach. Lyc. Lamium-A. Mur-Ac. Nat-M. Nat-S. Nit-Ac. Nux-V. Pæon. Petr. Rhus-T. Sep. Sil. Sul. Sul-Ac. Thy.*]

Anacardium & **Apocynum**

Anacardium: Internal piles. A sensation, as if a plug were being forced up into the anus.

Apocynum: A feeling, as if an wedge were being hammered into the anus.

Anacardium & **Lamium Album**

Anacardium: See above.

Lamium Album: External piles.

Carbo Animalis & **Carbo Vegetabilis**

Carbo Animalis: Piles, with weak digestion; oozing of a thin inodorous fluid from the rectum—but not marked.

Carbo Vegetabilis: Bluish protruding piles; oozing of a thin inodorous fluid from the rectum—marked.

Graphites & **Arsenicum**

Graphites: Burning and stinging pains; the anus is so extremely sore, that the patient is annoyed very much when sitting.

Arsenicum: Protrude at stool with burning. Intense irritability, mental anguish, and extreme prostration.

HÆMORRHOIDS *(contd.)*—

Lachesis & **Arsenicum**

Large protruding hæmorrhoids with stitches upwards at each cough or sneeze ; bluish ; pain in the sphincter ; torpidity with loss of vitality, but associated with nervous excitability ; intolerance of pressure. May be associated with constipation. Worse at the menopause or with scanty menses.

Hæmorrhoids of the dyspeptics or drunkards.

Hæmorrhoids of the drunkards.

See also above.

Lachesis & **Carbo Vegetabilis**

See above.

See above.

Lachesis & **Sulphuric Acid**

See above.

Hæmorrhoids of the drunkards—piles are moist, burning and may prevent defæcation.

Nux Vomica & **Æsculus Hippocastanum**

Itching, worse at night ; apt to bleed ; frequent ineffectual urging to stool. Relief from cold water.

A feeling of dryness in the rectum ; sensation as though little sticks or splinters were pricking the folds of the mucous membranes. Throbbing deep in the abdomen, particularly in the hypogastric region.

Nux Vomica & **Aloes**

See above.

Hæmorrhoids protrude like bunch of grapes and are greatly relieved by cold water.

Nux Vomica & **Collinsonia**

See above.

Sensation of sticks in the rectum. Constipation.

Nux Vomica & **Hamamelis**

See above.

Considerable hæmorrhage with marked soreness of the affected parts. The back feels, as if it would break.

Sepia & **Aloes**

Bleeding at stool, with a feeling of fulness in the rectum, as though it were distended with some foreign materials, which seems to excite an urging to stool.

See above.

HÆMORRHOIDS *(contd.)*—

Sepia	&	**Lycopodium**
See above.		Bleeding piles. Considerable hæmorrhage. Piles, which do not mature and remain hard as bluish lumps.
Sulphur	&	**Aloes**
Hæmorrhoids from abdominal plethora.		See above.
Sulphuric Acid	&	**Pæonia**
Dampness or oozing of moisture from the rectum. Burning. So large that they feel up the rectum		Enormous hæmorrhoids with great soreness and smarting.

INJURIES

[**Remedies.**—*Acon. Amm-C. Amm-M. Angus. Arn. Bell. Bov. Bry. Calc-P. Calend. Cepa. Cic. Con. Eup. Glon. Hyper. Lach. Led. Millef. Nat-S. Petr. Rhus-T. Ruta. Sil. Staph. Sul. Sul-Ac. Symph. Verat-V.*]

Angustura	&	**Ruta**
Injuries with incipient muscular contractions.		Injuries to the periosteum.
Arnica	&	**Calcarea Phos.**
Injuries of the soft parts. Injuries of muscles from a sprain or from sudden wrench and in hæmorrhages of mechanical origin. Bruises with well-marked ecchymoses. Concussion of the brain or spine. Compression of the brain. Fracture of bones—and swelling and tumefaction of the limbs, twitching of muscles.		Irritability of bone at the point of fracture, due to defective nutrition.
Arnica	&	**Calendula**
See above.		A torn or ragged wound—inflammation of the parts.

INJURIES *(contd.)*—

Arnica	&	**Hypericum**
See above.		Injury of the nerves along with the soft parts. Follows *Arnica* in concussion of the spine.
Arnica	&	**Ledum**
See above.		Injuries inflicted by pointed instruments. Punctured wounds. Follows *Arnica* when it fails to remove soreness of the injuries.
Arnica	&	**Rhus Tox.**
See above.		Injuries of the fibrous structures, ligaments of joints.
Arnica	&	**Staphisagria**
See above.		Smooth clean cuts.
Arnica	&	**Sulphuric Acid**
See above.		Injuries of the soft parts—follows *Arnica*. Long-lasting black and blue spots with soreness and stiffness.
Arnica	&	**Symphytum**
See above.		Bone injuries, injuries of the orbital plates of the frontal bones. Irritability of the bones at the point of fracture.
Conium	&	**Sulphuric Acid**
Injuries of the glands. Induration from contusions and bruises.		Bruises of the glands—follows *Conium*.
Glonoin	&	**Natrum Sulph.**
Pains and other abnormal sensations, following some time or long after local injuries. Retroversion of an old scar.		Chronic effects of injuries, especially to the head.
Ruta	&	**Sulphuric Acid**
See above.		Injuries of bones—follows *Ruta*. See also above.

JAUNDICE

[**Remedies.**—*Acon. Ars. Bry. Carduus. Cham. Chel. Cin. Dig. Hep Jug-C. Kali-C. Lach. Merc. Myrica. Nat-S. Nux-V. Phos. Pod. Puls.*]

Digitalis & **Myrica Cerifera**

Digitalis

Associated with cardiac diseases. The liver is enlarged and feels sore, as if bruised, somewhat indurated. The pulse is slow, even slower than the beating of the heart. The urine is high-colored from admixture of bile pigment. The tongue may be perfectly clean or whitish-yellow ; stools—ashy-white.

Myrica Cerifera

Functional. The eyes and sclerotic have a dirty, dingy, yellowish hue, the lids being abnormally red. The tongue—coated dirty yellow. Weak, sinking feeling in the epigastrium after eating. The pulse is slow but intensified. The urine dark and turbid. The stools—ash-colored.

The patient is weak and drowsy, and complains of muscular soreness and aching in the limbs.

Nux Vomica & **Aconite**

Nux Vomica

The patient has attacks of faintness, after which he feels very weak.

Aconite

Jaundice from fit of anger. *Mental symptoms* prominent.

Nux Vomica & **Arsenicum**

Nux Vomica

See above.

Arsenicum

Jaundice from abuse of Quinine. Mental irritability and thirst peculiar to this remedy.

Nux Vomica & **Bryonia**

Nux Vomica

See above.

Bryonia

Jaundice from abuse of Calomel or blue-mass. From fit of anger—associated with chilliness. The tongue—white.

Nux Vomica & **Carduus Marianus**

Nux Vomica

See above.

Carduus Marianus

White-coated tongue, especially in the middle, with the tips and edges red. Nausea with vomiting of an acrid green fluid. Uncomfortable fulness in the region of the liver. The stools are bilious and the urine golden-yellow.

Nux Vomica & **Chamomilla**

Nux Vomica

See above.

Chamomilla

Jaundice from fit of anger. Tongue yellow. Face pale with one cheek red. Associated with heat. The patient is cross and irritable.

JAUNDICE *(contd.)*—

Nux Vomica	&	**Chelidonium**
See above.		Pain under the right scapula.
Nux Vomica	&	**Cinchona**
See above.		Jaundice from sexual excess, loss of animal fluids or abuse of Alcohol. Surface of the body and sclerotica are yellowish. A feeling in the right hypochondrium as of sub-cutaneous ulceration. The stools are whitish, accompanied with fœtid flatus or else there is diarrhœa.
Nux Vomica	&	**Hepar**
See above.		Jaundice from the effects of Quinine
Nux Vomica	&	**Juglans Cineria**
See above.		Pain under the right scapula. The stools are bilious or yellowish green, burning the anus and associated with tenesmus.
Nux Vomica	&	**Mercurius**
See above.		Jaundice from effects of Quinine. The tongue coated dirty yellowish-white, and takes the imprint of teeth. The skin and conjunctiva have a well-marked jaundiced hue. The stools are either clay-colored, from absence of bile or yellowish-green, bilious and pass with a great deal of tenesmus and followed by a "never-get-done" feeling.
Nux Vomica	&	**Natrum Sulph.**
See above.		Jaundice from fit of anger, with pain under the right scapula. A great deal of flatulence.
Nux Vomica	&	**Podophyllum**
See above.		The liver is swollen and sensitive and the friction over right hypochondrium relieves this sensation; constipation or diarrhœa; stools clay-colored.

JAUNDICE *(contd.)*—

Nux Vomica & **Pulsatilla**

Nux Vomica: See above.

Pulsatilla: Jaundice from effects of Quinine. Mental symptoms characteristic.

Phosphorus & **Myrica Cerifera**

Phosphorus: *Functional*, but is indicative of organic disease ; associated with pregnancy or malignant diseases of the liver. The stools are apt to be greenish-white.

Myrica Cerifera: It is more superficial in its action. The stools are ash-colored.

See also above.

LARYNGITIS

[**Remedies.**—*Acon. Ap. Carb-V. Caust. Kali-Bi. Lach. Merc-P-I. Merc-V. Phos. Rhus-T. Samb. Sang. Sel. Spong. Sul.*]

Aconite & **Spongia**

Aconite: Caused by dry, cold winds.

In the beginning.

Spongia: Indicated after *Acon.*

Harsh, barking cough and suffocative spells during sleep arousing the patient.

Rawness in larynx ; larynx is extremely sensitive to touch ; simply turning the head, will bring on a suffocative spell.

< in cold, west wind.

Apis Mellifica & **Rhus Toxicodendron**

Apis Mellifica: Erysipelatous or catarrhal inflammation.

Larynx, as if scalded, worse in warm room ; takes cold in wet, cold weather.

Rhus Toxicodendron: Also rheumatic.

Larynx, as if raw and sore ; stuffed up, < in cold, even exposing hands ; takes cold in wet, *esp.* when warm or sweating.

Causticum & **Carbo Vegetabilis**

Causticum: Due to dry, cold severe winter weather.

Hoarseness, with aggravation in morning.

Carbo Vegetabilis: Caused by exposure to damp evening air.

Hoarseness, *agg.* in evening.

Causticum & **Phosphorus**

Causticum: Paretic symptoms, with rawness and burning in throat and trachea. Relief of symptoms from cold drinks.

See also above.

Phosphorus: Extreme sensitiveness of the larynx ; the patient dreads to talk and cough, because they *agg.* laryngeal soreness.

Hoarseness, with evening aggravation.

LARYNGITIS *(contd.)*—

Mercurius Prot. Iodatum	&	**Mercurius Vivus**
Ulcerated ; patches livid, purplish. Discharge : thin, offensive.		Ulcerated ; patches white. Profuse ptyalism.
Phosphorus	&	**Lachesis**
Hoarseness : more prominent ; burning rawness, most marked ; talking causes severe pain. Tightness across the chest, accompanied with a sense of weight and oppression. See also above.		Hoarseness ; attended by a feeling, as if something in larynx prevented clear speech—it cannot be hawked up. Suffocating spells in sleep ; the child arouses in agony, as if choking ; agg. of the symptoms after sleep.
Selenium	&	**Carbo Vegetabilis**
With congestion of the lining membrane of the larynx, with dark purplish spots, here and there, through it. Frequent necessity to clear the throat, by reason of the accumulation of clear starchy mucus.		See above.
Selenium	&	**Causticum**
See above.		See above.
Selenium	&	**Phosphorus**
See above.		See above.
Spongia	&	**Lachesis**
Extreme sensitiveness of the larynx to touch—when it is the result of the inflamed condition of the laryngeal cartilages. See also the above.		Extreme sensitiveness of the larynx to touch—when it is due to hyperæsthesia of the cutaneous nerves. See also the above.
Spongia	&	**Sambucus**
See above.		With frequent spasms of the larynx.
Spongia	&	**Sanguinaria Canadensis**
See above.		Aphonia. A feeling of swelling in the throat, as though the patient would choke.

LUMBAGO

[**Remedies.**—*Calc-Fl. Calc-O. Kali-C. Led. Nux-V. Petr. Phos. Pic-Ac. Rhus-T. Ruta. Sec. Staph. Sul. Valer. Zinc.*]

Rhus Tox. & **Calcarea Fluorica**

Great pains on attempting to rise; better from warmth and worse from cold.

Worse on beginning to move, improving on continued motion.

Rhus Tox. & **Calcarea Ostrearum**

See above.

Affections caused by working in water. Follows *Rhus* if that remedy fails.

Rhus Tox. & **Kali Carb.**

See above.

Sharp pains in the lumbar region, worse at 3 A.M., compelling the patient to get up and walk about. The pains shoot down the buttocks.

Rhus Tox. & **Ledum**

See above.

A feeling of stiffness after sitting still for a long time.

Rhus Tox. & **Nux Vomica**

See above.

The patient cannot turn over without sitting up. Worse at night when lying in bed. The longer he lies in bed in the morning, the more does his back ache.

Rhus Tox. & **Petroleum or Ruta**

See above.

Worse in the morning before rising.

Rhus Tox. & **Secale**

See above.

Sudden "catch" or "klink" in the back.

Rhus Tox. & **Staphisagria**

See above.

Compels the patient to get up early.

Rhus Tox. & **Sulphur**

See above.

Stiffness and sudden loss of power on attempting to move.

Rhus Tox. & **Valeriana**

See above.

Strained feeling in the lumbar region, worse from sitting and better from motion.

MENINGITIS

[**Remedies.**—*Acon. Apis. Ars. Bell. Bov. Bry. Calc-O. Camph. Canth. Cupr. Dig. Ferr-P. Gels. Glon. Hell. Hyos. Kali-H. Lach. Merc. Nat-M. Ox-Ac. Pic-Ac. Rhus-T. Sul. Zinc. Zinc-O.*]

Apis & **Arsenicum**

Apis: Nervous fidgetiness. Cri encephalique. Cerebral irritation. Adynamia.

Arsenicum: Anxiety and fear more marked.

Apis & **Belladonna**

Apis: Nervous agitation predominates, with the shrill cry, which betokens stabbing, piercing pains or excitement.

Increasingly indicated as long as symptoms of irritation obtain, and the cephalic cry is marked.

Belladonna: Every symptom appears suddenly and with great intensity.

More intense cerebral irritation. Violent congestions with throbbing of the carotids, flushed face, injected red eyes and drowsiness broken by starts and frightened outcries.

Decreasingly indicated as the symptoms of effusions increase.

Apis & **Bryonia**

Apis: Senses are perverted; when the sensorial depression amounts to *sopor* accompanied by cri encephalique—more shrill cephalic cry

Bryonia: Cerebral effusions following suppressed exanthemata. The sensation is benumbed. Constant chewing motion; the face is dark-red, the lips parched; when offered a drink, it is taken hastily and impatiently.

Apis & **Cuprum**

Apis: If convulsions occur, they are less violent, consisting of restlessness and twitching of one-half of the body; the other half is lame and trembles.

Cuprum: Loud screamings followed by violent convulsions, which usually starts from the brain, and especially of the flexor muscles; the thumbs are clenched, and the face is pale with blue lips; the eye-balls are constantly rotating; frothing of the mouth. The convulsions are followed by deep sleep.

Apis & **Glonoin**

Apis: See above.

Glonoin: Spasmodic vomiting of cerebral origin—most prominent, as also intense congestion and throbbing. A sensation, as if the head were expanded.

MENINGITIS *(contd.)*—

Apis	&	Helleborus
Cephalic cry is more marked ; and more excitement and irritation. Spasm of the flexors, so that the big toes are drawn upward.		Mental torpor with want of reaction. Sopor is complete. There are automatic motions of one arm and one leg ; the forehead is bathed with cold sweat. *Sensorial depression*—characteristic.
Apis	&	**Zincum**
See above.		The child awakes with fear ; rolls the head ; cries out and starts in sleep. Constant fidgety movement of the feet. Sharp lancinating pains through the head—worse from wine or anything that stimulates. Pressing, tearing pains in the occiput, particularly about the base of the brain, shooting through the eyes, and sympathetically into the teeth.
Belladonna	&	**Aconite**
Develops collateral symptoms only. Courting of death ; jerking in sleep, hallucinations and visions. See also above.		Absolute inflammation of the meninges with an increase of exudation. Meningitis from lying with the head exposed to the direct rays of the sun, especially when asleep. Anguish, fear of death.
Belladonna	&	**Bryonia**
See above.		The face is flushed red or alternately red and pale. Slightest attempt to move the child, makes it shriek with pain. Marked squinting with one or both the eyes ; the pupils do not react readily to light. The child moves the mouth, as if it were chewing or sucking. The bowels are constipated usually and the abdomen distended, and well-marked sensorial depression which seems to border on stupor. It follows *Belladonna*.

MENINGITIS *(contd.)*—

Belladonna	&	**Glonoin**
Relief from bending backward, from sitting up with the head erect. See also above.		Cephalic cry is more marked. Head seems, as if expanding. Head symptoms worse by bending the head backward. Relief from uncovering the head. See also above.
Bryonia	&	**Helleborus**
See above.		Follows *Bryonia,* when the sensorial depression is developed into sopor. See also above.
Helleborus	&	**Digitalis**
Automatic motion of one arm and one feet—which may occur at regular intervals. See also above.		Scanty albuminous urine. Characteristically slow pulse, which may be even slower than the heart-beat.
Helleborus	&	**Zincum**
See above.		The patient is so ennervated that he has not sufficient strength to develop the eruption ; he arouses from sleep, as if in terror. Constant fidgety motion of the feet. See also above.
Hyoscyamus	&	**Belladonna**
Relief from shaking the head or sitting with the head bent forward. The patient complains of pulsating waves through the head.		See above.
Lachesis	&	**Belladonna**
The patient is at first very drowsy, but unable to sleep ; followed by stupor—becomes heavy and sleepy and can be aroused only with difficulty ; trembling or palpitation of the heart. Follows *Belladonna.*		Evidences of irritation not wholly of depression. See also above.
Mercurius	&	**Belladonna**
Glandular swellings ; tendency to sore-mouth. May follow *Belladonna.*		See above.

MENINGITIS *(contd.)*—

Picric Acid & **Belladonna**

Associated with priapism. | See above.

Sulphur & **Apis**

Retroversion of an eruption before the disease. Follows each other well. | Follows each other well. See above.

Sulphur & **Belladonna**

Follows *Belladonna ;* when effusion within the ventricles or beneath the membrane commences. | See above.

NASAL CATARRH

[**Remedies.**—*Æsc. All-C. Alum. Ambra. Amm-C. Amm-Caust. Amm-M. Ant-C. Ars. Arum. Arund. Aur. Bell. Brom. Bry. Calc-O. Cinnab. Cist. Cor-R. Cycl. Euph. Grp. Hydr. Kali-Bi. Kali-C. Kali-S. Lach. Lith-C. Lyc. Merc. Merc-Cor. Nat-C. Nux-V. Penth. Phos. Pic-Ac. Puls. Senec. Sil. Spig. Stict. Sul.*].

Ammonium Carbonicum & **Ammonium Causticum**

Worse in winter ; nose stopped up, worse at night, awakes the patient from sleep with gasping for breath ; worse from 3 to 4 A.M. Cough dry, tickling, hoarseness, chest oppressed with mucus. The sputum slimy, contains little specks of blood. | Associated with *Aphonia,* with burning rawness in the throat.

Ammonium Carbonicum & **Ammonium Muriaticum**

See above. | Stoppage of one nostril ; both stopped up at night ; nostrils sore and raw ; discharge of bluish mucus or scalding coryza ; severe burning in the throat.

Ammonium Carbonicum & **Carbo Vegetabilis**

See above. | Catarrhal troubles provoked by warm moist atmosphere. Worse in the evening. Aphonia recurring regularly in each evening ; painless or associated with raw feeling down the larynx and trachea. Dry, tickling cough, at times quite spasmodic in character.

NASAL CATARRH *(contd.)*—

Ammonium Carbonicum & **Causticum**

See above.

Spastic symptoms. Hoarseness with aggravation in the morning. The sputum often tastes greasy and soapy. *Drinking cold water relieves the cough.*

Ammonium Carbonicum & **Kali Bich.**

See above.

Tickling in the nose and sneezing—being especially marked in the open air. The secretion from the nose is ropy and stringy and often collects in the posterior nares.

Bryonia & **Aconite**

Suppressed coryza—dull throbbing headache just over the frontal sinuses, aggravated from motion. The discharge is thick and yellow.

Suppressed coryza, due to dry cold winds and there is red face, fever, etc.

Bryonia & **China**

See above.

Suppressed coryza—headache worse from least draught of air and better from pressure.

Bryonia & **Lachesis**

See above.

Suppressed coryza ; the discharge is *not* yellow and aggravation from motion, less marked. Great relaxation of the whole system.

Calcarea Ostrearum & **Belladonna**

The wings of the nose are thickened and ulcerated; there is apt to be a moist, scurfy eruption about the nostrils. There is an offensive odor as of rotten eggs, gun-powder or manure from the nose. The nose is stopped up, with thick yellow pus. Nosebleed, in the morning—often.

Follows *Calcarea* well.

NASAL CATARRH *(contd.)*—

Graphites &	**Calcarea Ostrearum**
Extreme dryness of the nose. The sense of smell is too acute—the patient cannot bear the odor of flowers. The borders of the nostrils are sore and scabby and crack readily. There is cracking or roaring in the ears when swallowing or chewing. Sometimes the discharges are very offensive.	See above.
Ipecacuanha &	**Allium Cepa**
The nose feels, as if stopped up; there is often epistaxis, loss of smell, nausea, etc.	The nasal secretion is watery and acrid and the lachrymation mild. Raw feeling in the throat and cough provoked by tickling in the larynx.
Ipecacuanha &	**Arsenicum**
See above.	Follows *Ipecacuanha,* in catarrhs of fat, chubby children.
Ipecacuanha &	**Euphrasia**
See above.	The nasal secretion is watery, but the lachrymation is excoriating and the nasal discharge is bland.
Mercurius &	**Kali Sulph.**
Ripe cold ; the discharge from the nose is yellowish-green, thick and muco-purulent. The nose itches and burns, and feels stuffed up. Aching in the joints.	The discharge is more apt to be yellow.
Mercurius &	**Pulsatilla**
See above.	The discharge is never irritating, but is perfectly bland.
Nux Vomica &	**Mercurius**
Coryza caused by exposure to dry cold ; there are soreness, roughness and a harsh, scraped feeling in the throat.	*Mercurius* always has a smarting raw or sore feeling.
Phosphorus &	**Allium Cepa**
Green mucus and blood-streaked. It is also indicated when by the administration of *Cepa* the catarrh is driven to the chest.	See above.

NASAL CATARRH *(contd.)*—

Pulsatilla & **Cyclamen**

The nasal discharge is thick, muco-purulent, yellowish or yellowish-green and not in the least excoriating.

In chronic cases—loss of smell and taste in addition to the above.

In chronic cases—spasmodic sneezing and aversion to open air.

Pulsatilla & **Hydrastis**

See above.

The discharge is of a thin and watery character, and is attended with a great deal of burning and rawness, together with a sensation, as of a hair in the nostrils.

Pulsatilla & **Mercurius**

See above.

See above.

Pulsatilla & **Penthorum**

See above.

The patient complains of a constant raw feeling in the nose, but without coryza. Later, there is formation of thick purulent discharge.

Pulsatilla & **Spigelia**

See above.

Profuse discharge of mucus through the posterior nares; nasal mucus passes off only through the posterior nares.

NEURALGIA

[**Remedies.**—*Acon. Act-R. Amm-C. Amm-M. Amyl-N. Arg. Ars. Bell. Cact. Caps. Ced. Cepa. Cham. Chel. Chin-S. Cinch. Colch. Coloc. Cup. Cup-Ars. Dios. Ferr. Ferr-C. Ham. Hepar. Ign. Kalm. Kreos. Mag-C. Mag-P. Mez. Nat-M. Plat. Prun. Puls. Rob. Sep. Sil. Spig. Stann. Staph. Stront. Sul. Tab. Ther. Thuj. Valer. Verb.*].

Aconite & **Amyl Nitrite**

Neuralgia caused by exposure to dry cold winds. Violent congestion of the affected parts, which is usually the face. Tingling, usually in the affected part.

Prosopalgia with much local congestion.

NEURALGIA *(contd.)*—

Aconite	&	**Belladonna**
See above.		Pains come on suddenly, last a longer or shorter time, and then as suddenly disappear. In prosopalgia, the right side is mostly attacked, especially the infra-orbital nerves. Exacerbation at 2 or 3 P.M. and again at 11 P.M.
Aconite	&	**Colchicum**
See above.		Excited by washing in cold water, especially after being over-heated. Throbbing pain, worse at night.
Aconite	&	**Ferrum**
See above.		Left-sided prosopalgia with paralytic weakness of the muscles.
Aconite	&	**Kreosotum**
See above.		Neuralgia of the face with burning pains, increased by motion and talking. Nervous and irritable.
Aconite	&	**Spigelia**
See above.		Left-sided prosopalgia, with severe burning and sticking pains. The patient exhibits intense excitement and great intolerance of pains.
Actea Racemosa	&	**Cedron**
Sensation of heat on the top of the head just behind the centre. Sharp, lancinating neuralgic pains in and over the eyes, and supra-orbital pains shooting up to the top of the head.		Pains involving supra-orbital nerve and the eyes, *worse on the left side.* The eye burns, as if it were on fire. The pains recur regularly at the same hour every day.
Actea Racemosa	&	**Kalmia**
See above.		Supra-orbital pain, *worse on the right side.*

NEURALGIA *(contd.)*--

Actea Racemosa	&	**Spigelia**
Worse at night. Also see above.		Neuralgia comes and goes with the sun—*reaches its height at noon and subsides in the evening.* Pains begin in the back of the head and comes forward, settling over one or the other eye. Sensation, as if the eye-ball were enormously large.
Arsenicum	&	**Cactus Grandiflorus**
The pain usually affects one side of the face and seemed to be almost maddening, driving the patient from place to place. At the height of the attack there are nausea and vomiting and buzzing in the ears.		Neuralgic pains when the patient misses an accustomed meal.
Arsenicum	&	**Cedron**
See above.		Supra-orbital nerve. Pain appears at precisely the same hour each day, with clock-like regularity.
Arsenicum	&	**Cinchona**
See above.		Infra-orbital nerve. The symptoms are typical in their return; the slightest touch or draft of cold air aggravates the pain.
Arsenicum	&	**Chininum Sulph.**
See above.		Periodical attacks, relieved by hard pressure.
Arsenicum	&	**Kalmia**
See above.		Burning pains. Pains increase and decrease slowly—but less markedly.
Arsenicum	&	**Kreosotum**
See above.		Burning pains increased by motion.
Arsenicum	&	**Magnesia Phos.**
See above.		Regular night attacks, relieved by heat and pressure.
Arsenicum	&	**Mezereum**
See above.		Neuralgia in the cheek-bone or over the left eye. The pains leave numbness. Worse from warmth.

NEURALGIA *(contd.)*—

Arsenicum & **Platinum**

See above.

Cramping pains with numbness and tingling in the affected parts. Pain at the root of the nose, as though the part were squeezed in a vise. Pains increase gradually, and decrease just as gradually as they came.

Arsenicum & **Robinia**

See above.

Jaw-bones feels, as if disarticulated. Intensely sour taste and water-brash or sour vomiting.

Cinchona & **Cedron**

Neuralgia of the infra-orbital nerve on either side. The symptoms are typical in their return. Slightest draft of cold air makes the patient worse. The patient dreads the slightest attempt to approach him lest you touch him, yet firm pressure or rubbing relieves.

Usally supra-orbital.

See also above.

Cuprum & **Cuprum Arsenicum**

Sudden attacks with active congestion affecting the nervous supply of the involuntary muscles.

Neuralgia of the abdominal viscera.

Platina & **Belladonna**

Gradually increasing, and gradually decreasing pains.

See also above.

See above.

Thuja & **Mezereum**

If the patient sits up, pains almost drive him to distraction : they may even produce unconsciousness; he therefore maintains the horizontal posture. The pains seem to begin about the malar bones and eyes, and go back towards the head.

See above.

Thuja & **Spigelia**

See above.

The pains begin in the back of the head and come forward.

NEURALGIA *(contd.)*—

Verbascum & **Cedron**

Neuralgia of the left side of the face which appears periodically, generally twice a day, the same hour in the morning and afternoon, each day. Worse from every change of temperature, especially a change from warm to cold.

See above.

PARALYSIS

[**Remedies.**—*Acon. Ap. Arg-Nit. Ars. Bar-C. Cann-I. Carb-V. Caust. Cocc-I. Colch. Coll. Con. Cur. Dulc. Gels. Hell. Hyos. Ign. Naj. Nat-M. Nux-V. Olnd. Op. Phos. Phys. Pic-Ac. Plb. Rhus-T. Sec. Sil. Stan. Staph. Strych. Sul. Veratria. Zinc.*].

Aconite & **Cannabis Indica**

Paralysis, from exposure to cold, *esp.* dry, cold winds; accompanied by coldness, numbness and tingling.

Indicated in the beginning.

Tingling in the affected parts.

Aconite & **Causticum**

See above.

Indicated when the Paralysis has become chronic and refuses to yield to *Aconite*.

Aconite & **Rhus Tox.**

See above.

Preferable later; *esp.* in Paralysis from cold.

Aconite & **Staphisagria**

See above.

Tingling in the affected parts.

Aconite & **Sulphur**

See above.

Paralysis from overdose of *Aconite*.

Also indicated later, when *Aconite* fails.

Apis & **Sulphur**

Paralysis following devitalizing affections, such as, Diphtheria or Typhoid Fever.

Interpolation when the improvement temporarily ceases under *Apis*.

See also above.

PARALYSIS *(contd.)*—

Baryta Carbonica	&	**Causticum**
The patient is childish, has loss of memory, trembling of the limbs and well-marked Paralysis of the tongue. Paralysis following Apoplexy —immediate effects.		Has more contractures and spasms. Paralysis following Apoplexy —remote effects. See also above.
Baryta Carbonica	&	**Secale Cornutum**
See above.		The paralytic symptoms are apt to be associated with numbness and burning.
Causticum	&	**Carbo Vegetabilis**
Paralysis caused by deep-seated nervous disease or very characteristically by exposure to cold, particularly intense cold of winter, when the patient is of rheumatic diathesis. See also above.		Holds an inimical relation.
Causticum	&	**Dulcamara**
See above.		Paralysis of rheumatic origin, provoked by exposure to a damp and cold atmosphere, particularly when there have been changes from tolerably warm to cold and wet days—in the beginning, not when the trouble becomes chronic. < from every change of weather.
Causticum	&	**Rhus Tox.**
See above.		Paralysis of the same origin as in *Dulcamara*, but when the trouble becomes chronic. See also above.
Cocculus Indicus	&	**Aconite**
Paralysis originating in diseases of the spinal cord—in the beginning.		See above.
Cocculus Indicus	&	**Conium**
See above.		The paralytic state spreads from below upwards ; the lower part of the body giving out before the upper.

PARALYSIS *(contd.)*—

Cocculus Indicus	&	**Gelsemium**
Post-diphtheritic Paralysis. See also above.		Post-diphtheritic Paralysis of one side of the body, with sensation nearly perfect.
Cocculus Indicus	&	**Stannum**
Functional Paralysis; complete motor Paralysis. See also above.		Functional Paralysis which comes from fatigue or mental emotions. The *Stanum* patient is usually sad and lachrymose; crying usually makes the patient worse.
Dulcamara	&	**Rhus Tox.**
See above.		See above.
Gelsemium	&	**Natrum Muriaticum**
Paralytic state after emotions —of a depressing character Of the laryngeal muscles (aphonia). Also see above.		The arm almost loses its power, after a fit of anger. Partial Paralysis from weakness of the spine, *esp.* when it arises from grief, anger, etc.
Gelsemium	&	**Stannum**
See above.		Patients are so much affected by emotions as to lose their power of motion. Paralysis, mostly left-sided, after emotions, with perspiration of the affected parts. See also above.
Gelsemium	&	**Staphisagria**
See above.		Paralysis of one side of the body after anger. See also above.
Gelsemium	&	**Oleander**
Functional Paralysis. See also above.		Painless Paralysis, invading one or the other limb, and is usually preceded for a long time by vertigo. It implicates sensory, as well as the motor nerves.
Nux Vomica	&	**Phosphorus**
Tends towards partial Paralysis.		Tends towards complete Paralysis. See also above.

PARALYSIS *(contd.)*—

Phosphorus & Carbo Vegetabilis

Phosphorus

Threatened Paralysis of the whole system, as a sequel to severe diseases.

Paralysis due to loss of animal fluids, such as, blood, semen or milk or too frequent child-bearing or too rapid growth.

See also above.

Carbo Vegetabilis

Holds a complementary relation.

See also above.

Phosphorus & Causticum

Phosphorus

See above.

Causticum

Holds an inimical relation-marked.

See also above.

Physostigma & Strychninum

Physostigma

Spinal Paralysis, with diminished reflex action.

Strychninum

With trembling; so feeble that he can scarcely walk and finds difficulty in making the muscles obey the will.

Picric Acid & Sulphur

Picric Acid

Congestions followed by weariness, which progresses from slight feeling of fatigue to complete Paralysis.

Sulphur

Paraplegia from intense congestion of lumbar spine, with numbness and tingling. There is heat of the spine and retention of urine.

See also above.

Rhus Tox. & Sulphur

Rhus Tox.

Paralysis from over-exertion or exposure to wet, as from lying in the damp ground, in rheumatic patients.

Acute spinal Paralysis of the infants.

See also above.

Sulphur

Holds complementary relation to *Rhus*.

See also above.

Stannum & Natrum Muriaticum

Stannum

Functional Paralysis arising from onanism.

See also above.

Natrum Muriaticum

See above.

Stannum & Staphisagria

Stannum

See above.

Staphisagria

See above.

PARALYSIS *(contd.)*—

Zincum & **Cocculus Indicus**

Partial Paralysis from spinal irritation, with aching in the back at about the dorsal vertebræ, which is worse from sitting than from either walking or lying. With this there is weakness of the legs, *esp.* at noon, when the patient is hungry.

The spinal symptoms are made worse by wine.

Partial Paralysis in females with weak spine ; there is paralytic aching in the small of back—the patient feels, as if she could scarcely walk. With this there is an empty gone feeling in abdomen which feels, as if it were a hollow cavity.

See also above.

Zincum & **Phosphorus**

Paralysis from softening of the brain, following suppressed foot-sweat, with vertigo, trembling and formication, > by friction and greatly < by wine.

There may be marked Ptosis, with the Paralysis.

See also above.

It has not the *agg.* from wine or Ptosis.

See also above.

Zincum & **Plumbum**

See above.

It has impaired nutrition or atrophy of the affected parts.

There will be pain in the atrophied limbs alternating with colic.

PHARYNGITIS

[**Remedies.**—*Æsc. Ap. Chim. Hep. Ign. Kali-Bi. Kali-C. Kali-Chl. Merc-Iod. Nux-V. Puls. Sec. Sul.*]

Kali Bichromicum & **Æsculus Hippocastanum**

Ropy, stringy discharges.

Lacks the tenacious, stringy mucus and there is no swelling.

Kali Bichromicum & **Chimaphila Maculata**

See above.

Swollen tonsils and tensive pain on swallowing.

Kali Bichromicum & **Hepar**

See above.

A feeling as of a splinter in the throat, when swallowing.

Sensation, as of a fish-bone in the throat when swallowing.

PHARYNGITIS *(contd.)*—

Kali Bichromicum & **Ignatia**

See above.

Feeling as of a lump in the throat—globus hystericus, which is not felt during, but between the acts of deglutition.

Sensaton as of plug in the throat, < not when swallowing.

Kali Bichromicum & **Kali Chloratum**

See above.

A great deal of fœtor of the breath.

Kali Bichromicum & **Mercurius Iodatus**

See above.

The symptoms are < from empty swallowing, so that simple attempt to swallow saliva, is more painful than swallowing food.

Kali Bichromicum & **Nux Vomica**

See above.

Adherent mucus high up in the trachea and bronchi, inducing cough.

Soreness, roughness and a harsh, scraped feeling in throat.

Kali Bichromicum & **Secale Cornutum**

See above.

Hawking up of follicular exudates.

Kali Bichromicum & **Sulphur**

See above.

The more chronic the case the more it is indicated.

Pulsatilla & **Apis**

Marked redness of the tonsils and the fauces have a dark-red or purplish hue.

Stinging pains in the throat <usually from swallowing saliva or after taking food.

Stinging pains in the throat when swallowing.

PLEURISY

[**Remedies.**—*Abro. Acon. Ap. Arn. Ars. Ars-Iod. Asclep. Bell. Bor. Bry. Canth. Gaul. Gua. Hep. Kali-C. Kali-Iod. Phos. Ran-B. Seneg. Stan. Sul.*]

Aconite	&	**Bryonia**
In the beginning, when the fever is high, with restlessness and anxiety.		After *Acon.* when the high fever begins to decrease. The patient is quiet and full of pain ; he lies on the affected side.
Bryonia	&	**Arnica**
Sharp, stitching pain in the chest, < on motion. See also above.		After injuries to the chest-wall ; must often change position.
Bryonia	&	**Belladonna**
See above.		Right side. Great soreness. Cannot lie on the affected side. Worse from jar of bed.
Bryonia	&	**Guaiacum**
See above.		Pleurisy, during the second stage of Phthisis, with the peculiar putrid and muco-purulent sputum.
Bryonia	&	**Senega**
See above.		Violent attack, with *Bryonia*-symptoms, but < from rest. Feels, as if the chest were too tight.
Bryonia	&	**Sulphur**
See above.		Sharp, stitching pain through the left lung to the back,<lying on back and from least motion.
Stannum	&	**Kali Carb.**
Sharp, knife-like stitches in the left axilla, extending up into the left clavicle. Sometimes they extend from the left side down into the abdomen. They are < from bending forward, from pressure and on inspiration.		Stitches in the left chest (irrespective of motion), palpitation and dry cough. Pain, as if the lower lobe of right lung were adhering to ribs, < at 3 A.M. and on inspiration. Puffiness of the upper eye-lids.

PLEURISY *(contd.)*—

Sulphur	&	**Apis**
Cases that refuse to respond to the well-chosen remedies, particularly when there is well-marked pleuritic effusion. Plastic exudation. See also above.		Pleurisy, with exudation. It comes in when the fever has abated and the pains are very little if present, but there is great oppression (< at night and from warmth), and faintness from the quantity of exudates. Chronic or latent cases.
Sulphur	&	**Arsenicum**
See above.		Serous effusion. Painful asthmatic respiration. Dyspnœa. Diarrhœa, great thirst, dropsical swellings. Fear of death. Sweat. Insomnia. Pyo-thorax.
Sulphur	&	**Arsenicum Iodatum**
See above.		Pleuritic exudation, with great emaciation and prostration. Tuberculous cases.
Sulphur	&	**Asclepias Tuberosa**
See above.		Sharp, stitches through the part of the left chest, < from motion. Chronic Pleurisy in tubercular patients.
Sulphur	&	**Cantharis**
See above.		Profuse sero-fibrous exudation, excessive dyspnœa, stitches in the chest, dry, hacking cough, displacement of heart, palpitation. tendency to faint and profuse sweat ; scanty albuminous urine.
Sulphur	&	**Hepar**
See above.		Purulent, plastic or croupous exudation, often of long-standing, with hectic fever and emaciation. Chilliness ; sensitiveness to damp air, which brings on coughing.

PLEURISY *(contd.)*—

Sulphur & **Kali Iodatum**

Sulphur: See above.

Kali Iodatum: Pleuritic effusion ; great difficulty in breathing, with Hydrothorax ; cannot lie in comfort at all in the right side ; heart displaced ; absence of respiratory sounds in the affected side.

Sulphur & **Rananculus Bulbosus**

Sulphur: See above.

Rananculus Bulbosus: Effusion of serum ; acute stabbing pains ; dyspnœa, anguish, distress ; also stitches about the chest at every change of weather, often from pleuritic adhesions.

PNEUMONIA

[**Remedies.**—*Acon. Amm-C. Ant-T. Bell. Brom. Bry. Carb-A. Carb-V. Chel. Cupr. Elaps. Ferr-P. Hep. Hyos. Iod. Ipec. Kali-C. Kali-H. Lach. Laur. Lyc. Merc. Nit-Ac. Phos. Ran-B. Rhus-T. Sang. Sul. Tereb. Trifol. Verat-V.*].

Aconite & **Bryonia**

Aconite: First stage of Pneumonia, when the fever is high and has been preceded by *chill.* Symptoms of engorgement of the lungs. The cough is usually hard and dry with *frothy sputa* and rather painful. The expectoration is *serous and watery, and a little blood-streaked,* but never thick. The patient is full of anxiety.

Bryonia: Comes in to take the place of *Aconite,* when the hepatization has commenced. The cough is still hard and painful but loose and more moist, and is associated with *thicker expectoration,* either yellowish or blood-streaked ; oppression of breathing. *The patient prefers to lie still* rather than to toss about. Sharp pleuritic stitches in the chest, worse in the left side.

Aconite & **Veratrum Viride**

Aconite: See above.

Veratrum Viride: The pneumonic engorgement is severe, with violent excitement of the heart ; rapid, full pulse ; nausea, faintness on rising ; tongue—red, down the centre.

PNEUMONIA *(contd.)*—

Antimonium Tartaricum & **Bryonia**

Antimonium Tartaricum: Worse on the right side. Catarrhal Pneumonia—mucous rāles are heard distinctly in the chest; it seems, as if, there is an immense quantity of mucus there, and yet the patient can scarcely raise any portion of it. The cough ceases or becomes more rare and yet there is no diminution of mucus production itself.

Bryonia: See above.

Carbo Animalis & **Carbo Vegetabilis**

Carbo Animalis: Suffocating hoarse cough producing shaking of the brain, as if the brain is loose in the head. A cold feeling in the chest.

Carbo Vegetabilis: Threatening paralysis of the lung—coldness especially about the extremities, symptoms of collapse. Loose, rattling rāles when the patient coughs or breathes.

Chelidonium & **Antimonium Tartaricum**

Chelidonium: Bilious Pneumonia—marked pain under the angle of the right shoulder-blade. The stools are characteristically profuse, bright-yellow and diarrhœic or they may be clayey. Desire or craving for milk, which exceptionally agrees. Craving for acid and sour things.

Antimonium Tartaricum: Yellow skin, urine and vomit in bilious Pneumonia; stinging under the right false ribs; rattling in the chest with suffocation. Strong heart-beat.

See also above.

Chelidonium & **Mercurius**

Chelidonium: See above.

Mercurius: It differs from *Chelidonium* in the character of the stool more than in anything else. The stool is slimy and is attended with *great tenesmus* before, during and after the stool. Plastic exudation and the expectoration is apt to be blood-streaked.

Ferrum Phos. & **Aconite**

Ferrum Phos.: The pulse is full and round. The expectoration is scanty and blood-streaked. The fever is not sthenic.

Aconite: Pulse rope-like. Sthenic fever. See also above.

PNEUMONIA *(contd.)*—

Iodine & **Bromine**

Plastic exudation. A decided cough with great dyspnœa, difficulty in breathing as though the chest would not expand. Solidification of some portion of the lungs.

In the stage of resolution, instead of absorption and expectoration of the exudate, slow suppuration appears with hectic fever and emaciation. The patient feels better in the cool open air than in a warm room.

Lobar Pneumonia. The patient seems, as if he could not get enough air into the chest. While there seems to be plenty of mucus, the patient does not appear to be able to expectorate it. Often there is nose-bleed.

Iodine & **Mercurius**

See above.

See above.

Iodine & **Hepar**

See above.

Purulent exudation. Indicated in the stage of resolution.

Kali Carb. & **Chelidonium**

Stitching pain prominently located in the wall of the chest.

It is indicated not in the beginning, but later, when there is copious exudation into the lungs, with great rattling of mucus during the cough. The symptoms are worse towards 2 or 3 P.M. The expectoration contains little globules of pus.

See above.

Kali Hydriod. & **Bryonia**

Indicated when hepatization has commenced and the disease localises itself and infiltrations begin and as a result both lungs consolidate. At first the patient has a very red face, the pupils are more or less dilated, and is drowsy ; later the patient grows worse, breathing becomes more heavy and the pupils fail to react to light ; stitching pains through the lungs, particularly through the sternum to the back, worse from any motion.

See above.

PNEUMONIA *(contd.)*—

Kali Hydriod. & **Phosphorus**

Kali Hydriod.: See above.

Phosphorus: Indicated when the bronchial symptoms are prominent. There is great dryness of the air-passages, with burning, excoriating, raw feeling in the upper part of the chest.

Lachesis & **Phosphorus**

Lachesis: Indicated when the affection assumes a typhoid form. Low, muttering delirium and hallucinations. The sputum is frothy, mixed with blood and purulent, and the patient is bathed in a profuse sweat.

If tubercles form, it is the proper remedy.

Phosphorus: See above.

Lachesis & **Sulphur**

Lachesis: See above.

Sulphur: Slowness of speech, dry tongue. All sorts of rāles may be heard in the chest ; the expectoration is muco-purulent, hectic type of fever, emaciation.

It ceases to be the remedy, if Tuberculosis has been developed by Pneumonia.

Lycopodium & **Sulphur**

Lycopodium: Coldness of one foot, usually the right, while the other is warm.

Sulphur: Coldness of one foot, usually the left.

See also above.

Rhus Tox. & **Phosphorus**

Rhus Tox.: Indicated in Typhoid-Pneumonia.

Rāles are heard all through the chest, especially in the lower lobe of the lungs. The cough is at first dry and becomes more frequent and loose, with expectoration of blood-streaked sputum.

Phosphorus: Follows well, when *Rhus* fails.

The stools are yellow and diarrhœic, and blood-streaked, sometimes looking like "flesh-water."

See also above.

PNEUMONIA *(contd.)*—

Sanguinaria & **Antimonium Tart.**

Hectic fever. Sharp-stitching pains, especially about the right lung and in the region of the nipple. Rust-colored sputum with the cough. Very distressing dysponœa, hands and feet burning hot, or else just the reverse, icy-cold.

See above.

Sanguinaria & **Phosphorus**

See above.

See above.

Sanguinaria & **Sulphur**

The expectoration is very offensive even to the patient himself.

See above.

Sanguinaria & **Veratrum Viride**

See above.

Indicated before hepatization. More marked arterial excitement. Violent congestions preceding the disease.

See also above.

QUINSY

[**Remedies.**—*Bell. Fluor-Ac. Hep. Lach. Merc. Sil. Sul.*]

Belladonna & **Fluoric Acid**

The fauces inflamed and bright-red, the tonsils, particularly the right one, enlarged, with a tendency of the disease to extend towards the left; the tonsils rapidly suppurate; the glands in the neck, externally, are commonly involved and are to be felt as hard but very sensitive. Kernels in the neck. Sharp pains through the tonsils. The violence of the attack is its characteristic. The patient seems to be worse from swallowing the fluids.

Indicated when abscess has discharged but refuses to heal, in spite of the administration of *Silicea*. It has relief from cold.

QUINSY *(contd.)*—

Belladonna	&	**Hepar**
See above.		It should be administered when in spite of the exhibition of *Belladonna* pus forms in the tonsil; rigors and chills; lancinating pains with throbbing. It may still then prevent abscess formation.
Belladonna	&	**Mercurius**
See above.		Indicated in an advanced stage, when pus has already formed; the tonsil is enlarged and encroaches on neighbouring parts and the breathing is labored. It should be given *low* and repeatedly. *If administered at first, it will greatly lengthen the attack.*
Belladonna	&	**Silicea**
See above.		Indicated when abscess has discharged but refuses to heal. The pus keeps on forming and grows dark and fœtid and disagreeable to the taste. *It cannot bear any cold.* It follows *Hepar* and should be interpolated with *Sulphur* if the case is obstinate.
Belladonna	&	**Sulphur**
See above.		Like *Fluoric Acid* it should be interpolated when *Silicea* fails.
Fluoric Acid	&	**Silicea**
See above.		See above.
Hepar	&	**Silicea**
See above.		See above.
Mercurius	&	**Lachesis**
See above.		The pus degenerates and becomes of a dark, thin, offensive character, with sensitiveness to the touch.
Silicea	&	**Sulphur**
See above.		See above.

RACHITIS

[**Remedies.**—*Calc-P. Mag-M. Phos. Sil. Sul.*]

Calcarea Phos. & **Silicea**

The child is thin and emaciated, with sunken, rather flabby abdomen and predisposed to glandular and osseous diseases. Every little exposure produces a feeling of heat all over the body. The periosteum and articulations are irritated and inflamed.

The body is small and emaciated, with the exception of the *abdomen,* which is round and plump. The fibrous parts of the joints are inflamed, swollen or ulcerated—this gives the joints, especially the knees, a knob-like appearance.

Magnesia Mur. & **Silicea**

Indicated in the enlarged liver of children, who are puny in their growth and rachitic. They suffer from skin affections. The hairs drop out. Sweating of the feet, which is *not offensive.*

Offensive foot-sweat.
See also above.

Silicea & **Sulphur**

See above.

The child looks shrivelled and dried up, like a little old man; the skin hangs in folds and is rather yellowish, wrinkled and flabby. Voracious appetite. The child sweats about the head particularly during sleep.

RHEUMATISM

[**Remedies.**—*Acon. Act-S. Anac. Apis. Apoc. Arct-L. Arn. Art-A. Bell. Benz.-Ac. Berb. Bry. Calc-Fl. Calc-Ost. Calc-Ph. Caps. Caulo. Caust. Cham. Chin-S. Cinch. Colch. Coloc. Con. Dulc. Ferr. Gels. Guai., Iod. Kali-Bi. Kali-C. Kali-H. Kalm. Lac-C. Led. Lith-C. Lyc. Mag-C. Mang. Merc. Nux-M. Nux-V. Petr. Phos-Ac. Puls. Ran-B. Rhod. Rhus-R. Rhus-T. Sab. Sang. Sec. Sil. Sul. Thuj. Val. Verat-A. Viol-O. Zinc.*].

Actea Spicata & **Apocynum**

Rheumatism of the smaller joints, especially if the hands and wrists are involved.

Joints feel stiff, especially on moving in the morning.

RHEUMATISM *(contd.)*—

Actea Spicata	&	**Caulophyllum**
See above.		Phalangeal and metacarpal joints, particularly in females.
Actea Spicata	&	**Sabina**
See above.		Pains worse in a warm room. Rheumatism of the heels in plethoric women.
Actea Spicata	&	**Viola Odorata**
See above.		Right wrists.
Berberis	&	**Benzoic Acid**
The urine is yellow, turbid and flocculent; sometimes there is whitish sediment, later becoming red and mealy.		Urine smells strong, like that of the horse.
Berberis	&	**Calcarea Ostrearum**
See above.		Very offensive urine, with a white deposit.
Berberis	&	**Lycopodium**
See above.		Urine contains a lithic acid deposit.
Bryonia	&	**Actea Spicata**
The local inflammation is violent, the parts are very hot and dark or pale-red. Pains worse from motion. The bowels are constipated.		The patient goes out feeling tolerably comfortable, but as he walks the joints ache and even swell.
Bryonia	&	**Belladonna**
See above.		The affected joints are swollen, red, shining and often have red streaks, radiating from them along the limbs. Pains are cutting and tearing, running along the limbs like lightning.
Bryonia	&	**Colchicum**
See above.		Marked aggravation in the evening. The affected joints are swollen and dark-red. The pains are of a tearing or jerking character, and appear, as if in the periosteum.

RHEUMATISM *(contd.)*—

Bryonia	&	**Ledum**
Copious effusion. See also above.		Rheumatic inflammation of the great toe ; the effusion is scanty ; tends to harden into nodosities. Hot swelling of the hip and shoulder-joints.

Bryonia	&	**Rhus Tox.**
Muscular rheumatism. See also above.		Involves the fibrous tissues and sheaths of the muscles. Rheumatism after exposure to wet, especially when over-heated or perspiring. *Relief from moving about.*

Calcarea Ostrearum	&	**Rhus Tox.**
Rheumatic affections, caused by working in water. Rheumatism of the muscles of the back and shoulders, after the failure of *Rhus*. See also above.		See above.

Calcarea Ostrearum	&	**Nux Vomica**
See above.		Rheumatism of the back, when the patient is unable to turn over in bed, without first sitting up. Rheumatism of the trunk. The symptoms are almost always worse in the morning.

Causticum	&	**Colocynth**
Joints are stiff and tendons shortened, drawing the limbs out of shape. Articulation of the jaw particularly involved. Worse from cold and relieved by warmth.		Articular rheumatism—the joints remain stiff and unwieldy. Pains are *boring* in character.

Causticum	&	**Guaiacum**
See above.		Contractions of the tendons, drawing the limbs out of shape, aggravated by any attempt at motion. Follows *Causticum*.

Causticum	&	**Rhus Tox.**
Restlessness at night. Worse weather. See also above.		Restlessness all the time. Worse in damp weather.

RHEUMATISM *(contd.)*—

Chamomilla & **Colchicum**

Chamomilla: *Feverishness and excitement.* Pains drive the patient out of bed and compel him to walk about. Stitching pains jump from place to place, worse in the ankles and knees, and leave a sense of weakness. Sweat does not relieve him, but his *pains are better after sweat.*

Colchicum: Begins in one joint and travels thence to another, or in one side of the body and then flies to the other. The pains are worse in the evening. The joints are extremely sensitive to touch and the slightest motion. The patient is extremely irritable.

Metastasis of rheumatism to the chest. A sensation, as if the chest were being squeezed in a vise.

Chamomilla & **Ferrum Met.**

Chamomilla: See above.

Ferrum Met.: Rheumatism better from moving about slowly.

See also above.

Chamomilla & **Pulsatilla**

Chamomilla: The patient is cross and excitable.

Pulsatilla: The patient is mild and tearful.

The erratic pains do not leave any weakness.

Chamomilla & **Rhus Tox.**

Chamomilla: See above.

Rhus Tox.: Lacks the excitement of *Chamomilla.*

Chamomilla & **Veratrum Album**

Chamomilla: See above.

Veratrum Album: Lacks the feverishness and excitement of *Chamomilla.*

Dulcamara & **Calcarea Phos.**

Dulcamara: Aggravation from cold, damp weather or from changes from hot to cold weather, especially if these changes are *sudden.*

Calcarea Phos.: In *women*—joints ache in every change of weather.

Kali Bichromicum & **Actea Spicata**

Kali Bichromicum: Rheumatism of the smaller joints—particularly of the finger and wrists, in spring or summer weather when there are cool days or nights.

Actea Spicata: See above.

Kali Bichromicum & **Artemisia Abrotanum**

Kali Bichromicum: Gastric and rheumatic symptoms alternate.

Artemisia Abrotanum: Diarrhœa and piles alternate with rheumatism.

RHEUMATISM *(contd.)*—

Kali Carb. Stubborn rheumatism. Sharp stitching pains. 3 A.M. aggravation. Lumbago.	&	**Kali Hydriod.** Rheumatism of the joints, particularly of the knee. The skin above the affected joints is apt to be spotted and the pains are of gnawing, boring character.
Kalmia Rheumatism of the chest. Pains shift from joints to the heart, especially after *external applications* to the joints.	&	**Colchicum** See above.
Kalmia Rheumatism, usually travels downwards, *i.e.,* following the direction of its pains.	&	**Ledum** Follows the opposite direction.
Lithium Carb. Rheumatism of the finger-joints :— Tenderness with swelling and occasional redness of the last joints of the fingers. Pains.	&	**Calcarea Ostrearum** Gouty nodosities about the fingers. See also above.
Lithium Carb. See above.	&	**Kalmia** Tearing pains in the finger-joints. See also above.
Magnesia Carb. Rheumatism in the right shoulder. Rheumatic pains in the limbs, worse after a long walk, better from warmth, and worse in bed.	&	**Nux Moschata** Rheumatism in the *right* deltoid muscle.
Magnesia Carb. See above.	&	**Sanguinaria** Rheumatism in the *right* deltoid muscle.
Manganum In the rheumatism of the heels— The rheumatic symptoms come in dark almost bluish spots.	&	**Causticum** In the rheumatism of the heels— Symptoms are worse from cold and relieved by warmth.
Manganum Rheumatism of the heels, can not bear any weight on them.	&	**Ledum** Rheumatism of the great toes.

RHEUMATISM *(contd.)*—

Petroleum & **Kali Hydriod.**

Petroleum: In the rheumatism of the knees—

The knees are stiff and are associated with sharp stitching pains.

Kali Hydriod.: See above.

Pulsatilla & **Bryonia**

Pulsatilla: In rheumatism with erratic pains—

The tearing pains force the patient to move the affected parts. Pressure relieves. They are usually worse from warmth and are relieved by cold. They are worse in the evening.

Bryonia: In rheumatism with erratic pains—

See above.

Pulsatilla & **Chamomilla**

Pulsatilla: In rheumatism with erratic pains—

See above.

Chamomilla: In rheumatism with erratic pains—

See above.

Pulsatilla & **Kali Bich.**

Pulsatilla: In rheumatism with erratic pains—

See above.

Kali Bich.: In rheumatism with erratic pains—

See above.

Pulsatilla & **Lycopodium**

Pulsatilla: See above.

Lycopodium: Limbs easily go to sleep, with numbness and formication. Gastric symptoms. Better from warmth.

Pulsatilla & **Sanguinaria**

Pulsatilla: See above.

Sanguinaria: In rheumatism with erratic pains—

Sharp, stitching pains, with great soreness and stiffness of the muscles, especially those of the back and neck.

Pulsatilla & **Sulphur**

Pulsatilla: In rheumatism with erratic pains—

See above.

Sulphur: In rheumatism with erratic pains—

Inflammatory swellings ; seem to ascend. The pains are worse in bed and at night.

RHEUMATISM *(contd.)*—

Rananculus Bulb.	&	**Aconite**
Inter-costal rheumatism. Worse in damp weather and particularly from a change of weather or change of temperature.		Rheumatism due to exposure to cold after being over-heated.
Rananculus Bulb.	&	**Arnica**
See above.		Due to the combined effect of exposure to dampness and cold, and strain on the muscles from over-exertion. Aggravation from motion.
Rananculus Bulb.	&	**Bryonia**
See above.		See above.
Rhus Tox.	&	**Anacardium**
Relief by continued motion, while aggravation on beginning to move. Aggravation during damp weather or from dwelling in a damp place ; the patient cannot bear the least exposure to cool air. Prominent projections of the bones are sore to the touch. See also above.		Stiff-neck, worse from beginning to move.
Rhus Tox.	&	**Capsicum**
See above.		Relieved by moving about from the beginning. Worse from least draft of air, even though the air is warm.
Rhus Tox.	&	**Ferrum Met.**
See above.		Worse at night, relieved by slowly moving about.
Rhus Tox.	&	**Kalmia**
See above.		Tearing-down pains down the legs, without any swelling, without fever, but with great weakness. See also above.
Rhus Tox.	&	**Ledum**
See above.		The pains travel upward. Worse from warmth of the bed and ameliorated by cold applications. Drawing pains in the joints, aggravated by wine. The muscles feel sore, as if, out of place. See also above.

RHEUMATISM *(contd.)*—

	&	
Rhus Tox.	&	**Lycopodium**
See above.		Worse on beginning to move but better from slow motion. See also above.
Rhus Tox.	&	**Pulsatilla**
See above.		Worse on beginning to move, but better from slow motion. Worse from warmth. See also above.
Rhus Tox.	&	**Rhododendron**
See above.		Susceptibility to changes in the weather and to electric changes in the atmosphere. Pains in the limbs especially in the bones of forearms, hands and feet. Numbness. Formication.
Rhus Tox.	&	**Rhus Radicans**
See above.		Rheumatic pains in the back of the head.
Sanguinaria	&	**Ferrum**
Erratic pains. Rheumatism of the *right* deltoid muscle. The patient is unable to raise the arm to the head. See also above.		Rheumatism of the *left* deltoid muscle.
Sanguinaria	&	**Nux Moschata**
See above.		Rheumatism of the *left* deltoid muscle.
Secale	&	**Calcarea Ostrearum**
Sudden "catch" or "klink" in the back.		Rheumatism of the back. See also above.
Silicea	&	**Ledum**
The pains are predominantly in the shoulders and in the joints, worse at night and when uncovering.		Pains in the joints, extend from feet upwards. Worse from covering up.

SPRAIN

[**Remedies.**—*Amm-C. Amm-M. Arn. Calc-O. Petr. Rhus-T. Ruta. Stront. Sul-Ac.*]

Ammonium Carb. & **Ammonium Mur.**

The injured joint is hot and painful.

Chronic sprains. Symptoms are relieved by continued motion.

Ammonium Carb. & **Sulphuric Acid**

See above.

Long-lasting cases with soreness and stiffness.

Arnica & **Ammonium Carb.**

Considerable inflammation of the soft parts, other than the ligaments.

It follows *Arnica*.
See also above.

Rhus Tox. & **Arnica**

Inflammation of the tendons of muscles. The patient has relief of his symptoms by continued motion, while he experiences aggravation on beginning to move.

See above.

Rhus Tox. & **Ammonium Mur.**

See above.

See above.

Rhus Tox. & **Calcarea Carb.**

See above.

It follows *Rhus,* when that remedy has relieved, but fails to cure.

Strontiana Carb. & **Arnica**

Chronic sprains, particularly of the ankle-joints, with some œdema from long interference with the circulation.

It precedes *Strontiana.*

See also above.

Strontiana Carb. & **Ruta**

It follows when *Ruta* fails to cure.

It precedes *Strontiana.*
Worse in the morning before rising.

SYPHILIS

[**Remedies.**—*Asaf. Aur. Bad. Carb-An. Carb-V. Cinnab. Cor-R. Fl-Ac. Kali-Bich. Kali-H. Lach. Lyc. Mere-Bin. Mere-Cor. Merc-Prot. Merc-Viv. Nit-Ac. Plat-M. Staph. Stilling.*]

Aurum	&	**Asafœtida**
Syphilitic Iritis—sore, bruised sensation around the eyes. The eye is decidedly worse from touch.		Less marked. Bluish ulcers.
Aurum	&	**Mercurius**
See above.		Hypopyon.
Aurum	&	**Mercurius Cor.**
See above.		Symptons of violent character. Tearing pains in the bones around the eyes.
Aurum	&	**Nitric Acid**
See above.		Great soreness in the bones at night ; worse from every change of weather.
Carbo Animalis	&	**Badiaga**
Indurated buboes—hard like stones ; opened too soon—gaping wound which has partly healed, leaving the surrounding tissues stony hard.		Indurated buboes—mal-treated cases.
Carbo Animalis	&	**Carbo Veg.**
Coppery-red blotches on the skin particularly on the face. See also above.		Debility more marked.
Carbo Animalis	&	**Nitric Acid**
Constitutional and Tertiary Syphilis. See also above.		Secondary syphilis. Ulcers are characteristically irregular in outline. See also above.
Fluoric Acid	&	**Silicea**
Relief from cold.		Cannot bear anything cold.
Lachesis	&	**Hepar**
Chancre becomes gangrenous. Weakness.		A sore, bruised feeling, together with hyperæsthesia. No loss of vitality. A *concordant* of *Lachesis.*

SYPHILIS *(contd.)*—

Lachesis	&	**Lycopodium**
Small red blood-vessels shine through the yellow skin. See also above.		Ulcers on the throat dark-grayish-yellow, worse on the right side. Ulcers on the legs, made worse by poultices or by any attempt to dress them. The pus is often golden-yellow. Flatulent dyspepsia.
Lachesis	&	**Nitric Acid**
See above.		Irregular edges of the ulcer—present exuberant, easily-breeding granulations. The discharges are offensive, thin and excoriating. Cracks in the commissures of the lips ; sensations of a splinter in the throat. The ulcers are worse from the application of cold water. See also above.
Mercurius Cor.	&	**Mercurius Biniod.**
Symptoms of the most violent character. See also above.		Hunterian or hard chancre.
Mercurius Vivus	&	**Mercurius Cor.**
Soft chancre or chancroid. The ulceration is superficial and the base of the sore has a dirty lardaceous appearance. See also above.		The ulceration is very destructive. The ulcer is serpiginous; it has a rugged edge.
Staphisagria	&	**Platinum Mur.**
The discharge is thin and acrid. The bones are affected.		Caries of the tarsus. Necrosis.
Staphisagria	&	**Stillingia**
See above.		Long bones. The pains are worse at night and damp weather. 'Pains in and through the hips.

TOOTHACHE

[**Remedies.**—*Ant-C. Ap. Aran-D. Arn. Bry. Canth. Carb-An. Cham. Chel. Coff. Hep. Ign. Iod. Kali-C. Kali-I. Kali-Nit. Kreos. Lach. Lyc. Mag-C. Mag-Ph. Merc. Nux-V. Plant-M. Puls. Rat. Rhus-T. Sang. Sep. Sil. Staph. Sul. Zinc.*]

Antimonium Crudum & **Lycopodium**

Antimonium Crudum: In hollow teeth,<cold water, by least touch, > in open air.

Lycopodium: With gum-boils, swollen cheek ; < cold drinks, > warm applications.

Apis & **Rhus Tox.**

Apis: Congestive; with sore, bruised feeling, > from cold.

Rhus Tox.: Periosteal, rheumatic ; pains tearing, tingling, > by warmth, < from cold.

In jumping toothache, the pain is momentarily relieved by the application of a cold hand.

Aranea Diadema & **Mercurius**

Aranea Diadema: Sudden violent pains in the teeth of whole upper and lower jaw at night, immediately after lying down.

Esp. < in damp weather and when the patient gets into the bed.

Mercurius: Decayed teeth ; the pains are tearing and pulsating and shoot into face and ears.

< from warmth of bed.

Bryonia & **Antimonium Crudum**

Bryonia: In hollow tooth, but frequently in sound tooth, more than one tooth may be involved.

> lying on affected side, from firm pressure of the head against the pillow and cold applications.

Antimonium Crudum: Pre-eminently in hollow teeth.

See also above.

Cantharis & **Kreosotum**

Cantharis: Tearing in the teeth and gums.

Kreosotum: Tearing and burning.

Teeth at first become yellow, and then dark and decay.

Chamomilla & **Coffea Cruda**

Chamomilla: Cold application relieves for an instant.

Coffea Cruda: Cold application relieves permanently.

Chelidonium Majus & **Nux Vomica**

Chelidonium Majus: < in bed ; > cold water.

Nux Vomica: < from coffee ; > warm food.

TOOTHACHE *(contd.)*—

Chelidonium Majus & Sanguinaria Canadensis

Chelidonium Majus: See above.

Sanguinaria Canadensis: In decayed teeth; < cold water.

Coffea Cruda & Kreosotum

Coffea Cruda: Of children and nervous people.

In children from decayed teeth.

See also above.

Kreosotum: Nervous and irritable persons whose teeth decay rapidly.

Burning pains, < by motion and talking.

See also above.

Hepar Sulphur & Sulphur

Hepar Sulphur: With swollen gums; throbbing, as if suppuration had began.

< in warm room and at night.

Sulphur: With jumping pain; throbbing pain.

< in evening and in open air.

Iodium & Kali Iodatum

Iodium: Yellow teeth, gums full of blisters.

Kali Iodatum: With a feeling, as if a worm is crawling at the root.

Kali Carbonicum & Ignatia

Kali Carbonicum: With throbbing, while eating.

Ignatia: < between, than during eating.

Lachesis & Kreosotum

Lachesis: Throbbing pains; periodic; always come after waking from sleep, after eating, also from warm and cold drinks.

Gums swollen and bluish or tense and hot; and look, as if they would crack.

Kreosotum: Pains extend from teeth to the left side of the face; make the patient excitable and nervous, even throw into convulsions.

Gums bleed, blood being dark.

See also above.

Lachesis & Mercurius

Lachesis: See above.

Mercurius: Gums dirty, with white edges.

See also above.

Magnesium Carbonicum & Ratanhia

Magnesium Carbonicum: During pregnancy when the gastric and hepatic symptoms predominate, < at night.

Ratanhia: During pregnancy, at night.

Magnesium Carbonicum & Chamomilla

Magnesium Carbonicum: See above.

Chamomilla: It is complementary to *Mag-C.*

See also above.

TOOTHACHE *(contd.)*—

Mercurius & **Silicea**

Teeth hollow and dentine inflamed ; < by warmth of bed, open air and at night.

See also above.

Periosteum inflamed ; gums show, fistulous openings, oozing thin, offensive ichor.

Pulsatilla & **Plantago Major**

Nerve-pains (of head), when they go into face and teeth.

When associated with ear-ache.

Pulsatilla & **Zincum**

See above.

Pressing, tearing pains in the occiput, which seem to shoot through the eyes and sympáthetically, into the teeth.

TYPHOID FEVER

[**Remedies.**—*Absinth. Acon. Ail. Alum. Anac. Ant-T. Apis. Arn. Ars. Bap. Bell. Bry. Calc-O. Carb-V. Cast. Chlor. Cin. Cocc. Colch. Con. Cupr. Gels. Ham. Hell. Hyos. Lach. Lept. Lyc. Meph. Merc. Mosch. Mur-Ac. Nit-Ac. Nuphar. Nux-M. Nux-V. Op. Petr. Phos-Ac. Phos. Psor. Puls. Ran-S. Rhus-T. Selen. Stram. Sul. Sweet-Sp-O-Nit. Tarax. Tereb. Verat-A.*]

Baptisia & **Arnica**

Evident decomposition of vital fluids and rapid decomposition of tissues.

In the early stage—*always increase of temperature;* the pulse is usually accelerated in direct proportion to the intensity of fever. Yellow putrescent stools. Abdominal symptoms.

In the later stage—profound prostration. Stupor. Delirium. All the exhalations and discharges are exceedingly offensive.

A tendency to apoplectic congestion; the stupor is so profound that both stools and urine pass involuntarily. Loud, snoring respiration. Suggillation.

TYPHOID FEVER *(contd.)*—

Baptisia	&	Gelsemium
Deeper-acting remedy. Follows *Gelsemium*. See also above.		Indicated in the early stage. The relation between the two drugs is one of degree or intensity—it being the milder-acting drug of the two. Usually precedes *Baptisia* when there are malaise and muscular weakness, the patient feels sore and bruised all over, as if he had been pounded ; suffers from chills and creeps which go down the back ; the eye-lids are heavy, as though they could hardly be lifted. Gives place to *Baptisia,* if the case worsens despite its use.

Baptisia	&	Lachesis
See above.		Is called for in worse cases. Trembling of the tongue when attempting to protrude it ; the tongue catches on the teeth during the act—when he succeeds in getting it out, it hangs there tremblingly and he may not even have the sense enough to draw it in again. Hæmorrhages of dark or blackish blood from every orifice may be frequent. The sediment of the stools looks like charred straw. In severe cases, marked intolerance to pressure, even when the sensorium appears to be perfectly benumbed. Dropping of the lower jaw and involuntary discharges.

Baptisia	&	Muriatic Acid
A besotted look to the face ; the teeth are covered with black sordes, and the tongue is red on the edges and yellowish-brown down the centre. See also above.		Weakness is so great that the patient is unable to make the slightest exertion required to maintain his head on the pillow; he therefore slides down to the foot of the bed.

TYPHOID FEVER *(contd.)*—

Baptisia & Rhus Tox.

Baptisia

See above.

Rhus Tox.

Restlessness caused more by rheumatic pains than by muscular soreness alone. The tongue has a red triangular tip. Muttering delirium unaccompanied by delusions respecting personal identity. The discharges are less offensive. Diarrhœa progresses to a severer type—the stools being watery, sometimes bloody and involuntary.

Belladonna & Hyoscyamus

Belladonna

Indicated in the beginning of the disease when there is wild and furious delirium.

Hyoscyamus

Follows *Belladonna,* when the stupor becomes marked. The patient picks at the bed-clothes or his fingers in a somnolent sort of way and occasionally reaches out, as if grasping for something in the air. Tongue red and dry, speech difficult.

Bryonia & Belladonna

Bryonia

In the early stage—there is some confusion of mind; the sensorium is depressed, but there are no perversion of senses. Mild delirium. On closing his eyes for sleep, he thinks he sees persons who are not present ; on opening them he is surprised to find that he is mistaken. The patient has dreams, which have for their subject the occupation of the day. Splitting headache. Bowels are usually constipated—the stools being large, hard and dry and are either brown or dark in color. The patient desires to remain perfectly quiet.

In well-advanced cases—mushy stools. The patient expresses a continual "desire to go home"—he imagines he is not at home and longs to be taken there in order to be properly cared for.

Belladonna

Indicated in the early stage.

More cerebral erethism and more violent delirium. The patient jerks his limbs and starts during sleep. He springs up from sleep affright. As soon as he closes his eyes, he sees all sorts of persons and things, which disappear as the eyes are opened. Headache with throbbing pains and the patient may be obliged to sit up, rather than keep perfectly quiet.

See also above.

TYPHOID FEVER *(contd.)*—

Bryonia & **Rhus Tox.**

Bryonia

See above.

Rhus Tox.

Marked restlessness. Headache with a sensation as though a board is strapped highly across the forehead. The tongue is brown and dry and even cracked and has a red tip. There is frequent diarrhœa from the beginning.

See also above.

Calcarea Ostrearum & **Lycopodium**

Calcarea Ostrearum

In the early stage—the patient falls into a troubled sort of sleep and dreams of some perplexing subject which awakens him.

In the second week—the rashes do not appear, and the patient goes into a sort of stupor. There may be diarrhœa or constipation. More hallucinations.

Lycopodium

Complementary to *Calcarea*, but there is never any diarrhœa.

The tongue seems swollen and the patient cannot protrude it, or when the patient does put it out, it rolls from side to side like a pendulum. Almost always, too, the tongue is dry and has blisters on it.

See also above.

Cocculus Indicus & **Bryonia**

Cocculus Indicus

Nausea and inclination to vomit due to weakness of the cerebro-spinal nerves.

Bryonia

Nausea and vomiting due to intestinal causes.

See also above.

Cocculus Indicus & **Carbo Veg.**

Cocculus Indicus

The abdomen is greatly distended and tympanitic due to retention of flatus in the abdomen.

See also above.

Carbo Veg.

Tympanites when the flatus results from decomposition of the food.

Colchicum & **Arsenicum**

Colchicum

Restlessness, excessive debility and tympany. The chief symptoms are abdominal—great tympany, involuntary, forcible, watery stools, accompanied with nausea and frequent vomiting of bile.

Arsenicum

Restlessness and debility. A picture of complete exhaustion. The delirium is worse after 12 P.M. Sleepless at 3 A.M. Tympany is often absent.

TYPHOID FEVER *(contd.)*—

Colchicum & Carbo Veg.

Colchicum		Carbo Veg.
See above.	&	Giving out of the vital force—collapse ; the patient lies cold and almost pulseless. The pulse feels very much like a slight ripple beneath the examining finger; there is no decided pulsation ; the feet and legs, below the knees are cold or there may be coldness of the knees and feet, the parts between them not being cold. Watery stool is not so characteristic—the discharges being either absent or if present, horribly offensive. See also above.

Helleborus		Arnica
Complete sensorial depression. The patient cannot be easily aroused.	&	The patient may be temporarily aroused. See also above.

Helleborus		Opium
Pale face, which is often cold or at least cooler than natural, and at times hard and covered with a cold sweat. The pulse is small, weak and almost imperceptible. See also above.	&	The cerebral congestion is more profound. The breathing is loud and stertorous. *The face is dark, brownish-red* or often *blue.* The *pulse* is *full and slow.*

Helleborus		Phosphoric Acid
Marked *black soots about the nostrils.* Drowsiness from which the patient cannot be easily aroused. *Complete muscular relaxation.* See also above.	&	Drowsiness from which the patient is *easily aroused,* and then he is perfectly conscious.

Helleborus		Sweet Spirits of Nitre
Sensorial apathy most marked See also above.	&	Sensorial apathy in the lowest degree. The patient seems to be in a sort of torpor, from which he may, by exertion, be aroused, but he falls back immediately into the same indifference.

Lachesis		Agaricus
Loquacious, jumping from subject to subject. Also see above.	&	Loquacity—merry, incoherent talks.

TYPHOID FEVER *(contd.)*—

Lachesis	&	Arnica
See above.		Dark spots here and there on the body, irregular in outline and having a black and blue appearance—*ecchymoses.* See also above.
Lachesis	&	**Apis**
Dropping of the lower jaw marked. Hyperæsthesia. See also above.		A nervous fidgetiness with sleepiness, but inability to sleep. Muttering delirium; happy strange expression. *Abdomen swollen and extremely sensitive* (a bruised feeling). Dropping of the lower jaw—not marked.
Lachesis	&	**Hyoscyamus**
See above.		*Twitching of the muscles.* See also above.
Lachesis	&	**Lycopodium**
See above.		It is the complement of *Lachesis.* Rattling breathing. Rattling of phlegm in the throat during both inspiration and expiration, and the eyes are fixed and set, and are filled with mucus. See also above.
Lachesis	&	**Mephitis**
See above.		Loquacity, as if drunk.
Lachesis	&	**Muriatic Acid**
See above.		A *sunken* face, tongue smooth, as if deprived of papillæ or brown, shrunken and hard. Sliding in bed from muscular weakness.
Lachesis	&	**Opium**
See above.		Unconsciousness, stertorous breathing, and a *dark* or *brownish-red* hue of the face. *The darker-red the face more is Opium indicated.* The body is bathed in a hot sweat.

TYPHOID FEVER *(contd.)*—

Lachesis & **Paris Quadrifolia**

Lachesis: See above.

Paris Quadrifolia: A garrulity which is much like that produced by tea, a sort of vivacity with love of prattling.

Lachesis & **Rhus Tox.**

Lachesis: See above.

Rhus Tox.: Well-marked restlessness with relief from motion. Loquacity is not prominent. The tongue has a red, triangular tip. The discharges are never so offensive as of *Lachesis*.

Lycopodium & **Hyoscyamus**

Lycopodium: Meets in impending paralysis of the brain—the distinction is *one of degree*—it being the deeper-acting of the two.

Hyoscyamus: More pronounced afternoon aggravation and less nervous irritability.

Muriatic Acid & **Apis**

Muriatic Acid: The tongue grows more dry and seems to have actually shrunken and become narrow and pointed; so dry is it that when he attempts to talk, it rattles like a piece of wash-leather in his mouth.

Apis: The tongue is covered with little blisters, especially along the border. The patient cannot put the tongue out; it seems to catch on the teeth, or if he does get it out, it trembles.

Muriatic Acid & **Phosphoric Acid**

Muriatic Acid: Taciturnity. *Prostration.*

Phosphoric Acid: Apathy and indifference—indifferent to what may happen to himself or to others. Characteristic stupor.

Muriatic Acid & **Rhus Tox.**

Muriatic Acid: Debility more marked.

Rhus Tox.: It precedes the *Acid.*

Phosphoric Acid & **Arnica**

Phosphoric Acid: Pointed nose; dark-blue rings around the eyes. *Debility characterized by indifference or apathy.* The delirium is quiet, not violent—muttering, unintelligible speech. He lies in a stupor, or in a stupid sleep, unconscious of all that is going on about him; but when aroused he is fully conscious. May be indicated in the early stages.

Arnica: The *Arnica* condition is a *more advanced* state. The depression and stupor are *more profound*—the patient goes to sleep when answering questions put to him. Petechiæ or ecchymoses. Involuntary stool and urine.

TYPHOID FEVER *(contd.)*—

Phosphoric Acid & Opium

Phosphoric Acid: Face—pale, sunken and hippocratic.

Opium: Face—deeper-red, almost a *brownish-red.* The stupor is progressive; at first the patient can be aroused from sleep, but later, no amount of shaking can bring the patient to consciousness. The breathing grows more and more labored and stertorous.

Phosphoric Acid & Phosphorus

Phosphoric Acid: Watery diarrhœa, contains undigested food. There is copious escape of flatus with the stool. The tongue is dry and may have a dark-red streak down its centre, but it is apt to be pale and clammy.

Phosphorus: More sensorial excitement; all the senses are irritated; the patient cannot bear any noise or odor. If diarrhœa is present, the stools are blood-streaked and look like "*fish-water.*" More dryness of the tongue.

Phosphoric Acid & Rhus Tox.

Phosphoric Acid: In the early stage, epistaxis gives no relief.

It often follows *Rhus* when that remedy relieves the restlessness but not the diarrhœa, and the patient goes into quiet sort of stupor.

Rhus Tox.: Symptoms are relieved by epistaxis. Restlessness—marked.

Phosphorus & Arsenicum

Phosphorus: Diarrhœa as soon as he eats; the stools are flaky, dark and often bloody and there is extreme weakness after stool.

Arsenicum: Diarrhœa provoked by every attempt to eat or drink; the stool is yellowish and watery in character, horribly offensive and worse after midnight. Sometimes the stools contain blood, slime and pus.

Phosphorus & Carbo Veg.

Phosphorus: Acts more upon the cerebrospinal nervous system. Great cerebro-spinal exhaustion.

Carbo Veg.: Acts more upon the sympathetic nerves—particularly on the solar plexus. It follows *Phosphorus* very well in the stage of collapse.

See also above.

TYPHOID FEVER *(contd.)*—

Rhus Tox.		**Arsenicum**
Diarrhœa with yellowish-brown or greenish stools of a cadaverous odor.	&	Follows *Rhus* in erethistic form of typhoid fever. Notwithstanding great prostration, the patient is still irritable and anxious, even to the last hours of life. The profound weakness continues, the face grows blacker and the diarrhœa persists, notwithstanding *Rhus*. The thirst is intense. Pains are of a burning character. The stools are dark-brown, offensive and bloody, and more frequent after midnight.
Rhus Tox.		**Arnica**
See above.	&	Complete apathy.
Rhus Tox.		**Baptisia**
See above.	&	See above. Drowsy stupid state. The face presents a dark-red, besotted appearance, like that of one intoxicated.
Rhus Tox.		**Carbo Veg.**
See above.	&	Follows *Rhus*. The patient lies perfectly torpid, without any sign of reaction.
Rhus Tox.		**Muriatic Acid**
See above.	&	The prostration is great ; the patient is so weak that he slides down towards the foot of the bed.
Rhus Tox.		**Phosphoric Acid**
See above.	&	Follows *Rhus* when there is increased debility or prostration with perfect apathy. The stools are bloody and slimy. Nose-bleed brings no relief.
Rhus Tox.	&	**Phosphorus**
See above.		Follows *Rhus* well when the pneumonic symptoms have failed to yield to that remedy and when diarrhœa persists. The stools are yellow and blood-streaked, sometimes looking like "flesh-water."

TYPHOID FEVER *(contd.)*—

Rhus Tox. & **Taraxacum**

The tongue has, very often, a triangular red tip.

Mapped tongue.

Stramonium & **Belladonna**

Mania for light and company. The face is bright-red.

The face is deeply congested.

Stramonium & **Hyoscyamus**

The patient sees objects which seem to rise in every corner of the room and move towards him. The motions that he makes are quite graceful and easy, although they may be violent. The patient is bathed in a hot sweat, which does not give any relief to the patient. The desire to uncover—of the whole body. The tongue is often soft, taking the imprint of teeth; screaming in sleep, often with hiccough.

The movements are angular. Desire to uncover—particularly the sexual organs.

Terebinthina & **Lachesis**

Preponderance of tympanites, with burning, which is accompanied by a glossy, smooth tongue, as if it had lost its papillæ.

See above.

URTICARIA

[**Remedies.**—*Ap. Ars. Bov. Calc-O. Cop. Dulc. Kali-Brom. Medusa. Nat-Mur. Puls. Rhus-T. Sep. Tereb. Urt-U.*].

Apis & **Arsenicum**

Itching, burning and stinging, almost intolerable.

Burning, itching and restlessness.

Apis & **Bovista**

See above.

Urticaria attended with diarrhœa, the stools being followed by tenesmus and burning.

Apis & **Calcarea Ostrearum**

See above.

Chronic cases.

Apis & **Copaiva**

See above.

Urticaria after eating shell-fish.

URTICARIA *(contd.)*—

Apis	&	**Kali Bromatum**
See above.		Urticaria with nervous diseases.
Apis	&	**Pulsatilla**
See above.		Urticaria of gastric or uterine origin.
Apis	&	**Rhus Tox.**
See above.		Accompaniment .of ague or rheumatism.
Apis	&	**Rumex**
See above.		Worse in the open air and while undressing.
Apis	&	**Sepia**
See above.		Worse in the open air.
Apis	&	**Terebinthina**
See above.		Urticaria after eating shell fish.
Apis	&	**Urtica Urens**
See above.		The welts are smaller.
Natrum Mur.	&	**Apis**
Urticaria about the joints—particularly about the ankles. Suitable to chronic cases.		See above.
Pulsatilla	&	**Dulcamara**
See above.		Relief from cold air.

VERTIGO

[**Remedies.**—*Ambra. Apis. Arg-N. Arn. Ars. Brom. Camph. Caust. Chel. Con. Dig. Ferr. Hydr-Ac. Kali-C. Lach. Laur. Mosch. Oleand. Petr. Pic-Ac. Piper. Rhus-T. Sang. Sep. Sil. Therid. Thuja. Verat.*]

Ambra Grisea	&	**Argentum Nitricum**
Vertigo comes on when the patient moves about, and the legs are unsteady ; he totters when he walks.		The vertigo is associated with general debility and trembling from nervous weakness. The patient staggers and reels, as if he were intoxicated. It is so *severe* at times that the patient becomes momentarily blind, in association with mental confusion, buzzing in the ears, nausea and trembling.

VERTIGO *(contd.)*—

Bromine & **Causticum**

Vertigo worse from running water. Anything moving rapidly produces this vertigo. It is relieved by nose-bleed. *Anxiety*—the patient expects to see objects jumping about or he feels, as if on turning his head he must see something or someone.

After dinner there is sensation deep in the brain as though a fit of apoplexy were impending. The patient feels, as if he would lose his senses.

Vertigo with a tendency to fall either forward or sideways. It is worse on rising and on trying to fix the mind. The sight is bedimmed, as if the patient were looking through a fog. A constant feeling of anxiety and weakness of the head.

Conium & **Ferrum**

Vertigo—exacerbation on turning over in bed. Often associated with a numb feeling in the brain, as if that organ were stupefied.

Vertigo, worse when rising suddenly from a lying to a sitting posture. Walking over a bridge or by some running water or riding in a car or carriage also causes this vertigo.

Ferrum & **Bromine**

See above.

See above.

Kali Carb. & **Oleander**

Vertigo from turning the head rapidly or from riding in a carriage. The patient is anæmic.

Vertigo as the result of weakness. Weak memory, forgetfulness and slowness of perception.

Kali Carb. & **Ferrum**

See above.

See above.

Lachesis & **Theridion**

Vertigo worse on closing the eyes or on sitting or lying down. Deathly paleness.

Vertigo with pains and nausea; all of which are aggravated by noise. Also worse on closing the eyes, from motion or from noise; sensitiveness to noise.

Picric Acid & **Piper Meth.**

Vertigo, worse from stooping, walking or going upstairs.

Vertigo worse on closing the eyes or on directing the attention to any object.

VERTIGO *(contd.)*—

Rhus Tox. & **Sanguinaria**

Rhus Tox.: Vertigo when the patient rises from a sitting posture. It is associated with heavy feelings in the limbs.

Sanguinaria: The patient feels, as if he would fall when he will attempt to rise from a sitting posture.

Sanguinaria & **Silicea**

Sanguinaria: See above.

Silicea: Vertigo, which seems to rise from the spine to the head. Difficulty in balancing. The patient fears that he will fall, and always to the left.

WHOOPING COUGH

[**Remedies.**—*Ambra. Ant-T. Arn. Bry. Cina. Coccus. Cor-Rub. Cup. Dros. Ipec. Kali-Bi. Kali-C. Meph. Seneg. Verat-A.*]

Coccus Cacti & **Drosera**

Coccus Cacti: Worse towards the morning. Vomiting of *ropy mucus*.

Drosera: Worse after 12 P.M

Corallium Rubrum & **Coccus Cacti**

Corallium Rubrum: Minute-gun cough—paroxysms coming very close together During the day the cough is short, quick and ringing in character ; when night comes, decided paroxysms of whooping appear, worse towards the morning—so that he falls back completely exhausted.

Coccus Cacti: Paroxysm of whooping cough, ending in vomiting of clear *ropy mucus*, hanging in great long strings from the mouth. Morning aggravation.

See also above.

Corallium Rubrum & **Kali Bich.**

Corallium Rubrum: Expectoration is clear.

See also above.

Kali Bich.: The expectoration is stringy, but it is yellow in color and not clear. Dry, barking cough, worse in the morning.

WHOOPING COUGH *(contd.)*—

Corallium Rubrum & **Senega**

See above.

The cough is worse towards the evening. Tough expectoration—transparent like the white of an egg and difficult to raise. A crushing weight in the chest.

Mephitis & **Corallium Rubrum**

Hard cough, with well-marked laryngeal spasm and a distinct whoop. *The catarrhal symptoms are slight and the spasmodic whoop is marked.* The cough is worse at night and after lying down.

Smothering *before* the cough and great exhaustion afterwards.

See also above.

Mephitis & **Drosera**

See above.

Spells of barking cough, which come so frequently as not to give the patient an opportunity to recover the breath. They are especialy worse after 12 P.M. The child holds each hypochondrium during the cough, and if sputum is not raised, vomiting and retching ensue.

Ipecacuanha & **Cina**

When the cough relaxes, the patient vomits phlegm, which relieves.

Just after a paroxysm, a gurgling sound is heard. Grinding of teeth.

Ipecacuanha & **Cuprum**

See above.

Complements *Ipecacuanha.* Spasms of the flexors predominate.

COMPARISONS OF REMEDIES

ACTÆA RACEMOSA—CAULOPHYLLUM

Actæa Rac. (misnamed *Cimicifuga*) has many symptoms in common with *Caulophyllum.*

In uterine diseases, *Actæa* has the general character of *constant* pains, *tonic* spasms ; *Cauloph.* of *intermitting* pains, *clonic* spasms. *Actæa, ceteris paribus, renders labor easier when given in the last month. Crampy pains in the groins, stitches* (either as after-pains or with undilated os) ; *Cauloph. helps when the patient seems so weak, she cannot develop labor-pains. Actæa* causes a marked general soreness ; tenderness in the hypogastrium with *dysmenorrhœa ; Cauloph.* causes intermitting crampy pains all over, hypogastrium, bladder, chest, &c., with *dysmenorrhœa.*

Sleeplessness is well-marked, but only *Actæa* has numbness all over preventing sleep, *Cauloph.* causing intense atony, is preferable in sleeplessness from nervous relaxation.

Actæa excels in inflammations with nervous excitement ; though causing often weakness, it shows a tendency to keep up irritability ; nervous tremor; nervous chill (*many cases in the first stage of labor,* [*Gels.*]) before the menses; trembling from debility, yet cannot bear the least noise, touch or motion, &c. *Cauloph.* excels in relaxation with uterine displacement, resulting in paralysis; paralysis from enervation.

Leucorrhœa is cured by *Actæa,* with *continuous* bearing-down pains; by *Cauloph.,* (*often in pre-pubic cases*) when it is profuse, as if from *atony* of the mucous membrane. Similarly, *Actæa* causes diarrhœa with *tenesmus; Cauloph.,* profuse, watery, *painless.*

Rheumatism affecting the belly of the muscle, metastasis to the heart call for *Actæa;* of the small joints of the hand, metastasis to the nape of the neck, panting, delirium, call for *Cauloph.*

Papular eruptions appear under *Actæa ;* "moth" spots under *Cauloph.*

ACTÆA RACEM., rheumatism of the belly of the muscles or of the lower extremities; ACTÆA SPICATA, only of the small joints.

AILANTHUS	Mind, Sensorium	ARUM TRIPH
Low-spirited, depressed. Delirium continuous, *low muttering; insensibility.*		Irritability (1). Delirium with tossing about; *picking at the dry lips or at one spot; boring in the nose.*
Cannot concentrate the mind.		Forgetful.
Dizziness with great *confusion of mind;* apoplectic fulness; drowsy, as if *intoxicated.*		Dizziness with fulness of the head and absent-mindedness; not so stupid as *Ailanth.*; sleepy.

Head

AILANTHUS	ARUM TRIPH
Headache with dull, heavy sensation, disinclination to think; confusion of ideas and drowsiness; heat and redness of the face.	Headache with dull, heavy sensation, sometimes with absence of thought, but with *restless sleep;* more shooting pains as in catarrh.

Eyes

AILANTHUS	ARUM TRIPH
Letters look blurred, dance up and down; vertigo.	Dimness as from a veil before the eyes; not relieved by spectacles.
Eyes suffused; startled look when aroused; pupils dilated. Smarting, burning in the eyes; pus-like discharge.	Eyes cloudy, heavy, sleepy, lids (especially the lower) heavy. Smarting lachrymation, swelling of the margins of the lids.

Nose, Mouth, Throat

Both remedies attack the mucous membrane of nose, mouth and throat; but they differ in intensity. Here, too, it will be found that *Arum* causes more excoriation, more irritation; *Ailanthus* offers more symptoms of a typhoid state (see Teeth, Tongue).

AILANTHUS	ARUM TRIPH
Discharge from the nose, copious, ichorous; blood and pus.	Discharge *makes the nostrils and upper lip raw and sore; boring in the nose.*
Lips cracked; blisters or ragged little ulcers near the corners of the mouth.	Lips swollen, *corners of the mouth sore, raw, cracked and bleeding.*
Teeth covered with a brown sordes.	Inner mouth sore, *desire to wet it, but the child refuses to drink, cries when it is offered.*

(1) Irritability corresponds to the acrid *Arum;* low-spiritedness to the more toxical, stupefying *Ailanthus.* It is a distinction running through the whole pathogeneses that irritation predominates in *Arum,* torpor in *Ailanthus.* The lines between these remedies ought to be sharply drawn; for they meet in the severest forms of scarlatina and kindred diseases. A mistake here might prove fatal.

Nose, Mouth, Throat

AILANTHUS	ARUM TRIPH
Tongue dry, red, cracked; moist, white with *livid tip and edges;* white with a *brown centre.*	Tongue cracked, burning, raw spots; tongue red; the ***papillæ being raised; child will not open the mouth.***
Throat feels as after an astringent; feels sore on inhaling cold air; feeling of fulness above the sternum; tender and sore on swallowing, pains extend into the ears; throat livid, swollen, tonsils studded with deep, angry ulcers, fetid oozing; neck swollen; glands enlarged and tender.	Throat feels, as if constricted, with sneezing; sensation of something hot during inspiration; swelling over the larynx; swallowing and chewing almost impossible, mouth and throat are so sore; throat burning, raw; uvula dry; putrid throat *more burning than in Ailanthus; neck swollen;* glands swollen.

Stomach, Abdomen

AILANTHUS	ARUM TRIPH
Great thirst; or drinking only while eating.	Simply moistens **the mouth** or refuses water; **mouth sore**.
Food is repulsive; stomach inactive; great hunger during the chill; *goneness* in the stomach.	Loss of appetite; **qualmish feeling**; *burning heat* **in pharynx**, œsophagus and stomach.
Sleepiness, fulness of the head, after wine.	Headache, heat in the head, after coffee.
Sudden violent vomiting, or spitting up.	Feels sick, qualmish, burning heat in stomach.
Emptiness in the stomach; stomach *inactive,* does not *contract.*	Cramps in the stomach, *too great irritability of the stomach.*
Pain like a stricture under the short ribs; tenderness over the hepatic region.	Pain in the liver from front to back; pain under the left short ribs.

Rectum, Stool

AILANTHUS	ARUM TRIPH
Frequent painful stool, much bloody mucus; dysentery; tympanites.	Soft stool with much severe tenesmus; loud rolling in the abdomen.
Loose, watery stools, expelled **with great force;** ***weakness and burning*** **in the bowels.**	**Loose,** watery stools, yellow-**brown,** burning at the anus.

Urine

Both have scanty or suppressed urine (scarlatina) (2). *Ailanthus,* **true to its typhoid, torpid state, has urine passed unconsciously.**

(2) When in a scarlatina case after *Arum,* the urine escapes abundantly, the patient is surely improving.

AILANTHUS **Larynx, Chest** **ARUM TRIPH**

Arum has more action on the larynx; *Ailanthus more* on the bronchi and lungs.

AILANTHUS	ARUM TRIPH
Voice hoarse, fails sometimes.	Voice *uncertain* (singers, &c.), *cannot be controlled.*
Dry, hacking cough, sticky expectoration; oppression in the region of the *bronchi;* cannot expand the chest ; *feels, as if the air-cells were stuck together.*	Dry, distressing cough; *constant pain in the larynx* ; phlegm collects in the *trachea,* causing difficult breathing; *larynx sensitive; voice lost; after N. W. winds.*
Lungs sore, tender ; burning in the chest.	More rawness; burning from chest to stomach.
Pulse rapid, cannot be counted.	Pulse more frequent; circulation excited.

Neck, Back

AILANTHUS	ARUM TRIPH
Dorsal vertebræ ache, pressing feeling; pain in head, neck, back and numbness under the left scapula; pain through from left lung.	Atlas and deltoid vertebræ painful; headache and stiffness of the neck; pressing between the shoulder-blades.

Limbs

AILANTHUS	ARUM TRIPH
Tingling prickling of the left arm; numbness; headache.	Both hands feel stiff and more swollen.
Legs feel numb, tingling, as if asleep.	Cramps in the (r) leg, worse on awaking.
Feet pain, tension when walking.	Feet sting, sore; hurt when walking.

Sleep

AILANTHUS	ARUM TRIPH
Drowsy or very restless with delirium; *soon passes into insensibility.*	*Sleepless,* nervous, from *itching of the skin, from sore mouth;* drowsy but no stupor.

Fever

AILANTHUS	ARUM TRIPH
Chilly, with hunger and sense of emptiness.	Repeated chills, yawning, sneezing, same hour on 2 days.
Dry hot skin, morning until noon (lungs); flushes of heat after the chill.	Dry skin, intense heat with burning face 4 to 7 P.M. ; flushes.
Typhoid type of fever; *vomiting on sitting up ;* rapid, small pulse; face red and hot; great anxiety, restlessness; *later drowsy, unconscious, muttering delirium; sordes on the*	Typhoid symptoms not so prominent; but sometimes, restless, tossing about the bed, desire to escape; unconscious of what he is doing or of what is said to him ; *constantly*

AILANTHUS	Fever	ARUM TRIPH
teeth; tongue dry; *livid* or *brown down the middle* (see Skin); *torpor.*		*picking at the dry lips until they bleed; boring in the nose or at one spot;* urine scanty or *suppressed;* more *excitement* than in *Ailanthus.*

Skin

Ailanthus has very characteristic skin symptoms, which aid in its selection in scarlatina, especially in *malignant forms. An eruption* like miliary rash appears *before the chill;* it comes in patches. Between these points the skin is *dark, almost livid.* The rash is *dark, livid* (scarlatina) from the beginning. After passing the finger over it, the *livid color returns slowly.* The itching is all but intolerable. Sometimes bullæ, containing a *claret colored fluid,* appear; again *petechiæ* form. *Arum* develops an eruption like scarlet-rash. The itching is severe, causing *sleeplessness and restlessness;* but there is no evidence of the malignancy of the *Ailanth.* The skin *peels off in large patches,* so characteristic of scarlatina. Sometimes this occurs two or *three times.*

Generalities

AILANTHUS	ARUM TRIPH
Great exhaustion; cannot sit up (scarlatina); tottering gait; can not stand long; cannot guide the feet.	*Great exhaustion (mostly in the* last stage of typhus; probably uræmia); right side lame during dentition.
Cold inflames the eyes.	N. W. wind causes hoarseness.
Left side mostly.	Right to left.
Morning: Nervous symptoms worse, sore-throat; pus from eyes; nausea, diarrhœa; heaviness, *better.*	*Morning:* Cramps, heaviness, headache; mouth raw; diarrhœa; swollen hands, *better.*
Evening, night: Nervousness; neuralgia lying down.	*Evening, night:* Headache; drowsiness; throat burns more lying down.
Compare with *Arnica* (sore lungs); *Hydroc. Acid; Bryon.; Phytolac.; Nitric Acid; Baptisia,* &c. (scarlatina).	Compare with *Lycopod., Nitric Acid, Amm. C. et M., Silicea* (scarlatina, angina); *Calad., Nitric Acid* (typhus).
ANTIDOTES: *Aloes* (headache); *Nux V.*; stimulants.	ANTIDOTES: Butter-milk has been successfully used.

ALOES	SULPHUR
Mind	
Hypochondriacal humor; worse in cloudy weather, while in pain, when costive.	Hypochondriacal humor; worse all day, better in the evening (1).
Anguish with ebullitions—principally abdominal in origin; hates people, repels every one, peevish.	Anguish with hot head; præcordial or abdominal; concern about one's salvation, health, or family; weeping, peevish.
Children chat and laugh.	Children bold, quick or restless.
Vertigo makes everything seem insecure.	Vertigo, as if the ground were shaking.
Ailments from chagrin.	Ailments from mortification, with fear.
Head	
Congestion, with throbbing in the middle of the brain, cold feeling in the occiput; better from cold washing, and in the open air; worse in the warm room. Must sit up.	Congestion, with burning, throbbing, buzzing, coldness in the vertex; worse from cold washing, and in the open air; better in the warm room. Must lie with head high.
Every step causes stitches in the temples.	Every step causes pain through the head.
Scalp sensitive in spots.	Scalp tender on the vertex.
Eyes	
Half-shutting the eyes with headache.	*Closing eyes* with headache.
Eyes glittering, prominent.	Eyes generally sunken.
Ears	
Earache, with distress in the abdomen; congestion to the ears and head, with deafness from damp rooms (2).	Drawing in the ear during eructations; congestion to the ears, deafness preceded by too acute hearing.
Cracking in the ears when reading aloud.	Cracking when chewing; cracking like a cord breaking.

Both offer symptoms of congestion to the ears, with buzzing, burning, pulsating; especially is this true of those subject to hæmorrhoids.

ALOES	SULPHUR
Nose	
Nose red in the open air.	Nose red in warm room (3).
Epistaxis on awaking.	Epistaxis mostly afternoons.

---

(1) *Aloes* also has cheerfulness in the evening, but it is most marked in *Sulph.*

(2) The aggravation of the earache, with abdominal symptoms, shows wherein these remedies agree. They both cause abdominal congestion, portal stasis.

(3) *Sulph.* has congestion to the nose in the cold air. It has red nose of a scrofulous origin, less frequently, from intemperance.

ALOES	**SULPHUR**

Mouth, Throat

Lips dry, red, chapped, scurfy, in both.

ALOES	SULPHUR
Inflames uvula and *palatine arches;* worse yawning, empty swallowing, not from food.	Inflames uvula, *tonsils;* worse swallowing solids, and after eating.
Hawks mucus in jelly-like lumps. (Compare stool.)	Hawks up mucus in hard lumps.

Taste, Appetite

ALOES	SULPHUR
Taste earthy, like ink, bitter, sour, metallic.	Taste empyreumatic, bitter, sour, metallic.
Appetite for bread, beer, juicy things, apples.	Appetite for beer, brandy (4), liquid food; averse to bread.
Hunger after eating (5) 7 A.M., or 10 P.M., during diarrhœa.	Hunger all night, must eat, from 10 to 11 A.M.
If he cannot eat, weak with changeable pulse.	If he cannot eat, headache, weary, must lie down.
Nausea from motion.	Nausea riding.

Stomach, Abdomen

It is in the abdominal organs that *Aloes* and *Sulph,* display their greatest similarities. They cause portal congestion, congestion of the liver, intestines, uterus. Hence appear tension, burning, pulsation, fulness, heaviness, vomiting of blood, inflammation, and even ulceration. These give rise to flushed face, ringing in the ears, hot mouth, red tongue, *red lips,* aphthous or ulcerated mouth, and even spinal congestion.

ALOES	SULPHUR
Abdomen pains from a mis-step.	Abdomen pains from a strain (integuments).
Flatulence; gurgling in the abdomen like water running out of a bottle; running along the descending colon.	Flatulence; moving like the arm of a fœtus ; rumbling through abdomen, mostly in the sigmoid flexure.

---

(4) The *Sulph.* patient usually dislikes wine, because it is not "strong" enough. He is filthy, coarse in taste, as well as in habit. *Aloes* creates an unnatural appetite for beer, and is, hence, used in the adulteration of lager, ale, etc.

(5) The hunger after eating, in *Aloes* arises from the torpid state of the stomach ; it is not until *some time after a meal* that the nerves of the stomach are stimulated to the normal state, which would cause the impression of hunger.

ALOES — Stomach, Abdomen — SULPHUR

Alhough both remedies cause the passage of flatus, yet it is more characteristic of *Aloes*. The lower bowels, and especially the rectum, are full, heavy, and the stool is effected with much effort, resulting in a small escape of mucus or fæcal matter, and immense quantities of wind.

ALOES	SULPHUR
Stool contains jelly-like masses; stool like long, stringy bands, like pieces of flesh; bilious stool, bright, golden-yellow.	Stools consist of slimy mucus, or frothy, white mucus; changeable in color; bilious stools —greenish-yellow.
Musculature of the bowels relaxed; hard stool passes unnoticed; bowels move when urinating, passing flatus, moving, walking or standing. Sphincter ani insecure.	Musculature relaxed; stool involuntary or sudden, hurrying out of bed; stool when passing flatus; abdominal muscles weak, he cannot rise. Prolapsus ani.
Urging to stool, hurries out of bed or in evening; hungry; bowels feel, as if scraped.	Urging to stool, hurries out of bed in the morning; bowels feel, as if tied in knots.
Before stool: Colic about the navel; passing flatus; fulness and weight in the anus	Before stool: Cutting pains; rumbling of flatus, as if rectum would protrude.
During stool: Numbness and weakness of the thighs; coldness general; hunger; vomit slime.	During stool: Cramps in the limbs; chilly more in lower abdomen; hunger at all times; nausea.
After stool: Urging; weight in the anus.	After stool: Urging; prolapsus ani.
Stool worse hot, damp weather; staying in damp rooms; from chagrin; on awaking, 7 A.M. or 10 P.M.; ale relieves.	Stool worse in cold, damp weather; from evening air; early morning on awaking; at night (dysentery); ale aggravates.
Hæmorrhoids protrude like grapes; when urinating feeling as though bowels would move	Hæmorrhoids of all kinds; burning in the urethra during micturition.

Urine

ALOES	SULPHUR
Sediment yellow-red, mucous, or bloody.	Sediment dark-red, slimy, loamy or bloody.
Urine increased; must rise often at night.	Urine decreased; increased or involuntary at night.
Urine of an offensive, ammoniacal odor.	Urine fetid, greasy pellicle on the surface.

Genitals—Males

ALOES	SULPHUR
Erections after urinating; sexual desire increased; worse after eating (6). United the torn prepuce of a child.	Erections weak; sexual desire increased, but without physical excitement. Cured many cases of phimosis.
Testes cold, scrotum relaxed, penis shrunken, offensive sweat on the genitals; wakes with urgency to urinate, and erections (7).	Testes cold, scrotum relaxed, penis shrunken, sweat offensive; semen watery; headache, hungry, weakness of the legs.
Gonorrhœal sequelæ; sticking, burning in urethra as far as the bladder; penis when erect, bent; epididymitis; discharge thin.	Gonorrhœal sequelæ; scrofulous or psoric patients; strumming sensation in the testicles; epididymitis; discharge purulent or *white*.

Females

ALOES	SULPHUR
Fulness, weight, dragging in the pelvis; worse standing; better from cold washing.	Fulness, weight, etc.; worse standing; worse from cold washing.
Menses too early; earache, drawing, labor-like pains extend into the thighs; fulness in the rectum.	Menses *generally* too late (8); labor-like pains in abdomen and back; toothache; lassitude of the limbs; urging to stool.
Abortion, with copious mucous stools.	Abortion, with constipation; blenorrhœa.

Larynx, Chest

ALOES	SULPHUR
Difficult breathing, with weak limbs, anxious going up stairs; must sit and sleep; blood leaves the surface.	Difficult breathing from congestion, with trembling limbs fainting; worse at night when lying.
Wheezing from smoking tobacco.	Wheezing in a smoky atmosphere.
Voice hoarse, thick.	More a deep-toned voice.

(6) Probably one of the best remedies to repress a too lively desire, especially in children which only a few remedies do (C. Hg.). *Sulph.* on the other hand, is the best remedy for the ill consequences of onanism.

(7) *Aloes* gives the symptoms of sexual erethism with increased afflux of blood, and conversely with coldness, dwindling, etc., as results of venous stasis. The emissions are followed by increased excitement, micturition and stool; frightened at the least noise. *Sulph.*, with the same local weakness, gives us constitutional symptoms of more importance.

(8) That is, according to Bœnninghausen; but *Sulph.* is now and then indicated in premature, profuse menses.

ALOES	SULPHUR
Back, Limbs	
Lumbar pains, worse sitting, better moving.	Lumbar pains, worse walking than sitting.
Paralytic weakness of the limbs, with weight in the pelvis; torpid bowels; stool passes with urine.	Paralytic weakness of the limbs from spinal disease; no urine passes (9).
Sleep	
Sleepless, with *activity of body and mind;* brain excited, urging to urinate, to defecate, sexual desire; sleepless from cold feet.	Sleepless, or "cat-naps"; awakens *often, becomes wide awake;* sudden jerking of the legs on going to sleep; sleepless from burning feet.
Generalities	
Useful in severe, painful developments of chronic diseases.	The leading antipsoric remedy; helps the system to respond to medicine.
Hypochondriacal, sedentary, lymphatic, worse cloudy weather.	Hypochondriacal, sedentary, lymphatic, but quick in acting.
Lies on the side; worse when lying on the back.	Generally lies on the back, even if worse therefrom.
Antidotes: Vinegar, *Sul., Nux V.,* and *Lyco.* (earache).	Antidotes: *Puls., Sep., Merc., Chin., Nux V.*
Similar to: *Sul., Nux V., Lyco., Carbo V., Puls., Sab., Calc. C., Cham., Coloc., Jalap., Phos., Rheum.*	Similar to: *Puls., Lyc., Calc C., Sep., Sil., Acon., Nux V., Merc., Rhus T., Nit. Ac., Chin.,* etc.

Aloes and *Sulph.* are complementary; hence when the first partially cures, the second completes the cure. They have at least a hundred identical symptoms. In treating a chronic disease with *Sulphur* or allied remedies, *Aloes* does well to check acute symptoms appearing, after which *Sulph.* may be resumed. Many of the symptoms, specially those of the skin, are too near alike to bear differentiation.

(9) *Sulph., c.m.,* in repeated doses, every three hours for a month or more, caused paralysis of the legs (Macfarlan). Since then it has several times benefited cases of paraplegia from spinal disease. *Aloes* produces weakness of the thighs, with dysentery, apparently arising from pelvic pressure, and probably spinal congestion. Weakness of the wrists and ankles occurs in both remedies.

Mind

ANTIM. CRUD.	LYCOPODIUM
Melancholy about one's present **or future** ; woeful mood.	Melancholy about one's salvation; scrupulous conscientiousness.
Child will be neither touched nor looked at.	Child *suddenly* becomes obstinate; awakens cross.
Depression of spirits ; or ecstatic mood.	Depression of spirits ; or angry, proud, imperious.
Physical suffering produces a suicidal mood.	Physical suffering produces a disgust for life (1).
Mind weak, almost idiocy. So **apathetic, has no want and is unconscious of the voided still; sits speechless, aimlessly pulling his cravat** ; gastric weakness.	Mind weak as from over-taxing the brain. Indifferent ; talks well on abstract ideas, but forgets familiar objects ; misplaces letters and names; **great** exhaustion (2).
Vertigo with nausea; nose-bleed and intense prostration when ascending the stairs.	Vertigo with nausea, when looking at anything which turns or when walking by a rail fence (3).

Head

ANTIM. CRUD.	LYCOPODIUM
Stupefying headache, worse in the **evening** ; nausea.	Stupefying headache, worse from 4 to 8 P.M., dry mouth and lips.
Rheumatic **headaches, with tearing, boring or crampy pains into forehead, vertex or temples ; worse going up stairs** ; ***nausea.***	Rheumatic headaches, with tearing pains into the temples, face, eyes or teeth ; worse rising from bed ; fainting (4).
Losing hair from nervous headaches.	Losing hair from abdominal diseases, parturition.

(1) In *Antim. Crud.* we find colic headache and skin diseases, with propensity to shoot or drown oneself. In *Lycop.* the disgust is an element of hypochondriasis, so prominent in those who suffer from liver diseases.

(2) The *Antim. Crud.* state is one of fatuity; the *Lycop.* arises in constitutions greatly exhausted, after apoplexy, typhus, or in cases of incipient cerebral softening. It may also play a good part in aphasia.

(3) When looking at something new, as at new carpet with curious patterns, when rapidly passing a picket fence, when walking along serpentine **paths** cause vertigo, *Lycop.* helps.

(4) Both have relief in the cold like their co-relative *Puls.* If **gastric symptoms** predominate after *Puls.* has but partially relieved, *Ant. C.* may **follow.** If the pains still extend to the face after *Puls.* (which by the way **is** all but specific for these pains), *Lycop.* may be given.

ANTIM. CRUD.	LYCOPODIUM
Eyes	
Eyes inflamed, but in the canthi; outer canthus sore, moist.	Eyes inflamed, with pus too copious as to puff out the lids; eyelids ooze (5).
Worse from the glare of the sun or fire, or snow.	Worse from the light of a candle or lamp (after *Calc. C.*).
Ears	
Heat, swelling, pain; better from touch (otitis similar to *Puls.*).	More for *otorrhœa after* otitis or *exanthematic* fevers (6).
Nose	
Dry catarrh with nose obstructed in the evening and nostrils sore, *cracked and crusty.*	Dry catarrh, *cannot breathe at night with the mouth shut;* incrustations high up in the nostrils (7).
Face	
Eruptions on the face, scabs *yellow-green* and *hard, crack* and pus gushes out; *corners of mouth cracked, crusty.*	Eruptions on the face, scabs *thick* which ooze a fœtid pus; affects more the *lower* lip, but also the corners of the mouth.
Countenance sad, woeful, even stupid.	Countenance sad, deep furrowed or jaw dropped, eyes dim (8).
Facial muscles twitch, child delirious, drowsy, hot.	Facial muscles alternately expand and contract, also alæ nasi (9).

(5) Both remedies have an affinity for "corners"; corners of mouth, canthi, folds of skin, &c., but it is more characteristic of *Antim. Cr.* to give inflamed canthi, and more of *Lycop.* to produce purulent conjunctivitis.

(6) Both cause deafness from suppressed eruptions, ulcers; *Lycop.* more from checked otorrhœa. *Lycop.* also relieves a nervous deafness alternating with oversensitiveness to noises (*Sul.*).

(7) *Lycopodium* develops an acrid, corroding coryza with heat in the forehead and headache (scarlatina, &c.). This has not been noticed under *Antim. Cr.* The former proves curative in ozæna with orange-yellow discharge, the nearest approach to which in *Antim. Cr.* is a yellowish mucous hawking from the posterior nares. The latter has all the symptoms worse from *inspiring cold air.*

(8) *Lycopodium* gives us here the symptoms of incipient cerebral paralysis, which catastrophe it will prevent in typhus, scarlatina, apoplexy, &c. The dim, *watery eyes* and rattling breathing distinguish it from *Nux, Opium, Lach.*, &c.

(9) This far-famed "fan-like" motion of the nostrils must be distinguished from the expansive effort to get breath common to *Tart. Emet., Ars.*, and perhaps any medicine causing severe dyspnœa. In *Lycopodium* it is *an alternate contraction and expansion, a muscular oscillation* which runs through the whole pathogenesis. Thus interpreted it will prove a God-send in many alarming diseases.

ANTIM. CRUD.	LYCOPODIUM
Mouth, Throat	
Mouth dry or saliva flows : much thirst at night.	Mouth and tongue dry without thirst.
Ptyalism, saliva salty.	Saliva dries on lips and palate.
Toothache in *hollow teeth* ; worse from cold water ; better walking in the open air.	Toothache with gum-boils, swollen cheek ; better from warm applicatons.
Tongue, as if white-washed or blistered.	Tongue dry, blisters under the tip ; ulcers ; tubercles.
Like a plug in the throat; left side worse ; hawk yellow mucus.	Throat, as if contracted ; throat worse *right side ;* hawk bloody mucus (10).
Stomach, Abdomen	
Hungry even after eating.	Hungry soon afer a meal.
Worse from butter, fat, meats, especially pork ; long for acids (yet worse therefrom).	Worse from flatulent food; from oysters (yet great longing); long for sweets.
Adventitious appetite : Few longings, generally disgust for food. Tobacco causes headache, hiccough.	*Adventitious appetite* : Longing for tobacco or averse to smoking. Tobacco causes impotence.
Gastroses with agonizing burning in the pit of the stomach ; cramps drive to suicide ; cannot bear the least touch; worse or caused by wine, acids, bathing in cold water.	Gastroses with burning into throat or pain *into the back, alternate contraction and relaxation of the stomach* (9, 10), disgust for life (1); worse or caused by adulterated coffee, sour beer, wine, *oysters, heavy bread.*
After eating, *eructations tasting of the food;* inflated abdomen; hunger continues.	After eating, rumination; *full to the throat after a mouthful* (11); sensation, as if fasting.

---

(10) Here again comes the same alternation of contraction and expansion referred to in note (8). In *croup*, diphtheria, pneumonia, &c., we have *alternation of suffocation and free intervals ; loose cough by day, suffocation at night.* Among the tongue symptoms we find that this same tendency makes the patient say 'O' when he means 'A'. Again, he thrusts his tongue snake-like out of his mouth *and moves it to and fro, or like a pendulum.* Compare *Sulph., Cup. Acet., Cham.*

(11) It must be remembered that this fulsome condition is quite common, but is characteristic of *Lycopodium,* when bitter taste and pressure on the liver concur.

ANTIM. CRUD.	LYCOPODIUM
Stomach, Abdomen	
Not many liver symptoms; bilious vomit from regurgitant bile in the course of gastric irritation (12).	Many liver affections; gastric states associated with icterus, swollen liver, gall-stones, &c.
Colic, with *high colored* urine, *hard stool* (children); from over-eating; from lead; child will not be touched or looked at.	Colic with *crying before passing red, sandy urine* (children); from drugging the mother; child awakes cross, kicking.
Stool difficult from extreme size, much urging during stool; sensation, as of a copious stool when flatus passes, *later solid fæces.*	Stool difficult from constriction of the anus, urging long after stool; sensation, as if much remained with *painful accumulation of flatus.*
Stool *white,* dry, irregular in shape, solid particles floating in the liquid.	Stool *pale,* putrid-smelling, often mixed with hard lumps (13).
Diarrhœa during pregnancy, watery, morning and night; nausea and persistent vomiting.	Diarrhœa during pregnancy, worse from 4 to 8 P.M.; nausea when riding; earthy face.
Hæmorrhoids with much discharge of yellow mucus; so fidgety, can hardly keep still.	Hæmorrhoids, pain for hours after stool; pain worse when sitting.
Hæmorrhage from the bowels; blood dark; the discharge contains *solid lumps;* alternate diarrhœa and constipation.	Hæmorrhage from the bowels; blood bright; feeling, as of *fermentation in the bowels;* inveterate constipation.
Urine	
Frequent and copious urination at night, with mucous discharge; pain in the small of the back; catarrh.	Frequent at night, scanty by day; urging with flow of milky, purulent *offensive* urine, relieving all the symptoms (15); catarrh.
Urine involuntary with cough.	Incontinence at night.

(12) We find only tension in the right hypochondrium, which may indicate a slight hyperæmia, such as occurs physiologically after a meal or from over-eating.

(13) In *Lycopodium,* the pale hue denotes deficient bile, hence the odor; in *Antim. Cr.* the white is undigested milk, and, of course, occurs only in children. They also throw up a little sour milk after nursing.

(14) *Lycopodium,* is of great use in diseases of the urinary organs. We find backache, pressure on the bladder, renal colic with pain from right groin to bladder, &c., &c., *all relieved by urination.* In children, we find holding the hands to the lower abdomen, crying *impatiently, relieved by urination.* Both have red sandy sediment; but *Lycopodium* answers best for calculi, gravel.

Genitals

ANTIM. CRUD.	LYCOPODIUM
Atrophy of the testicles.	Indurated testicles.

Both have increased sexual desire or *impotence*.

Females

ANTIM. CRUD.	LYCOPODIUM
Menstrual blood dark or fluid, with lumps.	Menstrual blood bright at times, and again black; lumpy, fluid.
Amenorrhœa after a cold bath; after becoming over-heated.	Amenorrhœa *chronic*, after fright with anger.
Pressing in the uterus, as if something would come out.	Pressure on bladder or rectum, pressing in the vagina when stooping.
Ovarian region tender to touch; white tongue.	Boring, stitching pains in the ovaries; better after urinating.
Leucorrhœa of acrid water, containing solid lumps; causes smarting down the legs.	Leucorrhœa in *gushes, pains across abdomen from right to left*; jerking of the limbs causes itching of the labia
Alternate diarrhœa and constipation; gastric symptoms; ecstatic, sentimental mood, all with genital troubles.	Obstinate constipation with incarcerated flatus or flatus of the womb (15); temporal headache, as if screwed (8, 9); sad, tearful, all with genital troubles.

Larynx, Chest

ANTIM. CRUD.	LYCOPODIUM
Voice lost or weak, when overheated; rough voice.	Hoarse voice, sounds weak, husky (16).
Cough worse morning, in rays of sun, warm room, after exanthematic fevers; excited by irritation in the abdomen; expectoration of tenacious mucus mixed with dark blood, flat tasting.	Cough worse 4 to 8 P.M., in warm room, wind, after (membranous) croup; excited by irritation, as from Sulphur in the trachea; expectoration of bloody mucus or *lemon-colored*, green, tastes salty.
Breathing deep, sighing, suffocating; breath hot; suffocative catarrh, old people, burning in the chest.	Breathing *short, rattling* (*children*), oppressed; suffocative catarrh with danger of paralysis of the lungs.

(15) We find under *Lycopodium* circumscribed, *changing* tumors in the abdomen which may be caused by shifting flatus, but which may also answer for "phantom" tumors in hysteria.

(16) *Lycopodium* also offers difficult speech from thickness (nodosities), or paralysis of the tongue.

ANTIM. CRUD.	LYCOPODIUM
Back, Limbs	
Rheumatism with white tongue, nausea, great thirst at night; pains are worse from warmth, hot sun, working in water; muscles and tendons painfully shortened; especially the biceps flexor cubiti.	Rheumatism with sour belching, nausea in early morning, flatulence; pains worse at night, better in warmth (17); muscles and joints rigid, feel numb; especially finger-joints and *insteps.*
Soreness of the soles of the feet and heels from walking, especially on the pavement.	Soreness and swelling of the soles of the feet and ankles from walking.
Stiffness of the knee (fungus of the knee).	White swelling of the knee (Lippe).
Inflammation of the heel.	Rhagades of the heel.

Sleep

ANTIM. CRUD.	LYCOPODIUM
Drowsy, (child) hot, delirious, face red; worse after a cold bath. Drowsy in the *fore-noon.*	Drowsy, lies in a stupor, rattling breathing, (child) jaw dropped, face pale. Drowsy all day.
Dreams pleasant, amorous; or frightful, causing him to start.	Awakens with a *scream,* will not be left alone; jerks the limbs, asleep or awake (18).

Fever

ANTIM. CRUD.	LYCOPODIUM
Chill, with thirst (for beer); or thirstlessness; shivers over the back, feet icy-cold.	Chill preceded by thirst; chill accompanied by numb hands and feet.
Heat from the least exercise.	Sweat from the least exercise.
Morning sweat with shivering of the tips of the fingers.	Morning (and night), sweat with cold face.
Partial cold; nose internally icy-cold.	Partial cold; one-sided; *one foot cold, the other warm.*
In intermittents, mood woeful; vomit bitter.	In intermittents, mood tearful; vomit sour.
Measles, scarlatina, &c., preceded by convulsions, drowsiness; earache.	Measles, scarlatina, &c., with coma, threatened cerebral paralysis; otorrhœa and deafness.
Fever from over-heating or bathing; gastric type.	Fever from getting wet (feet); bilious type.

(17) Better from the warmth of the bed, but worse warm poultices.

(18) *Lycopodium* has legs involuntarily spread asunder and then pressed together; jerking arms or legs up and down; involuntarily nodding the head backward and forward. Compare (9, 10). The screaming mentioned above is very characteristic, even in hip disease (*Stram.*).

Tissues

ANTIM. CRUD.	LYCOPODIUM
Corns *horny*, hard, mostly on the soles.	Corns inflamed, pulsating tearing.
Eruptions green, *hard*, horny, purulent.	Eruptions with thick crusts which *crack ; fœtid.*
Horny warts.	Pedunculated warts.
Skin hardens, becomes *horny*.	Skin like parchment or *moist in the folds (intertrigo).*
Nails split, grow horny.	Hang-nails.
Ulcers around warts.	Ulcers from varicose veins.
Obesity or emaciation.	Upper part emaciated, lower part distended (19).
General dropsical swellings.	Dropsy, especially of the ankles, goes from r. to 1. (heart disease).
Venous hyperæmia ; pulsations in the veins.	Ebullitions ; circulation, as if stopped in the veins.

Generalities

ANTIM. CRUD.	LYCOPODIUM
Exanthema miliary, *pustular* ; like nettle-rash.	Exanthema moist, scurfy, suppurating; like nettle-rash (20).
Boils (perineum).	Boils point of nose, forearm (21).
Left side predominant.	Right side predominant.
Dark hair.	Light hair.
Worse in *moonlight*.	Worse at new moon.
Worse every two or three weeks; alternate days.	Worse on alternate days ; 4 to 8 P.M.
Worse in the sun and glare of snow.	Worse in snow air.

Antim. Cr. has *amelioration,* and *Lycop. aggravation* from ascending, stooping, eructations, uncovering.

Antim. Cr. has *aggravation,* and *Lycop. amelioration,* from wrapping up warm, sitting.

---

(19) *Antim. Cr.* prefigures a rather robust, corpulent patient, but predisposed to gastric disturbances. *Lycopodium* portrays a patient of keen intellect, but of feeble muscular development, lean and predisposed to pulmonary and hepatic diseases. In chest symptoms, it so favors *Phosph.*, that one might suppose it the preferable medicine when *phosph.*, though seemingly well-chosen, aggravates. With a sallow face, gray expectoration and neglected or maltreated pneumonia present, the choice for *Lycopodium* is certain.

(20) Hence *Antim. Cr.* corresponds to measles, small-pox, prickly heat, bites of insects, &c., *Lycopodium* to tetter, eczema, erythema. But of course the *subjective symptoms when present, must ever decide.* Thus in scarlatina, sopor, rattling breathing, &c., would indicate *Lycopodium,* no matter what was the eruption.

(21) *Lycopodium* cures large boils, especially when they do not mature but remain blue.

Mind

APIS	BELLADONNA
Hydrocephalic inflammation of brain, following suppressed eruption (urticaria, &c.); *stage of exudation.* Cry most marked; sweat on head, musk-like; snapping of teeth; urine though scanty, often milky; pulse intermits; is full and rapid only in beginning; limbs tremble; big toe turned up; spuinting; stiffening of body, if tonched or moved.	Hydrocephalic inflammation; *stage of congestion* or commencing exudation, less when exudation is established. Moaning or starts in sleep; sweat hot, pungent (sometimes cold on forehead); grind teeth; urine dark, fiery-red, turbid, scanty; pulse full, rapid; throbbing parotids; limbs jerk; convulsions of arms; eyes staring or red, wild, face glowing, later squinting. Screams, if touched or jarred.
Congestion cerebral or spinal; feels, as if must hold head and eyes down; head better uncovered.	Congestion better, throwing head backward, worse bending forward; better covered warm.
Delirium, muttering, stupor, drowsiness. Apathy more marked than with *Bell.*	Delirium, muttering, violent, alternate state of fury and coma. Apathy, indifference.
Dread of death.	Dread or *indifference.*
Anxiety felt in head.	Anxiety felt in præcordia.
Awkard, clumsily breaks things and laughs at the mishap.	Awkward gait; hurried manner; raises feet high when walking.
Constantly busy; changes occupation (hysteria).	Sits breaking pins all day (Hysteria).
Children imbecile; brain feels tired—emaciation.	Children precocious, timid; obesity.
Vertigo, worse sitting and lying, than walking.	Vertigo, worse walking.
When closing eyes, dizzy.	When closing eyes, visions.
Prosopalgia with impaired memory.	Prosopalgia with excitement of brain.
Erysipelas whitish or pinkish; puffy, œdematous under eyes; burning, stinging pains; little thirst. Œdematous form.	Erysipelas smooth, shining, scarlet; worse right side, great thirst; stitches in head. Erysipelas fugax.

Both have metastasis to the brain.

APIS		BELLADONNA
	Eyes	
Production of mucus in eyes. **Eye-lids puffy œdematous; granulated, worse on border.**		Dryness of eyes or scalding tears. Eye-lids interstitially distended; granulated lids, whole inner surface.
Twitching of eye-ball; squinting.		Twitchnig, spasms of eyes and lids; squinting.
Chemosis (1).		Ulceration of eye (1).
Staphyloma (2).		Fungus-medullaris.
Cornea gray, smoky, opaque; **"scrofulo-ribbon."**		Cornea specked or ulcers on the cornea; pannus (1).
	Face	
Swelling of upper lip with prickling pains; neuralgia; erysip., &c.		Swelling of upper lip, with swollen gums; struma, erysip., &c.
Face swollen œdematous (under eyes) or swollen with hives; pale, waxy or pinkish, purple.		Face swollen, **indurated,** as from congestion; scarlet, scarlet spots or yellowish-red, dark-red.
	Mouth	
Mouth and fauces inflamed, **rosy-red; blisters in clusters on back of tongue; burning, stinging pains; irritable, fidgety.**		Mouth and fauces **inflamed, highly injected, hot, dry; point of tongue feels, as if blistered;** whining mood, crying, hot head.
Mouth and tongue, as if scalded, burning, stinging.		Mouth and tongue parched, as if from something acrid or corrosive.
Tongue white **(diarrhœa); deep-red, coverèd with blisters** (scarlatina).		Tongue white in middle, red edges, red, raised papillæ (scarlatina).

(1) *Apis* tends to produce, besides a simple conjunctivitis, a superabundance of serous effusion, with relaxation of the various tissues of the eyes; thus we have puffed lids, chemosis, staphyloma. It is of little use compared with *Bell.*, in inflammation of the whole eye, tending to supuration, or in purulent ophthalmia. *Bell.* is bast-adapted to pannus, because this is so often a consequence of purulent ophthalmia. In mucous states, *Apis* is preferable; in intense inflammatory, *Bell.*

(2) Payr recommends *Bell.* as a preventive of staphyloma, but *Apis* is far preferable.

APIS	BELLADONNA
Throat	
Tonsils swollen, red (mostly from inflammation of mucous membrane covering them); contraction and rawness in the throat, worse morning; difficult swallowing from contraction, swelling or weakness of the muscles of the throat (diphtheria).	Tonsils swollen (inflammation of whole glands, even to suppuration) dark-red; constriction like spasm, worse 3 P.M. or 12 P.M.; difficult swallaoing from constriction of the fauces or pharynx, causing regurgitation.
Diphtheria, throat, as if varnished or mottled; exudate dirty gray; pains in the ears when swallowing; prostration from beginning; numb limbs; weak larynx; itchy, stinging rash.	Diphtheria, throat highly inflamed; tenacious mucus on the tonsils (not an exudate); pains shoot to ears, even when not swallowing; restless, brain excited; skin red or covered with scarlet-colored rash (3)
Ulcerated throat, erysipelatous (with undeveloped scarlatina).	Ulcerated throat, ulcers come quickly on the tonsils.
Goitre, with ovarian disease.	Goitre sensitive; with congestion to head.

Stomach, Etc.

Both have nausea, felt in the throat.

APIS	BELLADONNA
After eating or drinking, heat and burning in the stomach, nausea, eructations.	After eating or drinking, contractive pain in the stomach, sometimes causing vomiting.
Pit of stomach sensitive to the touch; burning; painless, yellow diarrhœa; drinking causes burning.	Least jar or touch is unbearable; slimy diarrhœa, burning with aching, clawing; water causes fulness and intense pain.

Both have drinking, little or often, or thirstlessness; only *Bell.* has burning first with aversion to water.

APIS	BELLADONNA
Appetite for sour things.	Averse, except during reconvalescence, when acids promote cure.

(3 Those who are guided by the symptoms, need not fear to use *Bell.* in diphtheria, even if it does not seem to correspond to the exudation, prostration and paralysis of the disease. It has been used by competent men in the stage of irritation or excitement, although not later, when the membrane is formed. It corresponds to many of the cerebral, febrile and skin symptoms. *Apis* has in *addition*, urinary symptoms and the intense debility accompanying or following diphtheria. The mucous covering of the tonsils in *Bell.* is more indicative of tonsillitis than diphtheria, where the exudation is albuminous.

APIS	Abdomen	BELLADONNA

Both have abdomen sensitive to touch, from pressure of bed or clothing ; distension.

APIS	BELLADONNA
Tendency to dropsy with swollen feet, scanty urine ; or if inflammatory, intestines feel bruised, sore ; diarrhœa painless. Sore pain superficial, as if beaten.	Tendency to suppurative inflammation ; supersensitive to least touch or jar ; diarrhœa painful. Sore pain *deep* in the abdomen, as if ulcerated.
Peritonitis, stage of exudation, with dropsy : dark, scanty urine ; metritis as a complication. Sharp, sudden pains; great prostration.	Peritonitis, stage of inflammation; with cerebral congestion; urine scanty, yellow ; pains come and go suddenly ; typhlitis, as well as metritis (4).
Acts more on the spleen than liver. Bilious diarrhœa ; also bitter fluid vomit.	Acts more on the liver than spleen. Many bilious symptoms : congestion of liver ; calculi, &c.
Piles protrude, anus swollen ; fidgety, restless, irritable ; scanty urine ; constipated.	Piles protrude and are constricted by spasm of anus ; feverish restlessness ; dysuria ; tenesmus even in back.
Dysentery—more urging than actual pain ; bloody stool with but little pain; rawness of the anus ; tongue dry, shining or white ; urine frequent, profuse or strangury ; skin hot, dry, yet little thirst ; disturbed sleep with muttering.	Dysentery, with tenesmus so severe as to cause shuddering; cutting, tearing pains ; burning of anus ; tongue dry, very red at the tip or two white stripes on a red ground ; urine profuse or suppressed ; dry, hot skin or hot sweat ; thirst, yet averse to drink ; starts in sleep ; stupor.
Cholera Inf. with tendency to hydrocephaloid ; stupor, start with a shrill cry ; hands cold and *blue;* stool green, yellow, slimy ; anus open ; worse morning.	Cholera Inf. with congestive symptoms of the brain ; stupor with frequent starts ; angry when awake; hands and feet cold. the head being hot ; stool clay color, green or with chalk-like lumps ; worse afternoon.

(4) *Bell.* has an especial affinity for the cæcum and its appendages ; thus we find it of service in ulceration of Peyer's glands in typhus. with delirium, &c. In peritonitis or enteritis, with or without suppuration, it becomes of the first importance, if the cæcum is the principal region attacked.

Kidneys, Urine

APIS	BELLADONNA
Bruised pain in the region of the kidneys ; worse stooping.	Stitching pains from kidneys along the ureters to the bladder ; renal colic.
Bright's disease, skin waxy, pale ; œdema, worse under eyes ; hydrothorax ; breathing oppressed, must sit up ; urine milky, scanty or like coffee-grounds (5).	Bright's disease, alternate red and pale face; neuralgia of the head ; spasm of the diaphragm ; urine scanty, bloody, fiery red (5).
Strangury, with pressing down in the region of the sphincter ; from enlarged prostate. Must press long before urine flows. Bladder feels bruised with stinging pains.	Strangury, bearing-down, as from something turning in the bladder; spasm of the sphincter, from alcohol, stricture, gout, prostatitis. Urine voided in drops with fear to strain from extreme cystic tenderness.
Involuntary urine with great irritation of the parts ; worse at night and when coughing ; urine clear, straw-colored.	Involuntary urine, night and day, in girls or scrofulous children ; urine contains white epithelia.
Urine profuse, afterwards scanty (6).	Urine scanty, afterwards profuse (6).

Sexual Organs

APIS	BELLADONNA
Sexual desire increased ; or, with widows decreased ; coition causes stinging in the ovaries.	Sexual desire lessened in males; nymphomania in females ; coition hindered by dry, hot vagina.

(5) *Bell.* corresponds to the congested kidney with albuminuria, scanty bloody urine and intense irritation, bordering on inflammation. In scarlatinal dropsy, it is of service when the inactive skin throws double work on the kidneys ; they become congested and so secrete less actively. But besides, there must be congestive symptoms elsewhere : as in the brain, liver, heart. Uræmia is not so marked as with *Apis ;* because the latter tends more readily to defibrinate the blood, while it also irritates the kidneys and retards the secretion of urea, which according to Buchner, frequently changes into *Carb. of Ammonia* under the fermenting influence of poor fibrin. Hence *Bell.* tends more to irritate the tissues, blood-poisoning being more remote ; *Apis* soon poisons the blood and adds to the danger. *Bell.* is preferable when gout, alcohol, spasms of the bladder or gravel are the apparent cause ; because they tend to congest the kidneys.

(6) This primary and secondary contrast of the two medicines, is given to show a probably different action on the kidneys. *Apis* seems to irritate the Malpighian tufts to increased excretion primarily, while *Bell.* congests them primarily, decreasing the excretion. The first, then, owes its scanty urine to secondary changes ; the latter, to simple congestion.

APIS	Sexual Organs BELLADONNA
Scrotal dropsy.	Induration of testicles.
Ovarian tumors mostly dropsical; burning, stinging pains; or intense bruised, sore pains.	Ovarian induration with crampy pains; bearing-down more than *Apis*; clawing, cutting pains.
Inflammation of the external genitals (females), stinging pains; erysipelatous; vesicular; gangrenous.	Inflammation with dryness and heat to the examining touch: erysipelas in rays; gangrene with throbbing and weight.
Inflammation of internal genitals (females); tendency to dropsy or gangrene. Metritis after confinement; sharp, stabbing pains.	Inflammation of internal genitals: tendency to induration, suppuration or gangrene. Metritis after confinement. Shooting or clawing pains.
Menstruation checked with cerebral congestion, delirium; back feels stiff or bruised; œdema of limbs.	Menstruation checked with cerebral congestion, delirium; back aches, as if broken; jerking of limbs.
Flow of blood scanty, dark, mixed with mucus; bearing-down, worse in ovaries; restless, yawning, change of place, but no relief therefrom (dysmen.); flow profuse, fluid (afibrinous) with faintness (metrorrhagia)	Flow profuse, bright-red; more neuralgia than *Apis*; bearing-down with heaviness most at the vulva; yawning; arms jerk; (dysmen.); flow profuse, bright red or fœtid and lumpy, faint, delirious (metrorrhagia).
Girls who are thin, jealous; frivolous levity; awkward; busy, but do nothing.	Girls with thin skin or plethoric; who are loquacious, hasty, suspicious.
Milk leg, restlessly change posture without relief; limb looks waxy, œdematous.	Milk leg, limb purple; restless, continually moving limbs; limb cold.
Mammæ inflamed, erysipelatous; burning, stinging pains.	Mammæ inflamed; throbbing, stitching pains.
Milk diminished.	Milk increased.

Bell. has also diminished milk, heaviness, headache, red eyes and other signs of cerebral congestion.

APIS	BELLADONNA
Leucorrhœa profuse, yellow or green and acrid, with painful urination; straw-colored, not so deep as with *Bell.*	Leucorrhœa, acute catarrh, white mucus; colicky pains; worse morning; strangury; urine stains linen yellow.

Larynx, Chest

APIS	BELLADONNA
Voice hoarse, rough, husky; phlegm difficult, scanty, clear, saliva increased; aphonia in consequence of diseases which poison the blood and paralyze parts (diphtheria, &c.).	Voice hoarse, rough, shrill or weak and wheezing; mucus rattling but little sputa; saliva increased and stringy, slimy; aphonia, catarrhal or in conjunction with hysteria.
Cough with tough, scanty sputa, which must be swallowed; worse from exposure to wet and cold.	Cough without sputa, spasmodic; or bloody sputa, worse from warm to cold.
Respiration difficult, worse leaning forward or backward; cannot see how she can get another breath.	Respiration irregular, labored, with moaning; better holding head back, or holding breath; difficult from mucus in the chest.
Tendency to serious infiltration in the chest.	Tendency to spasm of the chest; purulent infiltration.
Chest feels bruised, as if jammed; dryness of the air-passages, with sensation of burning, as if scalded.	Chest feels sore, as if raw; dryness of the air-passages, especially as far as the trachea, with tickling, as if from dust.

Heart

APIS	BELLADONNA
Heart: Pain arrests breathing; febrile excitement, anguish; restless, but no relief from change of position; hydropericardium; blowing sound with diastole.	Heart: Aching which takes breath, violent arterial pulsations, anxiety, cerebral congestion; stage of inflammation, no valvular lesion.
Pulse full and accelerated; thread-like; intermits, but is regular in volume (typhus).	Pulse full, accelerated and *hard*, soft and small, or slow and full (apoplexy), irregular and unequal (heart disease)

Sleep

Both have inclination to sleep with inability; perhaps *Bell.* has more drowsiness with jerking of limbs, crying out in sleep; *Apis* more so-called nervousness with less of the flushed face. The congestions of *Apis* are seldom as acute as those of *Bell.*, but vitality is lower and absorption less active.

Fevers

APIS	BELLADONNA
Chill with thirst.	Chill without thirst.
Chills on suffering part.	Coldness on suffering part.

APIS	Fevers	BELLADONNA
Chill commences in abdomen, hands, chest or knees; worse from heat; better uncovering.		Chill commences in the arms; better from heat and worse from cold or uncovering.
Chill 3 to 4 P.M.		Chill evening or morning.

Both have hot head with chills; chilly least movement.

APIS	BELLADONNA
Liver free, but sore pains in the region of the spleen; dropsy, feet swollen, waxy skin; diarrhœa; scanty urine; swollen abdomen.	Liver and spleen both swollen; incipient dropsy; cases mal treated with Quinine; constipation.
Heat with burning in the chest, which almost suffocates.	Heat with throbbing arteries, red face, delirium; choking sensation in the throat.
Sweat alternate with dry skin; sweat increased in room.	Sweat partial, mostly on head, or on covered parts; lessened in room.

Scarlatina.—Both have red, irritated skin, with restlessness, sensitive skin, sleepy but can't sleep; throat swollen; tongue red, &c.

APIS	BELLADONNA
Skin stings and burns, œdematous swelling of eye-lids, ulcers in the throat, erysipelatous or œdematous; tongue blistered; if eruption fails, throat inflamed, nose discharges thin ichor; murmuring delirium; great prostration, typhoid state. More allied to *Rhus* (yet inimical), Ars. (in scarlatina).	Skin hot, burning the examining hand; face and throat and neck swollen from congestive engorgement; "straw-berry" tongue; if eruption fails, furious delirium, restless; if soporous, snoring; jerks, twitches; best suited to smooth, scarlet exanthema. More allied to *Sul., Lach., Op., Stram.* (in scarlatina).

Measles.—Both have croupy cough, inflamed eyes, &c.

APIS	BELLADONNA
Eruption confluent with erysipelas or œdema; throat œdematous.	Eruption on a red skin; skin swollen, turgid; parotids swollen.
Typhus; useful in febris nervosa putrida, stage of debility; symptoms of decomposition of the blood.	Typhus; useful in inflammatory stage, when symptoms alternate between excitement and depression (7).
Apathy; stupor with murmuring delirium; hardness of hearing;	Profound coma, with snoring *or* furious delirium; deafness

(7) By noting the alternate symptoms connected by *or*, we see how two-fold are the indications for *Bell.*; hence its extensive range, and hence the more care in its use.

APIS	Fevers	BELLADONNA
expression pleasant, happy, with senseless apathy ; cannot talk or put the tongue out ; difficult swallowing; urine and stool involuntary ; slide down in bed—all signs of paralysis from decomposition of blood. Tongue cracked, sore, ulcerated, covered with vesicles ; tenacious mucus in the throat, difficult to remove; swallowing difficult from weak muscles ; dry, burning skin or partial, clammy sweats; urine involuntary, strong like horse urine, pupils dilated ; white miliary eruption ; abdomen distended and sore ; bruised.		*alternate* with acute hearing ; expression depressed ; glassy eyes, *or* staring, furibund delirium; tongue trembles, talk thick or speechless ; no stool, distortion of the mouth ; debility with sleepiness ; no stool —all as a result of irritation and congestion of the nervous centres. Tongue red, hot, dry, cracked or red margins; white centre ; stringy mucus, brown on the tongue and in the throat, *or* dry throat ; swallowing difficult from spasm *or* paralysis ; dry skin, hot, *or* hot sweat *or* cold sweat on the face ; urine bright yellow or scanty and red ; pupils contracted *or* dilated ; red eruption ; abdomen distended, pains worse in ileo-cæcal region.

Limbs

Apis	Belladonna
Rheumatic pains, burning, stinging ; or sore, bruised feeling in muscles. Arthritic nodes ; worse in wet weather ; after checked gonorrhœa ; chronic forms.	Rheumatic pains with stitching, red in streaks ; extreme sensitiveness to touch. Arthritic pains, boring, shooting like lightning from joints along bone ; worse changing warm to cold ; acute forms.

Skin, Etc.

Apis	Belladonna
Urticaria with uterine catarrh. Boils large ; mostly before suppuration begins.	Urticaria with profuse menstruation. Boils small ; worse in Spring ; throbbing, tendency to suppuration.
Punctured wounds with traumatic erysipelas.	Nervous symptoms from concussions ; inflammation from sprains.

Both have affections from stings, and contagious anthrax. Only *Bell.* has symptoms of hydrophobia.

Apis	Belladonna
Wounds become œdematous.	Wounds suppurate profusely.

APIS	Generalities	BELLADONNA
Inclination for open air. Blood black, viscous, non-coagulable (afibrinous).		Aversion to open air. Blood bright-red, clotted ; but later, as in destructive diseases, as cancer, &c., offensive, watery.
Left Side.—Complaints from *Iod.*, *Sul.*		Right Side.—Complaints from *Merc.*, *Plumb.*, *Iod.*, *China.*
Similar to *Ranunc.*, *Nat. M.*, *Rhus.*		Similar to *Hep.*, *Merc.*, narcotics, *Lach.*
Remission during the day.		Remission after midnight and in the forenoon.

Apis has *aggravation,* and *Bell. amelioration,* from warmth, lying in bed, stooping, sitting down, holding the breath, wrapping up.

Apis has *amelioration,* and *Bell. aggravation,* from open air, cold washing, rising from bed, uncovering.

APIS	Mind	CANTHARIS
Mental symptoms more those of deficient brain action—coma, imbecility—brain feels tired—hydrocephalus ; sero-tubercular deposit ; absent-minded.		Mental symptoms more hyper-action—fury, violent cries, insanity—wild look—cerebral inflammation with violent symptoms even if unconscious. Fancies. (See Sleep.)
Restless, with the meaningless, busy manner of the weak-minded : always at work, yet awkward, break things and laugh at the mishap. Sensitive to pains.		Restless, agitated, frantic, an inflammatory state of both mind and body; passions wild, parts burning. Frantic with the pains.
Coma caused by hydrocephalic effusion, sero-tubercular ; one side paralyzed, the other jerking ; shrill cry ; boring head in pillow ; squinting. Breathing oppressed, worse lying. Big toe is turned up.		Coma caused by internal erosions or suppurations; arms lie lifeless, with occasional starts; scowling, barking; eyes closed, or if open, expressionless. Breathing oppressed, better lying.

Throat

APIS	CANTHARIS
Erysipelas of face ; begins about eyes, temples ; blisters, if any, small.	Erysipelas, burning as though scalded; begins in dorsum of nose; blisters large; bleb-like.
Dryness of the nose (as in Scarlatina) or coryza dry in morning, fluent in the evening.	Difficult detachment of tenacious mucus from posterior nares, causing a burning, smarting sensation.
Involuntary snapping of teeth together (brain). Vesicles in clusters on root of tongue or along border; tongue swollen, burns, stings.	Grinding of teeth, hydrophobia ; spasms, lascivious mania. Vesicles in mouth, on tongue, burn, sore, suppurate; burning to stomach.

Face

APIS	CANTHARIS
Diphtheria, prostration constant from beginning; throat, as if varnished, rosy-red, mottled or gray deposit; saliva tough, stringy; rash; neck swollen.	Diphtheria, prostration, later, fainting spells, coldness ; throat excoriated, burns, dark red ; saliva frothy, bloody ; rash shines through epidermis; spasm in throat.
Tonsils swollen, red, highly inflamed ; erysipelatous.	Tonsils swollen dark-red, burn, suppurate.
Difficult swallowing of liquids or solids, because throat is swollen, contracted, or muscles are too weak.	Difficulty of swallowing liquids from spasms of the throat—often impossible ; even the sight of water causes choking.

Both have strangury in diphtheria.

Stomach, Abdomen

APIS	CANTHARIS
Inflammation of internal organs, parts feel sore, as if bruised ; dropsies follow.	Inflammation of internal organs with intense burning with the soreness ; more suppuration than in *Apis*.
Generally little thirst ; if any, drink often and little.	Thirst, drink seldom and much at a time, or aversion, because drink excites the pains.
Inflammation of stomach ; burning, stinging pains ; fever, dry skin, full pulse, restlessness.	Inflammation of stomach, agonized tossing about, burning like coals of fire, stomach, as if screwed together.
Peritonitis especially with exudation and prostration. Feet swollen, waxy. Abdomen so sore and bruised, it cannot bear pressure. Metritis as a complication.	Peritonitis especially with erosion or suppuration. Pains cutting, burning, agonizing. Despair; face sunken. Complicated with inflammation of serous covering of bladder.

Stomach, Abdomen

APIS	CANTHARIS
Costive, or stool painless yellow. Ascites may follow, with involuntary diarrhœa from relaxed sphincter ani.	Stool bloody, slimy, extorting cries. Suppuration may follow with coma, arms hang lifeless, pulse weak, hands cold, occasional starts.
Alvine discharges more from mucous state of intestines; sub-acute inflammation, vascular fulness. Hence painless, mucous; mucous with tenesmus or griping rawness, bruised soreness, bloody stools.	Alvine discharges more from intense, destructive inflammation, pains cutting, burning, with agony, destructive. Hence scrapings of intestinal mucous membrane; bloody, corrosive stool, scream with the tenesmus.
Indicated in hydrocephaloid stage of Chol. Inf. with coma; cold, blue hands. Similar to *Phos., Calc. C., Sul., Zinc.*	Indicated in collapse of dysentery, peritonitis, &c., sinking, death-like spells. Similar to *Camph.*
Affects more the spleen; hence diseases affecting the quality of the blood.	Affects more the liver; hence yellow skin, yellow sight, &c.

Kidneys, Urine

APIS	CANTHARIS
Kidneys (1). Bruised pains in kidneys, worse stooping.	Stitches in kidneys, arrest the breahting.
Pains from bladder to kidneys.	Pains from kidneys to bladder.

Both have strangury, irritation of neck of bladder, burning during and after micturition.

APIS	CANTHARIS
Urine copious with hemiplegia. Incontinence with great irritation of parts; worse at night and when coughing.	Urine copious, involuntary, after *long retention* or with paraplegia.
Urine scanty, bloody or like coffee-grounds or milky (Scarlatina).	Urine scanty, contains casts of epith. flaky, purulent.
Dropsy with scanty urine, thirstlessness, defibrinated blood (1).	Dropsy caused by cystic retention, atony of urinary organs.

---

(1) *Cantharis* is best adapted to nephritis vera with tendency to suppuration or croupcus exudation. In Bright's Disease, it owes its uræmic symptoms to destructive inflammation, thus preventing the functional action of the kidneys. In *Apis*, we would scarcely find a remedy for true nephritis, as it seldom acts on parenchymatous parts or causes suppuration or croupy (fibrinous) exudation. Its uræmia results from defibrinated blood, albuminuria. It claims precedence where the blood is the cause of the disease, Scarlatina, &c.

APIS	CANTHARIS
Sexual Organs	
Sexual desire may be strong; often lessened in widows.	Priapism, desire intense, most with inflamed bladder, &c., &c.

The lascivious symptoms of *Canth. render* it far superior in Nymphomania, although *Apis* also has eruptions and inflammation of external genitals, so often the apparent cause of this disease.

APIS	CANTHARIS
Inflammation more vascular, erysipelatous. Scratching raises lumps, like hives.	Inflammation of a destructive nature. Scratching (pruritus) raises little tumors.
Gonorrhœa, system contaminated—gonitis—fever—gleet. Answers to the hydrogenoid constitution of Grauvogl.	Gonorrhœa, inflammation intense, spreads to bladder, kidneys, prostate. Sometimes in secondary forms, when discharge increases again—seldom true gleet.
Ovarian disease, right side; burning, stinging; soreness upper left chest, numbness down thigh or up to ribs. Dropsy, pale complexion, waxy, œdematous limbs; scanty urine; constipation.	Ovarian disease; burning, pinching; stitches arrest breathing. Dropsy with sickly complexion; more strangury than *Apis;* tetanus of both rectum and bladder.
Abortion, direct congestion with bearing down; heaviness in abdomen; flow with yawning and faintness.	Abortion, strangury, especially when subject to moles or fœtus is dead; flow black, clotted.
Complaints among widows.	Complaints among the sterile (subject to moles).
Dysmenorrhœa, sharp, stabbing pains in head or uterus, congestion to head.	Dysmenorrhœa, membranous, burning; lancinating deep in brain.

Chest, Etc.

APIS	CANTHARIS
Dropsy of chest, no inflammation; cannot see how can get another breath. Restless, can bend neither forward nor backward.	Dropsy after pleurisy; chest so weak can make neither effort to breathe nor speak. Face expressive of despair, cold sweat; syncope.
Cough, awakes before 12 P.M., expectoration difficult, scanty, tough, clear.	Cough early on rising; expectoration difficult, tenacious, bloody.
Respiration hurried; painful, spasmodic, worse lying down (cerebro-spinal diseases, &c.).	Respiration oppressed, with crampy pains in chest; better lying down (cerebro-spinal diseases, &c.).

APIS	CANTHARIS
Chest, Etc.	
Weakness of air-passages in diseases which devitalize the blood. Diphtheria, &c.	Weakness of air-passages, as from exhaustive inflammation or suppuration, &c.
Soreness of chest, as if jammed, bruised.	Cutting, burning, stitches in chest.
Palpitation not marked. Pulse full, accelerated or intermittent, or thread-like.	Palpitation violent. Pulse full and *hard,* or intermittent and *hard,* or feeble, slow.
Back, Limbs	
Stiff back or weakness in the small of the back. (See kidneys.)	Stitches up the back to the axilla or into the abdomen (2).
Hands blue, cold, in diarrhœa.	Hands cold, in bladder diseases.
Sleep	
Sleepless from nervous irritation ; fidgety.	Sleepless from illusions of persons walking, striking bed, &c.

Fevers

Scarlatina.— Both have kidney affections, dropsy, strangury, uræmia, &c. (See note 1).

APIS	CANTHARIS
Throat sore, with non-development of eruption ; muttering delirium or sopor ; nose dry, or discharge of white or bloody mucus.	Throat covered with tenacious mucus ; vitiated, frowning look, sleepless, great distress ; nose dry, burning or discharge ichorous.
Chill, worse least motion ; face and hands hot. Worse, warm room.	Chill, worse rising from bed ; face pale ; sometimes resists warmth, but better therefrom.
Heat with muttering, unconsciousness ; drowsy or sleepless : thirstless mostly. Better from uncovering.	Heat delirious, talk of business or of the dead ; great thirst ; sometimes thirsty, yet averse to drink. Worse from uncovering.
Intermittents, all stages marked; thirst during chill.	Intermittents with strangury ; thirst after chill. Chilly stage predominates.
Better if sweat is checked.	Better *after* sweat.
Sweat not marked ; alternate with dry skin ; musk-like, in brain diseases.	Sweat profuse ; cold on hands and feet (collapse, &c.).

---

(2) *Cantharis* has the symptoms of neuralgia of kidneys, bladder, urethra, as well as of irritability. *Apis,* only those of irritability.

Skin

APIS	CANTHARIS
Skin, muscles : rigid.	Skin, muscles : lax.
Skin raises in welts ; feels sore, bruised ; burning, stinging. Hives.	Skin, as if blistered or actually blistered ; burns like fire. Blisters. Burns. Pemphigus.
Red areola around carbuncles, boils, ulcers ; (erysipelatous) with burning, stinging pains. Gangrene.	Red areola around pimples ; ulcers burn, tearing pains. Gangrene with vesicles.
Eruptions better washing.	Eruptions worse washing.
Inflammation of the periosteum.	Tearing in the bones.
Remission during the day.	Remission morning, evening until midnight.

Generalities

Apis has *aggravation,* and *Canth. amelioration,* from warmth, warm air, lying down, when growing warm in bed.

Apis has *amelioration,* and *Canth. aggravation,* from open air, cold washing, moistening the suffering part.

Mind

APIS	LACHESIS
Always busy, but awkward, break things ; change occupation. Overstrained merriment, happy expression. Typhus, muttering delirium, tongue dry, cracked, hard to put out, swollen ; slide down in bed ; eyes turn up, squinting or strange, happy look ; stool putrid, involuntary, urine involuntary ; speech impossible.	Hurried, awkward on rising, body bends to left ; changes subject to talking. Talk as in foreign language, or cry, whine, and then silly laugh ; expression vacant. Typhus, muttering ; tongue dry, cracked, *black,* trembles when put out, catches on teeth or rolls in mouth ; lower jaw hangs, eyelids droop ; eyes roll vacantly ; face sunken ; stool offensive ; speech, nasal or indistinct.
Absent-minded — brain feels tired.	Active mind—studies well at night.
Ailments from rage, vexation with fright.	Ailments from grief, disappointed love.

Head, Face

APIS	LACHESIS
Headache forehead ; better pressure.	Headache vertex ; worse pressure.
Staphyloma.	Pterygium ; fistula lachrymalis.
Erysipelas of face ; begins about eyes ; pale, pinkish.	Erysipelas of face ; begins on cheeks ; blue or purplish.
Coryza dry morning, fluent in the evening.	Coryza fluent ; pulsating headache precedes.

Mouth

APIS	LACHESIS
Tongue and mouth inflamed ; fauces, tonsils, rosy-red ; vesicles clustered on posterior of tongue, or whole border.	Tongue blistered on tip ; vesicles tend to ulcerate ; tingling pains.

Throat

APIS	LACHESIS
Diphtheria, weak from the beginning ; patches dirty-gray, or throat, as if varnished; voice weak, larynx numb ; worse swallowing liquids or solids ; legs numb ; skin waxy ; nose dry.	Diphtheria, throat purple, gangrenous ; worse left side ; larynx sensitive to least touch; worse swallowing liquids and *saliva* ; legs mottled, livid ; nose discharges thin, slimy fetor.
Hoarse, rough voice ; phelgm difficult, scanty, clear (1).	Hoarse voice, weak, low; phlegm difficult, watery, salty.

Both have contraction of the throat, rawness, stinging.

APIS	LACHESIS
Contraction less marked ; more like a tonic astriction ; swallowing difficult from diminished power over the muscles of deglutition. Feels, as if throat and mouth were scalded.	Constriction like spasm, *clonic* ; almost choke when swallow ; fluids escape through the nose. Dryness in spots ; less scalded feeling ; tingling pains.

Stomach, Abdomen

APIS	LACHESIS
Ascites from tumor (uterine, ovarian); abdomen sore, as if bruised.	Ascites from enlarged liver, spleen, heart ; worse least touch or feeling, as if ulcerated (2).
Inflammation of internal organs, dropsy following.	Inflammation of internal organs, suppuration or engorgement following.

---

(1) *Apis* has been given in Clergyman's Sorethroat after cauterization. (Compare *Nat. Mur., Ars.*).

(2) This distinction is important ; because *Apis* seldom causes suppuration ; *Lachesis,* often.

Stomach, Abdomen

APIS	LACHESIS
Burning in the stomach, worse eating; yellow, painless diarrhœa. More the acute symptoms of gastric catarrh.	Burning pressure, gnawing, better from eating; returns soon, more violent the emptier is the stomach; more the symptoms of chronic catarrh, gastralgia, &c.
Diarrhœa, yellow-green mucous; worse morning; hand blue, cold.	Diarrhœa yellow, fæcal, worse at night; alternates with constipation.
Dysentery, intestines feel bruised; tenesmus *after stool.*	Dysentery, stool cadaverous; abdomen feels, as if ulcerated; tenesmus *during* stool.
Costive; stool large, difficult; rawness at the anus.	Costive; stool natural or like sheep's dung; offensive; burning at the anus. Stool hindered by constriction.
Piles protrude; fidgety, restless, stinging soreness (vascular state); anus swollen.	Piles protrude; stitches when coughing; can't bear least touch (nervous state); prolapsus ani.

Kidneys, Urine

APIS	LACHESIS
Urine generally scanty, but frequent; straw-colored (not so deep yellow as sometimes in *Lach.*); more acute cystic symptoms; tenesmus vesicæ, urine mixed with blood. Not so much *pressure* as with *Lach.*, hence symptoms not so *chronic.*	Urine frequent and profuse; foamy (bilious state); with bad-looking mucus (cystitis); pressure on the bladder as from hæmorrhoids of bladder (after liquor). Blood sometimes, then it looks like charred straw, settling to the bottom.
Kidneys; sore, bruised feeling; back feels sore when stooping; stiff or weak feeling in the back. (See Scarlatina.)	Kidneys: Stitches; warmth; like a ball moving; drawing into hips, with urging to urinate; stiffness from the loins to the sacrum and thighs.

Genitals

APIS	LACHESIS
Complaints among widows.	Complaints at climacteric age.
Right ovary; pains up to ribs; tightness across hips; ovarian dropsy.	Left (3) ovary: Pain to liver, chest or genitals; ovarian suppuration.

---

(3) *Lachesis* has been given for tumor in the right groin; but its main action seems to be on the left ovary.

Genitals

APIS	LACHESIS
Menstruation: Heaviness in abdomen; bearing down, most right ovary; congestion to head constipation; legs œdematous, wax-colored; restless, uneasy; yawning.	Menstruation: Tearing in abdomen; bearing down, left ovary; congestion to head, nosebleed; diarrhœa; legs with ulcers, purple; chilly by day, flashes by night.
Sexual desire strong; sometimes in widows, weak; coition causes stinging in the ovaries.	Sexual desire strong, irresistible, often with functional weakness; pollutions or intercourse improves.
Milk diminished.	Milk spoiled.

Chest

APIS	LACHESIS
Cough; soreness upper left chest; worse before midnight, after lying down, after sleep; sputa tough, scanty, must be swallowed; sputa small.	Cough; ulcerative pain in chest; worse lying down, *during and after* sleep; sputa must be swallowed; expectoration all day.

Both have cough continuing until phlegm is loosened.

APIS	LACHESIS
Respiration difficult, leaning forward or backward; cannot see how can get another breath; restless, yet no relief from change of place; breathe quickly; asthma in Winter.	Respiration better sitting bent forward; awake suffocating, gasping, anxious; anguish worse from least motion of arms; breathe slowly; asthma in warm, wet weather (Spring).

Both have emotions affecting the heart.

APIS	LACHESIS
Pulse accelerated, full; or thread-like; if intermitting, regular.	Pulse full or small, **weak**; unequal.
External plethora (mostly).	Internal plethora **(mostly)**.
Feel sore all over superficially.	Feel sore **internally**.

Fevers

APIS	LACHESIS
Chill worse in a warm room; in the morning; burning in the chest; smothering feeling in the chest; begins in the chest stomach or hands.	Chill better in a warm room; in the afternoon, burning in the face; tearing, tightness in the chest; runs up the back.
Heat, wants to uncover.	Heat, averse to uncovering.
Sweat alternative with dry skin.	Sweat with heat; worse motion.
No thirst in the sweat.	None in the chill; mostly before chill.
Scarlaina; restless, agitated; irritation of the whole surface; erysipelas of the throat; *whole*	Scarlatina; tendency to gangrene in the throat; tonsils and glands suppurate; puffy in

Fevers

APIS	LACHESIS
neck swollen; saliva tough, **stringy**; dropsy with scanty, **milky** urine; skin waxy.	*front* of the neck; saliva copious, tenacious or slimy; dropsy with copious urine, black in spots.
If **rash recedes or fails, throat worse**; delirium, **bores head in pillow**, shrill **shriek; skin hot** and cold in **places**; face **œdematous.**	If rash recedes or fails; face and jaws sunken; skin cold, purple in spots.

Sleep

Both **cause sleeplessness** from nervousness with desire to sleep.

Skin

APIS	LACHESIS
Boils, abscesses, &c.; stage of inflammation (**Erysip.**) or gangrene.	Boils, abscesses, &c.; suppuration, pus laudable but retarded; later, bluish.
Panaritium, **burning**, stinging; erysipelas **far around.**	**Panaritium**, pricking, tingling, **more** than stinging; blue far around.
Skin peels.	Skin suppurates.
Cancers **and** eruptions **burn**, sting; yellow, **painless** diarrhœa.	Cancers with lancinating pains; eruptions more with constipation.
Varicose veins **burn, sting.**	Varicose veins ulcerate.
Skin and muscles **rigid.**	Skin and muscles lax.

Generalities

APIS	LACHESIS
Allied to *Ranvnc., Nat. Mur., Sulphur.*	Allied to *Merc., Solanaceæ, Hepar.*
Complaints from *Anthrax, Iod., Sul.*	Complaints from *Merc., Quinine.*
Remission during the day.	Remission midnight until noon
Inclination for open air.	Aversion to open air (mostly).

Apis has *aggravation* and *Lashesis amelioration* from motion, warmth, shaking the head, after rising from a seat, swallowing food, cold weather, inspiration.

Apis has *amelioration* and *Lachesis aggravation* from holding suffering part, assuming an erect position, rising from bed, open air.

Mind

APIS	NATRUM MUR.
Fear of apoplexy; apoplexy more than paralysis (1).	Fear of loss of reason ; paralysis more than apoplexy.

Both have ailments from fright with vexation ; rage.

APIS	NATRUM MUR.
If with jealousy.	If with reserved displeasure.
Fickle inconsistency ; foolish gaiety, overstrained gaiety.	Sad, tearful, or alternately sad and excessively merry (2).
Loquacious.	Taciturn.

Both have absent-mindedness, mental weakness, dulness, imbecility, weary feeling in the head.

APIS	NATRUM MUR.
Awkward ; breaks things from clumsiness.	Awkward ; hasty; drops things from nervous weakness.

Head

APIS	NATRUM MUR.
Vertigo when lying with closed eyes ; nausea and headache ; congestive from suppressed menses ; faint when stooping, with revolving vertigo ; evening vertigo after sleep ; from Sun or hot room; in the Spring.	Vertigo when rising, goes off if lie down awhile ; congestive from suppressed hæmorrhoidal flow or in pregnancy ; faint if move ; morning vertigo ; from spirituous liquors ; from straining eyes or close study (3)
Nervous headache ; must hold the head and eyes down ; better in cold air.	Same with constrictive pains, cutting ; worse in cold air and while walking ; eyes drawn together.
Congestion ; pressure in forehead, relieved by pressure of the hand; throbbing and burning; worse, moving or stooping (4).	Congestion ; like little hammers beating; pressure both sides of head like a vice; worse, rising or moving; (worse, waking); better from sweat.

---

(1) *Apis* seldom causes paralysis, except from blood-poison (Diphtheria, &c), or from causes within the brain (tumors, apoplexy, &c.).

Nat. Mur. causes paralysis from emotions, pains, onanism, excesses in liquor ; hence from direct nervous exhaustion.

(2) The alternation of symptoms in *Nat. Mur.* is very characteristic, and shows its efficacy in nervous diseases ; especially hysteria.

(3) The sun's heat seems to aggravate all symptoms of the *Natrum Salts*. *Nat. Mur.* gives us, especially, weak, fainting feelings in chest and head when walking in the sun and not so much vertigo as *Apis or Natr. Carb.*

(4) Generally, *Apis* feels better if sweat is lessened. Perhaps this will be true of headaches.

Eyes

APIS	NATRUM MUR.
Staphyloma corneæ.	Suppuration of cornea.
Vesicles on the cornea ; cornea smoky; profuse lachrymation ; twitching of the ball ; lids granular. Scrofulous ophthalmia from suppressed (itch) eruption ; hence like *Sulph.*	Acrid, corroding tears from the eyes ; twitching of the balls and spasmodic closure of the lids. Dermoid tumor on edge of lid. Scrofulous ophthalmia, abused with Nitrate of Silver (5) ; like *Ars.*
Obscuration of sight, with blind staggers or from opaque cornea. *Lachrymal sac* inflamed (like *Puls.*).	Obscuration amaurotic, from debilitating, nervous losses. Fistula lachrymalis.

Ears

APIS	NATRUM MUR.
Erysipelatous, redness of the ears.	Ears red from congestion, together with otorrhœa, beating, throbbing.

Nose

APIS	NATRUM MUR.
Dryness of the nose, or white, thick or acrid, bloody, fetid mucus.	Thick mucus with loss of smell and taste. Membrane thickened.
Dry coryza, morning ; fluent, evening.	Alternate dry and fluent coryza.
Erysipelas of nose ; œdematous.	Red and swollen nose; numb.

Face

APIS	NATRUM MUR.
Neuralgia with or followed by impaired memory (6).	Neuralgia after Quinine ; pains produce paralytic symptoms.
Face pale, waxy or purplish.	Face shining, yellowish or livid; one cheek red.

Mouth

APIS	NATRUM MUR.
Upper lip swollen, feels stiff.	Upper lip swollen, feels numb.
Mouth inflamed, rosy-red; dry as **if burned**; or vesicles mostly **along the** edge of the tongue ; prickling in the tongue.	Mouth inflamed, tongue and gums swollen, blisters ; ulcers form more than in *Apis;* gums bleed ; ptyalism ; one side of the tongue numb (7).

(5) Yet *Apis* has cured sore-throats after cauterization, and it may be, that is will apply equally well to the eyes.

(6) *Apis* has blind staggers, revolving vertigo, neuralgia with deficient memory and hemiplegia, all symptoms of cerebral tumors. Will it be of use in their treatment ? Many of the *Apis* symptoms point to organic brain changes

(7) *Nat. Mur.* has scorbutic symptoms, and always produces more excoriated, raw sensations than *Apis.*

Mouth

APIS	NATRUM MUR.
Tongue dry, white.	Mapped tongue.
Saliva, tough, frothy.	Saliva, copious, bloody or limpid.

Throat

APIS	NATRUM MUR.
Swallowing difficult from contractive sensation in the throat; from swelling; or from diminished power over the muscles of the throat (Diphtheria).	Swallowing difficult, as from a plug in the throat; from spasm of the pharynx (8); food goes down "the wrong way" or not at all; muscles of swallowing weak; speech impaired.
Throat dry, glistening; or œdematous; or gangrenous ulcers (Scarlatina).	Throat dry, yet constantly hawking mucus; putrid, ulcerated patches in the throat and on the gums (Scorbutus).
Goitre, with ovarian disease.	Goitre, with chronic sore throat; glands worse coughing, swallowing.

Stomach, Etc.

APIS	NATRUM MUR.
Nausea felt in the throat.	Nausea felt in the stomach.
Longing for sour things.	Longing for bitter things.
Thirstless (dropsy), or drink little and often; drinking causes burning and nausea.	Thirst constant; nausea after drinking.
Eructations bitter.	Empty eructations; sour.
Appetite less (with diarrhœa).	Hunger increased, often with lessened appetite. Hungry for supper.
Symptoms of acute catarrh of the stomach; burning, sensitiveness to least touch; soreness; diarrhœa, painless, yellow.	Symptoms of chronic catarrh; cramp-pains; burning alternating with coldness; pressure, with nausea and sudden sinking of strength; sleepy after eating.

Abdomen

Both have a tightness of the skin across the abdomen from hip to hip:

---

(8) *Nat. Mur.* always gives us crampy, colicky, spasmodic pains in nearly every locality. *Apis* offers more symptoms of vascular irritation. Both may appear in the treatment of hysteria, but *Nat. Mur.* must ever cover the majority of cases.

APIS	NATRUM MUR.
Abdomen	
—worse raising the arms ; ovarian.	—must loosen the clothes.
Abdomen feels sore, bruised, worse walking, or from least touch.	When walking, abdominal viscera feel, as if loose, dragging.
Abdomen distended, œdematous.	Abdomen distended, with flatus (9).
Bowels	
Constipation, stool very large ; sensation as though something tight would break if too much effort is used.	Constipation, stool hard, dry ; crumbling, fissures the anus, sensation of pressure from navel downwards, with leaden heaviness across the bladder and pelvis (10).
Diarrhœa painless, bloody (dysenteric) or painless, yellow ; worse in morning ; emaciation with anasarca, indescribable weakness; hands blue and cold (Cholera Infantum), ascites.	Diarrhœa green, watery, bloody; worse during the day; emaciation most about the neck ; eat well, yet grow thin ; alternation of constipation and diarrhœa ; abdomen sunken or distended. (9).
Hydrocephaloid symptoms, with Cholera Infantum.	
Hæmorrhoids small, protrude, cause smarting and much fidgetiness ; urine very scanty.	Hæmorrhoids, with protruding rectum and much smarting ; cutting in the urethra after micturition ; herpes around anus.
Swelling of anus.	Prolapsus ani.
Kidneys, Urine	
Sore, bruised feeling in region of kidneys; painful stiffness, worse stooping ; urine scanty, red, bloody.	Tension and heat in region of kidneys, even while sitting ; walking soon tires ; urine with brick-dust sediment.

(9) *Nat. Mur.* causes emaciation, with hunger ; constipation alternate with diarrhœa, etc., because the glandular system is diseased. *Apis* tends to produce dropsies, albuminuria, etc., because the blood is defibrinated.

(10) Crumbling of the stool seems to be the especial property of the *Muriates* ; at least *Mag. Mur.*, *Amm. Mur.*, *Nat. Mur.*, representatives of three different bases, have it ; and *Kali Chlor.* (*Mur.*) has hard, *dry* stool, a favorable pre-disposing state.

Kidneys, Urine

APIS	NATRUM MUR.
Incontinence at night, and when coughing, with great irritation of the parts (11).	Incontinence night and day when coughnig, walking or laughing.
Burning before and after urinating ; strangury.	Stitches in the bladder, burning during urination ; cutting in urethra, after.
Urine scanty, albuminous, often like coffee-grounds.	Urine generally profuse or like coffee-grounds, black.
Gleet, with gonitis (rheumatic subjects). Compare note (5).	Gleet, green (females), intensely itching; genitals (male) smell strong, humid, itching ; herpes scroti et ani. After *Nitrate of Silver*.

Genitals

APIS	NATRUM MUR.
Sexual desire increased or, with widows, decreased.	Excitement physical ; weakness of the parts ; impotence.
Embrace (female) causes pains in ovarian regions.	Embrace weakens, coldness of joints (12) (male); feels easy and light-hearted at first, later, ill-humored (females) (13).
Menses suppressed, cause congestion to head, vertigo, delirium ; awkward, constantly busy, but do nothing.	Menses delayed, cause bloody saliva, heat in face, heavy abdomen ; congestion of head more *after* menses ; hasty, impatient.
Vulvitis, erysipelatous ; or eruptions stinging like bee-sting.	Vulvitis with falling off of the hair ; pimples on mons veneris, and on border of hair, nape of neck.
Leucorrhœa profuse, yellow ; green and acrid, with dysuria.	Leucorrhœa with colic, white, thick, transparent, or green ; when walking causing smarting and itching (8).

(11) *Apis* suits vesical irritability, with accompanying enuresis. *Nat. Mur.* develops more a paralytic state, hence, no irritation. *Apis* may, perhaps, cause profuse paralytic enuresis with hemiplegia.

(12) This sensation of coldness, compared with similar sensations, in other parts, will be found to run through the whole pathogenesis of *Nat. Mur.*

(13) But, after the menses, *Nat. Mur.* gives us aversion to embrace, which has become painful from dryness of the vagina. The sadness so characteristic at this time, also helps to induce the aversion.

APIS	NATRUM MUR.
Genitals	
Bearing-down mostly in region of ovaries (congestive).	Pressing from sides of abdomen in morning, must sit to prevent prolapse.
Tendency to dropsy, with uterine (and ovarian) diseases.	Chlorotic symptoms with uterine diseases.

Larynx, Lungs, Heart

APIS	NATRUM MUR.
Hoarseness, rough voice, husky; phlegm difficult, scanty, clear; clergyman's sore-throat.	Hoarseness, with dryness in larynx and nose; accumulation of mucus mornings; in chronic cases, with sensation of swallowing over a lump.

Both have been successfully used after abuse of *Lunar Caustic.*

APIS	NATRUM MUR.
Cough worse evening until 12 P. M.; after lying down; after sleep.	Cough worse evening after lying down; from motion.
Expectoration tough, scanty, must be swallowed. Cough causes soreness left pectoral region.	Expectoration yellow, blood-streaked, flat or sourish, seldom salty. Cough with cutting (14), tearing in chest, bursting pain in head.
Breath fetid (with headache).	Breath—hot.

Both have oppression of chest worse in the room.

APIS	NATRUM MUR.
Dyspnœa; does not see how he can breathe again. (Pneumothorax.) Pain near heart almost arrests breathing.	Dyspnœa from manual labor; [Emphysema. (Hysteria?)].
	Pains generally take away breath, and almost paralyze.
Must sit up; worse bending backward or forward.	When sitting erect, cough comes.
Suffocative fulness in larynx and chest, less constriction.	Oppression, as if constricted or lungs were too tight, burning hands.

Both have bruised feeling in the chest (15), and both have emotions affecting the heart.

---

(14) As comparable, we note cutting as a characteristic sensation in headache, cough, backache, urination. It is often combined with crampy pain.

(15) The bruised pains of *Nat. Mur.* differ from those of *Apis,* lacking the extreme sensitiveness to touch, so characteristic of the latter.

Larynx, Lungs, Heart

APIS	NATRUM MUR.
Valvular diseases of the heart; febrile excitement, distress, anguish, restlessness, get no relief from change of position. Blowing with diastole.	Valvular disease; chronic forms, with weak, faint feeling, must lie down; fluttering heart (16), worse lying on left side; cold feeling about heart from mental exertion; worse from least motion.
Pulse accelerated, full, or thread-like; if intermittent, it is equal in volume.	Pulse at one time rapid and weak, at another full and slow; feel pulse all over least motion, irregular, intermittent, trembling (16).

Back, Limbs

APIS	NATRUM MUR.
Flashes of heat over the back, as though sweat would break out, with pain in the left ileo-sacral articulation.	Throbbing in the small of the back; whole spine is over-sensitive to touch or pressure.
Spasmodic, rapid, painful respiration, with congestion of head and spine.	Sensation of weight in back and shoulders, with dyspnœa. Spinal irritation.
Muscles of back feel stiff or weary; weak, must lie down.	Paralytic weakness in the lumbar region.
Stiffness and swelling of the limbs (œdema).	Stiffness, rigidity of a paralytic nature.
Rheumatism, inflammatory; worse in damp, cold weather; burning, stinging pains.	Rheumatism, with less inflammation, but marked contraction of muscles, and especially of hamstrings.
Tingling, with fiery burning at the points of the fingers.	Tingling over all limbs; worse in tips of fingers.
Panaritium, burning, stinging.	Panaritium starts from a hang-nail.
Hands blue, cold.	Hands burn or are sweaty.

Both have suppressed foot-sweat.

Sleep

Both have sleeplessness from nervous restlessness, yet with *desire* to sleep; awaken agitated; awaken unrefreshed. The restlessness of *Nat. Mur.* is most marked in the legs.

---

(16) As comparable, mark under *Nat. Mur.* trembling pulse, fluttering heart, trembling hands when writing, limbs tremble when walking, trembles after siesta, fluttering in ear, tremor of lids, letters run together.

Sleep

APIS	NATRUM MUR.
Awakens with a shrill shriek ; hydrocephalic (17).	Awakens as from fright, with throbbing all over ; *headache*.

Dreams. frightful, with disturbed respiration. occur in both. Only *Nat. Mur.* has the true *incubus* and the symptom : "Dreams of robbers; on awaking, will have house searched."

Fever

APIS	NATRUM MUR.
Chill, afternoon (3—4 P M.) ; begins in the chest.	Chill, morning (10 A. M.) (18) ; begins in *back*, hands, feet, right side.
During chill, thirst; burning and oppression of the chest, as though he would smother.	During chill, persistent vomiting, debility, pale face (C. Pearson).
Heat, with inclination to uncover.	Heat, with aversion to uncover.
During heat, delirium and muttering, unconsciousness ; diarrhœa ; short breath ; drowsy or sleepless.	During heat, violent headache, stitches in the head ; unconsciousness, blindness, or blurred sight.
Sweat, scanty or alternate with dry skin. Urticaria.	Sweat copious, relieves all symptoms. Hydroa.
During apyrexia, pain under short ribs ; sore limbs and joints; large abdomen; swollen feet, scanty urine.	During apyrexia, yellow face, stomach disordered ; swollen liver, stomach ; drawing in limbs.
Typhus, enteric ; exanthematic ; cerebral. Delirium, slides down in bed. Generally thirstless ; if drink, takes only small quantities at a time ; unconsciousness.	Typhus versatilis; gastric symptoms; on getting up sink down to the floor. Unquenchable thirst, dry tongue ; water tastes spoiled ; nausea from drinking ; unconsciousness.

Skin, Bones, Etc.

Both develop an urticaria, worse from violent exercise ; with red spots on abdomen; stinging pains; lichen; prurigo; also eruptions with thin, scaly scabs. Impetiginus and other pustular eruptions belong more to *Nat. Mur.*, as do also raw, excoriated eruptions.

---

(17) The adjective, *Hydrocephalic,* is used, because the symptom has occurred in children who had no real dropsy of brain, but were predisposed to that disease.

(18) *Nat. Mur.* has also an evening chill, internal, as from want of animal heat. This often occurs in Chlorosis and kindred diseases.

APIS	**NATRUM MUR.**
Skin, Bones, Etc.	
Boils large; before suppuration (19).	Boils small, especially blood-boils; corners of mouth.
Punctured wounds become erysipelatous.	Wounds become painful, suppurate; pain in old scars.
Arthritic nodosities.	Arthritic contractions.
Muscles, as if jammed, bruised.	Muscles, as if torn from the bones.
Ulcers gangrenous.	Ulcers fistulous, phagedenic.

Erysipelas appears in both, but predominantly in *Apis*.

Generalities

APIS	NATRUM MUR.
Complaints of children, women (widows).	Complaints of old people.
Paralysis from pressure (in ovarian dropsy); from blood changes (diphtheria); hemiplegia (from serous effusion in brain); not so predominant as with *Nat. Mur.*	Paralysis from intermittents; from sexual excesses or other nervous exhaustion; from diphtheria; from anger or emotions; even from pains.
Spasms from cerebral effusion; starting from sexual organs (in females). Hysteria, Mania of women.	Spasms, chronic or hysterical. Come at full moon. Mania, especially when accompanied by paralytic debility (20).
Spasms with unconsciousness.	Spasms with full consciousness.
Left side predominantly affected.	*Right* side predominantly affected.
Remission during day.	Remission afternoon.
Sensitive to touch; over-sensitive to pain.	Sensitive to touch, but numbness predominates.
Worse in heat of sun.	Worse in sultry weather (3).
Worse lying down; better rising from bed.	Better lying down; worse rising from bed.
Worse drinking cold water.	Better drinking cold water.
Better from wine.	Worse from spirituous liquors.
Better uncovering; from wet applications.	Better from wrapping up.

(19) According to Virchow, the degeneration necessary for suppuration must occur in deep parts. Now, as **Apis** seldom influences parenchymatous parts, it seldom produces suppuration. (See Gross, *Apis-Lach.*).

(20) *Nat. Mur.* produces alternate heaviness and lightness of the limbs; parts of the body move involuntarily, or move further than intended: in walking, one side seems to advance further than other. These point to disordered nervous centres; the latter, especially, to the cerebellum.

APIS	Generalities	NATRUM MUR.

Apis and *Nat. Mur.* are complementary. First noticed by Dr. Hering, this has been confirmed by Drs. Raue, Lippe and many others. Chronic symptoms resulting from bee-stings, will be cured by *Nat. Mur.*, in a very high potency. Cases relieved by *Apis,* will be completely cured by *Nat. Mur.* when the symptoms concur.

APIS — Mind — RHUS TOX.

APIS	RHUS TOX.
Irritable, irascible, morose, fickle, foolish gaiety.	Usually sad, despairing, easily vexed but undemonstrative.
Anxiety felt in head, fears apoplexy.	Anxiety præcordial, fears being poisoned.
Consequences of fright, rage, vexation, jealousy, hearing *bad news.*	Consequenes of vexation with *fear,* all ailments worse from least annoyance.
Dread of death, or sensation, as if he should not breathe again.	Dread of death with sighing, vertigo; desires death in Melancholia.
Memory weak, with or after prosopalgia.	Slow, difficult thought, memory weak from damp weather, congestion, injuries.
Suppressed eruptions followed by hydrocephalic congestion.	Suppressed eruptions followed by melancholy, anxiety, paralysis.

Both depress the sensorium with absent-mindedness, apathy, stupor, low muttering delirium, confusion of mind, dulness of head.

APIS	RHUS TOX.
Brain feels tired; imbecility; always busy yet does nothing; awkward, drops things.	Brain shakes when jarred, almost unconscious if even turn head; disinclined to work or think.
Vertigo when closing eyes, nausea.	Vertigo after a meal, chilliness.
Delirium, muttering, indistinct loquacity, stupor, senseless apathy or pleasant, happy expression.	Delirium mild, murmuring or chats to himself or seemingly roams far and wide; stupor, as if intoxicated.

Head

APIS	RHUS TOX.
Pressing in forehead; worse, from warmth.	Pressing outward, temples and sides, better, warmth (1).

---

(1) Except the sensitive scalp, which in *Rhus* is worse from becoming warm in bed.

APIS	RHUS TOX.
Burning, stinging in head or scalp; better, cold washing.	Burning, tingling (2) or stinging in head, face, jaws; worse, walking.
Hydrocephalus; for horses that kick and try to run off.	Hydrocephalus; horses jerk the head.

Eyes

APIS	RHUS TOX.
Burning, stinging in eyes; stiffness.	Burning, cutting, pressures; heavy lids.
Lids swollen, œdematous; turned inside out; lashes fall out; edges granulated.	Lids swollen, œdematous; lids show tylosis, hence eye-lashes turn in.
Conjunctiva swollen, mostly around cornea, chemosis.	Conjunctiva dark red, protrudes between the lids like a pad.

Both have cured ophthalmias from scrofula, rheumatism, gout; blepharitis, profuse lachrymation; erysipelas; herpes corneæ.

APIS	RHUS TOX.
Mucous states, agglutination.	Purulent discharges; agglutination.
Eyes tender to even a compress.	Eyes feel sore when turned.
Twitching of eye-ball.	Twitching; spasm of lids.
Staphyloma.	Traumatic suppuration; iritis.
Herpes corneæ, conjunctiva injected, forming a band like pterygium; burning, stinging, photophobia; after suppressed itch (which it restores).	Herpes corneæ, conjunctiva congested, forming a network; burning, smarting; swollen axillary glands, parotids; vesicles form on cornea.
Blindness with staggering; opaque cornea.	Blindness with rheumatism; nervous headaches.

Nose

APIS	RHUS TOX.
Discharge from nose, white, thick, or acrid, bloody, fetid mucus. Eruptions on nose and lip, burning, stinging; nostrils red, burn; lip swollen, prickling.	Discharge green, offensive, pus, or thick, yellow mucus, blood. Eruptions under nose; fever-blisters, crusts; nostrils sore to touch; lip cracked, crusty, burning, tingling.

Face

APIS	RHUS TOX.
Erysipelas begins about temples or eyes; forms reddish bags under eyes; vesicles, if any, small; best before pustulation.	Erysipelas begins on nose or on ear, spreading across face to other; large blisters, confluent; pustules may form.

---

(2) This tingling is important as expressing the paralytic tendency of *Rhus*, a property not prominent in *Apis*, except from intense blood-poison, (after typhus, diphtheria, &c.) or as hemiplegia, and hence intracranial in origin.

APIS	RHUS TOX.

Face

Both appear in erysip. with œdema, gangrene; erysipelatous eruptions; phlegmon. erysip. Only *Rhus* has the fugax. *Apis* is best-adapted to metastasis to brain. *Rhus* exhibits the drowsy, languid state, so common in erysip. of scalp when the brain sympathizes.

APIS	RHUS TOX.
Lip (upper) swollen; dry; peels.	Lips dry, parched, covered with brown scurf.

Mouth

APIS	RHUS TOX.
Tongue dry, cracked, sore, covered with blisters or ulcers, rosy red, swollen, white all over.	Tongue dry, cracked tip, covered with brown mucus, feels hard as a board, red triangular tip, red, smooth, white one side.
Gums, inflamed, swollen, throb, numb.	Gums stand off from the teeth.
Toothache, congestive, sore, bruised feeling, better from cold.	Toothache, periosteal, rheumatic, pains tearing, tingling, better warmth (3).
Mouth, inflamed, dry, but little thirst.	Mouth dry, thirst unquenchable (4).
Saliva, tough, frothy.	Saliva bloody, runs out while asleep.

Throat

Both have stinging in throat when throat is dry, contraction of throat, tough mucus.

APIS	RHUS TOX.
Sore, as if scalded; tonsils inflamed; mucous coat.	Sore, as if strained; deep tissues involved (fibrous, muscular).
Swallowing difficult from swollen tongue; from diminished power; worse from drinks or food.	Swallowing difficult from strained feeling; from paralyzed state of epiglottis; food enters larynx; worse from saliva or food.
Fetid breath (with headache).	Putrid taste after eating; from teeth.

Stomach, Etc.

APIS	RHUS TOX.
Nausea felt in throat.	Less in throat, more in chest.
Violent eructations.	Water-brash.
After eating, burning in stomach.	After eating, pressure like a stone; colic.

(3) The darting, cutting, when the nerve is affected, is better from cold touch in *Rhus*.

(4) Stomatitis is not characteristic of *Rhus Tox.*, but is of *Apis*. *Rhus Ven.* is here very similar to *Apis* but only the latter has great difficulty (not pain) in swallowing.

APIS	RHUS TOX.
Stomach, Etc.	
Vascular irritation or inflammation of mucous coat of stomach ; sensitiveness to least touch.	Tingling in stomach ; bad effects of cold drinks ; ulcerative pains ; throbbing in stomach (5).
Abdomen, Etc.	
Abdomen sore to least touch, even in sneezing; bruised feeling in bowels.	Liver sore to touch ; abdomen sore when stretched.
Abdomen bloated, sore.	Abdomen distended, fetid flatus.
Peritonitis, tendency to serous effusion ; death-like appearance ; cough and vomiting ; diarrhœa ; stabbing pains ; burning, stinging ; metritis.	Peritonitis, tendency to typhoid state ; pale face ; despairing look ; oozing ulcers on œdematous legs ; pressing, clawing pains ; metritis.
Dysentery, tenesmus, yet little pain ; bloody stools.	Dysentery, tenesmus; tearing in thighs ; stools also jelly-like.
Diarrhœa, painless, yellow ; greenish, involuntary (7) ; thirstless, or drink little and often, worse in a warm room, morning, motion.	Diarrhœa usually thin, painful ; frothy, slimy stools, involuntary at night; thirst unquenchable ; worse, in cold, damp ; better, from warmth; worse, at night ; better, on motion.
Chol. Infantum, tendency to hydrocephaloid.	Chol. Infantum, tendency to a typhoid state.
Constipation, urine scanty.	Constipation alternate with diarrhœa (6).
Hæmorrhoids cause fidgets, irritability.	Hæmorrhoids ; restless, better on moving.
Kidneys, Urine	
Kidneys sore, bruised ; stiff back stooping ; œdema general ; after scarlatina ; sleepy yet cannot sleep.	Kidneys, tearing pains ; œdema general ; after scarlatina ; restless, tossing, after midnight.
Urine, albuminous, scanty, turbid, red, like coffee-grounds ; strong smell, involuntary. Urine pale, straw color.	Urine albuminous, dark, frequent ; less, though drink more ; involuntary at night. Urine white, flocculent.

(5) *Rhus* is the principal remedy in œsophagitis, even if caused by a foreign substance. It involves the muscular and fibrous parts. This *Apis* could never do. *Apis* most resembles gastritis, cancer of the stomach, &c. *Rhus*, dyspepsia, gastrosis from rheumatism, getting wet, mechanical injuries, &c.

(6) Hence *Rhus* is better adapted to tabes-mesenterica.

(7) In typhus, *Apis* has involuntary, *painful* stool ; *Rhus* involuntary at night.

APIS	RHUS TOX.
Kidneys, Urine	
Dysuria, pressure on sphincter; scalding pains, bloody.	Dysuria, turbid, drops of blood.
Scrotum œdematous.	Testes dark red; hydrocele, left half of scrotum.
Female Genital Organs	
Metritis; tendency to dropsy; lower limbs numb from pressure; stabbing pains in head.	Typhoid symptoms; lower limbs powerless from paralytic tendency; bursting pains in head (Comp. Peritonitis).
Coitus causes stinging in ovaries.	Coitus hindered by soreness in vagina.
Catamenia too soon.	Too soon, profuse, protracted.
Before and during menstruation eruption, worse on abdomen; bearing-down mostly in ovarian regions.	Bearing-down mostly in uterus; worse, standing, or from straining; red rash on chest.
Discharge profuse, with heaviness in abdomen; faintness; yawning; nervous restlessness.	Discharge profuse, more coagula than *Apis;* restlessness more at night.
Amenorrhœa, congestion to head.	Amenorrhœa from getting wet.
Dysmenorrhœa, congestive type.	Dysmenorrhœa, membranous type.
Abortion from uterine congestion; second to fourth month.	Abortion from muscular exertion or strain.
Ovaries diseased with numbness, worse right side; with tendency to dropsy; worse, on motion.	Ovaries less affected than uterus; right leg numb; after a strain; better, moving about.
Milk diminished.	Milk increased or suppressed, with burning all over body.
Tightness in ovarian region when raising the arms.	Drawing, strained feeling when raising arms; like a band in hypochondria.
Milk leg, high fever; restless, yet not relieved by change of posture.	Milk leg, burning all over; restless, relieved momentarily by change.

Larynx, Chest

Both have hoarseness, rough voice; erysipelatous or catarrhal inflammation.

APIS	RHUS TOX.
Larynx, Chest	
Larynx, as if scalded; worse warm room; takes cold in wet, cold weather; skin dry or foot-sweat checked.	Larynx, as if sore, raw; stuffed up (influenza), worse in cold, even exposing hands; takes cold in wet, especially when warm, sweating.
Cough incessant all night, ceases when least phlegm is loosened; soreness, upper left chest; painful concussion of head; *expectoration* difficult, clear, tough, must be swallowed; mostly evenings.	Cough at sunset, lasts until midnight, periodically returning each evening; tearing loose in chest; concussion of head and chest; *expectoration* difficult, bloody or purulent; mostly mornings.
Adapted to *clergyman's sore-throat,* after cauterization (*Nat. Mur.*).	Adapted to rheumatic catarrhs or to *influenza* (*Bryon.*).
Does not see how he can get another breath; short oppressed breathing with catarrh; breathing possible only when sitting erect; respiration hurried, abdominal; worse in warm room.	Apprehensive that unless relieved, he could breathe but a short time; short breath with catarrh; breathes better when moving; always worse after a meal and exertion; respiration quick, thoracic; better in warm.
Heart, Pulse	
Heart diseases with hydropericardium; blowing with diastole.	Chronic forms after rheumatism, with numbness left arm; with relaxation of heart muscle.
Pulse full, accelerated; or, if intermittent, never irregular.	Pulse weak, soft, irregular; trembling about heart (8).
Back, Limbs	
Bruised, stiff feeling in back (region of kidneys); worse on pressure, stooping, moving.	Bruised pain; better from walking (not from exertion) and lying on hard couch; hence, pressure.
Flashes of heat, as though sweat would break out over back.	Creeping in back, or sensation of cold water poured over it.
Rheumatism; burning, stinging, pains; great soreness to touch; joints swollen, tense, pale or	Rheumatism, more of the fibrous parts with tearing, tensive, burning pains; pains, as if

(8) *Rhus* can seldom be of use in sthenic inflammations with high fever, *full* pulse, &c. *Apis* may. *Rhus* becomes of use when typhoid or asthenic symptoms appear, or when the patient was previously weakened by over-exertion.

APIS	RHUS TOX.
Back, Limbs	
erysipelatous. Has tingling, only when swelling compresses nerves. Pains are worse from motion (except dull pains in bones).	sprained; stitches in joints when touched; red streaks. Has tingling from paralytic tendencies. Pains better from motion, or compel motion.
Cold applications relieve pains.	Warm, dry, applications relieve.
Sleep	
Sleepless, drowsy, yet cannot sleep, because fidgety; nervous restlessness.	Sleepless, with restlessness caused by bodily pains, heat, &c., must move about.
Dreamy sleep; awakens with a start, agitated; breathing oppressed.	Dreams of wearisome journeys; starts when going to sleep, as if he dropped something; short breathing.
Skin, Etc.	
Eruptions dry; scabby, laminæ thin, straw-colored or brown. Best adapted to itch (after abuse of *Sulph.*); lichen, especially when conical; prurigo.	Eruptions moist; scabs moist, thick. Best adapted to eruptions which pustulate; impetigo, &c.; lichen if eczematous, cracked.
Urticaria, stinging, burning; croupy cough; uterine catarrh. Eruptions with painless, yellow stools.	Urticaria, burning, stinging, tingling; fever; rheumatic. Eruptions with dysenteric stools.
Carbuncle; erysipelatous far around—or bluish.	Carbuncle, red streaks or black.
Run-arounds; pains burning, stinging; sensitive to touch; after abuse of *Sulph.*, bright—red or pale.	Run-arounds and whitlows (tendons involved); red streaks up arm (lymphatic vessels); shooting pains; after or before *Bry.*, dark-red.
Wounds punctured, erysipelas.	Wounds with vesicular erysipelas.
Sphacelus, bluish.	Gangrene of exanthema, black.
Suppuration rare; causes inflammations, which tend toward serous effusion or degeneration into ulcers, gangrene, &c.	Suppuration common; sometimes laudable; always copious; often low graded; ichor, bloody serum, &c.
Fever, Etc.	
Chill begins in front of chest.	Chill begins in hands or right side.
During chill: Oppression and burning in chest as though would smother.	During chill: Cough: tearing in hips, limbs, back; restless,

APIS	RHUS TOX.
Fever, Etc.	
Chill 3 to 4 P. M.; least motion, chills with heat of face and hands. Worse near warm stove (chill).	Chill evening, lasts all night; motion makes cold with hot face, cold hands. Better, warmth.
Heat in chest, pit of stomach, abdomen, hands. Better uncovering.	Heat forepart of body, cold head, back and hands. Worse uncovering.
Sweat alternate with dry skin; sweat scanty.	Sweat profuse, often with flushes of heat.
Apyrexia: Pain under short ribs; soreness, limbs and joints; swollen abdomen; dropsy; scanty urine.	Apyrexia: Pain in joints, chest; dropsy; burning eyes; diarrhœa; urine scanty, frequent; cold hands.
Drowsy during fever.	Drowsy before paroxysm.
Swollen abdomen (ascites).	Pit of stomach swollen; palpitation.

Both have debility, dropsy, soreness of joints; scanty urine during apyrexia.

APIS	RHUS TOX.
Scarlatina: Skin very red, sensitive; better, cold applications; thirstless; scanty urine; eruption thick, with cerebral excitement, boring head in pillow, &c., sopor. Eruption bright red, confluent. Tonsils swollen; erysipelatous ulcers in throat.	Scarlatina: Skin peels. better from scratching, worse from cold or wet; great thirst; ischuria; eruption vesicular, or like millet seeds; restlessness. Eruption dark red with nose-bleed at night, sopor, &c. Parotids suppurating (left to right), discharging bloody ichor.

(Compare also Typhus. Brain. &c.)

APIS	RHUS TOX.
Variola: Eruption stings, burns, red.	Variola: Eruption sinks, looks livid.
Typhus: Best adapted to exanthematic, *enteric*, cerebral forms, less to pneumo-typhus.	Typhus: Best adapted to exanthematic, enteric, cerebral, mucous, pectoral, putrid forms. Also cursory stages.
Delirium low, muttering, talks indistinctly; thinks he is dead; stupor with senseless apathy or a happy expression; congestion to head with moderate delirium; brain excited; fidgety.	Delirium mild, talks incoherently, disconnectedly or answers short, angrily; stupor, as if intoxicated, with brown mucus in mouth and on lips; congestion with red face, nose-bleed; heat in head; dulness of thought.

APIS	Fever, Etc. RHUS TOX.
Tongue cracked, sore, ulcerated, covered with vesicles ; white all over ; inability to put it out or talk.	Tongue cracked ; triangular tip of red, covered with brown mucus ; feels hard ; white on one side.
Abdomen bloated, sore to least touch ; eruption, white miliaria ; diarrhœa bloody, painful, involuntary, or painless, yellow ; no stool for a long time ; stage of ulceration of Peyer's glands with purulent, involuntary stool ; bloated abdomen, urine smelling strong like horse's, involuntary.	Abdomen sore ; sensitive over the liver, rash red ; diarrhœa slimy, involuntary at night ; sudden, thin, yellow, frothy, odorless ; stage of abdom. inflammation and ulceration with colic, tearing in limbs, involuntary stool ; papescent stool, which affords relief (stage of inflammation), urine and stool involuntary at night.
Cough from tenacious mucus in throat.	Cough dry, or sputa covered with blood ; bloody.
Pulse intermits, weak, feeble. Over-estimates strength, tries to get up and fails. Wants to lie quietly, but is nervous, restless, no better from change of position. Slides down in bed. Sweat partial, clammy ; mostly burning skin; thirstless or drinks little and often ; removes the tenacious mucus from throat (in malarial typhus).	Pulse irregular, weak, small, trembling. Worse from any over-exertion ; wants to lie (in beginning). Pains intolerable in rest, better changing position. Great debility of mind and body, as if paralyzed ; settles down in bed ; open mouth. Head hottest ; sweat all over except face; thirst unquenchable ; brown coated tongue, lips, mouth.

Generalities

Burning, stinging pains.	Burning, stinging, tingling.
Cutting internal parts, fulness internal.	Cutting external, internally, as if something were torn loose.
Symptoms go from left to right.	Symptoms go from right to left.

Apis has *aggravation,* and *Rhus amelioration,* from warmth, wrapping up, motion.

Rhus has *aggravation,* and *Apis amelioration* from cold, uncovering, washing in cold water, spirituous liquors, during rest, when assuming an erect position.

Worse in heat of sun.	Worse in snowy air.

BADIAGA & BELLADONNA

BADIAGA	BELLADONNA
Mind almost always is clear, active.	Not inclined to talk or *fast* talking; nervous anxiety.
Headache unchanged by posture.	Headache worse lying; better bending head backward.
Pains in the eye-balls.	Photophobia.
Sounds as of distant artillery.	Humming and roaring in the ears.
Fluent coryza.	Bleeding from the nose.
Face ashy or lead colored; blue under the eyes.	Face red or pale or alternating.
Mouth dry with thirst.	Mouth dry, without thirst.
Cough spasmodic with forcible expectoration flying out of the mouth; better in the warm room; excited by a tickling as from sugar dissolving in the larynx; worse afternoon and evening.	Cough spasmodic, dry, worse at night and on the slightest motion; excited by tickling in the throat, as if from down or as if from constriction of the larynx (1); worse evening and just after 12 P. M.
Palpitation of the heart *from the least elating thought or emotion* (2).	Palpitation of the heart after sleeping, after 12 P. M. with loud pulsations in the temporal arteries.
Worse while swallowing solids, on moving the eyes, in the afternoon.	*Worse* while swallowing liquids, looking at bright things, afternoon and after 12 P. M.

(1) *Bellad.* is one of the few medicines having relief from sweets; sugar lessens the burning in the œsophagus. *Spongia* has the sore-throat worse from sweets, and here *Badiaga* gives us the sensation of melting sugar, a by no means uncommon symptom. I agree with Dr. Bell, who asserts that *Bellad.* is more frequently indicated in spasmodic croup than the famous trio *Acon., Spong., Hepar.* The child awakens about 11 P. M., face red, eyes suffused, expression anxious, there is *constriction* of the *glottis, crying with the cough which frequently ends with a half-suppressed sneeze.* Soon the the little patient drops off to sleep, to shortly awaken with the same symptoms. If with these symptoms the cough is *brassy*, simulating membranous croup, *Kali Brom.* But we just as often have a croup with swelling of the mucous membrane, when neither Bœnninghausen's three, nor *Bellad., Kali Brom.,* will do much good. The spasmodic form generally follows dry, cold (north-west) winds; the others occur in damp, wet weather. The choice then falls on such medicines as *Iod.* (black eyes, moist but deep cough, Wheezing); *Brom.* (blue eyes, suddenly awaken, hoarsely cry for water, which relieves); *Ipecac.* (in changes in winter from north-west to warm south winds, rattling cough, &c.; child fat; *Arsenic* (hives suppressed by damp, croup), &c.

(2) No medicine acts so well here as *Badiaga.* Compare *Coff., Acon., Phos.*

BADIAGA	**SPONGIA**
Headache severe yet mind unaffected; better in the morning and worse after breakfast.	Headache with moroseness; worse in the morning and better after breakfast.
Headache with inflamed eyes.	Headache and the eyes feel cold.
Noise like distant artillery.	Hardness of hearing.
Coryza fluent; or sneezing; worse left side.	Coryza dry, hoarseness.
Sore throat, worse from swallowing solids.	Sore throat, better from swallowing.
Diminished appetite.	Ravenous appetite.
Urine high colored and reddish.	Urine frothy or saffron-colored, yellow, white red.
Cough spasmodic, caused by tickling in the larynx as from melting sugar; expectoration of a viscid mucus flying out of the mouth, afternoons; better in a warm room.	Cough deep, hollow, caused by feeling of a plug in the larynx; expectoration tough, yellow, hardened, mucus generally swallowed, mornings; better after eating.
Palpitation of the heart, sitting or lying, *from any elating thought.*	Start up with palpitation, *anguish, bellows murmur with each beat.*
Glands enlarged, hard, inflamed or suppurating. Inguinal glands; left side.	Glands enlarged, but generally little pain or inflammation. Testes and cord enlarged.
Indicated in fat children.	Indicated in children and women.
Aggravation 1 to 8 P.M.	Aggravation afternoon and before 12 P.M.
Worse lying on unpainful side.	Better lying on unpainful side.
Position does not affect the head or chest symptoms.	Better lying flat, (head); better sitting (chest).
Worse lying long in one position.	Better lying in the horizontal position, head low.
Worse moving the eyes.	Worse looking intently.
Worse stormy weather.	Better in stormy weather (1).

(1) *Spong.* requires that the patient shall feel better in wet weather and worse in dry, cold weather.

BAPTISIA &	**ARNICA***
Anxious, certain of death.	Indifference.
Falls asleep in the midst of his answer.	*Falls asleep, forgetting the words for his answer.*
Lies with head thrown back, lower jaw dropped; slides down in bed.	Lies quiet, *no complaint*; *says he is well*; lower lip trembles.
Vertigo, worse stooping.	Vertigo raising the head.
Gasping; breathing, as if he could not draw a long breath.	Loud, blowing inspiration and expiration in sleep.
Can swallow only liquids; spits out the water taken.	Pharynx seems "lame"; a gurgling noise when swallowing.
Stool involuntary, fetid.	*Stool and urine involuntary.*
Pulse *full* and slow; variable.	Pulse frequent, sunken.
Nervous symptoms predominant.	Stupefaction from the very beginning.

BAPTISIA &	**MURIATIC ACID**
Goes to sleep while answering.	*Forgets what he has said.*
Delirium; cannot sleep, because *she must toss about to get the pieces of her head together.*	Delirium; would sleep, but cannot; vivid hallucinations of changing images from past to present.
Soreness, as if in the frontal brain; wild feeling.	*Brain feels sore, as if it was torn or had been beaten.*
Senses generally blunt; *besotted, heavy expression.*	Senses generally too acute; *distant talking gives headache.*
Dull hearing during and after typhus.	Dull hearing, with dryness of ears, or dark wax.
Cheeks, *dark red,* yellow ground. *Aphthæ putrid, dark, ulcerating*; thick, viscid saliva.	Circumscribed *glowing red cheeks. Aphthæ putrid, small, bluish, deep.*
Tongue dry, *brown down the centre;* feels numb or scalded.	*Tongue small, bluish or rattling like leather; heavy, as if paralyzed.*
Goneness; sinking at the stomach.	Emptiness all over the adomen.

* *Arnica* has but little resemblance in the beginning of typhus; but when stupor and petechiæ appear, we find in common, such symptoms as: Must move the bed feels so hard; brown tongue; putrid breath; goes to sleep while answering; stupid, heavy look, etc.

BAPTISIA	MURIATIC ACID
Stool involuntary, *putrid ;* occasional diarrhœa or costive (beginning).	Involuntary *stool while urinating;* putrid; during crisis, papecent stool relieve.
Urine *offensive, alkaline.*	Urine acid ; *difficult to expel.*
Heart-beats seem to fill the chest.	Heart-beats seem to be felt, in the face.
Pulse full and slow ; variable ; thread-like.	Pulse irritated, but without energy ; *omits every third beat.*
Slides down in bed ; lower jaw dropped ; *putrid breath.*	*Slides down in bed ; lower jaw hanging ; moaning.*
Scarlatina with fetid *dark, ulcers in the throat ;* great prostration; petechiæ ; stupor.	Scarlatina with *blue feet ; dark bluish fauces ; scanty eruption ; sudden red face ; petechiæ ; stupor.*
Stupor resembling that of *Arnica, Opium.*	Stupor and nervous weakness after *Rhus, Bry.* fail.

BAPTISIA	RHUS TOX.
Anxious, certain of death.	Faint, timid, fear of death.
Delirium constant, low ; *thinks her head is scattered over the bed, and that she must toss about to get the pieces together.*	Delirium mild, low ; *thinks that he is roaming over fields, swimming or engaged in some other physical work.*
While answering a question, goes to sleep.	Answers correctly, but in a hasty manner.
Mentally restless, yet too lifeless to move; confused, as if drunk.	Mentally restless ; slow flow of ideas ; *better moving.*
Feels, as if the top of the head would fly off.	Feels, as if a board were bound across the forehead.
Expression besotted; cheeks yellow, with a deep central flush.	*Expression listless ;* or anxious appearance ; cheeks dark red.
Teeth covered with sordes ; mouth full of *ulcers, fetid* breath, aphthæ.	Teeth and mouth covered with *thick, hard, brown mucus ; vesicles.*
Jaws rigid ; pain.	Jaws-crack ; feel stiff.
Tongue white, dry yellow centre (early stages of typhus).	Tongue white on one side, dry (early stages of typhus).
Tongue dry, dark red, shining, cracked, *ulcerated ;* or, dry,	Tongue dry, hard as a board, *hardened, dirty phlegm ;* or,

BAPTISIA &	**RHUS TOX**
with a *brown streak down the centre,* edges clean, red.	*red, triangular tip,* cracked, shows imprints of teeth.
Saliva viscid, thick.	Saliva bloody, *runs out in sleep.*
Dry mouth, great thirst ; spits out the liquid put into his mouth.	Dry mouth, unquenchable thirst; repugnance to either food or drink.
Uvula long; mucus in the throat, cannot raise or swallow it ; *can only swallow liquids.* Putrid, *painless,* dark ulcers (1).	Throat sore, as if strained; swallowing difficult from paralyzed epiglottis; œsophagitis, cannot swallow solid food.
Stool yellow, involuntary *horribly fetid;* sour belchings.	Stool yellow, slimy, involuntary at night, *almost no* fetor ; empty belchings.
Dysentery, great tenesmus with *discharge of pure blood, no mucus.*	Dysentery, tenesmus, discharge of *transparent lumps of mucus.*
Urine alkaline, *offensive,* dark red.	Urine albuminous ; *involuntary at night.*
Cannot draw a full breath, gasping ; tightness across the chest.	Difficult breathing referred to the lower chest and pit of stomach.
Heart throbs audibly ; seems to fill the chest.	Heart beats feebly ; *trembling* about the heart.
Pulse *full,* whether hard, slow or quick ; variable, thread-like.	Pulse small, *weak* and quick, weak and small, thread-like.
Cannot lie long anywhere ; *yet motion is painful.*	Cannot remain quiet ; *motion of the limbs improves* (2).
Must change position, *the bed feels so hard.*	Must change to relieve *the pains in the limbs.*
Feels, as if *sinking away ;* lies with the head thrown back ; jaw dropped ; sliding down in bed, putrid breath.	Feels, as if paralysis were coming on; mouth open; lies, as if intoxicated ; involuntary stool and urine (3).

(1) The painlessness may decide for *Baptisia* not only in typhus, but in scarlatina, putrid sorethroat, &c., when the suspicious odor and general weakness, offer a dangerous reason for the absence of pain. The ability to swallow only liquids distinguishes it from *Lach., Apis, Canth. Rhus Tox.;* has not so marked a tendency towards putrid ulcers. In œsophageal spasm, both can only swallow liquids ; but with *Baptisia* solids simply cause gagging ; with *Rhus vomiting.*

(2) *Rhus,* in the beginning of typhus during profound weakness, has an exceptional symptom : *Wants to lie still in one spot.*

(3) It would be premature to characterize *Baptisia* while so imperfectly proved. But in general, it shows a heavy, besotted face ; fetid breath, stool and urine ; dyspnœa from weakness ; in the beginning, *nervous restlessness. Rhus* shows a bland expression, pale, waxy skin : hepatization of lower lobes (hence dyspnœa is referred to the stomach and hypochondria) ; in the beginning, *erethism* (hence the nose bleeds, *which relieves*).

Mind, Head

BROMINE	IODINE
At first gloomy, later cheerful, disposed to mental labor.	Irritable, excitable, constantly on the move; feeling of melancholy.
Feels, as if on turning around he must see some one; expects to see things jumping about.	Fears every little thing will result in some trouble; anxiety, shuns even the doctor.
Running water causes giddiness; giddy and nose-bleed.	Less true vertigo; sometimes a half-sided vertigo.
Headache, as of a band around the head; dizziness, which increases the more marked is the band; worse in the sun; headache after milk; headache during and before catamenia.	Headache, as of a band around the head; forgetful, continual feeling, as if he had forgotten something; worse in warm air; headache mostly on the left side with paralytic feeling in the arms.
Sensation deep in the brain with fear of apoplexy.	Brain feels, as if stirred up; fears he will go crazy.

Eyes, Ears, Nose

BROMINE	IODINE
Flashes through the eyes; dilated pupils (see Chest).	Small sparks before the eyes, while sewing.
Lachrymation and inflammation of the right eye; fistula lachrymalis.	Œdematous swelling of the eye-lids; candle-light dim; twitching of the lids.
Coryza with stoppage of the nose and sneezing.	Fluent coryza, hot water drops out; general heat.

Face, Mouth, Throat

BROMINE	IODINE
Face pale. Spider-web feeling over the face when moving the nose.	Face pale or yellow, changing. Twitchings of the facial muscles.
Yellow spot on lip (cancer).	Lips dry, peel off.
Affections of the *lower jaw*; toothache, worse cold water; lower jaw, bone feels, as if being sawed.	Toothache with bleeding of the gums; little blisters on the gums.
Aphthæ with *affection of the eyes.*	Aphthæ in the mouth, but no smell.
Salivation; much frothy mucus in the mouth.	Salivation after abuse of *Murcury.*
Enlarged tonsils; net-like redness of the throat; *raw spots;* spasm of the glottis (see Chest).	*Enlarged tonsils;* elongated uvula; torpid cases when there is no pain or spasm.
When stooping feel, as if the fauces would drop out.	Nostrils feel widened; weakness of the chest.

Stomach, Abdomen

BROMINE	IODINE
Nausea, retching, better from eating.	Vomiting renewed by eating.
Emptiness in the stomach; contractive spasm of the stomach, both relieved after eating.	*Great hunger; must eat; anxious, if do'nt eat; desire to cry during digestion; eating renews the spasm.*
Enlarged spleen.	Sore in region of the liver.
Black fecal diarrhœa; painful blind varices with black stools.	Whey-like diarrhœa in the morning; *piles protrude, burn, worse from heat.*
Milk causes headache.	Milk opens the bowels.

Urine, Genitals

BROMINE	IODINE
Testicles swollen, smooth, hard, painless; worse from riding.	*Swelling and induration of the testicles and prostate; offensive sweat.*
Menses bright red, profuse; *membranous catamenia*; headache.	Menses premature, copious; *great prostration; pains in the mammæ.*
Dull constant pain in the left ovary.	*Dropsy of the ovaries*; leucorrhœa corroding the linen.
Loud escape of air from the vagina. Not yet studied in cancer uteri.	Uterine hæmorrhage at every stool; cancer uteri.
Contractive pains during the menstrual flow; soreness of the abdomen afterwards.	Cutting in the abdomen, bearing-down, sharp pains in the loins and back.
Scirrhus of the mammæ with drawing like a string into the axilla; lancinating pains at night.	*Dwindling of the mammæ; at first they feel heavy, later they lose their fat.*

Tissues

BROMINE	IODINE
Glands indurated, generally painless. Also intense glandular inflammation; the gland suppurates; throbbing and warmth even with thin excoriating discharge. Ovarian inflammation (because inflammation is more common in the young, and *Brom.* is adapted to young pregnant females).	*Glands indurated, painless.* More torpid, sluggish, rather than intense; the so-called cold-swellings, hard, painless; glands tend to soften and dwindle (mammæ, testes); corroding discharges. Ovarian dropsy (hence more adapted to older females).

Tissues

BROMINE	IODINE
Ulcers with greenish hue of the surrounding skin ; smell like carrion (1).	Ulcers ; scrofulous ulcers with spongy edges.
Emaciation less marked ; debility noticed especially after breakfast.	*Emaciation and yet hunger* ; debility, *chest weak* ; extensors weak in the morning.

Generalities

BROMINE	IODINE
Worse from evening until midnight.	*Worse* after midnight and in the afternoon.
Worse in cold weather, uncovering, inspiration.	*Better* in cold weather, uncovering, inspiration.
Better rapid motion, riding on horseback, expiration.	*Worse* from walking rapidly, and on expiration.

BRYONIA — Mind — ANTIM. CRUD.

BRYONIA	ANTIM. CRUD.
Irascible ; easily angered ; wants to quarrel.	Disposed to be sad; impressible; weeping mood.
Concerned about pecuniary or household affairs ; *dreams of the affairs of the day.*	Sentimental, woeful mood; concerned about the present or future; *ecstatic* love.
Dread of death ; timid.	Desire to shoot oneself.
Children cross, irritable ; want to be kept still.	Children will neither be touched nor looked at.
Intellect weak ; so forgetful, he drops what he holds.	Intellect weak ; threatened dementia, with complete apathy.
Vertigo, as if rocked ; vertigo when rising from bed, with nausea and fainting.	Vertigo when going up stairs ; vertigo with nausea, nosebleed and intense prostration.

Head

The forehead is the common seat of headaches ; fulness, as if it would burst ; nausea, loathing, white tongue. As exciting causes, both have : Exposure to heat, taking cold, debauchery, rheumatism.

BRYONIA	ANTIM. CRUD.
Headache from washing the sweating face ; from ironing in the sun; in sultry weather (1).	Headache from bathing ; from the sun's rays, a warm room.

---

(1) *Bromine* is an excellent disinfectant and also cures offensive ulcers, threatening gangrene.

(1) *Bryonia* has aggravation from heat, especially from moist, hot, or *foggy* air. Such an atmosphere prevents the evaporation of the sweat ; hence, *Bryon.* is worse from suppressed sweat ; therefore, cold washing, by checking the sweat, aggravates. One element in the headache following ironing, is probably the steam rising from the hot iron when applied to the "sprinkled" clothing.

BRYONIA	ANTIM. CRUD.
Head	
Stitches in the forehead, or one side ; worse from any motion (rheumatic).	Boring, crampy pains in the forehead, temples or vertex ; worse ascending (probably in gout).

In gastric headaches, *Bryon.* gives tongue white in the centre, or yellow ; aggravation after awaking on beginning to move ; *Antim. Cr.* tongue, as if white-washed all over, time less marked.

BRYONIA	ANTIM. CRUD.
Eyes	
Eye-lids inflamed, sore from moving, or the least touch.	Eye-lids inflamed, moisture and gum *only in the canthi.*
Eyes red, conjunctiva puffed, dark-red ; pus. Worse in the sun.	Eyes red, dreads light on awaking ; worse in glare of snow.
Glaucoma (2).	Blindness ; lids partly open.
Ears	
Earache worse *moving* or stooping; of best use when cold has checked an otorrhœa, headache following (after *Bell.*).	Earache with redness, heat and swelling ; hence more like *Puls.;* pains are better from touch (3).
Deafness, rheumatic; but oftener oversensitiveness of hearing.	Deafness caused by suppressed ulcers or eruptions (*Sulph.*).
Nose	
Nose sore to touch, swollen ; nostrils ulcerated, hardened crusts of mucus in the nose.	Nose sensitive *to inhaled air ; nostrils* and *corners of mouth sore, cracked, crusty.*
Nose-bleed morning ; after suppressed menses ; headache.	Nose-bleed evening ; after congestive headache and vertigo
Face, Mouth	
Lips dry, chapped.	Lips sore, crusty in the *corners* (4).
Toothache in hollow teeth, but oftener in sound teeth ; better lying on painful side, from pressure, from *cold water ;* worse at night.	Toothache, pre-eminently in *hollow teeth ;* worse from the least touch, from cold water ; better walking in the open air ; worse at night.
Saliva increased ; f r o t h y, soapy.	Saliva increased, saltish.

(2) The puffed conjunctiva and suppuration of *Bryon.*, correspond to ophthalmia neonatorum. *Bryon.* serves after operations on the eye when burning pains and vomiting follows. It is recommended in glaucoma ; probably useful because of its reabsorptive power. *Antim. Cr.* on the other hand, by reason of its aggravation of eye symptoms after awaking, deserves consideration in ophthalmia scrof., but only when the lids show the gumlike deposit in one or other canthus.

(3) In *Bryon.*, touch generally aggravates, pressure relieves. Similarly we find that an almost unbearable soreness remains after pains cease.

(4) Compare eyes and mouth, and we see the *corners* attacked in both ; canthi inflamed ; commissures of the mouth inflamed.

BRYONIA — Face, Mouth — ANTIM. CRUD.

Dry mouth, though occurring in *Antim. Cr.*, belongs more to *Bryon.*, especially when associated with dry lips and throat, with thirstlessness and constipation.

BRYONIA	ANTIM. CRUD.
Sore throat worse turning the head (5); or touching the throat (3); sticking pains.	Sore throat left side; hawking of mucus in the morning.
Voice rough, hoarse, nasal, after measles, croup.	Deep bass voice, or aphonia.

Appetite, Stomach

BRYONIA	ANTIM. CRUD.
Wine agrees; longs for acids.	*Wine aggravates;* longs for acids (6).
Worse from meat, if it causes flatulence; better from cold things; worse from vegetables.	Worse from fat meat, especially pork; worse from cold things; from butter.
Adventitious appetite (7); wants uneatable things, things that cannot be had, or are not wanted if procurable; tobacco aggravates the toothache.	*Adventitious appetite;* few symptoms of abnormal craving; more commonly a disgust for all food; tobacco causes headache, hiccough.
Drinks seldom, but much at a time.	Drinks a good deal at night, less by day.

Both have loss of appetite, even with empty stomach: the need of food is felt, but no desire. *Bryon.* also has canine hunger, demanding food little and often (*the opposite of the thirst*). *Ant. Cr.* has a false hunger, not relieved by eating.

BRYONIA	ANTIM. CRUD.
Nausea when drinking water; when sitting up (with faintness); after eatings, even when food was relished; with anxiety, from eating too much.	Nausea after drinking wine; after smoking tobacco; repugnance to food; with vertigo; from eating too much.
Vomiting, with tongue white in the middle; dry mouth and no thirst; face bloated; yellowish; anguish; dry stools.	Vomiting continues, nausea ceases; tongue white; delirious; red, hot face; drowsy, (child), hard stools.

---

(5) Worse turning, because there are rheumatic pains in the muscles of the neck, hence it is very characteristic, *Bryon.* being a rheumatic remedy, worse from motion.

(6) Yet sour wine, vinegar, etc., always disagree; *Bryon.* has aggravation from sour-kraut or cabbage howsoever prepared.

(7) *Adventitious* in the sense of *acquired.* It is an unconscionable mistake to insert tobacco among the foods. Wine possessing nutritive properties may be termed a food.

BRYONIA — Stomach — ANTIM. CRUD.

Both have cutting pains in the stomach, soreness to pressure, contractive pains. In *Bryon.*, the soreness is most acute, being worse from a *false step,* touch or coughing. We also find the characteristic pain as from a stone, worse from any motion ; in *Antim. Cr.* the pain is spasmodic and almost drives the patient to suicide (8).

Stool, Etc.

BRYONIA	ANTIM. CRUD.
Constipation, stool too large, hard, as if burned, brown, worse after castor oil.	Constipation, stool (large) hard or watery with solid lumps ; worse in old people (9).
Stool dirty, watery, undigested ; worse in changes from cold to warm ; in the morning when *beginning to move;* from taking cold ; after fruits ; from a cold drink when heated.	Stool watery, undigested; worse if overheated ; at night and *early* morning ; from bathing, especially in cold water ; from cold water or cold food.
Stools loose, brown (children) ; worse from *moving,* even turning in bed ; tongue yellow or white centre, blistered ; vomit solids and drink immediately.	Stools white, dry, irregular in shape (children); tongue white all over, blistered ; after nursing child throws up a little sour milk.
Bilious symptoms predominate. Liver diseases.	Gastric symptoms predominate (10).

Antim. Cr. also cures a flatulent state, when with the sensation of a copious stool, flatus passes, succeeded by solid fæces.

Bryon. has putrid stools, stools smelling like old cheese.

Urine

BRYONIA	ANTIM. CRUD.
Urine dark, red, hot, but no sediment.	Urine dark, deposits a red, sandy sediment.
Affects more the urethra.	Affects more the bladder (11).

(8) This spasm is in keeping with the prevailing action of *Antim. Cr.* ; thus we see why the nausea may cease, while the vomiting (spasmodic) continues (compare vomiting).

(9) *Bryon.* has a nightly involuntary stool in typhus, and with old people.

(10) It may at times be of service to compare the organs affected by these two remedies. The bitter taste and vomit, brown offensive stools, yellow tongue, stitches in the liver, infra-scapular (right) pain, &c., point to the action of *Bryon.* on the liver. In *Antim. Cr* we have bitter taste. bitter vomit, loathing ; but they evidently arise from the stomach, the spasmodic action of which may have caused a reverse motion, throwing the bile into the pylorus. Boenninghausen does not mention the *Antim. Cr.,* as acting at all on the liver. Hence we have : Predominant liver symptoms, *Bryon.* ; predominant gastric symptons, *Antim. Cr.*

(11) *Bryon.* has burning in the urethra when *not* urinating, constriction during urination, passage feels too narrow, stitch pains, feeling, as of a drop

BRYONIA — **Genitals** — **ANTIM. CRUD.**

Both give us tenderness in the ovarian region worse from touch. *In Bryon.* it co-exists with, or follows shooting pains.

Bryonia	Antim. Crud.
Metritis, stitch pains, sometimes there are ulcers, which feel cold (subjectively).	Uterine ulcers when there co-exists a discharge of *acrid water with lumps of pus* (12).
During pregnancy, abdominal pains; burning in the uterus.	During pregnancy, troublesome diarrhœa.
Leucorrhœa; pains in the limbs, mucous discharge.	Leucorrhœa watery, causes smarting down the thighs.
Menses early and profuse, blood dark-red; burning in the uterus; tearing in the limbs (13).	Menses profuse, blood dark; a peculiar pressure in the uterus, as if something would come out.

Larynx, Chest

Bryonia	Antim. Crud.
Cough excited by irritation in the *epigastrium;* worse going into a warm room; in a damp room; becoming cold after being heated; after measles; vomits solid food as soon as he eats.	Cough excited by irritation deep in the *abdomen;* worse going into a warm atmosphere; in the burning sun; from the glare of the snow or fire; after measles, variola, varicella, etc.; vomits only liquids.

Expectoration is nearly the same in both; the mucus in *Bryon.* is difficult; in *Antim. Cr.*, tenacious or *watery.*

The spasmodic coughs are very different. In *Bryon.*, the patient has a dry cough coming in *spasmodic shocks* as though striking the upper part of the windpipe; or, a *suffocating sensation forces him to spring up in bed and cough.* In *Antim. Cr.* the cough begins hard, and comes so rapidly that the spells grow *weaker and weaker, as if the fauces were closing.*

---

remaining after urinating; hence Wahle recommends it in gonorrhœa. *Ant. Cr.* gives burning during urination, but it co-exists with mucous urine, copious at night, backache, "mucous" piles; hence, we find its use in catarrh of the bladder.

(12) See how this compares with the characteristic constipation.

(13) *Bryon.* represents the congestive type; hence. have burning in the uterus, headache, etc.; and if amenorrhœa obtains, nose-bleed, blood spitting, drowsiness, etc. By virtue of its power to form false membranes, we find it numbered among the remedies curing membranous dysmenorrhœa. In *Antim. Cr.*, congestions are rare, and we have symptoms of pressure, etc., expressing a spasmodic tendency which runs through the whole remedy.

BRYONIA	Larynx, Chest — ANTIM. CRUD.
Difficult respiration, the chest scarcely moves; worse from any motion; in foggy weather. Asthma.	Difficult respiration, with hot breath, burning pains; worse from raising the arms (14). Asthma.
Pulse full, hard, quick; seldom intermitting.	Pulse irregular, now quick, now slow.

Back, Limbs

BRYONIA	ANTIM. CRUD.
Rheumatism worse from warmth, motion, change of weather; parts red, shining or pale swelling; metastasis to chest, head, eyes.	Rheumatism worse from warmth and hot sun, working in water; parts swollen, red; metastasis to stomach, bowels, eyes (15).
Prickling, stitches in the soles and heels when walking; they feel swollen, *tense*.	Soles and heels very sensitive when walking, especially on the pavement.

Sleep

Sleepiness in the daytime appears strongly marked in both. In *Ant. Cr.*, it is more in the *forenoon.* A comatose state characterizes both. We see it in *Bryon.* in many inflammatory diseases of chest, abdomen, etc., when the brain, sympathizing, induces a drowsiness, and the patient wishes *to lie perfectly quiet.* We see it in *Antim. Cr.* expressed as drowsiness, with delirium, nausea, red face, the child worse *from cold bathing.*

Bryon. possesses, likewise, sleeplessness from ebullitions or pain; restless tossing, yet much worse from motion. Sleeplessness is less marked in *Antim. Cr.* (16).

Fevers, Etc.

BRYONIA	ANTIM. CRUD.
Intermittents, gastric symptoms; much thirst; low-spirited and impetuous; chill in the evening, with heat of the head,	Intermittents, gastric symptoms; little thirst; melancholy, woeful mood; chill in the day, about noon; shivering in the

(14) *Antim. Cr.* seldom causes ebullitions of blood as does *Bryon.* In the lungs we note venous hyperæmia; hence the hot breath; deep breathing from the sluggish circulation; pulse irregular, now fast, now slow, from the same cause.

(15) *Antim. Cr.* has more symptoms of gout; *Bryon.* more of acute rheumatism. Both have gastric symptoms as concomitants. With *Antim. Cr.* we note white tongue, alternate diarrhœa and constipation, spasms of the stomach, vomiting; gout from rich food. With *Bryon.*, we have constipation, tongue white in the middle, nausea, etc. In deciding between the two, the character of the disease, whether gouty or rheumatic, may decide, although the symptoms are ever paramount.

(16) It must be borne in mind that in the restless, sleepless state, so common in inflammatory fevers, *Bryon.*, when well chosen, will speedily induce a tranquil sleep, to disturb which, by unwarranted repetition, would be to spoil the cure.

BRYONIA	ANTIM. CRUD.
Fevers, Etc.	
and cheeks ; chill right-sided ; heat, dry burning; sweat profuse, grows worse from the least motion.	back, with icy-cold feet, the body being sweaty; heat with sweat, which drying, leaves the skin hot ; sweat periodical (17).
Sweat day or night, oily, sour.	Sweat every other night, inodorous (17); same hour.
Measles, with inflammatory symptoms if the eruption delays.	Measles, with vomiting, if the eruption delays.

Skin

BRYONIA	ANTIM. CRUD.
Induration of cellular tissues (as after boils, abscesses, &c.).	Skin tends to thicken and harden (as in corns, &c.) (18).
Corns with tearing pains in change of weather (rheumatic, as it were).	Corns, *horny,* hard, mostly on the soles of the feet.
Swellings, (abscesses, tumors, &c.). tense, pale or red, shining.	Swellings, hot, smooth, hard or *spongy* (as in fungus artic).
Emaciation.	Obesity (19).
Petechiæ.	Gangrene.
Tends more to dry scaly eruptions (dandruff, &c.) (20).	Tends more to pustular eruptions.
Nettle-rash, worse in change of weather ; pains in the legs.	Nettle-rash ; gastric derangements ; cramps in the legs.
Eruptions (in measles, scarlatina, &c.), suppressed or retarded, cause *dyspnœa,* bronchitis, meningitis, &c.	Eruptions (in measles, &c.), if suppressed, cause *nausea,* vomiting, headache, &c.
Light hair.	Dark hair.
Burning in the veins.	Pulsations in the veins.

(17) Periodicity is marked in *Antim. Cr.* Complaints return after weeks, every other day, etc. In ague, *Antim. Cr.* resembles more *Puls. ; Bryon,* more *Cham.*

(18) Similarly, *Ant. Cr.* develops a polypus (of the bladder) and attacks the nails, making them grow in splits with *horny* spots.

(19) The *Kalis* produce a bloated, flabby state ; *Calc C., Sil., Caust., Baryt.,* &c., present enlarged abdomens ; *Senega, Ipec., Kali Bich.* are adapted to fat children ; but few medicines suit general adiposis better than *Ant. Cr.*

(20) Yet so superficial a comparison should not prevent one from using *Bry.,* if weightier symptoms concur, as in small-pox, &c.

BRYONIA **Skin** **ANTIM. CRUD.**

Both suffer from the sun ; *Antim. Cr.* from its heat or glare ; *Bryon.,* especially when the weather is sultry and hot.

Both are adapted to the diseases of old people.

BRYONIA	ANTIM. CRUD.
Worse bathing, when over-heated ; *better,* warm baths.	*Worse* from cold bathing ; not worse from warmth.

Bryon., has *aggravation,* and *Antim. Cr. amelioration* from cold air, after rising from bed or from a seat, walking in the open air.

Bryon., has *amelioration* and *Antim. Cr. aggravation* from pressure, lying on the painful side, in wet weather.

CALC. CARB. Mind CALC. PHOS.

CALC. CARB.	CALC. PHOS.
Like mental work, but unable to perform it.	Indisposed to mental work.
Self-willed (children).	Fretful (children).
Bad news, vexation with dread or fear, cause return of catamenia ; also heavy feet.	Bad news causes sweat, indigestion. Vexation with vehemence causes *lameness,* loose bowels.
Anxiety more *mental* (horror at twilight, conscience-stricken, dread disease, insanity, etc.).	Anxiety more *physical,* with sweat, bellyache ; desire to change place ; in change of weather.
Fears being alone (must *see* his wife in the room).	Likes to be alone.
Imbecility; silly or sad.	Cretinism ; indifferent ; stupid.
Forgetful; chooses wrong words.	Forgetful; writes the same word twice.
Vertigo worse ascending, walking in open air ; looking upward; vertigo in young people.	Vertigo rising from a seat, with leucorrhœa before catamenia ; in old people ; in the wind.
Heat on vertex, coldness on one (right) side; face pale, puffed.	Heat on vertex running down to feet (from the *Phos.*), coldness occipital, with crawling.

Head

CALC. CARB.	CALC. PHOS.
Headache worse from mental labor ; washing in cold water.	Headache better from mental labor and cold washing.
Sweat mostly on occiput and neck.	Sweat mostly on brows and eyelids.
Eruptions spread from scalp to face; itching.	Eruptions, ulcers on vertex, with cold crawling.

CALC. CARB.	CALC. PHOS.
Head	
Hydrocephalus and -oid ; fontanelle (anterior) open ; head grows larger.	*Hydrocephaloid* or -us ; fontanelle (posterior) open ; bones thin, brittle (1).
Hair falls off, mostly on temples.	Hair poor in quantity or falls off.
Nose	
Epistaxis worse morning.	Epistaxis worse afternoon.
Coryza predominates, dry or obstructed, with pus ; stench before nose ; smell of brimstone.	Coryza mostly fluent ; fluent in cold, dry in warmth and outdoors.
Face, Mouth	
Face, pale, bloated.	Face pale, sallow, earthy.
Dentition slow from beginning, or irregular ; fat or, if emaciated, stomach remains bloated.	Dentition slow, especially later teeth ; emaciation; stomach flabby.
Sore throat, must swallow the saliva ; worse from warm drinks.	Sore throat worse swallowing saliva ; better from warm drinks.
Sensation of lump in the left side of the throat.	Uvula, tonsils, etc., feel weak, empty (2).
Abdomen	
Hunger, morning.	Hunger afternoon (4 P.M.).
Better after breakfast (weakness).	Worse after breakfast.
Cold food relieves.	Icecream, cold food, aggravate.
Enlarged abdomen in mesenteric tabes predominates.	More frequently flabby abdomen, with mesenteric tabes.
Cholera infantum worse from smoked meat ; long for eggs.	Cholera infantum; long for ham-fat, bacon, corn-beer (3).
Stool white, sour.	Stools green, much fetid flatus.
Hard, undigested, hot stools every day.	Watery, hot stools every day.
Anal troubles (piles) alternate with head.	Anal troubles (fistula) alternate with chest.

(1) *Calc. Phos. has* much more marked than *Calc. Curb.* a weak condition of the neck in children, head totters. Compare *Natri. Mur.*, summer-complaint ; *Verat.*, whooping cough ; *Lyc.*, *Sul.*, etc.

(2) This sensation of emptiness, weakness, runs through the whole remedy. It is probably due to the influence of the combining *Phos.* We find it in throat, abdomen, stomach, genitals : male and female.

(3) In tumors, ulcers, etc., which bear the closest resemblance, the *Phosphate* is best when they appear on the occiput ; the *Calc. Carb.*, when on the sinciput.

CALC. CARB.	Urine	CALC. PHOS.
Urine deposits white (calcareous).		Urine flocculent (phosphatic).
Hæmaturia from checked piles.		Diabetes when chest is involved

The *Calc. Carb.* does not materially alter the *quantity* of urine. The *Calc. Phos.* causes copious emission, with weak sensation (Diabetes).

Sexual Organs

Erections too short during coition.	Erethism, intense during coition.
Sexual excitement predominates, moral.	Sexual excitement predominates, physical.
Amorous dreams before the menses.	Nymphomania, erethism, before the menses.
Milk changed in quantity.	Milk changed in quality.
Prolapsus uteri (like *Bell.*), with bearing-down pains.	Prolapsus uteri (like *Phos.*), with weak, sinking feelings.

Both appear in rheumatism, but only *Calc. Phos.* has uterine displacement with rheumatic pains, worse in damp weather, or in changes from warm to cold; also dark catamenia in rheumatic females.

Menses too early, too profuse, lasting too long; amorous dreams; throbbing in the head when ascending; anæmia; congestion of the head and chest.	Menses every two weeks, black, clotted; sexual desire; stiff all over when ascending; stitching pains in the left side of the head; griping and rumbling in the bowels.

Calc. Phos. may serve in menstruation during lactation.

During pregnancy: Pelvis feels lame all over; limbs feel heavy.	During pregnancy: Pelvis painful in the sutures; limbs feel weak, trembling.

Calc. Phos. has "heartburn up into the throat; soreness right groin; kicking, quivering over the os pubis; pressing; aching in the neck of the bladder; drawing in the region of the navel to the sacrum;" hence, symptoms of pregnancy. *Calc Carb.*, on the other hand, seems to suit better the period of parturition,—"labor-pains when the uterus goes upward," etc.

Larynx, Chest

Cough with rawness in the chest; tearing, as if something were being torn loose.	Cough with stitches in the chest, burning rising up into the throat (4).

(4) These burning sensations are more marked in the *Phosphate*, and tend to spread over considerable surface; but start in spots.

Larynx, Chest

CALC. CARB.	CALC. PHOS.
Asthma worse lying.	Asthma better lying (5).
Phthisis pulmonalis, second stage, or even first stage in plethoric young. Coldness between the shoulder-blades; night-sweats in the *first* sleep.	Phthisis pulmonalis, incipiens, burning *in spots,* hawking causes gagging; burning from the vertex down the whole spine; sweat towards morning awakens him.

Back

CALC. CARB.	CALC. PHOS.
Spine curved; worse in the dorsal region or neck. Stool white, sour.	Spine curved; worse in the lumbar region.

Limbs

CALC. CARB.	CALC. PHOS.
Hip-disease, second stage; sweat on the head during sleep; scratches head impatiently when waking; desires boiled eggs; abdomen hard, bloated; diarrhœa, especially towards evening; glands of neck swollen.	Hip-disease, third stage; it puts an end to the further destruction of the bone, stops suppurations, and promotes new organization. (Raue's Pathology.)
Rheumatism from getting wet; from working in water, or from long continuance in the water.	Rheumatic pains erratic; from wet or windy weather; from every cold; especially in females with prolapsus uteri, etc.

Sleep

CALC. CARB.	CALC. PHOS.
Child awakes suddenly, and points to some imaginary object on the wall (fontanelles open).	Child awakes cold, screaming, grasping in agony toward the mother (fontanelles open).

Bones, Skin

CALC. CARB.	CALC. PHOS.
Bones diseased, mostly in the whole epiphysis.	Bones diseased in symphyses or sutures (6).
Rachitis, head sweats profusely; child fat or, if emaciated, stomach large; stools white, sour; legs deformed.	Rachitis, child thin, flabby all over; stool green or watery; legs bend outward.
Bones of the head (after injury) grow larger.	Bones of the head grow soft, crackling, brittle.

---

(5) *Calc. Phos.* ought to be considered in cyanosis neonatorum. It has many chest symptoms, worse when rising.

(6) The *Calc. Phos.* causes so much irritation in sutures that we may here find a reason why it so often assists in forming a callus after fracture, by irritation (formative, Virchow) of the fracture, a sort of artificial suture.

CALC. CARB.	Skin	CALC. PHOS.
Skin pale, watery, bloated or flabby.		Skin dark-brown, yellow, flabby, (more like *Sulph.*)
Warts turn into ulcers.		Furuncles become ulcers.

Both appear in scrofulous, sluggish ulcers. The *phos.* is preferable in ulcers from poultices of *Mustard.*

Generalities

CALC. CARB.	CALC. PHOS.
Child makes an anxious face when raised from the cradle (Cholera infantum).	Child has suffocating spells, turns blue, bends head back when raised from the cradle (5).
Resembles, *Bell., Sul., Iod., Nit. ac.*	Resembles *Carbo An., Berb., Sul., Ruta, Sil.*
Exhausted, *dizzy,* walking up stairs.	Exhausted, trembling, walking up stairs
Best in early childhood.	Best in second dentition; old age (7).
Better lying on the back.	Worse lying on the back, (twitchings).
Better being touched.	Worse from slight touch.
Better after breakfast.	Worse after breakfast.
Better on rising.	Worse on rising.
Better often from cold food.	Worse cold food (ice-cream, jellies, cold water).
Worse from mental work.	Better from mental work (8).
Worse washing.	Better washing (head).
Worse lying on side.	Better lying on side.
Worse cold, wet weather.	Worse same, and in wind.

Extract of letter from Dr. Neidhard.—"*Calc. Carb.* is used by me in diseases of infancy and childhood, particularly in enlargements and indurations of the sub-maxillary and cervical glands, as well as those of the mesentery; marasmus, tendency to hydrocephalus; innumerable cases of neuralgia affecting the head, worse cold air. *Calc. Phos.* suits diseases of youth and middle age when the respiratory functions are chiefly affected. Bronchial coughs, and incipient tubercles are benefited more than by any other remedy. Attendant diseases of spine; fistula in ano. In the advanced stages of consumption, *Calc. Hypophos.* is our only hope, and often relieves."

---

(7) *Calc. Phos.* like *Phos.* has many symptoms of old people; hence, *also children, who appear too old from disease. Calc. Carb.* cannot be repeated with advantage in affections of the aged (Hahnemann), except the potency be a very high one. (C. Hg.).

(8) *Calc. Phos.* has complaints among school-girls, *growing* children (like *Phos. Ac.*). They get anxious, restless, want to go home when at school, and to school, when at home; sighing, etc.

CALCAREA CARB. & SILICEA

Calcarea Carbonica and *Silicea* have many symptoms in common. They frequently meet in scrofula, ulcers, bone diseases, gland affections, nutritive defects, as, emaciation, defective osseous growth, retarded dentition, toothache from caries of the teeth, blennorrhœa, hip-disease, convulsions, paralysis, neuralgias, muscular weakness of children, hectic fever, consequences of suppressed discharges, etc.

Constitution

The *Calcarea* patient is described as leuco-phlegmatic, of a light complexion, fair skin, blue eyes, blonde hair, lax fibre. He is plethoric, and exhibits a tendency to early obesity. The activity of the lymph-glands is not proportional to the capacity for assimilation ; oxidation is imperfect ; hence there is a rapid deposit of fat in cellular tissues, especially about the abdomen ; but tissues are imperfectly nourished. Thus, though apparently robust, he is really sickly. His plethora is apparent; his blood is watery and contains too many white blood-corpuscles.

Anæmia and Chlorosis are but a step further on in this condition of hydræmia. Continued defective nutrition or protracted loss of animal fluids are sufficient causes. At puberty Chlorosis appears, still under the mask of plethora ; but the pale, flabby face, palpitation on ascendnig, craving for chalk, coal, etc., weak muscles, cold hands and feet, disgust for meat, show plainly enough the true state of the system.

This constitution is generally inherited, or belongs to childhood and youth, when such

The *Silicea* patient is described as nervous, irritable, with dry skin, pale face, light complexioned, lax muscles. He is imperfectly nourished, not from want of food, but from imperfect assimilation. He exhibits but little tendency to corpulence or plethora. In him defective nutrition has permitted a marked debility of the cerebro-spinal nervous system. Thus he suffers from what is called nervous weakness. He is costive from enervation ; whenever he is sick, spinal symptoms appear and qualify every other. He is emaciated, there is none of the bloat which so characterises *lime.*

His erethism has less vascular excitement than that of *lime.* While he is exhausted, as

CALC. CARB.	Constitution	SILICEA
disturbances of nutrition are quite common. But there are many causes which may develop it, such as long-continued loss of animal fluids; anæmia. milk, mucus, semen, etc.		shown by his many symptoms of weakness, paralysis, etc., there is an exhausted susceptibility to nervous stimuli, which may be termed "irritable weakness", as well described by Dunham.

Thus, then, the *Calcarea* patient has decreased bodily irritability; the *Silicea,* increased.

Blood Changes

We have seen that there is a hydræmic condition produced by *Calcerea. Silicea,* however, exhibits symptoms of more malignant blood-changes :

Face pale, bloated, or emaciated, with deep-set eyes, surrounded by dark rings ; as if from loss of animal fluids; anæmia.	Face pale, earthly, ashy ; skin waxlike, or a cadaverous expression; all indicating cachexia, as from cancer, or exhaustion from long-lasting suppuration.

TUBERCULOSIS comes within the range of both remedies. Thus, with Gross, classing white-swelling, hip-disease, with tuberculosis of lungs :

Especially suited to the plethoric young who have long suffered from copious mucous expectoratoin (thus losing much albumen) ; or, after protracted nursing ; or, at puberty when the menses set in with profuse and long-lasting flow ; congestions to head and to chest ; chest extremely sore to touch ; also later cavities have formed ; much mucous rattling on the chest ; loud breathing through the nose ; profuse yellow-white or purulent expectoration ; hæmorrhages from the cavities.	Especially suited to the mucopurulent catarrh of old people; loose, rattling cough day and night with dyspnœa, vomiting up of tenacious mucus or yellow-green expectoration; it is generally indicated later in phthisis than *lime; viz.,* in the stage of ulceration with induration and shrinking of the lung-tissue around the cavities. It controls the disease by its power to diminish suppuration, while *lime* has more effect on the tubercular deposit itself.
Tight breathing, tension across the chest as from rush of blood ; relieved by raising the shoulders ; icy-cold between	Asthma worse lying down ; spasmodic cough with spasm of the larynx ; cannot bear the slightest draft on the back of

Blood Changes

CALC. CARB.	SILICEA
the shoulder-blades; tuberculosis of young plethoric people.	neck; catarrh of aged people.
Night-sweats; limbs cold; sweat during the first sleep; sweat clammy, causes anxiety.	Night-sweats; mostly after 12 P.M., towards morning; sweat sour, offensive smelling.
Face pale, with frequent flushes.	Face, pale, waxen.
Hip-disease; evening diarrhœa; constitutional symptoms; scratching head impatiently when awaking; limping; pain on inner side of knee.	Hip-disease; watery, exhausting diarrhœa, constitutional symptoms, limping, but generally later, with evidences of caries.
White-swelling of the knee-joint; knee spongy; pressing, stinging intermitting at night and when at rest; worse from flexion, as from going up and down stairs; mostly at inner and lower side of the knee. See also Scrifulolsis.	White-swelling. *Silicea* is particularly distinguished by its tendency to cause indurations of cellular parts; thus, between the fistulous ulcers there are irregular, hard elevations, reddish but transparent, as if filled with glue; the pains are lancinating; caries of the bone is present.
GANGRENE has been cured by *Calcarea*. Thus, in the mouth we find gangrene following canker-sores or stomatitis. Again, an allied condition is decribed under that doubtful name, gastromalacia; red, raw tongue, emaciated neck, thirst, but no appetite; vomiting of all food; green, watery stool, with little lumps. Cancer uteri and scirrhus of the mammæ have been treated with the *lime*, constitutional symptoms agreeing.	*Silicea* is more specifically adapted to malignant diseases; gangrenous inflammation and ulcers; fungi which readily bleed; cancerous ulcers; thus ulcer on right border of tongue eating into it, discharging much pus; brown, profuse, fetid ichor from uterine cancer. Akin to this is the lupus which *Silicia* cures; serrated ulcers with grayish surfaces corroding the cheek, threatening perforation, the surrounding parts being indurated. See also Carbuncle, under cellular tissue.

Tissues

CALC. CARB.	SILICEA
Calcarea has nutritive action on nerves, mucous membranes, glands, skin, cartilages and bones.	*Silicea* acts on nerves, fibrous structures, cellular tissue, skin and bones.

CALC. CARB. **Mind** **SILICEA**

Lime has running through all its symptoms a peculiar anxiety of both mind and body. *This condition is not so marked* in *Silicea.* Thus we find as characterising the *lime* :—

Fear of going crazy with great anxiety lest others shall observe it.

Anxious, timid, full of fear; cannot bear to be alone, or in the dark; hence always worse at night and twilight.

Emotions, excitement cause anxious sweat; flying heat through the body. Anxious if he listens to tales of cruelty.

Fright with præcordial anxiety.

Sudden blindness with anxious sweat.

Anxiety, as if from the stomach, with nausea and vomiting.

Anxious dread of disease; is in constant dread of heart-disease.

Anxiety abdominal, when standing.

Anxious thoughts with fear of death, before sleep.

Awakens with anxiety and heavy breathing.

Cardiac anxiety with suicidal mood; wants to stab herself.

Silicea also gives us a suicidal mood, with anxiety referred to the epigastrium, desire to drown oneself. But anguish is not so interwoven through symptoms of all parts of the organism as with the *lime.* Sometimes while sitting, the patient is attacked with anguish, which forces him to rise and walk about. Palpitation after dinner; after anxious dreams. These few symptoms of *Silicea* depend upon its action on the abdominal ganglia, especially the solar plexus, as will be seen under "Convulsions". Akin to this state is a condition of mental concern; melancholic, despairing mood.

Under *Calcarea,* we find the greatest possible fearfulness, dread, timidity. The patient :—

Despairs of recovery; fears loss of reason; dreads some imaginary impending calamity; as evening comes, he is filled with awe, shudders; his imagination is so excited that he pictures visions of rats and mice; thinks some one is

Silicea differs here materially. It has equally marked gloominess, despair, weeping, but the mood is different :—

Dread of disease; great solicitude concerning his spiritual welfare; compunctions of conscience about trifles.

CALC. CARB. **Mind** **SILICEA**

walking by his side; converts articles of furniture into animate objects, which alarm him.

Yielding mind, faint-hearted, showing the depressing character of *Silicea*. Fear is not so marked a characteristic as with the *lime*. The imagination is weak, not excited ; it forms few or no delirious fancies. At night, under the stimulus of vivid dreams, however, the *Silicea* patient awakens with horrible imaginings or falls into a distressing state of nightmare. But this phenomenon is not so much owing to a primarily excited brain as to a diseased condition of the abdomen ; the solar plexus is the nervous centre whose deranged action is reflected to the cerebrum.

Thus the *Calcarea* patient is excitable, predisposed to delirium. Alcoholic liquors develop readily a delirium tremens with the above symptoms of an excited mind. In typhoid states, it is an invaluable remedy in the beginning when :—

Thus the remedy has no place in hallucinations, and cannot cure mania-a-potu like *lime*. Wine, in fact, only causes ebullitious of blood, not delirium.

On closing the eyes he sees visions of persons or horrible fantastic forms. Sleepless, the same thought continually runs through his mind, keeping off sleep.

The mental aberrations of *Silicea* are more allied to imbecility than to insanity:

She sits playing with pins; is afraid of their sharp points ; she is under the delusion that they are in her throat ; they occupy her mind constantly.

Obstinacy, wilfulness, characterises both remedies and is common enough with children. The differences are only in degree, *Silicea* more marked.

Mind

CALC. CARB.	SILICEA
Under *Calcarea* there is no aversion to mental labor, but it fatigues, causing :—	Under *Silicea* there is a condition which Dunham well describes :—
Hyperæmia of the brain; chorea ; trembling spells ; headache, the pains changing about ; dyspepsia. Especially is it useful for school-children who are growing rapidly.	Fatigued, dreads labor, yet there is a nervous erethism which makes him work well when once he has commenced.
	Mental labor causes nervous weakness; dizziness; pressing frontal headache.

Vertigo

Both appear in vertigo from excessive use of the eyes; from study; with rachitis; with nausea; from suppressed discharges; from loss of animal fluids.

CALC. CARB.	SILICEA
Calcarea represents vascular erethism.	*Silicea* represents a spinal origin ; its forms are more purely nervous :
Vertigo when ascending a height, as going upstairs.	Vertigo rising from dorsal spine, spreading thence to nape of neck and head.
Vertigo with cerebral hyperæmia from suppressed menses; from checked hæmorrhoidal flow.	When of vascular origin it is more from venous stasis:
The pneumogastric sympathises, for nausea is soon produced.	Vertigo with constipation, venous stasis, deficient peristaltic action ; but here, too, the cause of this state is in spinal enervation.
	Silicea is peculiarly obnoxious to anything which jars the nervous system, causes concussion ; hence, vertigo when riding.
Vertigo with tendency to fall backwards or sideways.	Vertigo with tendency to fall forwards or sideways.

We can appreciate the value of thus noting the direction of real or apparent falling, when we remember that vertigo is frequently caused by partial cerebral anæmia. This results from sudden constriction of vessels from local vaso-motor irritation. Thus ensues loss of equilibrium and consequently a sense of falling. The direction differs according to the parts of the brain so affected.

CALC. CARB. **Head** **SILICEA**

Congestion to the brain figures in both, but under quite different circumstances.

CALC. CARB.

Under *Calcarea* the determination of blood is profound. There are hammering, thumping, boring pains; the head feels, as if it would burst through the skull; buzzing, roaring in the ears; throbbing in the very centre of the brain; red, puffed face. In fact there is a state of plethora—not perhaps from absolute excess in quantity: but the lax fibre of the *Calcarea* patient permits these rapid congestions, when an exciting cause exists, as alcoholic drink, suppressed menses, severe mental labor, etc. Thus apoplexy may be produced, especially as *lime* favours degeneration in the coats of blood-vessels.

Feeling of icy-coldness, mostly right side of head; face pale, puffed.

Apoplexia sanguinea.

Migraine, from occiput to vertex; feels, as if brain was dissolving, and she was becoming insane; wild feeling; brain very sensitive to shrill noises; roaring, buzzing in the ears, better with eyes closed; dim vision, especially after a full meal; nausea, vomiting at the height of the attack; worse from alcohol, from study after dinner, from

SILICEA

Silicea, on the other hand, has not plethora as a determining cause; suppressed discharges, as checked foot-sweat, talking, study, may develop congestion towards the head.

But the cerebro-spinal system is again at fault:

Rush of blood to the head, coming up from the spine into the back of the head.

Feeling of coldness from nape of neck to vertex; head heavy.

Apoplexia nervosa.

Migraine, from nape of neck to vertex; loss of reason; or a peculiar exaggeration of mind; must restrain himself to prevent committing violence; worse from noises, jarring the head; roaring in the ears as from something alive in them; eye-balls sore when revolved; loud cries; nausea to fainting; dim sight after headache, worse from study; with great nervous

CALC. CARB.	SILICEA
Head	
suppressed menses; suddenly checked hæmorrhoidal flow; scalp covered with dandruff.	exhaustion; better while eating; worse after; from suppressed foot-sweat; straining to stool; scalp sensitive, covered with papulæ.
Headache, with boring in left temple.	Headache.
Headache better from tying something around the head.	Headache worse from pressure even of the hat.
Special Senses	
Amaurosis from suppressed menses, hæmorrhoidal flow, etc.	Amaurosis from suppressed mucous or purulent discharges or foot-sweat.
Amblyopia, with headache; with abdominal complaints.	Amblyopia after the nervous headache.
Mist before the eyes after eating, after reading; anxious sweat; nausea; bright flashes.	Letters run together; look pale after reading a short time; lightning-like flashes; nervous feeling in the head.
Dilated pupils.	Contracted pupils.
Sees only one side of an object.	Day-blindness.
Short-sightedness; or long-sighted.	Only long-sighted.

We have seen that only *lime* causes mania-a-potu; both however, have amblyopia from excessive use of alcoholic liquors, but with differences in temperament:

CALC. CARB.	SILICEA
Sight impaired by excessive drinking of alcohol; face red, bloated; sluggish.	Amblyopia from abuse of stimulants; sensitive, nervous persons.
Hardness of hearing, of rheumatic origin, abuse of Quinine; beating in the head and ears; hence vascular erethism predominates. Better from sweating; worse in the open air.	Hardness of hearing, more of nervous origin; deaf to the human voice; during changes of the moon; suddenly after a faint; ringing in the ears and deafness with the paralysis.
Cracking in ears when cheering.	Report in ear when blowing nose, then better.

Nervous System

CALC. CARB.	SILICEA
Calcarea has not such extreme nervous susceptibility as *Silicea*. It is more characterised by torpidity, while *Silicea* only exhibits torpidity in its attack on the lower tissues: Abscesses, for instance.	The action of *Silicea* on the nervous system is at once peculiar and important. It seems to correspond to nervous phenomena which usually arise from organic changes in nerve structure. Defective

CALC. CARB. **Nervous System** **SILICEA**

Lime, it is true, has brain excitable, sensitive to shrill noises, alternate acute and dull hearing ; but these are not so marked or general as in *Silicea.*

nutrition is here felt profoundly ; but withal there is an over-excitability already, in part, referred to. There is an over-susceptibility to nervous stimuli. The senses of vision, hearing and smell are at first sharpened when neuralgia begins, but later, become dull. This erethism enables the *Silicea* patient to work on in spite of his increasing exhaustion.

He feels an ennui and dread of mental and physical exertion, but when "wormed up", goes on with an alacrity which amounts to overdoing. This has been well-illustrated by Dunham. So, too, in consumption, he does not feel badly while walking, but when he stops to rest, dyspnœa, and cough, and sweat, and almost fainting exhaustion attacks him. Sight is good enough during his nervous headache, but afterwards he is almost blind.

So again with spasms, Dunham has shown that they may be provoked by fatigue, muscular exertion, etc., as for instance, cramp in the feet after walking, writer's cramp, etc.

This irritability gives us a valuable hint : Touch cannot be tolerated ; parts rested on go to sleep ; jarring or noise cause intolerable headache. Riding, which is a passing motion with jarring, causes distress, and further,—

Riding in a carriage produces momentary unconsciousness.

Nervous System

CALC. CARB.	SILICEA
Spasms ; aura, like a mouse up the arm, or from pit of stomach through abdomen to feet ; cold thighs before attack, chewing motion of mouth, stretching of the limbs. Worse during full moon, protracted intermittents, etc.	Spasms ; aura, like a mouse running through the limbs, or from solar plexus to the brain, left side cold; left arm twists ; starts in sleep; moaning, loud groaning. Worse during new or full moon ; after vaccination.
Chorea from fright ; muscular twitchings ; throws herself about, tries to grasp clothing of bystanders, bites, spits, eyes wide open ; also in hysteria.	Dissipation, hard work, with close confinement, cause obstinate neuralgias, hysterical attacks or paralysis.
Awkward ; clumsy.	Cannot hold things ; spine-disease.
Weak and faint before breakfast ; better after eating ; loss of fluids.	First on leaving the bed in the morning, cannot walk, so weak ; spine-disease.
Muscular debility ; feels sore ; stiff when beginning to move ; muscular atrophy ; parts feel subjectively cold ; trembling of inner and outer parts.	Weakness from spine ; legs tremble, with great nervousness; feeling of loss of power, buzzing in the ears, head heavy, can hardly raise it, as if cervical muscles failed ; muscles atrophied ; numb feeling.
Gressus Vaccinus; weak feeling in the back; worse from mental annoyance, can hardly rise ; softening of the spine, with contraction of limbs.	Gressus Gallinaceus; spasmodic pain in small of back, can hardly rise ; spinal irritation.

Male Genital Organs

CALC. CARB.	SILICEA
Spermatorrhœa ; complaints from coition, from onanism ; limbs weak, especially about the knees ; lassitude, hands tremble, chorea ; palpitation, epilepsy ; pressure in head and back; angry, discontented, excitable after coition, which was imperfect.	Spermatorrhœa ; complaints from coition ; emissions, followed by sensation, as if right side of head were paralyzed ; limbs feel bruised ; right arm and wrist weak ; burning in the feet ; with sweat sacrum aches ; nervousness, often emission.

Modalities

CALC. CARB.	SILICEA
Calcarea has decided aggravation from :—	Silicea, more than the *Lime*, suffers from electric changes :—

Modalities

CALC. CARB.	SILICEA
Electric and barometric changes, etc. Cold air, drafts, especially if cold and damp. North-east winds, because they are usually damp.	Worse in dry, rather than wet weather. Worse in west or south-west winds; in stormy, windy weather; in changeable weather, when electric variations are marked.
Worse from washing; eruptions, rheumatism, ischias; pains in the limbs; rhagades; ulcers cannot tolerate wet poultices. Washing does not so disagree as with *Silicea*. It may produce: Heavy feeling in the hands (here again showing the nervous influence); abscess from getting the feet wet, sitting with the feet in water.	Worse during a thunder-storm; great debility.

Silicea more than *Calcarea* has desire to be magnetised.

CALC. CARB.	SILICEA
Worse from cold air; it seems to go right through her; worse from a draft of air.	Worse from least exposure of the feet; a draft on the back of the neck causes pain and nervousness.

Typhoid conditions may be classed here.

CALC. CARB.	SILICEA
First stage, when on closing the eyes, sees persons and things, the same idea haunts him all night, keeping him awake; on the 14th day, rash does not appear; anxiety, delirium, red face, diarrhœa, short cough.	Great debility, profuse sweat; desire to be magnetised; sleepless; sometimes when thus prescribed it develops superficial boils and abscesses, thus determining the disease to the surface.
Paralysis. *Lime* causes paralysis of parts as a result of exhausting sweats, loss of animal fluids; it acts mainly on arms, fingers, with great coldness; spinal paralysis from frequently getting wet.	Paralysis. *Silicea* develops a paralytic difficulty in swallowing; paralysis of the limbs of spinal origin, with constipation; paralysis as a sequel to convulsions; paralysis affecting prominently the sensory nerves.

Both produces a paralytic state of internal organs; but only *Calcarea* has cured impending paralysis of the lungs in scarlatina:

Loud rattling in the wind-pipe, hot breath; præcordial anguish; no cough; rattling mostly noticed during expiration.

CALC. CARB.	Mucous Membranes	SILICEA

Calcarea has a more marked action on mucous membranes; blennorrhœas are more general. It increases the secretion of mucus.

CALC. CARB.	SILICEA
Mucous membrane inflamed; mucus increased.	Inflamed, with no secretion or with serous secretion.

Nasal Catarrh

Nasal catarrh, especially when there is a scrofulous tendency to frequent attacks may call for both as follows:—

CALC. CARB.	SILICEA
Sudden, violent, fluent coryza; dropping of water from the nose; much sneezing; heat in the head; mouth dry; palate rough with a stinging, pricking cauisng cough; chill and heat alternately; pain over root of nose; neck stiff; inertia.	Alternately dry and fluent coryza; with every fresh cold stoppage and acrid discharge from the nose; frequent but ineffectual sneezing; makes inner nose sore and bloody; dryness of the throat; rough cough; itching in the Eustachian tube; often useful in rose cold.
Chronic cases: Smell before the nose as of manure or gunpowder, or putrid eggs; discharge thick, slimy, mixed with blood; edges of nostrils sore; swelling of nose, especially at the root, frequently going and coming; discharge stops in the morning and thus causes a dull, stupefying headache. There are painless hoarseness; and accumulation of mucus in the throat. Sometimes there is purulent, fetid, yellow-red discharge, making the lip sore; itching red pustules on the cheeks; tip of nose swollen; red; becomes scurfy.	Chronic cases: Smell before the nose as of recently slaughtered animals; discharge slimy, tough, or acrid, bloody, making inner nose and edges of nostrils sore and bloody; face-ache; pain in the nose and antrum of Highmore; discharge stops in the morning, and thus causes pounding, throbbing in frontal sinuses, which are also affected; there is husky voice or nasal voice; hawking of green, fetid mucus in the morning. Indurated mucus in the nose; curdy secretion; tip of the nose red, itches intolerably; tetters on the nose.

Throat

CALC. CARB.	SILICEA
Uvula swollen; dark-red; covered with little blisters; aphthæ, on roof of mouth; hawks saltish mucus, or in early morning profuse phlegm is raised.	Uvula sore, pale-yellow in color; swollen; throat very dry; ulcers which seems to perforate the parts; hawks tough slime, or thick, green, fetid mucus.

Throat

CALC. CARB.	SILICEA
Feeling of a lump in the left side of throat; compelled to swallow saliva often, which seems to cause the lungs to descend.	Feeling of a lump in left side of throat; swallows with great difficulty; chronic tonsillitis; see also below.
Tickling in the throat, as from a feather.	Like a feather on the tongue; pricking in the throat as from a pin.
Throat feels narrowed; he must swallow frequently; pharynx spasmodically contracted; food seems to remain sticking in œsophagus, with a sort of nausea.	Throat sore, as if the food glided over sore spots; swallowing forces food up through the choanæ; or painful, difficult swallowing as from paralysis; the food goes down slowly.
Tonsils swollen, chronic cases; palate elongated; pains extend to ears when swallowing; whitish-yellow ulcers on tonsils.	Tonsils swollen, chronic cases; also in quinsy to hasten the abscess, or stop the purulent discharges when too long-lasting; swallowing distorts the face; deep ulcers, even gangrene.

Scrofulosis

Calcarea has more action on glands and their functions, *Silicea* more on bones and fibrous structures. We shall see whatever affections depend upon hypertrophy of cellular tissue or of fibrous or conversely depend upon destructive changes in these parts, are better cured by *Silicea.* In nature and art, *Silicea* seems to give hardness and stability to bodies. Thus, flint, quartz, glass, the covering of some seeds, the stalks of plants, and the bones of animals.

CALC. CARB.	SILICEA
Difficult dentition; child fat, fair, plump; face often red; or emaciation general, except abdomen, which is large, hard and swollen; head too large, with open fontanelles; sweat on the scalp in large drops, wets the pillow far around, during sleep; gums pale, shiny; threatened hydrocephalus; glands swollen about the neck; loose, rattling cough; stool like lumps of chalk; sleepless after 3 A.M.; feet cold, damp; child sweats	Difficult dentition; child emaciated, but head is too large; face pale, waxen-hued; abdomen hard, swollen, hot, fontanelles open; profuse sweat only on the head; profuse salivation; gums sensitive; child frequently grasps at the mouth; blisters on the gums; feverish every evening and night with hot head, restlessness; costive, the stools partly expelled slip back; usually very dark, loose, and offensive; feet sweat, especially

Scrofulosis

CALC. CARB.	SILICEA
easily and takes cold; convulsions.	between toes sweat is fetid, makes toes sore. (See Guernsey's Obstetrics).

Eyes

CALC. CARB.	SILICEA
Ophthalmia ; stinging pains ; sweat on the forehead ; keratitis pustulosa profuse lachrymation, excessive photophobia, lids red, swollen ; sticking pains ; ulcers on cornea highly vascular ; spasmodic closure of the lids.	Ophthalmia ; especially useful when ulcers or abscesses form on iris or cornea, sloughing ulcers followed by corneal fistula; hypopyon; biting pains in the canthi.
Dry scurf on the lids during the day.	Cystic tumors on lids, suppurating; edges of lids ulcerate.
Induration after styes.	Styes which becomes filled with pus.
Eyes worse morning, changes to damp cold weather, in the gaslight.	Eyes worse from gaslight, and from daylight which dazzles the eyes.
Cornea ulcerating, bland pus; or opacity of the cornea, milky-white or bluish in color.	Cornea thick, rough, wartlike, as if hypertrophied ; scales off ; cicatrices corneæ ; opaque after small-pox.
Cataract.	Cataract after suppressed foot-sweats.
Traumatic ophthalmia ; feels, as if a foreign substance were in the eyes.	Traumatic ophthalmia, suppuration.
Fistula lachrymalis; thick yellow bland pus ; itching, humid eruption on lids.	Fistula lachrymalis, gnawing pains ; thin, offensive pus, bones have become caried.

Ears

CALC. CARB.	SILICEA
Otorrhœa muco-purulent ; ulceration of meatus ; granulation ; then polypus ; scurf or boils about ears.	Otorrhœa purulent ; also from caries; catarrh of the middle ear ; caries of the mastoid process.

Face, Mouth

CALC. CARB.	SILICEA
Swelling of the upper lips as in scrofula.	Lips swollen, ulcerated, even cancerous.
Parotid gland swollen, especially in scarlatina ; it suppurates and discharges an ichor ; great prostration; throat sore; cervical glands swollen.	Parotid gland swollen, indurated ; or suppurating when the process is too slow, is painless, and healing is too tardy ; even in scarlatina.

Face, Mouth

CALC. CARB.	SILICEA
Caries of the teeth; pains, especially around loose stumps, throbbing pains with great rush of blood to the head; gum-boils, bleeding of gums; fistula dentalis.	Caries, especially with coaffected periosteum; throbbing, as if in the jaw-bone; pains shooting into the antrum; gum-boils; fistula dentalis with caries of jaw-bone.

Stomach

CALC. CARB.	SILICEA
Appetite ravenous; or fastidious, longing for boiled eggs; scrofulous children.	Appetite ravenous; or fastidious, craves dainties; scrofulous children.
Children refuse the milk of the mother; it is watery, nauseating.	Children have an aversion to mother's milk.
Vomits milk as soon as taken, sour, curdled.	Vomits the mother's milk as soon as taken.
Calcarea, acting more on mucous surfaces, cures mucous polypi—in the ear, nose, bladder, uterus.	*Silicea,* as we have several times observed, acts more on connective tissue; hence it is more often indicated in indurations—hard scars or indurations after boils, abscesses; arm and hand swollen, cellular tissue indurated; thigh twice its natural size, indurated, etc.

Bone Diseases

Both cure caries, curvatures of bones, rachitis; but *Silicea* is preferable in periosteal diseases; in necrosis, with fistulous openings, and fetid ichorous pus.

CALC. CARB.	SILICEA
Useful in the beginning of rachitis, when the child refuses to move about, lies down almost all the time, the joints begin to swell, but are still normal in color. Here *Calcarea* is indicated, because *lime* acts on the epiphyses, and it is their tumefaction which produces the enlarged joints. It is at this stage that a white frothy diarrhœa often appears, also pointing to *lime.* There are incrustations on the face; voracious appetite, yet the	*Silicea* generally suits after *lime* in rachitis. There is the same large head, bulging forehead, emaciation; but there is a much more marked

CALC. CARB.	**Bone Diseases** **SILICEA**
child wastes; the skin becomes flabby, harsh, wrinkled; the child looks like an old man.	tendency to ulceration; slight scratches refuse to heal; glands suppurate.
Arthritic nodes. Rheumatism from working or standing in water.	Rheumatism rare; felt in change of weather; hereditary forms.

Skin

Ulcers, with red, hard, swollen edges, high and feeble granulations, without much pain, or tearing throbbing pains; ulcers whitish or yellow; pus sour, scanty, or profuse and bland, albuminous; sometimes offensive; worse from wet poultices.	Ulcers with hard edges indurated far around, proud flesh; stinging, burning, itching; edges sometimes spongy, ulcers black, cancerous, gangrenous; pus thin, ichorous, offensive; perforating ulcers; phagedenic, fistulous, from bones; ulcers in membranous parts; better from warm applications, wet or dry.
Warts, small, soft.	Warts hard.
Hang-nails, nails ulcerate; rough skin between the fingers.	Nails rough, thick; or brittle, ulcerate; in-growing toe-nails; sore between toes.
Rhagades, worse from working in water; cracking, bleeding.	Rhagades not common except on face and arms; elephantiasis; callosities.
Skin dry, parched.	Skin like parchment, thick.
Erysipelas in repeated attacks.	Erysipelas after suppuration; deep-seated phlegmonous erysipelas.
Acne simplex, after sexual excesses; at puberty.	Acne indurata; acne simplex, burns all day, not at night.
Suppressed itch followed by otorrhœa.	Scabies papuliformis; especially if ulcers form.
Eruption of white spots, and scattered red patches on wrists, hands, thighs, legs, with violent irritation.	Eruption of acne on backs of hands; phagædenic blisters on the fingers; burn more by day.
Eczema; thick scabs, bleeding when picked; pus yellow, bland; eruption spreads to the face and ears.	Eczema, moist or dry, more offensive, scabby, burning-itching, scratching makes worse; spreads from back of head; discharges pus; pustules form.

CALC. CARB.	Skin	SILICEA
Eruption in the form of ringworm ; small white patches of thick scabs here and there on the face and scalp.		Ringworm, with formation of pustules.
Variola during dentition.		Variola ; desiccation delayed, suppuration exhausts ; bone diseases as a sequel.
Swellings pale ; shining (as in tumor albus), cold swellings.		Swellings bluish-red; hot swellings.
Bad effects from strains ; backache, headache, stiffness in lumbar region; strains, after the failure of *Rhus*. Brain symptoms after a fall or blow on the head, especially after *Bellad.*		Strains, wounds, with suppuration and tardy healing ; bursa mucosa of knee-pan from long working on the knees ; anthrax ; non-malignant carbuncle.
		Splinters, with festering; foreign bodies under the skin ; brings them to the surface.
Prevents return of felons, of boils ; also in tardy suppuration, especially when worse from wet poultices ; rheumatic diathesis.		Felons, bone-felons, boils; tardy or long-lasting suppuration ; pains unbearable, causing fainting ; pains worse when warm in bed.

CAUSTICUM — Mind — PHOSPHORUS

Common to both remedies are: Melancholy, sorrowfulness; timidity especially evening and night; anxiety with cardiac oppression. But *Causticum* adds *weak memory,* weak feeling in the brain on exerting the mind. There is seldom present an opposite state of mental excitement, mental activity. The *face is yellow, especially about the temples*, and there often concur *ptosis, facial paralysis,* &c. *Phosph.,* on the other hand, is as well characterized by excitement as *Caust.* is by depression of mind. Weak memory, promiment in the latter, is rare in the former and when present has generally followed abnormal activity. In *Phosph.* the melancholy and tearfulness often alternate with *spells of laughter;* and any vehemence is sure to display itself at times. The face is more frequently *pale, sunken, with dark rings around the eyes. Somnambulism* and clairvoyance could only belong to the exciting *Phosph* Thus, *depression* predominates in *Caustic., excitement* in *Phosph.*

CAUSTICUM **Mind** **PHOSPHORUS**

Remembering this we may understand why ailments from grief or care, real or unfounded, find a remedy in *Caustic.;* fright or fear with anger and vehemence in *Phosph.*

Vertigo is very characteristic of *Phosph.,* less so of *Caust.* The former proves curative in many forms: In *anæmic,* as after loss of fluids, too protracted thinking, senile cerebral atrophy with its ever-present staggering, uncertain step, dizziness when turning around, dizziness on rising from bed with fainting, blindness, or muscæ volitantes; also in vertigo from a *too great susceptibility to external impressions,* as in dizziness and fainting from odors, from music, &c., (1), feeling as if very tall, or as if the chair was rising; likewise in vertigo from *hyperæmia and stasis,* as in congestion of the brain with heat ascending from the spine, pulsation in the brain, *worse about the ears,* with nausea and vomiting after eating; again, as in dizziness from heart-disease, from tumors, from pressure of the uterine tumor in pregnancy, &c.

Caustic. has vertigo with a *paralytic weakness of the brain,* dizzy on awaking, redness of the face and hot head; vertigo with paralysis; after seminal emissions; with *sensation of a film before the eyes;* rheumatic patients.

Causticum	Phosphorus
Tension and tightness of the scalp (forehead and temples); worse on awaking and in the evening.	Tension in the skin of the forehead and face; worse from change of weather, while eating; better from eating.
Sensation in the forehead as of a space between brain and bones; better from warmth.	Empty sensation in the head, vertigo; cold and stiff sensation mostly in the cerebellum; worse from warmth.

In eruptions on the scalp they concur in tinea capitis. *Caustic.,* it is well-known, selects the *occiput and nape of neck;* especially in children with large abdomen; weak ankles. *Phosph.* is less prominent in eczema (2), but more so in pityriasis when *"clouds of dandruff"* can

---

(1) Here by reflex irritation, the cerebral vessels are contracted, vasomotor spasm, the resulting symptoms being the same as though the anæmia were actual want of blood.

(2) A prover of *Phosph. 2c.* after taking it in repeated doses, developed an eczema spreading from the nape of the neck over the scalp to the vertex and behind the ears. The scabs were thick, yellow, the discharge glutinous. She never had such symptoms before. Lice took up their abode, the young lady refusing longer to tolerate her loathsome burden, *Lycopod. 2c.* was successfully administered as an antidote. The prover was tall, slim, gracefully built. A few years since she lost a sister from consumption.

CAUSTICUM **Mind** **PHOSPHORUS**

be brushed out; itching relieved immediately by scratching, but soon worse with burning super-added. The hair falls out in bundles, giving the characteristic appearance of tinea decalvans; denuded spots on the scalp, clear, white and smooth.

Eyes

So far as vision is concerned, both develop symptoms of amblyopia. *Caustic.* causes a paralytic state of the optic nerve and also some of the muscles. It is especially useful after *neuralgic headaches, the blindness increasing with each attack* of headache; also in rheumatic patients. *Phosph.* causes amblyopia, glaucoma, having but little effect on the external parts. It is especially useful in blindness from lightning, asthenopia in anæmic, debilitated persons, as after seminal emissions, &c.

Causticum	Phosphorus
Dim-sightedness as from a film before the eyes; sudden blindness; *black threads before the eyes.*	Dim-sightedness often with sensitiveness to bright light; *sudden blindness and fainting; black motes.*
Feeling of pressure in the eyes *momentarily relieved by rubbing; ptosis; paralysis of abducent muscle.*	Aching pains in the eye and orbit, *burning spots* on the eye-ball; no symptoms of muscles.

Ears

Deafness characterizes each. Sounds reverberate in the ear, especially words; hence the patient finds it difficult to appreciate the human voice:—

Causticum	Phosphorus
Hardness of hearing in *rheumatic patients*; worse from cold winds.	Hardness of hearing, especially after *typhus;* better in clear, dry weather.
Otorrhœa (in scroulous children), discharge thin, bloody, watery, *fetid;* external meatus swollen; cracking in the ear; *sore behind the ears* (3), *tinea capitis.*	Otorrhœa not so characteristic; discharge with throbbing in the ears, bloody, purulent, thin; the consequent deafness *better from pressing on the ear.*

Nose, Mouth, Throat, Larynx

Only *Phosph.* has prominently nose-bleed, indicating it in vicarious menstruation, nose-bleed during stool, *polypi easily bleeding. Caust.* rather dulls the sense of smell; *Phosph.* corresponds to acuteness of smell, *strong odors cause fainting; headache with acute smell.* In catarrhs they are more similar.

---

(3) Intertrigo is well-marked in *Caust.* and places it with *Graph.* and *Sulph. Phos.* has more dryness of the skin.

CAUSTICUM Nose, Mouth, Throat, Larynx PHOSPHORUS

CAUSTICUM	PHOSPHORUS
Coryza, hoarseness, nose obstructed; *morning aphonia,* with rawness *and soreness of the larynx and trachea, burning in the throat; influenza with rheumatic pains* (*Rhus*) *and weakness of the limbs; cough with involuntary escape of urine.*	Coryza fluent or dry; *sneezing causes laryngeal pain; smell often over-sensitive; evening aphonia; burning in larynx; coughing or talking causes pain in the larynx; trembling with the cough; great weakness; remarkably clear scleroticæ.* (See Record 1874.)
External nose pimply, *warts* on the nose; scabs about the nose, raw behind the ears, eyes inflamed; mucous expectoration (scrofulous children).	*External nose swollen, smooth, red;* nasal cavities painfully dry; discharge greenish-yellow, blood-streaked; nasal polypus frequently bleeding.
Chronic aphonia with weakness of the laryngeal muscles, glossal or facial paralysis; hoarseness and cough worse stooping; rheumatic patients.	Chronic aphonia, larynx sensitive, great nervous weakness, tightness across the chest; cough and speech hurt the larynx; tuberculous patients.
Spasmodic or catarrhal croup; excellent to check the disease (4); worse from dry, cold winds; rawness in the larynx.	Membranous croup to remove hoarseness, prevent return and also when paralysis threatens, with suffocation, cold clammy sweat, small pulse.
Cough with rawness, burning and soreness of throat and chest; spurting of urine during cough; pain over one hip; cough relieved by a swallow of water; sputa cannot be expectorated, must be swallowed. Adapted to phlegmatic patients, subject to rheumatism, to catarrhs of the respiratory tract; to paralysis; well-marked scrofulosis; yellow complexion; yellow, especially about the eyes.	Coughs of many kinds: from laughing, talking, strong odors, appearance of strangers; tightness across the chest; blood-streaked, purulent, rust-colored sputa; trembling with the cough. Adapted to tall, slender, tuberculous patients, with pale complexion, clear scleroticæ (Holcombe), weak nervous persons; great nervous irritability and sensitiveness to external impressions; pale, waxy face, sunken eyes.

(4) Dr. Heerman, of Paris, informed me while I was visiting his city, that he preferred *Caust. to Aconite* in spasmodic croup. The same information seems to have been communicated to Dr. Prige. (See *Am. Observer.*)

CAUSTICUM	Stomach, Abdomen PHOSPHORUS
Tongue white down either side.	Tongue uniformly white.
Greasy taste in the mouth; *sensation, as if lime were slaking in the stomach,* (heartburn) after fat, starch or saccharine food. (Often accompanying bronchial catarrh).	Sour or saltish taste in the mouth; *burning in the stomach and pharynx often extending into the chest; vomiting of drinks so soon as they become warm; goneness in the stomach.* (Often tuberculosis.)
Violent thirst for cold drinks. easily quenched; vomiting not marked.	Thirst for cold or refreshing drinks, relieved thereby until they become warm, when they are vomited.
Desire for beer.	Desire for wine.
Colic (similar to *Coloc., Coffea, Staph.*), bending double relieves; worse after food; pressure, as if the abdomen would burst; better while lying down.	Spasm of the stomach especially *at the cardiac extremity;* "nervous" colic not marked; flatulent colic, worse while lying down; belching in large quantities after eating.
Abdomen hard, swollen, painful; general emaciation (scrofulous children).	Abdomen flaccid, sore when walking; debility, emaciation (consumption).
Constipation with intense spasm of the rectum, causing *great urging with red face, anxiety;* stool at first in hard pieces, later soft and as thin as a goose-quill.	Constipation when the stool is *small-shaped, hard, expelled with difficulty; "dog-stools;"* painful cramps in the rectum after stool.
Hæmorrhoids with stinging burning pains *worse at every attempt to walk and when thinking of them;* oozing and moisture at the anus, stools often mucus-coated.	Hæmorrhoids with frequent bleeding; they protrude while passing flatus; *hæmorrhoids and discharge of blood from the bowels in consumptives;* discharge of mucus from a wide open anus.
Diarrhœa not so well-marked as in *Phosph.* Scrofulous children, scrofulous adults with consumption or dyspepsia who get a diarrhœa *every time they eat fresh meat.*	Many forms of diarrhœa. Cholera infantum with cough and golden-yellow stools; watery diarrhœa with abdominal burning; morning green diarrhœa (as in cholera times); diarrhœa while coughing; great debility, emaciation, &c.

CAUSTICUM	Urine, Genitals — PHOSPHORUS
Involuntary urination *while coughing;* also in children during the first sleep; *incontinence of urine day and night in cold weather;* children are weak, weak-minded, totter while walking.	Involuntary urination during typhus; sometimes also at night, in children who correspond to the *Phosphorus*-build; children who grow too rapidly. Profuse pale urine of nervous women and in diabetes mellitus.

Paralysis of the muscular coat of the bladder, belongs to *Caustic.* especially when a result of too long retention of urine. In great debility, as after typhus, *Phosph.* may be indicated when the bladder is full, but urine does not flow because of absence of urging.

Hæmaturia belongs only to the blood-decomposing *Phosph.*

CAUSTICUM	PHOSPHORUS
Sexual desire (male and female) too weak; emissions are followed by vertigo.	Sexual desire (male and female) too strong; nymphomania; shameless exposure. Spermatorrhœa.
Menses bright red, generally profuse and too late; preceded by melancholy, disposition to view the dark side of things; yellowness of the face. Labor-like pains in back and abdomen; menstrual colic, as *if the pelvic contents were being squeezed;* flow ceases on lying down.	Menses generally pale, profuse and long-lasting, preceded by tearfulness, nymphomania; face pale, blue around the eyes; pains cutting, go up even into the chest, great emptiness in the abdomen; heat up the spine into the head; cold feet and hands; sometimes vicarious through urethra or from the lungs.
Disposed to chafing between the thighs; to sore, cracked, nipples with small pustules around.	Disposed to mastitis, to ulceration of the mammæ, to erysipelas even after pus has formed.
Secretion of milk lessened.	*Increased secretion of milk,* great debility.

Heart

Caust. fades into insignificance when compared with *Phosph.* in its action on the heart. The former remedy possesses palpitation with cardiac anxiety as a part of its well-known melancholy, and as a symptom in paralysis.

Phosph. has palpitation of nervous origin *from every motion,* in anæmia, with tightness across the chest, dyspnœa and nervous weakness. But *Phosph.* plays a part in inflammatory affections; as an extension of pneumonia, as secondary to Morbus Brightii and blood

CAUSTICUM **Heart** **PHOSPHORUS**

dissolution; as a result of rheumatism (symptoms agreeing). It also applies to fatty degeneration of the heart.

Spine, Nerves, Etc.

CAUSTICUM	PHOSPHORUS
Spinal irritation (often from rheumatism or uterine disease), tearing, drawing pains with hardness of the muscles; internal parts, as if squeezed (pelvis); spasmodic colic; *nape of neck stiff with twisting of neck to one side and tearing over the head to the face.*	*Spinal irritation* (often in chest diseases, confinement, reflex uterine, caries, &c.), the pains are more *burning, burning in spots, better from rubbing*; more congestion than in *Caust.*; *throbbing and burning in the neck, thence over the head to the forehead, with burning on the vertex.*
Backache worse rising from a seat; better after; bruised feeling and bearing down in the lumbar region during menses.	Backache worse when rising from stooping; pain in the sacral region after confinement; pain, as if broken, cannot move about.

Phosph. applies to spinal diseases from inflammation of the vertebræ; here, *Caust.* is unknown.

CAUSTICUM	PHOSPHORUS
Neuralgia of the face, pain from the cheek to the mastoid process; *chilly*; scanty or suppressed menses; worse at night; face yellow; *rheumatic patients.*	Facial neuralgia especially involving the jaw; pains go to the root of the nose, temples; *hot bloated face; worse from talking, eating; caries of the lower jaw.*

Phosph., holding as it does, a nutritive relation to nerve-tissue, presents all phases of nervous debility, from simple weakness to complete paralysis. Often in pneumonia, typhus, exanthematic diseases, croup, bronchitis, vitality reaches its lowest ebb, the cerebro-spinal system is depressed, *the surface is cold, pulse like a thread, breathing rattling, trembling of the whole frame*—in just such cases *Phosph.* acts with astonishing rapidity.

In milder forms of nervous weakness, *Phosph.* is characterized by debility with increased susceptibility to external impressions, the so-called "irritable weakness."

Its paralysis may often be traced to cerebral or spinal softening, or atrophy—states which were preceded by *over-excitement*, as shown by the history. The accompanying concurring, we may employ it in progressive muscular atrophy, *the intellect remaining clear.* Paralysis of spinal origin frequently calls for *Phosph.* There are *tingling and formication in the limbs, better from friction; heat in the paralyzed part; anæsthesia; caused* by onanism, chlorosis, Bright's disease, etc.

CAUSTICUM Spine, Nerves, Etc. PHOSPHORUS

Caust. cures a *one-sided facial paralysis, glossal paralysis, ptosis*. Exciting causes are different from those of *Phosph.*

Rheumatism stands foremost and for similar reasons, *exposure to dry, cold winds.* The mind is always compromised. There are *hopelessness, fear of death, weak memory.* Scrofulous children, *weak-minded, totter and fall,* not so much from muscular, as from cerebral weakness.

But *Caustic.* claims precedence in spasms. It pictures epilepsy perfectly : Headache, heat, sweat, pressure in the stomach and chest, causing dyspnœa. If now, *a glass of water is taken,* the whole may be aborted. If not, the spasm develops, frothing at the mouth, biting the tongue, &c. Afterwards sopor. Exciting causes are suppressed itch,. delayed menses, fear, &c. Paralysis may be a sequel. *Phosph.* has no such range. Spasms with consciousness are noted ; hence more likely of spinal rather than of cerebral origin. The relation of *Phosph.* to albuminuria, however, makes it even superior to *Caust.* in *puerperal eclampsia.* Here it is allied to *Zinc.* The attack is preceded by a *hot rush up the spine into the head.*

In *Chorea, Caustic.* suits when the patient cannot sleep; *cannot sleep* because of the contortions ; tongue heavy, words are jerked out: twitching of the mouth. *Phosph.* suits the spinal form ; walks, as if paralyzed; makes mis-steps from weakness; indicated when the *child grows too rapidly.*

Rheumatism

Causticum	Phosphorus
Rheumatic diathesis ; flexors contracted ; shortening from contracted tendons ; *stiffness and swelling of joints ;* worse from cold, better from the warmth of the bed. Rheumatism attacks the head, with roaring, burning in the ears, deafness, nausea.	Rheumatism not so well-marked, drawing, tearing, *tight* feeling in the affected part ; worse from cold weather. Rheumatism always affects the chest with oppression, cough, dyspnœa forcing the patient to sit up (endocarditis).

Fever

Causticum	Phosphorus
Chill mostly left-sided ; better from drinking, in bed, in warm room ; worse after eating.	Chill right-sided ; better from drinking and from eating (the accompanying debility); worse in bed and in a warm room.
Heat from 6 to 8 P. M. ; flushes of heat followed by chilliness; heat descends. Heat not so prominent as the chill.	Heat predominates ; *anxiety ;* burning hands ; *heat ascends ; heat from the stomach into chest and throat ; heat causes frequent waking.*

CAUSTICUM	Skin	PHOSPHORUS
Sweat often directly follows the chill; profuse while walking outdoors; sour, 4 A.M.; increased when eating.		Sweat on head, hands, face, with increase of urine, *followed by great debility;* lessened from eating.
Thirst before the chill; thirst with aversion to drink.		Thirst in the heat; desire for drink without thirst.
Varicosities; net-like appearance of the capillaries.		Distended veins; red spots; petechiæ; hæmorrhages.
Pulse not much altered; sometimes frequent towards evening.		Pulse accelerated, full, hard; weak, small.
Orgasm of blood; congestions not marked (5).		Orgasm of blood; blood *excited by sensual impressions.*
Hæmorrhages of dark blood.		Hæmorrhages of bright red blood.

Sleep

CAUSTICUM	PHOSPHORUS
Sleep disturbed by colic or *spasmodic jerks of head and limbs.*	Sleep disturbed by *heat of the body;* or by oppression of the chest.

Skin

CAUSTICUM	PHOSPHORUS
Eruptions moist; *itch after abuse of Mercury* and *Sulphur; especially with large pustules;* eczema ani, *intertrigo.*	Eruptions dry; dry herpes; *eruption scaly, as psoriasis;* dry even if pustular.
Injuries of the skin which have been healed, suppurate again.	Injuries of the skin which have been healed, bleed; *small wounds bleed much.*
Warts, suppurating; warts on the *nose,* eye-lids.	Polypi; fungus hæmatodes; blood boils.

Blisters appear in the provings of either remedy. Under *Caust.* they resemble *burns, pemphigus.* Under *Phosph.* vesicles form in clusters *about the joints.*

CAUSTICUM	PHOSPHORUS
Superficial suppurations; as in run around (*Graph.*); ulcers *after burns* with throbbing, burning pains and watery pus.	*Phlegmonous inflammations;* chronic suppurating openings *with hectic* (*Silicea*); ulcers often with caries, painless or with a "festering" sensation; *bleeding.*

(5) *Caust.* has red face, congestion to head with roaring, as during stool; flushes after walking; *film before the eyes, blindness, hot head, during pregnancy.* But *Phosph.* has the circulation disturbed by the slightest external impression as well as by emotional causes. Congestions with stasis are common in all vascular parts. Characteristically, *Caust.* has predominant *chilliness; Phosph.* predominant *heat.*

CAUSTICUM	Generalities	PHOSPHORUS
Restlessness of the legs in the evening; anxiety, afraid of the dark.		*Restless moving because of burning heat; anxiety at twilight.*
Pains better *in bed* and in wet weather.		Pains better in dry weather; worse in *change of weather.*
Cold air aggravates the colic and paralysis; sensitive to cold air.		Cold air relieves the head but aggravates the chest symptoms; sensitive to cold air.
Washing improves.		Washing aggravates.
Colic better, throat and chest worse, from bending forward.		Generally worse from bending forward.
Abuse of *Euphras., Asaf., Plumb., Coloc., China, Sulph.* and *Merc.* (itch).		Abuse of *Iodine, Nat. Mur.* (excessive salt eating), *Turpentine,* over-doses of *Camphor.*
Compare with *Coloc., Cham., Staph., Cupr., Lach., Sepia, Graph., Sulph., Rhus, &c.*		Compare with *Nux V., China, Camph., Petroleum, Carbo Veg., Kali. C., Sulph., Calc. C., Rhus, Silicea, &c.*

Frequently agreeing in symptoms, but, for some unknown reason, *found to be* INIMICAL.

COFFEE, TEA, COCA *

Coffee increases the intellectual activity; congestions. *Tea* does the same with excessive garrulity; nervousness.

Coffee renders the arteries tense; tense fibre; stomach feels tight after food; pulse quick but *force* lessened. *Tea* renders the arteries lax, stomach, as if it would sink; pulse intermits.

Give *Coffee* as a drink when weary from travel in the heat, *with deprivation of food;* also in diarrhœa from overwork with *too much care.*

Give *Tea* as a drink for the bad effects of a walk in the sun, especially when followed by difficult breathing.

Give *Coca* in fatigue from climbing mountains, especially in old, short-breathed persons, and in states of the atmosphere when *the barometer stands low.* All three increase the nitrogenous bodies by

---

* These comparisons of some hygienic value, are taken from the N. A. J. H., Vol. III. No. 11, with some additions. The *Coca* must not be confounded with cocoa. It is the plant used by the natives to aid them in the ascent of the Andes, not a beverage.

COFFEE, TEA, COCA

diminished tissue waste (less urea, uric acid, &c.). Hence *Tea* and *Coffee* are injurious to the young but beneficial to the old.

Coffee should be used by wine drinkers; *Tea* by beer drinkers (C. Hering).

Coffee and *Tea* stimulate the intellect ; *Coca*, the motility.

CHELIDONIUM		NUX VOMICA
	Mind	
Low spirited, weeps yet knows no reason ; must move about. Sometimes violent bursts of anger.		Fearful, hypochondriacal, but more uniformly irascible, cross. *Over-sensitive to external impressions.*
	Head	
Heaviness of occiput, can scarcely raise the head; *pains thence to left ear,* headaches worse sneezing, coughing ; better *while eating, but worse after.*		Bruised, aching in the occiput ; *feeling, as of a nail driven in the head ;* headaches worse *stooping,* moving, even moving eyes ; *after eating, especially dinner.*
	Eyes, Face, Ears	
Face yellow, conjunctivæ yellow ; or face sunken, gray, eyes surrounded by blue borders.		Conjunctivæ yellow ; face yellow, and *at the same time, florid,* pale, sunken face, blue or yellow around the eyes.
Supra-orbital right-sided neuralgia; *lachrymation.*		Supra-orbital left-sided neuralgia ; eyes injected.
Inflames the lachrymal sac ; epiphora ; lachrymal fistula.		Inflames the inner canthus, circumscribed extravasations of blood.
Roaring like wind in the ears ; *sensation, as if wind were rushing out ; pressure in the occiput towards the left ear;* tearing from the ear into the teeth ; ears obstructed during cough.		Reverberation of sounds in the ears ; otalgic pains extending to the forehead and temples ; pains into the middle ears, tympana feel, as if pressed outward, while swallowing.
	Mouth, Throat	
Toothache worse in bed, better from cold water.*		Toothache better from warm food ; worse from coffee.
Tongue narrow, pointed, thickly furred.		Tongue white or yellow, especially on the base.

CHELIDONIUM	Mouth, Throat — NUX VOMICA
Tightness around the neck, as if constricted; hinders swallowing; feeling as after swallowing too large a morsel.	Throat feels scraped, raw, and as if too narrow; sensation, as of a plug in the throat.

Stomach, Abdomen

CHELIDONIUM	NUX VOMICA
Taste bitter; but food tastes natural.	Taste mostly sour; food tasteless.
Desire for wine, coffee, milk; they agree; aversion to cheese cold food, boiled meats.	Desire for fats; they disagree; for brandy; aversion to coffee, it disagrees; coffee, milk, beer, water, do not taste right.*
Pains like gastralgia *relieved while eating.*	Pains like gastralgia *worse from food or drink.*
Stitches through the liver to the back; pain under the angle of the right scapula; powerful palpitation.	Pressure and stinging in the region of the liver; cannot bear clothing tight; stitches worse from motion or contact.
Costive, stools like sheep's dung, but more frequently *bright-yellow, thin diarrhœa.*	*Costive with ineffectual urging, or stools small, frequent; dysenteric, mucous stools.*

Urine, Genitals

CHELIDONIUM	NUX VOMICA
Urine rather profuse, frequent; dark or reddish, uric acid sediment.	Urine seldom and scanty; generally light-colored, sediment reddish.*
Daily burning in the vagina at the same hour.	Swelling and burning of the vagina.*
Menses retarded, but last too long.	Menses too early and too profuse.

Chest

CHELIDONIUM	NUX VOMICA
Pneumonia, capillary bronchitis, dark red face, great oppression with fan-like motion of the alæ nasi, *bright yellow diarrhœa.*	Pneumonia not characteristic, but sometimes with prominent bronchial catarrh, *in drunkards,* gastric symptoms; *costive.*
Palpitation forcibly lifting the clothing.	Anxious palpitation; heart feels tired.

Back, Limbs

CHELIDONIUM	NUX VOMICA
Pain under the angle of the right shoulder-blade.	*Tension and aching between the shoulder-blades.*
Tearing in the lowermost lumbar vertebra extending to the iliac bones (Guernsey).	Lumbar spine aches, *worse when attempting to turn over in bed.*

CHELIDONIUM	NUX VOMICA
Back, Limbs	
Rheumatism, cannot bear the least touch; sweat but no relief.	Rheumatism mostly of large muscles; *cannot bear the least jar.*
Sleep	
Wants to sleep, but cannot; very drowsy all day (jaundice).	Goes to sleep late, *awakens* 3 A.M., *falls again asleep awaking feeling tired.*
Dreams of corpses, journeyings, music, *vivid.*	Dreams sad or frightful mutilations, confused.*
Fever	
Chill begins in hands and feet; wakeful during the chill.	Chill begins in the back or limbs or whole body, not lessened by warmth; *sleep between chill and heat.**
Shaking chills while walking out, even in summer; better in warm room.	Chills just as soon as he moves the bed-clothing.
Heat not characterized.	*Chilly, if move* during the heat.
Generalities	
Pricking pains now here, now there.	Numbness in different parts.
Itching changing place and finally relieved by scratching.	Burning itching or stinging after scratching.*
Worse afternoon, evening and night.	Remission evening until 12 P.M. *

Chelidon. is predominantly *better* and *Nux worse* after eating, wine, sour things, milk, coffee. *Chelidon.* is predominantly *worse* and *Nux better* from chilly weather (damp), in bed.*

CHELIDONIUM	SANGUINARIA
Mind, Head	
Anxiety, must move about; *weeps and knows not why.*	Anxiety, *irritability; cannot bear to hear persons walk across the room.*
Occiput *so heavy he can hardly lift his head;* pressure to the left ear; head worse from sneezing, stooping, open air; *better from eating.*	*Headache from occiput to forehead, over right eye; periodical;* worse from *noises,* light, stooping, motion, eating, better from lying still and after sleep.

---

* From a contribution by Dr. J. B. Bell. Other symptoms from this kind of fever are so incorporated as to render distinction impossible.

CHELIDONIUM Eyes, Face, Ears SANGUINARIA

CHELIDONIUM	SANGUINARIA
Pupils contracted.	Pupils dilated.
Profuse lachrymation with neuralgia, using eyes, and as a result of fistula lachrymalis.	Burning lachrymation as a symptom of catarrh, coryza, raw throat, cough, diarrhœa.
Rushing as of wind out of the ears. Deafness during cough.	Tinnitus from congestion ; ears hot ; *oversensitive to noises.*
Mostly dry coryza, one side obstructed ; or fluent with thick blood in the morning.	Mostly fluent right-sided coryza; hot discharge, eye waters, throat raw finally diarrhœa. Polypus.
Face yellow ; gray, sunken, blue around the eyes. Face *dark-red in pneumonia, capillary-bronchitis.*	Face pale, swollen around the eyes ; *bright red circumscribed cheeks; or, livid in typhoid pneumonia. Veins swollen.*
Supra-orbital neuralgia ; worse right side, copious lachrymation.	*Supra-orbital right-sided neuralgia ; relieved only by holding the head to the floor.*

Mouth, Throat

CHELIDONIUM	SANGUINARIA
Toothache worse in bed, better from cold water.	Toothache, decayed tooth, worse from cold drinks.
Tongue *narrow, pointed* (dyspepsia) ; furred.	Tongue, *as if scalded;* coated white, (loss of appetite).
Taste *bitter ;* food tastes natural.	Fatty, slimy, taste ; sweets taste bitter.

On the throat the two remedies have but little similarity of action. *Chelidonium* inflames the fauces, but, as will be seen, its main action is on the larynx. *Sanguinaria,* on the other hand, causes ulceration of the mouth and fauces:—Mouth, gums and roof sore, burning ; throat feels, as if scalded, tonsils swollen, worse the right: pearly diphtheritic exudation : worse from swallowing sweets ; throbbing in the head, red cheeks ; distended temporal veins.

Stomach, Abdomen

CHELIDONIUM	SANGUINARIA
Longs for milk, hot drinks, coffee ; they agree.	Loss of appetite with craving for piquant food.
Aversion to cheese, boiled meats.	Aversion to butter.
Gastralgia with gnawing pains in the stomach made better from continued eating.	Gastric catarrh, burning; tongue and lips red ; throat hot ; eating relieves the sensation of nausea.
Hepatic congestion with sharp stitch pains, pains under the right scapula; clay-colored or	Hepatic symptoms less marked; *like a hot stream from breast to liver ;* yellow stools less

CHELIDONIUM	SANGUINARIA
Stomach, Abdomen	
bright yellow, thin stools; colic from portal congestion, with great heat, contraction of the navel; headache behind the eyes and in occiput.	characteristic than in *Chelidon.;* colic with much flatulence and torpor of the liver; *sick headache over the right eye,* nausea, vomiting of bile.
Stool *bright yellow, thin;* or dry, in hard lumps; white, clay-colored.	Stool yellow, thin, undigested; *much offensive flatus; terminotes the catarrh.*
Urine, Genitals	
Sharp spasmodic pains in the kidneys and bladder; urine greenish (bile) or deposits red sediment.	Pain in the left hypochondrium with copious, pale, urine; urine yellow, (bile); reddish sediment.
Menses too late, profuse and last too long; pain under angle of right scapula.	Menses too early, black offensive blood; sick headache from occiput over right eye.
Burning in the vegina periodically at the same hour.	Discharge of flatus from the vagina; climacteric changes.
Milk vanished.	Nipples sore, burn.
Larynx, Chest	
Hoarse periodically every day 5 P. M.; *dry, hard, spasmodic cough* as from dust in the larynx; spasm of the glottis in expiration; constriction across the upper part of the larynx; worse in the morning, (cough).	Aphonia wih swollen larynx; *rawness, burning; ulcers;* dry, cough ceases when flatus is passed up and down; *or as soon as diarrhœa ensues; wheezing, whistling cough;* worse at night and lying with the head low (1).
Pneumonia or capillary bronchitis with bilious complications; loose rattling cough; *bright, yellow, thin diarrhœa;* in severe cases, dark-red cheeks, great dyspnœa with fan-like motion of the alæ nasi; *one hot and one cold foot.*	Pneumonia with marked vascular disturbance; rust-colored sputa; little pain or simply burning; *circumscribed red cheeks;* great dyspnœa; in severe cases, livid face and hands; quick, small pulse, weak feeling at the heart; extensive hepatization (2).
Heart beats so forcibly as to raise the clothing, (bilious complaints).	Palpitation violent, felt in the head, constriction of the stomach, *deathly nausea.*

---

(1) *Sanguinaria* corresponds more to inflammation and ulceration; *Chelid.* offers more spasmodic symptoms. *Sanguin.*, with its peculiar cough has cured croup (J. B. Bell) and is similar in pseudo-membranous croup to *Kali Bich.* (*Nichol.*)

(2) It is now known that one great danger in pneumonia is heart-failure. The symptoms of *Sang.* point to its use in just such an emergency.

CHELIDONIUM	SANGUINARIA
Larynx, Chest	
Pulse full, hard but not much accelerated; or, small and rapid (cap. bronchitis).	Pulse frequent, full; or quick, small; frequency and force reduced (pneumonia).

Back, Limbs

CHELIDONIUM	SANGUINARIA
Pain under the angle of the scapula.	Pressure and pain along the inner border of the left scapula.
Rheumatism not so well-marked as in *Sanguin.* Tearing pains, parts will not bear the least touch; sweat gives no relief.	Rheumatism especially of the *right deltoid,* muscles of the back; parts sparely covered are sensitive to touch; sweat relieves the pains; pains shift (3).
Nails blue, joints of the fingers yellow, cold.	Livid hands (pneumonia); roots of the nails ulcerate one after the other.
One foot cold, one hot (pneumonia).	Feet generally burn.

Sleep

CHELIDONIUM	SANGUINARIA
Sleepy yet cannot get to sleep.	Restless, dreamy sleep; awakens frightened, as if falling.

Fever

CHELIDONIUM	SANGUINARIA
Irregular circulation; dark-red face; one cold, one warm foot; one ear cold, one warm; palms hot; veins of hands and arms swollen.	Irregular circulation; hectic red cheeks; hot streaming from chest to abdomen; flushes of heat at climaxis; feet, hands burn; veins swollen, especially temples.
Chilly in the open air, even in summer.	Chilly and hot alternately.
Heat with the colic; heat with *dark-red* cheeks; cold feet; short breath, nausea.	*Flushes of heat; hectic with bright red cheeks;* nausea, sick headache; dyspnœa.
Sweat ceases on awaking.	Profuse sweat; cold sweat.

Generalities

CHELIDONIUM	SANGUINARIA
Itching with jaundice.	Itching precedes the nausea (4).
Old, putrid, spreading ulcers (Lippe).	Indolent ulcers, no pain, dry, sharp cut edges (W. Wesselhœft).

---

(3) *Sanguin.,* is an excellent remedy in acute rheumatism, worse from motion at night; pains are throbbing, burning and there are spasmodle pains in the joints. When metastasis to the heart occurs from external application to the affected joint, *Sanguin.* or *Kalmia* (according to Hering) will be of great service.

(4) Bute proposes *Sanguinaria* as the quickest antidote to *Rhus.*

HEPAR	SULPHUR
Mind	
Malicious mood.	Changeable mood; hypochondriacal.
Irritability; vehement, *hasty speech and hasty drinking.*	Irritable, peevish; *restless,* hasty temper; *haste in working or walking* (1).
Anxiety in *the evening driving to suicide; after abuse of Mercury.*	Anxiety with *doubts about his salvation;* with desire to escape.
Apprehensive about his relations.	Thinks only of himself; cares nothing for the salvation of others.

Sulphur is by far the most important in weak memory. *Hepar* has weakness of thoughts, sits speechless in a corner, *worse when out of humor. Sulph.* has *misplacing or misapplication of words; answers are given slowly, as if comprehension was difficult;* or the words spoken to him are repeated, as if difficult of comprehension. Here we find a well-confirmed indication for *Sulph., when a typhoid state is impending.*

The imagination is active in *Sulphur.* The patient fancies that *rags are fine dresses,* that he is happy, contented; this state may alternate with sadness. *Hepar* preserves unchangeably a despondent mood.

Head

HEPAR	SULPHUR
Vertigo from riding in a carriage; reflex from the abdomen, with diminished peristaltic action; in hysteria with hyperæsthesia of smell.	Vertigo worse sitting; crossing a stream; on rising from bed; with nose-bleed; with increased peristaltic action (Kafka); with chronic irritating discharges.

Sulph. has a wide range. Thus, it cures congestions to the head: *throbbing deep in the brain; throbbing of the heart and carotids; humming in the head; headache with throbbing, increasing with the increase of fever.*

Gastric headaches, periodically returning every week. Nervous forms, with stitch, pains over the left eye, setting in during the evening and reaching an acme during the night.

Hepar has less to do here with congestion. In nervous forms it attacks the *right* temple and supra-orbital region, causing a sensation as of *a nail boring* in the head; better from *binding the head tightly; worse in the morning.* Like *Sulph.,* there is sensitiveness to

(1) The *Sulph.* patient is often full-blooded, fat, but always nervous, hasty in temper and motion, thus contrasting with its near relative *Calc. Carb.*

HEPAR	Head	SULPHUR

cold air and aggravation from motion or touch; but in *Hepar* the soreness is a characteristic *bruised feeling, as though a boil were forming—sore as a boil.* In catarrhal headaches, *Hepar* is most important. Uncovering the head, every exposure to cold, especially *to dry, cold, west winds* causes headache, coryza, &c. *Sulph.* might be preferable if change of weather, evening air, getting wet or checking sweat was the cause.

HEPAR	SULPHUR
Nodosities on the head, sore to touch, better from covering the head warmly.	Inflammation of the bones and caries, with a feeling of a band around the head.
Eruption on the scalp *moist,* fetid; itching *worse on rising in the morning.*	Eruption on the back part of the head and behind the ears, *dry;* scratching relieves; skin *rough, dry.*

Ears

Sulph. has more action on the optic nerve, amblyopia from inveterate use of alcohol; from suppressed eruptions; after onanism.

It is in scrofulous affections of the eyes that the two remedies most intimately resemble each other.

HEPAR	SULPHUR
Eye-lids *feel sore, as if bruised;* patient dreads to have them touched.	Eye-lids swollen, conjunctiva *protruding like a bag.*
Edges of the lids swollen, studded *with pustules: pimples around the eye.*	Edges of the lids swollen, *red, covered with dry scurf,* itching continually.
Right eye; preferable when *suppuration with throbbing pains predominates; better from warmth.*	*Left eye;* preferable when the eye is *painfully dry;* worse in a *warm room* or in *warm weather.*

Eyes

In catarrhal deafness both are valuable. In the congestive forms of deafness, *Sulph.* is the remedy. It is associated with tendency of blood to the head; abdominal plethora, piles, &c.

In nervous forms *Sulph.* gives us deafness *preceded by oversensitiveness to noises.* Sometimes as with earache, there is sensitiveness to sounds, *music nauseates.*

HEPAR	SULPHUR
Deafness of catarrhal origin; after suppressed itch, scarlatina.	Deafness of catarrhal origin after *suppressed itch;* variola.
Earache, the external ear *sensitive to the least touch, feels bruised;* throbbing and stitching pains, indicating approaching suppuration (after *Bell.*)	Earache with stitches into the throat and head; great *burning heat; congestions to the head;* slightest sounds produce nausea.

HEPAR	SULPHUR
Ears	
Otorrhœa, fetid or purulent; mastoid cells involved. *When after Bell., &c., suppuration threatens or begins.*	Otorrhœa, chronic, bloody, fetid; mostly from the left ear. *When after otitis the discharge will not yield.*
Face	
Face yellow; blue around the eyes; eyes prominent.	Face yellow or pale, blue around the eyes; eyes sunken.
Face hot and fiery red.	Circumscribed red cheeks; *face blotched, red.*
Erysipelas of the face coming early in the morning, disappearing rapidly; *eyes remain bluish red, and feel sore to pressure.*	Erysipelas of the face beginning by a redness of the right ear and spreading thence over the face; excellent to prevent relapses.
Eruption on the face, corners of mouth, &c., of yellow vesicles very painful, *sore as a boil.*	Eruption dryer than in *Hepar*; skin of the face *rough, red*; lips dry, rough or *bright-red.*
Prosopalgia worse from dry, cold, west winds; associated with coryza, hoarseness, rheumatic pains; worse on the right side; after *Bell.* or abuse of *Merc.*	Prosopalgia, especially in chronic cases after other remedies fail; associated with scanty menses, constipation; worse on the left side; after *Merc.*
Nose, Mouth, Throat	
Smell sometimes too acute with vertigo; generally blunted.	Smell too sensitive; or subjective smell as of human fæces.
Coryza one-sided *with headache at every exposure; after Mercury; dry, cold west winds; croupy cough* (2).	Burning coryza in the open air, stopped up in the room; *rough screaming cough, raw throat, deep voice.*
Catarrh from every cold wind, *borders of the nostrils become sore, swollen; throbbing "cold sores" on the lips.*	Chronic catarrh, discharge yellow, thick or green; through the posterior nares; dry ulcers and scabs; smell as of old catarrh.
Nose red swollen; *sore, as if a boil were forming.* Small boils form in the nose, especially after abuse of *Mercury.*	External nose swollen; *often redness of the nose, worse in warmth.* Hepatic saddle across the nose; freckles; comedones.
Toothache with swollen gums, *throbbing, as if suppuration*	Toothache with "jumping" pain; throbbing pain, swelling

(2) *Hepar,* unless indicated by abuse of *Mercury* or accompanied by a croupy cough, has better not be given in the beginning of a cold. It is best adapted to the later symptoms, especially after the cough becomes loose.

HEPAR	Nose, Mouth, Throat — SULPHUR
had begun; worse in a warm room and at night.	around old stumps; worse in the evening and in the open air.
Offensive smell from the mouth after abuse of *Merc.*	Putrid smell in the morning; also after *Merc.*
Taste sour.	Taste sour, saltish, putrid.
Tip of tongue feels sore and as if burned, awaking him.	Tip of tongue red; dorsum dry and usually white.
Ulceration of mouth and throat after *Mercury;* ptyalism, ulcers with a lardaceous base.	Aphthæ, with bleeding gums, ptyalism; often after *Merc.* and in children when the stools *excoriate the anus.*
Tonsillitis when *pus begins to form.*	Tonsillitis when the abscess has broken but does not heal.
Sensation, *as of a splinter* in the throat, stitches into the ears; worse from swallowing soliva solids and after eating.	Sensation, as of a *plug* or of a *hair* in the throat; worse from swallowing saliva and from solids.

Stomach, Abdomen

HEPAR	SULPHUR
Longing for sour things, wine, pickles, for condiments; for brandy; they relieve the goneness and produce a feeling of strength.	Longing more for beer than for wine; great aversion to milk, it causes vomiting; especially inebriates, filthy in habits.
Eating relieves pains in the stomach; but is followed by fulness and pressure demanding the loosening of the clothing.	Eating produces pain, better bending double; fulness and pressure as in *Hepar* with a weight on the chest, making breathing diffiiult.

Sulph., far more than *Hepar,* deranges the portal circulation. It will cure *hard, swollen* liver with jaundice, vomiting of food and sometimes of blood; piles; bloated abdomen. It will relieve colic, abdominal tension after eating, headache, dizziness, palpitation, &c., caused by a *suppression of hæmorrhoidal discharges.*. *Hepar,* as well as *Sulph.,* has sharp stitching pains in the region of the liver, worse from motion. It suits in *hepatic abscess; Sulph.* in chronic hepatitis.

HEPAR	SULPHUR
Stool passed with much urging, even though papescent; insufficient peristaltic action.	Stool passed with difficulty; *much urging, tenesmus; urging continues after stool.*
Diarrhœa green, slimy, sour; the *child smells sour.*	Diarrhœa green, slimy or watery, sour, putrid, purulent; tenesmus an hour or so after.
Diarrhœa with weak digestion after *Mercury and Quinine;*	Diarrhœa hurrying the patient out of bed in the morning;

HEPAR **Stomach, Abdomen** **SULPHUR**

HEPAR	SULPHUR
weak empty feeling, longing for strong food ; better after eating (stomach).	weak, hungry, about 11 A.M.: pains are worse after eating (colic).

Urine, Genitals

HEPAR	SULPHUR
Frequent desire to urinate but the bladder is so weak he must wait long ; water drops perpendicularly.	Frequent urging from catarrh affecting the neck of the bladder ; urine passes in drops ; urging continues after.
Sediment whitish ; urine flocculent, turbid (3).	Sediment more often reddish, sandy.
Gonorrhœa when the discharge is purulent after abuse of *Mercury*.	Gonorrhœa with a whitish, mucous discharge ; also after the failure of well-chosen remedies.

Sulph. has more influence over the sexual organs. Seminal emissions often yield to it ; and it also has a remarkable effect in curing the tendency to masturbation. Both have relaxed organs, prostatorrhœa.

Larynx, Chest

Hoarseness with *deep, bass-voice,* belongs rather to *Sulph.*; especially if caused by *damp, evening air or damp, cold weather.* Hoarseness from *dry, cold winds,* belongs to *Hepar ;* morning aggravation.

HEPAR	SULPHUR
Cough, dry, hoarse or a *combination of rattling with croupy cough ; worse towards morning.*	Cough, dry, short, hacking ; spasmodic with constriction of the chest ; worse in the evening.
Sneezing and crying after cough.	Coughing preceded by sneezing.
Pneumonia (children) in the stage of resolution; with suffocative accumulation in the chest.	Pneumonia; especially indicated in the *stage of exudation* and when resolution delays.
Tuberculosis of the lungs ; especially first stage ; *croupy, rattling* cough ; disposed to bronchitis with loud mucous rattling ; the least *exposure of a part of the body causes cough ; mucous accumulation in the morning when going into the cold air ; sweats easi-*	Tuberculosis of the lungs, especially indicated as a *preventive, when there are congestions to head and chest ; dry, teasing, night cough ;* breath hot ; *pain like a rivet through the upper third of the left lung to the scapula ;* sweats ; flashes of heat ; *burn-*

(3) Kafka proposed *Hepar* in Bright's disease because it has a relation to croupuus exudations. Buchner denies that the exudation can be fibrinous and prefers remedies which produce an afibrinous state of the blood. Still several post-scarlatinal cures with *Hepar* are reported, and we must not neglect it on pathological grounds.

HEPAR **Larynx, Chest** **SULPHUR**

HEPAR

ly and turns *pale* from exertion, followed by burning of the cheeks and palms of the hands.

Asthma in *croupy* patients, must sit up with the head *thrown back ; swelling under the larynx ;* suddenly aroused from sleep after midnight; *little or no vascular excitement ;* often in catarrhs during the accumulation of *tenacious* mucus.

Pleurisy with fibrinous exudation.

Catarrhs are best cured by *Hepar* when exudation has taken place; given too soon, it often retards cure.

Whooping cough with great susceptibility *to cold air ;* pains in one spot in the larynx; suffocation compelling to sit upright and *throw the head back ;* anxious, *whistling respiration ;* weakness of the chest, making speaking difficult; throbbing of the carotids; swelling *about the ankles* with difficult breathing; sweat on the head and face; *hastiness ; crying after ;* eyes *protruding; sneezing after ;* worse after *cold* drinks; cough in paroxysms which follow each other rapidly. Applicable to those dangerous cases which become complicated with *croupous exudation.*

SULPHUR

ing of the feet; desire to uncover.

Asthma arising from suppressed eruptions, *especially itch ; or* from suppression of *chronic discharges;* periodical, spasmodic stinging in the back; *congestion to the chest; comes on in sleep,* when turning over in bed or in the evening.

Pleurisy with more serous than fibrinous exudation.

Catarrhs which come to a standstill, have resisted other medicines; organic changes threatening (4).

Whooping cough in children *who dread being washed ;* are worse or have relapses in *damp weather ;* difficult respiration at night, *constriction worse bringing the arms together ; burning* from chest to face; feeling, as if the lungs *touched the back ;* palpitation of the heart; *lump in the abdomen;* feet cold, cold sweat; *cold sweat on face ; hasty temper;* crying; eyes *sunken ;* nose-bleed; worse after food or drink; cough in *two paroxysms* following each other quickly. Applicable in the most serious forms; also as an *intercurrent when others fail to act.*

Sulph. far more than *Hepar* disturbs the circulation. It may be assumed as a general characteristic that *Sulph.* causes congestion to all parts, scarcely ever being of use unless the vascular system' is deranged. See headache; eyes (congestion in warm room, hot weather); ears (external ears red, &c.); face (red blotches, &c.);

(4) *Sulph.* is an admirable remedy when a cough becomes chronic, mucous rales through the chest are heard; the patient loses appetite, sweats at night and fears phthisis. Expectoration may be purulent or even bloody. *Sulph.* 2c. or higher, three or four doses daily for a week, will generally restore health.

HEPAR	Larynx, Chest	SULPHUR

nose (red, whether or not caused by alcohol ; nose-bleed) ; chest (asthma, hæmoptysis, pleurisy with congestion of the lungs, pneumonia, palpitation towards evening from rush of blood) ; abdomen (plethora, portal fulness, hæmorrhoids, hæmorrhages from the bowels, &c.) ; genitals (exciting to onanism, emissions, sweat of the parts ; congestion to the uterus, &c.) ; limbs (congestion, varices). See also Fever.

Hepar causes an orgasm of blood, throbbing of the blood-vessels ; congestions following exposure to dry, cold winds.

HEPAR	SULPHUR
Palpitation of the heart with a feeling of debility about the heart; stitches in the heart and left chest, worse in the cold air and from uncovering. Hypertrophy, relieving the weakness of the chest and anxiety.	Palpitation from climbing hills ; from congestion to the chest ; the heart feels, as if too large for the chest ; stitches in the side after vigorous exercise. Pain through the left chest to the back ; red lips ; sleepiessness ; after suppresed itch.

The pulse is almost identical. *Sulph.* claims precedence in the beginning of inflammatory diseases with pulse full, hard ; skin dry, hot.

Neck, back

HEPAR	SULPHUR
Symptoms of the back worse from *contact ; bruised feeling, as if a boil were forming.*	Bruised feeling, stiffness ; more a sensation, as if *the back had been sprained.*
Weakness of the whole spine.	Weakness, paraplegia ; urine retained (5).

Limbs

HEPAR	SULPHUR
Rheumatism, parts hot, swollen, red ; strained feeling ; profuse sweat ; nocturnal pains worse during the chill or when becoming cold. Excessive susceptibility to pain.	Rheumatism, with or without swelling ; erratic pains ; shortening of the tendons ; pains worse in dampness, after working in water ; after washing. Loss of power, numbness.
Cramps in the thighs or calves and pelvis when the limbs are drawn up.	*Cramps in the calves, mostly at night; also with loose bowels* (cholera).
Soles of the feet sore when walking.	Cramps of the soles of the feet when walking.
Soles of the feet burn ; must uncover ; anxiousness (6)	Soles of the feet burn ; puts them out of bed, tries to find a cool place for them.

---

(5) See note (9), page 106.

(6) Uncovering with relief is exceptional here. The anxiousness is characteristic, being a part of the *Hepar* susceptibility to pain.

Sleep

HEPAR	SULPHUR
Twitching of the body after lying down; must move the limbs to and fro ; sadness.	In going to sleep one leg is suddenly drawn up and shot out again.
Starts up from sleep, as if in a fright, *suffocating*.	Sleeps in "*cat-naps*" : starts up from congestion, fright, &c.
Profound sleep *with the head thrown back*.	Profound sleep, *eyes half open* (cerebral diseases).
Changes sides because the parts feel bruised, as if a boil were forming.	Turns on his back during sleep; yet it may cause rush of blood to the head.

Fever

HEPAR	SULPHUR
Before and during the chill, nettle-rash, *fever-blister*, tetter on the chest ; excitable.	Before the chill, thirst ; during the chill, pale, cold face ; or heat of the face, *delirium*.
Chill from 4 to 8 P. M. ; or in the night aggravating all complaints.	Chill from 5 to 8 P.M. ; or in the forenoon; begins in the feet or runs up the back; chill in bed.
Dry, burning heat, redness of the feet and violent thirst all night ; flushes with sweat. *Worse from uncovering*.	Intense heat at night without thirst ; frequent flushes of heat ; cold feet, hot vertex. Not worse from uncovering.
Sweat day and night, without relief.	Worse with and after sweat.
Sweats offensive, sour ; on the chest and forehead.	Sweat sour, empyreumatic, *with itching;* on the hands ; one side ; or only on body.
Sweat day and night ; sweat on the back after worrisome dreams.	Night-sweats mostly on the occiput and neck; worse A. M. *after awaking*.
Intermitting type of fever with nettle rash ; with coryza, cough, distress in the chest; or with bitter taste, bilious vomiting, diarrhœa ; weakness of the stomach from abuse of *Mercury*.	Intermitting type of fever or a remitting type with continued dry heat, harsh skin, no sweat; or no reaction, stupid ; slow in answering questions; after suppressed itch ; chronic cases.

Tissues

HEPAR	SULPHUR
The child exhales a *sour smell* ; with diarrhœa.	The child *has an offensive smell* not removable by washing.
Dropsy of cellular tissue and serous cavities is not marked; except perhaps after scarlatina.	Dropsy prominent ; after *Mercury*, after chills and fever, enlarged liver, &c. ; excellent in *absorption after pleurisy*.
Fibrinous exudation on serous membranes ; sensitive.	More serous than fibrinous exudation.

Tissues

HEPAR	SULPHUR
Croupous formations on mucous membranes; purulent mucus; *profuse secretion* of mucus; offensive mucus.	Thickening of mucous membranes; *purulent mucus;* or thick, viscid mucus; greenish-colored; smell *as of old catarrh.*
Weakness, *faint with the pains;* limbs weak and feel *bruised;* paralysis rare, except after *abuse of Mercury.*	Weakness; *walks stooped;* trembles; limbs give away; ***hungry*** 10 to 11 A.M.; *faint; flashes of heat; hot vertex, cold feet; paralysis marked.*
Itch with fat, *pustular* crusty eruption, after *Mercury.*	Itch, tingling, burning soreness; *dryness of the skin;* after *Mercury.*
Eczema and eruptions in general, usually moist, *pustular.* Scabs *dry in some parts, moist in others.*	Eczema and eruptions in general, usually dry; scaly. *Scabs dry,* cracked, itching, ***bleeding.***
Itching in the bends of the joints; eruptions *worse in the morning and after the use of salves,* worse from the *least touch.*	Itching general; scratching relieves the itching, but *causes burning, soreness and numbness; worse after washing.*
Ulcers *sensitive to contact,* easily bleeding, corrosive pains, burning, stinging; profuse suppuration; smell *like old cheese, lard-like base* (after *Merc.*).	Ulcers usually not sensitive; thus often in the beginning to prepare the way; suppuration thick yellow like *Hepar;* or thin offensive pus.
Abscesses (boils, &c.) large and extremely sore; throbbing, lancinating; thus *when pus begins to form; also after salves.*	Abscesses (boils, &c.), small chronic abscesses; in acute cases to expel the core after pus has formed; to destroy the tendency.
The slightest injuries produce suppuration and ulceration; pimples around the main diseased part.	Skin, rough, dry; or in chronic cases when slight wounds will not heal; rawness in the folds following erythema.
Superficial erysipelatous onychia around the nail or under, when suppuration threatens.	Beginning onychia under the suppuration to make the new nail, boring pains; also after nails grow rightly.
Panaritium with violent throbbing; it promotes suppuration.	Panaritium sometimes in the beginning, to prevent further progress.

HEPAR	**SULPHUR**
Tissues	
In scarlatina when croupous symptoms appear ; swelling and suppuration of the glands; also later when dropsy and albuminuria ensue ; with nose-bleed, bloated face, convulsions ; also for subsequent crops of boils.	In scarlatina when the body looks red, like a boiled lobster or red coalescing spots ; cerebral complications ; stupor, sudden starting, face bloated, shining, red ; nose and mouth dry, tongue-tip red ; later the eruption turns purple, diarrhœa, sopor.
In variola during the suppurating stage.	In variola when during suppuration delirium ensues.
Croupy, rattling cough, cannot raise the phlegm ; measles.	Catarrhal symptoms increase, the rash being tardy; severe cases, moist cough, raising pus ; measles.
Generalities	
Is best adapted to slow torpid constitutions ; lax fibre, light hair.	Best adapted to those who are quick, restless, even if fat ; dark or light.
Motion aggravates the pains ; better when at rest.	Worse beginning to move, from running ; better from continued moderate motion.
Worse from uncovering, especially uncovering *a part of the body.*	Generally better from uncovering ; pre-eminently *worse from washing.*
Worse from *dry, cold winds ;* from the least cold air ; improvement in damp weather, from warmth, wrapping up, from the warmth of the bed.	Worse from *changes of weather;* from cold air ; from *damp, evening air ;* often better in dry weather ; worse from the warmth of the bed, wrapping up, being near the fire.
Remission of complaints, afternoon.	Remission of complaints after noon and before midnight.
Not many symptoms return periodically See Chill, Fever.	Periodicity marked ; during full moon ; every spring, every 7 days ; neuralgia, &c.
Compare with: *Bellad.* (in inflammations, neuralgia, cough, erysipelas, toothache, after getting hair cut, headache, sleep, &c.) ; *Laches.* (dyspepsia, tonsillitis, croup, &c.) ; *Merc.* (anguish, crusta lactea, pustular eruptions, suppuration, otorrhœa, pimples	Compare with: *Bellad,* (in scarlatina, hydrocephalus, spasms, congestion of the brain &c.) ; *Merc.* (*Merc.* is a Hahnemannian intercurrent when *Sulph.* ceases to act; especially in the treatment of itch ; also compare iritis, eruption, abscesses, salivation, dysentery, bone and

HEPAR **Generalities** **SULPHUR**

and around ulcers, coryza, toothache, ulcers with lardaceous base, excessive sweats, glandular enlargements, salivation, bone-pains, &c.) ; *Spong.* (in croup, suffocation, aggravation from dry, cold winds, glandular swellings, &c.) ; *Nitric Acid* (ophthal. neonat., as *an antidote to Mercury,* &c.) ; *Silicea* (in nervousness, suppurations, boils, abscesses, bone affections, glandular diseases, unhealthy skin, felons, &c.); *Iodine, Metals, Kali Hyd., Cham.* (stools, skin) ; *Rheum.*

ANTIDOTES : *Bell., Cham.* Complementary to *Calend.* (in wounds).

glandular diseases, &c.) ; *Calcarea* (useful after *Sulph.* when the pupils grow large ; scrofula, ophthalmia, otorrhœa, foreign bodies in eye, chronic sore throat, aphthæ, hydrocephalus, congestions, asthma, diseases of the bones, burning or sweaty feet, flashes of heat, night-sweats, eruptions, &c., &c.) ; *Lach.* (dyspepsia, liver, &c.) ; *Acon.* (dry hot skin, sthenic fever); *Rhus* (*rheumatism,* getting wet, &c.) ; *Apis* (brain, urticaria, dropsy); *Puls.; Metals; Lycop.; Silicea ; Sepia ; Psorin.*

ANTIDOTES : *Puls., Cinchon., Rhus, Merc., Sep.* Complementary to *Aloes; Calc. C.*

IODINE **Mind** KALI HYD.

IODINE

Anxiety, *constantly on the move,* cannot even sleep ; *anxious, if he cannot eat.*

Shuns people, *especially the doctor;* want to cry during digestion.

KALI HYD.

Anxiety, *starts at the least noise ;* torturing anguish prevents sleep ; frantic ; *with catarrh or headache* (1).

Less sensitive to external impressions ; whining mood.

Head

IODINE

Pain like a tape drawn around the head.

Headache, as if the brain were stirred up ; fears he will go crazy.

KALI HYD.

Pain, as if the temples were *screwed in* (2).

Violent headaches, hard lumps on the cranium ; pains intense.

---

(1) This tendency to start belongs to all the *Kali Salts.* The frantic state is a part of the well-known "*Iodine* intoxication" ; but it is common enough after *Mercury,* when the dura mater and perhaps the brain itself are irritated. It will be well to compare note (8), and remember this symptom in pneumonia as there described.

(2) Quite a characteristic sensation.

IODINE	**Eyes**	**KALI HYD.**
Sparks before the eyes when sewing.		Screens the eyes, and yet light does not affect him.
Eyes protrude (as in Basedow's disease).		Eyes prominent from œdema, chemosis.

In scrofulous ophthalmia, the *Iodide* is preferable; when chemosis forms, and when *Mercury* has been abused.

Ears

Iodine	Kali Hyd.
Over-sensitive hearing, followed by deafness; deaf from Eustachian catarrh.	Sensation of a leaflet over the ear, yet not deaf; catarrhal deafness.

Nose

Iodine	Kali Hyd.
Coryza fluent in the open air; dull head; *cannot think;* posterior nares feel expanded.	*Coryza from abuse of Mercury;* comes from the least cold; *frantic excitation.*

Face, Mouth

Iodine	Kali Hyd.
Face pale, *yellow; frequently changing.*	Face pale (with the spasmodic attacks), *bloated.*
Toothache, with *yellow teeth;* gums full of blisters.	Toothache; feeling of a *worm crawling* at the root (3).
Aphthæ, no fetor; saliva profuse, watery (4).	Aphthæ; as if the mouth was coated with milk; saliva *viscid.*
Goitre *painless.*	Goitre *sentitive.*

Stomach, Bowels

Iodine	Kali Hyd.
Cold milk opens the bowels.	Cold milk aggravates the symptoms.
Better from eating a full meal (5).	Empty feeling not removed by eating.
Diarrhœa watery, foamy, *wheylike; fatty* (6).	Diarrhœa of serous mucus; *back feels, as if in a vise* (2).

Urine

Iodine	Kali Hyd.
Urine scanty; milky, variegated cuticle.	Urine copious, pale (7); scanty and bloody.

---

(3) A marked subjective sensation. It will be remembered that the root of the tooth is often the seat of decay in sycosis, indicating *Thuja,* and here *Kali Hyd.*

(4) *China* is preferable to *Iodine,* in salivation, after *Mercury;* salivation is not marked in the *Iodine.* Extreme fetor points more to *Kali Chlor.*

(5) A strong characteristic is this hunger of *Iodine.* The patient feels anxious if meals are not ready. He can eat often, yet he may be very thin,

(6) From its action on the glands, from this fatty diarrhœa, we know *Iodine* will render service in pancreatic atrophy.

(7) The *Kali Hyd.* may, other symptoms agreeing, cure diabetes mellitus. The *Iodine* has only scanty urine, according to Bœnninghausen. If Kafka, recommending *Kali Hyd.* for Morbus Brightii, because of its tendency to croupous formations, had advised it rather from its tendency to œdema, serous diarrhœa, &c. concur, and if gout or syphilis underlie the disease.

Genitals

IODINE

Sexual desire too strong.

Before menses, pressure on the bladder; during menses, pains in the back and ovaries; *weakness going up stairs.*

KALI HYD.

Sexual desire too weak.

Before menses, pressure on the bladder; during menses pains from groins into thighs; *thighs feel, as if squeezed* (2); chilly, head hot.

Larynx, Chest

IODINE

Hoarse, deep voice; cough from *tickling all over the chest;* dry cough or expectoration of clear mucus, or of *blood-streaked mucus;* worse during motion; emaciation with *morning* sweats, chest *intolerably weak* (8).

Croup with torpidity; child grasps the throat; wheezing, moist breathing; voice *deep;* worse in morning (9).

Palpitation from any exertion or after exertion; fainting, heart and chest feel weak; heart feels cramped.

Cardiac disease with purring feelings; worse when just rising or after exercise.

KALI HYD.

Hoarse, nasal voice; cough from roughness in the throat; dry or profuse expectoration of *greenish pus or like soap-suds;* worse during rest; emaciation with exhausting *night-*sweats and loose stools; *great oppression.*

Croup with hyperæthesia, awakens about 5 A.M. *with* great oppression, *loss* of voice, smothering.

Palpitation when walking; fluttering on awaking, giddy, must get up or smother.

Cardiac disease with darting pains; after the abuse of *Mercury* (10).

Back, Limbs

Rheumatism and gout belong to both; the pains are *worse at night, after Mercury,* jerkings. *Iodine* is preferable in gout after rich living; the *Iodide* in combinations of syphilis, rheumatism and mercurialization; the limbs are contracted.

---

(8) Such symptoms distinguish the two in pneumonia, phthisis, &c. When œdema occurs *Kali Hyd.* is preferable, (hence the *soap-suds sputa*). When suppuration occurs the *Kali Hyd.* is preferable, (night-sweats, alternate dry and sweaty skin, sputa are *green, purulent*). Again, when hepatization is so extensive as to seriously impede respiration, or when co-existing œdema renders breathing difficult, and we find bluish, bloated face; urine suppressed, apoplectic symptoms, dilated pupils, *Kali Hyd.* may save the patient. Here *Bell.* would certainly fail.

(9) *Iodine* cures croup in black-eyed children; this is not yet noticed under the *Iodide.*

(10) *Iodine* gives us the symptoms of functional and incipient organic heart disease. It is the character of the *Iodide* to produce *repeated attacks;* thus rendering the disease chronic; the remnant of each inflammation forming a salient point for subsequent attacks. See Rindfleish.

IODINE	KALI HYD.
Back, Limbs	
White swelling, second and third stages; fistulous openings discharging a thin, watery ichor, and surrounded by pale, spongy edges, which bleed easily; restless, continually moving.	White swelling, doughy (11), spongy, no fluctuation, skin tense, red in spots, hot. Internal feeling of heat; gnawing, boring pains at night forcing a change of position (*Raue*).
Sleep	
Dreams of *eating;* awakens weary, extensors ache; jerking.	Dreams vivid, cause him to start in his sleep (1) ; jerking.
Fever	
Thirst during the sweat.	Thirst during the chill.
Chill better arising from bed. Cold feet.	Chill, better in bed. Chilly up the back.
Fever with sallow face, *great languor, trembling hands, grasping* at flocks; great excitation or drowsiness (12).	Fever with ascites (11), starting, jerkings; great excitation or extreme drowsiness.
Tissues	
Emaciation with good appetite; glands atrophy (13).	*Emaciation with loss of appetite; glands atrophy.*
Chorea, very excited, zigzag motions; emaciated.	Chorea, when of a rheumatic origin.
Syphilis with salivation, skin *rough, dry, dirty, yellow;* after *Mercury.*	Syphilis with *deep ulcers;* skin covered *with thick scabs, rupia; after Mercury.*
Diseases of the periosteum; bones curve.	Caries, *necrosis,* exostosis; *bones swell.*
Glands enlarge or *dwindle.*	Glands enlarge, dwindle, grow *doughy* (11).
Pus thin, ichorous.	Pus thin or *curdy.*
Itching nettle rash on the thighs.	Itching herpes on the face; papulæ (14).

(11) The *Iodide* tends everywhere to infiltrate the cellular tissues with serum; pul. œdema, myelitis with effusion, pneumonia with œdema, Bright's Disease, *doughy* swellings.

(12) *Iodine* may be used in typhus. The starting, ascites and drowsiness under the *Iodide* are symptoms of dropsy; the first and third of cerebral effusion noticed in pneumonia, hydrocephalus, &c.; the second, a concomitant of intermittents.

(13) Atrophy is more characteristic of *Iodine* than hypertrophy.

(14) Papulæ also occur in *Iodine,* but they are characteristic of *Kali Hyd.*

IODINE **Character** **KALI HYD.**

The *Iodine* patient is *sallow, emaciated, hungry, restless, suffers from palpitation and intolerable weakness of the chest ; better lying.*

The *Kali Hyd.* patient is *bloated, emaciated, empty but not hungry, suffers from smothering spells and œdema ; must get up.*

LEPTANDRA & IRIS VERSICOLOR

LEPTANDRA	IRIS VERSICOLOR
Stupor ; shivering or dry, hot skin ; *stools tarry,* black.	Muttering ; chilly or *hot* and *sweaty skin ; stools black, watery or yellow.*
Tongue coated yellow down the centre.	Tongue coated uniformly white.
Taste bitter.	Taste greasy or sour.
Nausea, *deathly faint on rising,* vomiting of bile.	Nausea compels lying down ; sour vomit ; traces of bile ; or *sweetish.*
Burning in the *posterior of the liver,* or the region of the gall-bladder.	Burning in the throat, stomach, *pancreas,* intestines.
Headache dull, constant, right temple ; costive, bitter taste.	*Sick headache, nausea, vomiting ; worse right side ; sight fails.*
Stool tarry, black ; cutting above the navel after stool, worse afternoon and evening, from damp weather.	Stools mushy, bilious, with much fetid flatus, burning at the anus ; *worse at 2 or 3 A.M.,* worse in hot weather.
Stools of muddy, dirty water ; profuse, running as from a spout ; worse A.M. after beginning to move.	Stools watery, profuse, with vomiting and cramps (cholera, chol. morbus) ; worse 2 to 3 A.M. ; rumbling of gas in the abdomen (1).

(1) *Iris* irritates the whole alimentary canal; hence burning, serous diarrhœa, even rice-water from the epithelial exfoliation; cramps, purging and vomiting. Thus it corresponds to many of the summer diarrhœas. In cholera morbus or infantum coming at 2 or 3 A.M., it is far superior to *Veratrum.* It produces an inflammation of the pancreas, *Leptand.* acts more directly on the liver, causing black, pitch-like stools. Chronic cases of liver complaint, with a muddy, watery morning stool find here an excellent remedy.

LEPTANDRA & MERCURIUS VIVUS

LEPTANDRA	MERCURIUS VIVUS
Prostration, stupor; skin dry, burning; or extremities cold; tongue *yellow or black down the centre*; discharge of fetid, tarry, bloody stools; jaundice, (as in low bilious fevers).	More excitability; sleepy, but cannot sleep; extremities burning, dry; or *clammy*, cold sweat; tongue *thickly coated yellow, taking imprint of teeth*; or dry, clean; costive, or pitch-like stool, or *green-yellow, slimy stool* (1).
Nausea, deathly faint on rising.	Nausea, with *sweet taste*, headache, heat.
Weak, sinking sensation in the pit of the stomach.	Stomach feels, as if hanging down heavily after even light food.
Distressing pains, sharp, between umbilicus and epigastrium ; hot burning feeling ; burning distress in the region of the gall-bladder or posterior of the liver near the spine; tongue yellow down the centre; chilly along the spine.	Contractive pains, with swollen, hard, tender abdomen; burning, stinging pains, intense soreness in the region of the liver and duodenum, worse lying on the right side; tongue large, shows prints of teeth; chilly between stools.
Stools clayey, *tarry*, fetid; followed by *griping in the abdomen, but no tenesmus.*	Stools clayey, black, *green, slimy*, sour, excoriating; *tenesmus after stool* ; *cannot "get done"*.

LILIUM TIGRINUM Mind SEPIA*

Mental symptoms almost identical.

Head

LILIUM TIGRINUM	SEPIA
Headache from forehead to occiput.	Headache from occiput to forehead.
Fear of insanity.	Fear of apoplexy.
Taciturnity.	Loquacity.

---

(1) *Mercurius*, seldom admissible in Typhus, resembles *Lept.* in the preponderance of icteroid symptoms. Its mental phenomena are, however, not so much the stupor of *Lept.*, but simulate the excitability of *Bellad.* There is a desire to go away from the house, talking of robbers; sleepy, but cannot sleep, etc.

(*) It is not little singular that the isomorphic group, of which *Sulphur* is the type and *Sepia* an analogue, should find such similar drugs in the *Liliacæ* and analogues; thus *Sulph.* and *Aloes*; *Phos.* and *Cepa*; *Ars.* and *Allium Sativum* ; and here, *Sepia* and *Lilium*.

Stomach, Abdomen

LILIUM TIG.	SEPIA
Drinks often and much.	Usually thirstless.
Longs for meat.	Averse to meat.
Smarting after stool, (like a cathartic).	Tension ani after stool.
Urine retained causes oppression of chest.	Urine retained; anxiety; pressure on bladder.

Female Genital Organs

LILIUM TIG.	SEPIA
Absence of feeling in head; wild looks when menses cease to flow.	Mania caused by too profuse menses.
Menses generally scanty; cease when sitting down, flow while moving about.	Menses generally profuse; they flow only in the morning.
Leucorrhœa, *brown,* yellow, excoriating; worse after menses.	Leucorrhœa green or milky, excoriating; worse before menses.
Bearing down, funneling toward the vulva or anus; better from support.	Bearing down over whole pelvis; must cross the limbs.
Burning (less stinging), cutting in the ovaries; congestion.	Stinging in the ovaries; congestion.
Slow rccovery after confinement ; lochia too long; uterus remains large; must support the vulva to prevent everything from escaping; at times better, at other times, worse, from riding.	Slow recovery after confinement; lochia very fetid; become "pot-bellied"; must sit down and cross legs to prevent prolapsus; always worse riding (horse-back).
Mammæ tender ; *cutting through to left scapula.*	Mammæ sore, hard lumps ; stinging pains; cracked nipples.

Male Genital Organs

LILIUM TIG.	SEPIA
Sexual excitement; emissions followed by difficulty in fixing the mind; choose the wrong word; irritable; blurred sight.	Emissions followed by vertigo, irritability, sensitiveness to damp weather; *mental exhaustion.*

Chest, Heart

Both affect similarly the venous system; both cause congestive asthma, pulsations all over the body;. congestion to heart, worse from motion, better from pressure and rubbing; in both is there chilliness combined with internal heat in the chest.

LILIUM TIG.	SEPIA
Becomes worse if retain urine; sighing relieves; uterine trou-	Comes on when awaking from sleep; uterine and hysterical,

LILIUM TIG.	Chest, Heart	SEPIA
bles, pain through, left mammæ to back; dragging of all the viscera,		followed by jerking on one side. Hard, teasing cough.
Heaviness in the region of the heart, worse after eating (2).		Intermitting beats of heart after eating.
Pain, as if the *heart were alternately squeezed and relaxed.*		Palpitation with intense stitching pains in the left chest.
Congestion to the heart; pulse weak; heart feels *full to bursting;* taste of blood; faint; chills run down from face to chest; heart feels cold in the open air.		Congestion to the heart; bubbling in left chest, as if hæmoptysis were coming on; burning in the face; beating felt in the pit of the stomach.

Generalities

Both suit the weakened system, especially that of the female; fearful about one's health; hurried, nervous, fidgetty; so nervous the least excitement causes cold, clammy hands, palpitation, &c. In both the cause of the debility seems to consist in a relaxation of the ligamentous structures, serous sacs (3) and veins. The first two causes account for the empty, gone feelings; weak knees (even cracking in *Lilium,* from deficient synovial fluid) ; prolapse, &c. The last explains the readiness to portal stagnation (*Sepia*), fulness of the chest, heart and veins of the extremities. The most important distinction besides those already given is the following; because so characteristic of the respective remedies :—

Lilium	Sepia
Remission *forenoon.*	Remission *afternoon.*

LYCOPODIUM & NATRUM MUR.

The relation between *Lycopodium* and *Natrum-muriaticum* is one of opposites. Their comparison is ably given by Goullon, in which he shows that the former is more allied to *Sulphur* and the latter to *Sepia.* The differences pointed out below are intended to exhibit their opposite polarity, if one may use so doubtful a phrase.

---

(2) The heart symptoms of *Lilium* occurred late in the proving and are hence very characteristic. They seem to be mostly attended with congestive symptoms, and are linked with the uterine disturbances. But they occurred in both sexes and exhibit strong resemblance to organic disease.

(3) Dr. Hering taught long ago that serous membranes, containing little or no air in their sacs, acted by suction in keeping viscera in place. *Acon.,* seems to excite them, *Sepia, Iodine, &c.,* relax them.

LYCOPODIUM & NATRUM MUR.

When the influence of the atmosphere, electricity, seasons, and other natural phenomena, seems characteristic, then the subjoined remarks may be of diagnostic value.

Goullon's comparison shows their respective analogues, which continue the treatment in the same line of action; what is here added may mark their relation when just the opposite line of action is required.

According to Boenninghausen, *Lycopodium* and *Natrum-mur.* are especially indicated in diseases marked by periodicity.

LYCOPODIUM has aggravation when the barometer stands lowest and the diurnal electric tension is at its minimum, *viz.*, at 4 A.M.

NATRUM-MUR. has aggravation when the barometer stands highest and the electric tension is highest, *viz.*, at 10 P.M.

LYCOPODIUM is worse in snowy air, for then the barometer is low. But there is a kind of snow-storm, the weather being frosty, when the barometer rising causes snow. The wind is then N.E., and *Lyco.* will not be of service.

SEPIA is here needed, and probably *Natr-mur.*, as it is worse when barometer stands high, which always occurs with N.E. wind.

LYCOPODIUM is worse in a S. E. wind, because the barometer always stands low in wind from this quarter.

LYCOPODIUM is worse in those seasons in which the electric tension is lowest, hence in spring,

NATRUM-MUR. is worse in summer (July) and during a thunder-storm, when the opposite condition obtains.

LYCOPODIUM has the symptoms of the abdomen, colic, diarrhœa etc., worse in the morning; the chest, throat, and fever in the evening.

NATRUM-MUR. is the reverse in the case. Thus, in the former, the action is upward during the day; in the latter, downward.

They are certainly similar in many of their prominent symptoms of the mind, disposition, spine, chest, genitals, urinary organs, and also in hysteria, notwithstanding Goullon's remarks to the contrary, although it must be confessed that *Sepia* and *Natrum-mur.* are more allied in this disease.

MERCURIUS BIN-IOD.		MERCURIUS PROT-IOD
	Mind	
Ill humor.		Destructive disposition.
	Head	
Pains in the head from below upwards.		Pains in the head from above downwards.
Pulsations and heat in vertex.		Increased throbbing, more in forehead.
	Eyes	
Dimness of sight.		Black clouds float before the eyes.
Eyes inflamed, especially the right; bright light irritates so that must keep eye closed; psorophthalmia.		Inflammation of Meibomian glands, with ulceration and adhesion of the lids in morning; inflammation and ulceration of the conjunctiva and sclerotica, elevated, granular surface.

Both may be used in conjunctivitis.

MERCURIUS BIN-IOD.		MERCURIUS PROT-IOD
	Nose	
Coryza with profuse sneezing; right nostril worse; crusty eruption on the wings.		Coryza discharge white or bloody, mostly from posterior nares; turbinated bones diseased.
	Ears	
Catarrhal deafness improves.		Right ear feels closed, yet hears well.
	Face, Mouth	
Heavy, dull aching; first in the upper, then in the lower jaw.		Soreness in the inferior jaw bone.
Unusual afflux of saliva.		Mouth, gums dry, sticky.
Small, sore spots on the lower lip, and soreness in the thin part of the cheek.		Eruption, fine and of a bright-red color; worse on the root of the mouth.
Blisters on point of tongue.		Blisters back part of tongue.

A yellow or yellow-white coat on the back part of the tongue, with tip and edges clean, is characteristic of *Merc. Proto-Iod.*

MERCURIUS BIN-IOD.		MERCURIUS PROT-IOD
	Throat	
Diphtheria, with livid, purplish patches; discharge thin, offensive.		Diphtheria, with feebly organized patches, and great gastric, hepatic or intestinal disturbances.

Throat

MERC. BIN-IOD.	MERC. PROTO-IOD.
Hawks up hard, green lumps.	Mucous expectoration.
Left tonsil swollen, velum elongated; scalded sensation; must swallow, from a collection of saliva and a feeling of a lump.	Both tonsils; mostly the right; burning sensation; must swallow, from a constant sensation, as of a lump in the throat.

Taste, Appetite, ctE.

MERC. BIN-IOD.	MERC. PROTO-IOD.
Wants food salted more.	Wants acids, sour things.
Wants to drink in small quantities.	Wants to drink large quantities.
Pains about the navel.	Burning about the navel.
Slight tenesmus after a thin, loose stool; urine hot.	Dysentery when the stool is of a grass-green color.

Urine

Both have copious, red urine.

Genitals

Both have seminal emissions. In the *Proto-Iod.*, the patient may dream of urinating, and an emission follows. In the *Bin-Iod.* there is increased sexual desire, particularly on going to sleep.

Chest

MERC. BIN-IOD.	MERC. PROTO-IOD.
Dry cough evenings; expectoration white, scanty.	Slight, hacking cough when inspiring; sputa not observed.
Sticking in the region of the heart.	Heart gives an occasional spasmodic jump.

Back, Limbs

MERC. BIN-IOD.	MERC. PROTO-IOD.
Rheumatism worse mid-day, motion, putting on one's coat; less in the evening and night; pains more in the muscles.	Rheumatism worse at night in bed; worse writing, passive motion; pains deep-seated in the bones.

Skin

MERC. BIN-IOD.	MERC. PROTO-IOD.
Itching not marked.	Itching very persistent.
Small fissures and cracks.	Sore spots which itch.

Generalities

Aggravations are nearly the same in both. *Merc. Proto-Iod.* has more similarity with *Mercurius*; the *Merc. Bin-Iod.* with *Iodium.*

MERCURIUS VIVUS & CINNABAR

MERCURIUS VIVUS	CINNABAR
Fretful, malicious.	Fretful.
Forgetful ; headache—sinciput.	Forgetful ; headache—vertex.
Symptoms predominate, left eye.	Symptoms predominate, right eye.
Coryza anterior nares.	Coryza posterior nares.
Ophthalmia, pustules on and around eyes ; pustules on tarsi.	Condyloma of iris on border of pupil or eye-lids.
Salivation, with sore gums.	Saliva, with increased urine.
Catarrhs ; sensation of lump in the throat ; rawness in throat and chest ; nose runs a burning water ; pain like a stitch through right chest.	Catarrhs ; contraction in throat ; dryness at night so can't sleep ; nose discharges, posteriorly, a dirty, ropy mucus in morning ; pain from ensiform cartilage diagonally, through chest.
Dry, conical fig-warts.	Fan-shaped fig-warts.
Chancres simple. uncomplicated ; soft, free, thick pus.	Chancres neglected, badly treated, indurated ; exuberant granulations ; raised edges.
Bubo discharging thick pus.	Indolent bubo.

Cinnabar cures when there is a combination of scrofula with syphilis, or syphilis and tuberculosis.

MERCURIUS VIVUS	CINNABAR
Worse after stool, tenesmus.	Pinching before stool, better after.
Anus burns.	Pimples around anus burn, itch.
Painful diarrhœa at night.	Painless diarrhœa at night.
Eruptions painful, on palms of hands.	Eruptions on elbows, knuckles red.
Itching when warm in bed.	Itching all over, no eruption.
Pulse slow by day, increased at night.	Pulse slow forenoon, increased afternoon.
Sweat night, front of body.	Sweat at noon, between thighs.
Worse when alone.	Worse in company.
Worse cold air, evening air.	Worse in heat, better cold air.
Worse stretching.	Better stretching.

MERCURIUS VIVUS Mind, Head MERCURIUS CORR.

Forgetful.	Stares at people, don't understand them.
Vertigo ; things look black.	Vertigo, deafness, cold sweat.

Eyes

MERC. VIV.	MERC. CORR.
Pupils dilated.	Pupils contracted or angular.
Ophthalmia, catarrhal ; exanthematic, when pustules form ; pimples around inflamed eye ; relapses from every cold.	Ophthalmia, gonorrhœal, better than the *Vivus ;* iris irregular, pink line around cornea ; pus in ani. chamber ; phagedenic inflammation.

Face, Mouth

MERC. VIV.	MERC. CORR.
Lids closed, with pustules on tarsi.	Upper lid overlaps lower.
Nasal discharge anterior ; watery, corrosive.	Nasal discharge posterior ; discharge dries up, gluey.
Saliva profuse, fetid.	Saliva *acrid*, rarely ptyalism.
Ulcers in mouth, white, lardaceous ; breath not so offensive as *Merc. Corr.*	Ulcers phagedenic ; very offensive breath.
Upper lip swollen, dry, rough.	Lower lip everted, dark red.
Sweat on the forehead ; cold, oily or sour.	Sweat on forehead ; anxiety ; fetid towards morning.

Throat

MERC. VIV.	MERC. CORR.
Sore throat ; uvulitis, tonsils contain pus ; saliva copious, stringy.	Sore throat ; uvulitis ; when parts are *dark red*, burning ; tendency to phagedena.
Of little use in diphtheria.	Albuminuria after diphtheria.
Vomit bitter mucus ; slimy, bloody.	Vomit tough, stringy, albuminous mucus ; dark blood.
Dysentery ; when tenesmus is worse after stool ; urine frequent and scanty.	Dysentery, with more *burning* and bile ; tenesmus vesicæ, hot or suppressed urine ; cramps in calves.
Proctitis, typhlitis, etc. when abscess has formed.	Same when, during stool, discharge of urine is impossible.
Chronic diarrhœa (high potencies).	Constipation (highest poten cies).

Urine

MERC. VIV.	MERC. CORR.
Urine sour, pungent ; mixed with blood, white flakes or pus, soon becomes fetid.	Urine hot, bloody, contains, brick-dust sediment ; or purulent sediment.
Gonorrhœa when discharge is yellow-green, purulent.	Gonorrhœa, when phagedenic inflammation ensues.

It is probable that in Phimosis, when the parts become dark red, burning, *Merc. Corr.* will be the better remedy ; and as this state oftenest occurs in Paraphimosis, it will be preferable here.

Urine

MERC. VIV.	MERC. CORR.
Chancres simple, soft, superficial, regular, free and thick pus.	Chancres assume a phagedenic form, and secrete thin, ichorous pus (Raue).

Female Genitals

MERC. VIV.	MERC. CORR.
Leucorrhœa purulent, acrid, flocculent, lumps of mucus.	Leucorrhœa smelling sweetish, pale-yellow.
Menses profuse—too late.	Menses too early and profuse.

Chest

Merc. Viv. is by far the better proved medicine in coughs, influenza, etc. But *Merc. Corr.* is the remedy when, in bronchitis, there are severe, cutting pains in larynx ; fauces dark-red, tightness across the chest, can hardly breathe. If fauces are involved, *Merc. Corr.* is to be preferred when swallowing is not so painful as is depressing the tongue, putting the tongue out ; because the base is more affected than in *Merc. Viv.*

Extremities

MERC. VIV.	MERC. CORR.
Limbs cold, clammy ; or so sore can scarcely move them.	Limbs cold, muscles relaxed ; purplish, with small, spasmodic pulse.

Fever, Pulse

MERC. VIV.	MERC. CORR.
Sweat cold, sour ; often burns the skin.	Sweat cold, with anxiety ; fetid towards morn.
Pulse generally full, fast, sometimes tremulous.	Pulse always weak, intermitting, tremulous.
Small-pox, with dysenteric discharge, great salivation ; suppurative stage.	Small-pox when throat is so swollen and inflamed almost suffocate.

Skin

MERC. VIV.	MERC. CORR.
Caries mostly.	Narcosis.
Suppurations generally profuse ; laudable pus predominates.	Suppurations ichorous always ; phagedæna ; gangrene.
Nails yellowish.	Nails grayish.
Similar to *Aur.*, *Narcotics*, *Lach.*, *Sul.*, *etc.*	Similar to *Kreos.*, *Arg. Nit.*, *Arum*, *Ars.*, etc.
Complaints of women and children.	Complaints of men (Burt).

MERC. VIVUS — Mind, Head — MERC. PROTO-IOD.

Both have anxiety, restlessness, etc.

MERC. VIVUS	MERC. PROTO-IOD.
Longs to go abroad for relief.	Other symptoms better during care and anxiety.
Headaches, catarrhal, rheumatic, etc., worse open air.	Headache from catarrh, etc., better open air.
Vertigo lying or walking.	Vertigo when riding.
Discharge from nose, anterior nares.	Discharge from posterior nares, mostly.
Catarrhs : Discharges watery, excoriating, scurfy nostrils, bleed when cleansed ; green fetid pus ; nose red, shining, swollen.	Cattarhs : Discharge whitish or bloody, posterior nares ; nasal bones diseased, turbinated bones swollen, worse right nostril.
Catarrh of conjunctiva of eyes ; relapses from cold ; exanthema conjunctiva.	Catarrh of eyes, indicated in conjunctiva membranacea.
Tongue flabby ; dry, coated black.	Tongue yellow base ; bright-red tip.
Sore throat ; tonsillitis with suppuration, or slowly forming ulcers : best when pus has formed.	Diphtheritic sore throat (1) ; patches limited, easily detached ; ulcers on tonsils ; tubercular sore throat.

Merc. Viv. produces ulceration of mucous membrane, but *Merc. Iod.* seems to alter more the follicular glands so that their secretions are tough, opaque ; while those of the *Vivus* are tenacious, viscid. *Merc. Iod.* cures tubercular sore throat because of its action on follicles ; cheesy masses in sputum.

Stomach, Bowels

MERC. VIVUS	MERC. PROTO-IOD.
Nausea with vertigo.	Nausea with suffocation about heart.
Whitish, watery stools.	Thin, brown stools, much froth.
Dysentery, much tenesmus, especially after stool.	Best when there is griping, with little blood but much grass-green mucus.
Stool tenacious or crumbling.	Stool tenacious like putty.

Urine, Genitals

MERC. VIVUS	MERC. PROTO-IOD.
Urine copious, dark, sour.	Urine copious, dark-red.
Emissions at night, bloody.	Emissions when dream of urinating.
Chancres soft, pus free.	Chancres indurated, scars hard.

(1) *Merc. Proto-Iod.* may, perhaps, be of use in genuine diphtheria, but it is certainly the best remedy in the diphthertic sore throats so common every winter. It differs from *Lach.* in being darker, more livid ; like *Lach.* the swelling is worse left side, and from empty swallowing ; but it lacks the extreme sensitiveness to external touch about neck.

Chest

MERC. VIV.	MERC. PROTO-IOD.
Ulcerated laryngitis, with profuse ptyalism ; white patches.	Ulcerated laryngitis, patches livid, purplish ; discharge thin, offensive.
Bronchitis, bloody sputa ; symptoms of influenza.	Bronchitis, bronchial glands swollen ; sub-acute cases.

Sleep

MERC. VIV.	MERC. PROTO-IOD.
Sleepless before 12 P. M.	Sleepless before 1 A. M.

Fevers

MERC. VIV.	MERC. PROTO-IOD.
Scarlatina, consecutive anasarca, ascites ; genitals sore, inflamed.	Scarlatina, loose voice, fauces purple, ulcerated ; after *Lach.*

Merc. Proto-Iod. is the better medicine in Scarlatina, Measles, etc., when parotids, cervicals and tonsils are indurated. (See Burt.)

MERC. VIV.	MERC. PROTO-IOD.
Seldom useful in typhus, except with sore, fetid mouth ; pain in liver, with green-yellow stools, dark urine, yellow skin.	Typhoid fevers with enlarged liver or spleen ; torpor ; paralytic languor ; coma, even spasms, suppressed urine.

Skin

MERC. VIV.	MERC. PROTO-IOD.
Itching when warm in bed.	Itching all over, no eruption, comes in successive spots.

Generalities

MERC. VIV.	MERC. PROTO-IOD.
Worse during Fall.	Worse in thaws, hence Spring.
Worse swallowing saliva, liquids.	Worse saliva, or empty swallowing.
Averse to open air.	Often better in open air.
Pains worse on motion.	Pains better on motion.
Better in warm room, (not bed).	Worse in warm room.

Merc. Iod. has aggravation from passive motion, but relief from active exercise.

MERCURIUS VIVUS — Mind — SILICEA

In both remedies is found a desponding, melancholy mood. Anxiety, in *Mercury* seems to be caused by ebullitions, by alcoholism, &c. ; the patient wants *to escape from the house, to go abroad.* Under *Silicea* it is a part of *nervous weakness,* which cannot bear even normal stimuli. But under *Mercury* we find an irritability, even vehemence, and a *malicious, suspicious* state contrary to *Silicea,* which represents a *bland,* tearful *yielding* mind.

MERC. VIV. — Mind — SILICEA

The sensorium is weakened even to dementia. Under *Mercury*, weak memory results from congestions, from abuse of spirits or external injuries, or from syphilis. In extreme cases, the patient does all sorts of foolish things, laps his own spittle, takes people by the nose, &c., &c. Under *Silicea*, weak memory results from nervous weakness, exposure to wet, excessive study, &c. In some cases, the patient sits counting pins, thinks he is in two places at the same time, &c.

Head

MERC. VIV.	SILICEA
Headaches generally worse in bed at night, from sweat; pains like a *hoop* around the head.	Headaches generally, better warm in bed; worse at night; seem to *ascend the spine* into the head.
Head-sweat oily, sour; forehead icy-cold; worse *in the heat of the bed.*	Head-sweat sour, profuse, general over the head; *better covering the head.*
Eruption mostly fore-part of head scratching causes bleeding. (See Tissues.)	Eruptions back part of head and behind the ears; scratching causes burning.

Eyes

MERC. VIV.	SILICEA
Amblyoptic symptoms from inflammations, congestions, &c.; letters move when reading; using the eyes causes stinging soreness; worse from the glare of the fire.	Amblyoptic symptoms reflex nervous, &c.; from the uterus, lungs, suppressed discharges; letters look pale; using the eyes causes vertigo; worse from day-light.
Paroxysms of blindness; pupils dilated.	Momentary blindness; pupils contracted.
Inflammatory affections when pus or pustules form; pimples far around; pains are cutting, stinging.	Inflammatory affections; threatened perforation of the cornea; *fistulae*; pains like stitches from the forehead into the eyes.

Ears

MERC. VIV.	SILICEA
Deafness with roaring in the ears; swallowing or blowing the nose relieves; meatus always moist.	Deafness with gurgling, fluttering in the ears; relieved sometimes by a loud report in the ears; meatus red, swollen.
Otitis when ulceration has begun; tearing pains (1); inner ear feels cold; purulent otorrhœa.	Otitis with stitches *out* of the ear; *itching* of the middle ear; otorrhœa with caries. Otitis interna (often in scarlatina).

---

(1) Tearing must ever be a characteristic here; for it expresses the same tenesmus feeling so marked in the *Mercury* dysentery.

Nose

MERC. VIV.	SILICEA
Fluent coryza, discharge excoriates (influenza) ; chronic forms with green pus, inner surface of *wings* red, scabs ; pains, fever, &c., Eustachian tubes obstructed.	Nose generally *dry*, obstructed (chronic forms) ; *acrid, corroding discharge* (as in scarlatina) ; scabs *high up* in the nostril ; Eustachian tubes *itch.*
Nose red, swollen, *shining* with itching.	Point of nose *itches intolerably* without swelling.

Mouth, Throat

MERC. VIV.	SILICEA
Toothache ; dentine inflamed ; gums swell, become white, suppurate, bleed ; gum-boils.	Toothache ; periosteum inflamed ; gums show fistulous openings, oozing thin, offensive ichor.
Upper lip swollen (as in scrofula).	Upper lip hard (as in cancer).
Glossitis ; white tongue inflamed, even suppurating.	One-half swollen ; indurated ; as in carcinomatous disease.
Tongue black ; shows prints of teeth.	Tongue coated brown ; sensation of a hair on the tip.
Tonsillitis, &c., when ulcers form slowly, *when pus is present, and the abscess needs maturing* ; worse, swallowing liquids and saliva.	Tonsillitis, &c., *when the abscess will not heal*, or when each effort to swallow involuntarily distorts the face ; swallowing pains when there is no inflammation (2).
Fetor from the mouth.	Fetor in the morning (3).
Parotids swollen ; *pale* ; stinging pains.	Parotids swollen ; *hard* ; indolent.

(2) This dysphagia is a part of the general characteristic of *Silicea* ; the patient is weak, mentally and physically ; he has not strength of mind to resist, hence is yielding ; swallows slowly ; is tired ; drags the limbs ; his fæces are expelled with difficulty, even slip back ; as a child, he is slow in learning to walk in a word, he is in a semi-paralytic state.

(3) Clinically, these remedies differ greatly here ; *Merc.* presents a picture of scurvy, aphthæ, &c. ; tongue shows imprint of teeth ; when indurated, it is the result of inflammation ; gums are ulcerated, white, &c., hence the fetor. In *Silicea* the induration of the tongue is indicative of carcinoma, &c. ; the gums, though affected, are diseased in connection with the periosteum ; aphthæ are less marked ; hence the fetor is symptomatic of disordered stomach, disturbed sleep, and so comes in the morning.

MERC. VIV.	Stomach	SILICEA
Vomit *mucus*, *bile*, food ; sweetish rising, faint (as from worms).		Vomit *drink*, food ; nausea when over-heated ; vomits as soon as he drinks (4).
The child *becomes yellow ; vomits bile ;* rejects the milk.		The child *refuses mother's milk*, or *immediately vomits it* (4).
Pressure, as if the stomach were *hanging down heavily*, after a meal.		Pressure, as from a *heavy stone* after eating ; especially after *raw vegetables* (4).
Colic (as from worms), with *cold, clammy hands ;* slimy stool ; worse, 12 P. M.		Colic (as from worms), with yellow hands and blue nails ; constipation ; worse, new moon (4).
Discharges from the bowels, slimy, bloody, pitch-like,bilious, green, clay-colored, sour ; *much straining, tenesmus* ; uncovering even a hand, causes pains in the bowels.		Discharges from the bowels, slimy, bloody, of a cadaverous smell ; *difficult, but painless* ; uncovering causes pains and makes the general condition worse.
Stools tenacious and crumbling ; *require much straining to pass them.*		Stools too large ; *slip back when but partially expelled.*

In the treatment of hæmorrhoids which tend to suppurate, great care must be used in the choice of these remedies. In *Merc.* there co-exists a *prolapsed rectum, black and bloody* (5) ; production of slime ; in *Silicea*, only the hæmorrhoidal knobs protrude, with pains extending into the rectum and testes ; fistulæ.

---

(4) Such symptoms show but little similarity in the action of these remedies on the gastric organs, yet in actual practice, especially in the treatment of psoric children, they often clash. They seem to present a resemblance which is, however, deceptive. *Merc.* causes the so-termed bilious symptoms with *mucous derangements* ; and in the intestines, *slimy* diarrhœa and *dysentery.* In dyspepsia we always find co-existing, *yellow face, soft tongue,* bilious or clay-colored stools ; stomach and hypochondria *feel inflated.* or it *drags heavily,* as do also the abdominal parietes in walking. In *Silicea* the complexion is *earthy* or *waxy* ; vomiting occurs immediately after *drinking* or nursing, and shows an irritability of the stomach, as seen in gastralgia, cancer, &c. The bowels are inactive, rather than dysenteric. Despite these differences, both meet in *swollen liver* ; *hard, hot, tender abdomen* (as in children) ; *worm colic* ; *tender liver, worse lying on the right side, &c. Mercury,* however, promotes the formation of pus ; hence suits in *acute hepatic abscess* ; *Silicea* retards suppuration : hence suits in *chronic hepatic abscess.*

(5) Note how this compares with phimosis ; such analogies confirm the characteristic action of a drug.

Stomach

MERC. VIV.	SILICEA
Worms ; sweetish risings ; putrid breath ; hunger, yet great weakness ; fever ; escape easily at night ; *cause inflammation of the vulva ; of the genitals* (6).	Worms ; continuous water-brash ; fever becomes constant, almost like hectic ; hunger, yet nausea if attempt to eat ; symptoms *worse at new moon.*

Urinary Organs

The *Mercury* urine contains blood, pus, mucus ; is turbid, sour, or putrid. The *Silicea* urine deposits a yellow or reddish, sandy sediment. Both have frequent urination ; but with *Merc.* it is also *copious ;* with *Silicea, scanty.*

Genitals

Merc. corresponds to many forms of syphilis ; *Silicea* only to the bone affections ; open, stubborn chancres, buboes, &c., where *Mercury* has been used in excess. (See Ulcers, Bones.) Both produce spots, humid eruptions and itching of the genitals, especially of the corona glandis.

MERC. VIV.	SILICEA
Gonorrhœa thick, *green*, puriform, worse at night.	Gonorrhœa thick, *fetid*, pus ; worse exerting to sweating.
Emissions cause burning in the spine ; icy-cold hands.	Emissions cause a sensation of one-sided paralysis of the brain.
Leucorrhœa *green*, flocculent, with lumps the size of hazel-nuts ; *genitals inflamed* (6).	Leucorrhœa *milky, watery*, brown ; *instead of the menses ;* after acids.
Menstruation : Congestive type ; scorbutic patients ; whimsical, anxious ; hands, feet and face œdematous ; mucous stool, urging ; *urine excoriates the parts ;* sore spots on the tongue.	*Menstruation* : Nervous type ; chlorotic patients (7) ; melancholy ; icy-cold all over ; always great constipation before menses ; eruptions on inside of thighs ; cuts fester ; paronychia.
Vagina feels *raw*; prolapsus feeling, as if the abdomen would drop when walking.	Vagina feels *very tender* to the touch ; pressing down in the vagina when walking.

(6) The influence of *Merc.* on the genitals is remarkable. Often in scarlatina, measles, worms, &c., co-existing inflamed genitals point to *Merc.* as the cure all. In a great variety of complaints when the patient (child) is *continually pulling at the penis, Merc.* is the remedy. In delirium, stupor, &c., this same symptom points to *Merc., Canth., (Hyos.), Bufo.*

(7) Let it be remembered that in *no instance is it recommended to prescribe pathologically.* Whenever such comparisons are drawn the intent is brevity only. It would take a page to express in symptoms what is here stated in few words.

Genitals

MERC. VIV.

Fainting; *cold sweat on the forehead,* with metrorrhagia; especially among aged females.

Mammae, inflamed, feel raw, hard shining, swelling; *pus formed*; *milk spoiled, so that the child refuses it.*

SILICEA

Momentary blindness with metrorrhagia, uterine cancer, &c., blood flows while nursing; also between the periods.

Mammae: Chronic *fistulous openings,* callous edges; hard (scirrhus) lumps; *child refuses the milk or vomits it at once.*

Larynx, Chest

MERC. VIV.

Cough; chest seems to contract causing dyspnœa; comes in two paroxysms; causes a bursting pain in head and chest; sore over sacrum and between scapulæ; worse from worms, from teething; from lying on the left side; from cool evening air, damp weather (8).

Expectoration *watery*; of coagulated blood; of yellow mucus; of pus, tasting putrid or salty.

Dyspnœa worse ascending; better from tobacco-smoking.

Awakens with trembling and thumping at the heart; *feels, as if life was ebbing away* (9).

Pulse full and accelerated.

Ebullitions and trembling from the *least exertion.*

SILICEA

Cough short-breathed seems to arrest the breath; hollow, suffocating; causes protrusion of the hernia; pains like jerks over the sacrum; worse after rapid walking, from eating hastily; from lying on the back; from change of weather; thunder-storm.

Expectoration clear, profuse, viscid; of pale, frothy blood; or milky, acrid, ichorous or purulent mucus, tasting greasy.

Dyspnœa worse resting, *after* running or walking fast.

Violent, dangerous thumping of the heart; worse *after* any violent exertion.

Pulse small, hard and quick.

Ebullitions from *wine*; easily excited.

---

(8) *Mercury* gives us burning, rawness, pains in the bones, watery blennorrhœa such as we see in influenza. In suppuration of the lungs the resemblance between *Merc.* and *Silicea* is often perplexing. *Merc.,* however, is preferable after *hæmorrhage,* after acute inflammation, pneumonia, &c., soft, quick pulse, anxiety, weight on the chest, stinging pains, *cold sweat on the forehead*; *face yellow, bilious. Silicea* compares with *Calc. in cavities of the lungs*; rattling, panting, breathing; milky, purulent sputa, *hectic fever, pale, waxy face, night-sweats, fetid sweat on the feet.* Clinically, *Silicea* palliates the sleeplessness of consumptives. *Mercury* the diarrhœa and occasional catarrhs from evening exposure.

(9) A group common enough in debility, as well as organic disease. Compare *Merc. Præc. Rub., Kali Hyd., Lach.,* &c.

Fevers

MERC. VIV.	SILICEA
Chilliness, as from cold water poured over the body.	Chilliness, as from cold air blowing around the waist (10).
Chilly *after stool* (11), at night, with frequent micturition.	Chilly, from *want of animal heat.*
Heat with anxiety, constriction of the chest, faintishness ; chilly, if he moves	Heat with headache, appearing in flashes, worse in the face (10).
Sweat general, except the head ; or on the front of the body (10).	Sweat absent, except on the head ; or on the back of the body.
Sweat *never relieves* (12) ; sour, oily, clammy, burns the skin.	Sweat sour or offensive ; *foot-sweat offensive, about the toes.*
Hectic fever, worse all night ; sweat cold, skin feels clammy, especially on forehead and thighs.	Hectic fever, worse at night, especially towards morning ; sweat periodical ; feels cold.
Variola, stage of maturation.	Variola, *for the sequelae.*
Scarlatina with anasarca (6).	Scarlatina on a scrofulous basis. (See Ears, Nose.)

Sleep

MERC. VIV.	SILICEA
Sleepless from ebullitions, with *anxiety* ; as from alcohol, from a fright, home-sickness, &c.	Sleepless from ebullitions, as from *nervous excitement*, fantasies, crowding of ideas, &c.
Moaning continuously in sleep ; terrifying visions awaken ; fear of being alone.	*Screaming* in sleep, (night-mare) ; clairvoyant visions ; somnambulistic state.
Deep sleep, mouth open, coma (as in low fevers). Sleepy by day ; sleepless at night ; prostrated.	Coma vigil, jerks in sleep (as in typhus, &c.). Sleepy and prostrated during a thunder-storm.

---

(10) Neither remedy occupies a very prominent position in intermittents. Still, when they are indicated, there are resemblances enough to necessitate a differential study. In *Merc.*, the pains are referred to the liver ; the sweating stage is the worse, with palpitation of the heart, nausea and indescribable malaise, diarrhœa and dropsy. In *Silicea*, the pains are referred to the stomach, cramp pains ; the apyrexia gives us the most symptoms, mainly, because *Silicea* is indicated as a constitutional remedy, correcting psora. We find constipation, dry coryza, *want of animal heat and backache, with a sense of paralysis of the limbs.*

(11) This chilliness occurring in syphilis indicates mercurialization.

(12) Often a guide to *Merc.* But in typhus it rather leads to *Stram., Lach., Phos. Mercury* can only be used here when *pitch-like stool. great urging, soreness of the liver, icteroid skin, &c.*, point to hepatic complications. Then there co-exist indifference, deep sleep, *nose-bleeds at night, wants to go away from the house*, talks of robbers, does not know where he is, *sleepy but can not sleep, &c. Silicea*, with a similar state of debility and profuse sweat, comes into play *when there is a desire to be magnetized* ; the patient thinks he is in two places at once, &c.

Skin

MERC. VIV.	SILICEA
Abscesses, boils, &c., *when pus has formed.*	Abscesses, boils, &c., *when they will not heal ; cellular tissues.*
Ulcers spread *superficially*; feel raw; excoriated ; *lardaceous* surface ; worse from either warmth or cold.	Ulcers extend in *depth* ; very tender to the least touch ; *blackish* surface ; better from warmth ; worse from cold (13).
Erysipelas smooth, red, œdematous ; *with eruptions.*	Erysipelas, smooth ; mostly *with bone diseases.*
Scars redden.	Scars pain and break open.
Skin dirty, yellow, rough, dry ; or bloated, *flabby.*	Skin delicate, pale, earthy or waxy ; pale and bloated.
Glands inflamed, red, *painful,* hot.	Glands swollen, hard, *painless,* cold.
Skin unhealthy ; *discharges* (stool, urine, &c.) *excoriate.*	Skin unhealthy ; festers as from splinters ; *difficult to heal.*
Tumors, swellings, &c., smooth, *shining*, pale or red.	Tumors, swellings, &c., smooth or *spongy.*
Eruptions greasy, *yellow*, *thick, crusts* ; itching worse in bed ; scratching causes *bleeding.*	Eruptions *furfuraceous,* oozing black ; itching at night, as from ants crawling.
Run-arounds or whitlows (tendons).	Whitlows and felons proper (bone) (14).
Nails yellow, pain, as if sore.	Nails blue ; *grow into the flesh.*
NERVES : Pains *tearing,* like a *band* ; part affected is cold and clammy ; red spots on the cheeks ; sweats without relief ; worse every cold change, in damp evening air ; worse from warmth of bed.	NERVES : Pains *throbbing* (15) ; like *shocks* ; part affected is cold ; white or burning spots on the cheeks ; cannot sweat ; worse least draught (on back) ; change of weather, thunderstorms ; better from warmth of bed.
Paralysis agitans ; spinal paralysis, *membranes inflamed* ; *limbs rigid but can be moved by others* (16).	Tabes dorsalis ; spinal paralysis with *constipation and increased sexual desire* ; *caries of the vertebrae.*

(13) *Silicea* answers for almost any kind of pus ; but the thin pus is *not* offensive, while the thick pus *is.*

(14) *Silicea* is the remedy when felons seem to start from splinters, &c., it will also bring foreign substances to the surface.

(15) *Merc.* is not so much as *Hepar* the remedy when throbbing, rigors, &c., show that pus is about to form ; but it is the remedy when pus has formed, and then matures the abscess rapidly. *Silicea* has throbbing pains with neuralgia, hence not necessarily indicative of suppuration.

(16) *Mercury* gives us paralyzed bladder ; *pain in the spine when moving ; occasional contractions of the limbs* ; a perfect picture of meningitis spinalis ; hence curative *when concomitants concur.* *Silicea* often appears in scrofulous children, with spina-bifida, &c., &c., and is well characterized by the constipation, and in adults by increased sexual desire.

Skin

MERC. VIV.	SILICEA
Spasms with constant drivelling (17) ; mostly in the extremities ; at night with much thirst, bloated abdomen, itching nose, (worms).	Spasm with lachrymation ; start and spread from the solar plexus ; at night during sleep ; *worse during the new moon*, (worms).
Faint, with vertigo and sweetish risings.	Faint, if attempt to lie on the side.

Muscles

Mercury appears mostly in rheumatism ; *Silicea*, chiefly in chronic arthritic nodes ; *Mercury* serves when children suddenly begin to limp ; *Silicea*, when they are slow in learning to walk.

Bones, Etc.

Generally speaking, *Mercury* involves more the *glands and periosteum* ; *Silicea*, more the bones. It is true that *Merc.* cures caries, bone-pains, &c., but this is because of the periosteum. Only *Silecea* cures necrosis, osteitis, re-unites fractures, heals chronic abscesses, otorrhœa with caries, &c., &c.

Dropsy in *Merc.* is developed in almost any locality ; in amenia, *Merc.* offers œdema of face, hands and feet ; under *Silicea* dropsy is found principally in the joints ; also as *hydrocele* in scrofula. In anæmia feet swell in the morning (18).

Generalities

MERC. VIV.	SILICEA
Heat causes profuse sweat which weakens ; blood becomes so heated cannot "get cool".	Heat causes great dyspnœa ; nausea from the least rise of temperature.
Prostration after storms.	Prostration during thunder-storms.
Resembles *Bell.*, *Lach.*, *Hep.*, *Nit. Ac.*, *Mez.*, *China*, *Dulc.*, *Kali Hyd.*, *Sulph.*, &c.	Resembles *Sul.*, *Graph.*, *Ars.*, *Lyc.*, *Hep.*, *Phos.*, *Puls.*, *Calc. C.*, &c.
Remission during the day.	Remission before 12 P.M.
Worse in the Fall.	Worse in the Spring.

Mercurius has *aggravation*, and *Silicea*, *amelioration* from wet weather, warmth of bed or stove (19) ; empty stomach (20) ; lying on the *right side*.

---

(17) When in teething children the salivation suddenly ceases and spasms result *Merc.*, as well as *Kali Brom.*, are often curative.

(18) Of course, if the symptoms call for *Silicea* it will cure, even if not a prominent dropsy medicine. What is here meant is that in the absence of higher symptoms, *Merc.* has the preference in dropsies. This is the only use of these external contrasts.

(19) *Merc.* is better wrapping up like *Silicea*. These remedies so inimical, are perplexingly similar in modalities. They have at least twenty precisely alike. So much the more need for studying their differences.

(20) *Silicea*, like *Lycopod.*, has headache if the patient does not eat ; but is always worse from a satisfying meal.

MERC. VIV. **Generalities** **SILICEA**

Mercurius has *amelioration*, and *Silicea*, *aggravation* from dry weather, standing, smoking after breakfast, lying on the back, lying on the left side, assuming erect position.

Character

The *Mercury* patient is irritable, malicious, suspicious ; he is coarse in manners and tastes ; likes beer, not wine ; presents a dirty, rough, yellow face ; is scorbutic, scorfulous or syphilitic ; cannot bear damp, cold winds or the evening air ; contracts catarrhs, rheumatism ; sweats easily. As a child, he has open fontanelles, anxiety when alone ; restless during sleep, with clammy thighs and cold, icy forehead ; large, tender abdomen, and readily contracts dysentery.

The *Silicea* patient is more bland, yielding ; he is more refined in tastes and appearance ; his skin is *delicate*, pale or waxy ; he cannot bear thunder-storms ; takes cold when his feet get wet, and, because of his weak spine, is very susceptible to draughts on the back. As a child, he presents open fontanelles, large, sweaty head, body small but abdomen swollen ; cannot walk ; is always costive.

MYRICA CERIFERA & DIGITALIS

Digitalis, according to Hale, antidotes the jaundice caused by *Myrica*.

By diminishing the secretion of bile, both develop symptoms of cholæmia ; drowsiness, stupor, languor, slow pulse, jaundice, yellow eyes, swollen, heavy lids, clay-colored stools, frothy, brownish-yellow urine, &c.

In both we find indifference, sadness, irritability. Only *Myrica* has, "thinks hlmself better than any one else."

Digitalis causes serous or jelly-like secretions from the mucous membranes, *easily detached*. Ahpthæ, stomatitis with fetid or sweetish saliva. *Myrica* causes thick, vitiated mucous secretions, *difficult to detach*. Stomatitis with spongy gums, fetid mucus, mouth coated with an *adhesive coating difficult to loosen*.

Both give weak, sinking feeling in the epigastrium after eating ; *Digitalis*, specifically *after breakfast* ; *Myrica*, better from rapid walking.

In *jaundice*, *Myrica* has ash-coloured stool, drowsiness, slow pulse, but increased in intensity ; dull aching liver ; dragging in back ; tongue dirty, yellow ; catarrh of posterior nares. *Dlgiialis* differs in having clean tongue or tongue covered with easily detached slime ; pulse slower than the beating of the heart ; hardness in region of liver ; yellow in corners of eye-lids.

MYRICA CERIFERA & DIGITALIS

Both cause palpitation while lying on the left side ; constriction of chest ; tickling cough, made worse by lying or talking. But *Myrica* produces an audible pulsation (more like *Chelidonium*) ; *Digitalis* exhibits the quick, but small pulse of the weakened heart, laboring under the superadded pressure of the body.

Myrica, with its slow but intensified pulse, shows the system temporarily weakened by blood poisoned with bile, health returning with the resumption of hepatic activity ; *Digitalis* gives us an enlarged liver made so by organic heart disease, the enervating bile, but intensifying the weakness of organic defect.

PHOSPHORUS & ZINCUM

PHOSPHORUS	ZINCUM
Mind	
Sad at twilight ; alternate laughter and crying.	Sad at noon ; calm in the evening.
Easily angered ; *trembling, hot afterwards.*	*Easily angered* ; *trembling, as if chilly afterwards.*
Memory generally quick.	Memory weakened.
Indifferent.	Taciturn.
Anxiety, as if about to die.	Fears death (hypochondriac) ; thinks calmly of death (when exhausted).
Head	
Vertigo ; sensation, as *if ihe chair were rising* ; worse mornings ; revolving vertigo.	Vertigo ; sensation, as *if the seat were rocking* ; worse evenings ; revolving vertigo (1).
Hemicrania, forehead or occiput swollen ; *pulsations in the head* ; face congested.	Chronic, *maddening pain deep in the brain* ; face rather pale ; *eye-lids bluish.*
Headache, better for awhile after dinner (2).	Headache worse after dinner, after *wine.*
Itching of the scalp, worse from scratching (3).	Soreness of the vertex, better from scratching.
Hair comes out in bundles, over ears.	Hair comes out leaving vertex bald.
Softening of the brain ; incipient hemiplegia.	*Softening of the brain* ; distressing vomiting.

(1) *Phos.* and *Zinc.* both may be indicated in cerebral tumors ; for revolving vertigo is a symptom of their presence.

(2) But worse during mastication.

(3) *Phos.* is generally better from scratching.

PHOSPHORUS	ZINCUM
Eyes	
Glaucoma ; objects look green or gray.	*Pterygium* ; objects appear blue, yellow, green.
Burning *spots* on the eye-ball.	*Intense burning after operations.*
Ears	
Hearing too acute ; *deaf to the human voice.*	Hearing impaired, yet intolerance to the least noise.
Otitis ; throbbing in the ears.	*Otalgia* (among boys).
Nose	
Smell too acute (headache).	Loss of smell.
Point of nose red, shining.	Point of nose cold.
Face	
Circumscribed red cheeks.	Livid face.
Sick look, *puffed under the eyes* ; pale, flushes from the least emotion.	Sick look, face pale, waxy, yellow ; *alternately red and pale* (brain).
Mouth	
Tongue red, stinging tip, middle white.	Tongue blistered, swollen on one side.
Velum palati affected more than the tonsils ; worse, swallowing fluid or solids, pains after eating.	Blue herpes on the tonsils (suppressed gonorrhœa) ; worse, empty swallowing ; cramps in the neck, when drinking.
Stricture of the œsophagus ; *rumination.*	Stricture of the œsophagus ; *worse from wine.*
Stomach, Abdomen	
Eructations cause oppression of the chest, coming from the cardiac orifice.	Eructations cause a pressure in the middle of the spine.
Aversion to boiled milk, salt fish, beer ; longing for refreshing things.	Aversion to fish ; longing for beer.
Canine hunger after a meal ; at night she must eat or faint ; empty feeling, at about 11 A.M.	Canine hunger, hungry even when full ; sudden weakness of the limbs at noon, tremor.
As soon as water gets warm, it is thrown up.	*As soon as the first spoonful reaches the stomach it comes up.*
Contractive pain in pit of stomach extending to left hypochondrium, later to the heart and left shoulder ; better from warmth.	Screwing pain in the stomach, pinching deep in the region of the heart, extending to hypochondria ; warm all over ; worse wine.
Vomit blood, pure or brown ; bile ; feet and hands numb ; cold, cold sweaty forehead ; better lying down.	Vomit bitter mucus ; blood ; chilliness on the arms ; sweat ; tremulous feeling (subjective) ; better sitting, bent forward.

PHOSPHORUS — **Stomach, Abdomen** — **ZINCUM**

They differ widely in their action on the liver. *Phos.* causes jaundice from catarrhal inflammation of the duodenum ; also jaundice with the coma and collapse, belonging to atrophy of the liver or fatty degeneration, (not infiltration) ; also with Bright's Disease, with atrophy of the brain or heart disease ; dropsy ; hepatic congestion with pneumonia. *Zinc.*, on the other hand, behaves more like *Plumb.*, giving us indurations here and there in the abdomen, enlarged left lobe of liver ; the consecutive dropsy of the feet comes from pressure and retarded circulation, rather than from albuminuria and poisoned blood. The stool is lumpy, hard, difficult (like *Plumb.*) or pitch-like, involuntary, and hence indicative of obstruction, rather than suppression of biliary secretion.

Both meet in *colica flatulentia,* with consequent asthma ; but in *Zinc.*, the wind does not relieve when passed ; worse from wine, in the evening or after 12 P. M. *Phos.* finds some relief from flatus, which is not offensive, as in *Zinc.* ; generally wine does not aggravate ; worse after supper and first on lying down. *Zinc.*, like its relative *lead*, causes retraction of the abdomen, hence, may serve in lead colic. *Phos.* appears in the tympanites, attending typhoid states with symptoms of dissolution of the blood.

Phosphorus	Zincum
Inguinal hernia with relaxed abdomen ; *protrudes even with soft stool* ; sensitive.	Inguinal hernia with pains, as if *strangulated.* (*Comp. Nux Vom.*).
Stool *long, dry, difficult,* "*dog stool*".	Stool difficult, insufficient, *lumpy, hard, dry.*
Polypi recti wlth proctitis.	Leucorrhœa during stool with proctitis.
Blood from the rectum during stool ; blood dark.	Blood from the rectum ; blood pale.
Fatty degeneration of pancreas or spleen.	Sago-spleen with chlorosis ; crampy pains.

Kidneys, Urine

Phosphorus	Zincum
Hæmaturia from general dissolution of the blood ; after sexual excesses.	Hæmaturia, vicarious from suppressed menses ; diarrhœa, night cough (Raue).

Phos. is a leading remedy in the complications of Morbus Brightii, bearing no resemblance to *Zinc.* In renal calculi, *Phos.* suits more the congestive and inflammatory symptoms, with purulent, chalky or sandy sediment. *Zinc.* gives us a pure neuralgia ; vesical irritation, crampy, colicky pains, spasm of the bladder ; difficulty in beginning to pass water ; loamy or sandy sediment ; cannot pass urine unless sit bent backwards.

Urine

PHOSPHORUS	ZINCUM
Urine impeded by pain in the hypogastrium (fundus vesicæ).	Pressure on bladder, *sits with the limbs crossed, bladder full, yet none passes* (cervix vesicæ).
Urine ammoniacal ; with variegated cuticle ; white and flocculent sediment.	Urine yellow, depositing flocks ; loamy.

Genitals

PHOSPHORUS	ZINCUM
Gonorrhœa, gleet, hypertrophy of the prostate.	Gonorrhœa ; *bubo, left groin ; constriction in the testes.*

In both, the sexual desire is increased with local excitement ; strong erections. In spermatorrhœa, they are equally adapted to the nervous exhaustion ; pale face, weakness, sunken eyes, melancholy, &c. *Phos.* is preferable when the *lungs are involved, memory weak, diarrhœa ; locomotor ataxia.* Locally, we have interiorly an irritation of the genitals ; *impotence, feeble and too rapid emission of semen. Zinc.* is the remedy when the patient *torments everyone with his complaining, hypochondriacal ; spinal irritation, with pains only when sitting ; spine better for a few days after an emission.* Locally, there is an itching of the scrotum, not relieved by scratching (*Staph.*) ; emission absent during coition from failure in testicular secretion.

PHOSPHORUS	ZINCUM
Testes sore ; cord swollen, painful.	Testes inflamed ; orchalgia; *strangulating pain ; jerks in cord.*
Menses generally too early ; *relaxation, weakness felt in the abdomen* ; cramps in the calves.	Menses generally late ; *weakness felt in the hands and feet*; cramps in the hypochondrium or knees.
Ovarian pains during menses.	Ovarian pains *better* during menses.
Most complaints during menses.	Generally better during menses.
Amenorrhœa, stitches in the mammæ ; *eye-lids puffed.*	Amenorrhœa, mammæ swollen, painful, eyes sore.
Menorrhagia, blood pale or bright.	Menorrhagia, blood in clots.
Erectile tumors on the external genitals.	*Varicose veins* of the external genitals.
Leucorrhœa corrosive ; precedes menses.	Leucorrhœa causes itching ; in place of menses.
Mammæ inflamed, even threatened ulceration.	Mammæ painful ; nipples sore, excoriated.
Galactorrhœa ; weak therefrom.	Agalactia ; fever, nymphomania may follow.

According to Dr. Guernsey and others *Zinc.* has cured obstinate puerperal convulsions when *Phos.*, though indicated, failed.

PHOSPHORUS	ZINCUM
Genitals	
Sexual mania with *lasciviousness, obscene talk,* (male or female); after *Hyosc.* fails (4).	Sexual mania, more in females, caused by pruritus vulvæ; or by suppressed milk, lochia, menses.
Chest	
Hoarse; *voice lost* or altered from catarrh or laryngeal pain.	Hoarse; voice weak from use, as if the muscles were weak.
Cough, *tightness across the chest*; *larynx sensitive*; veins of hand swollen; sacrum feels, as if broken; *trembling all over.*	Cough, as if *chest would fly to pieces*; spasm in the suprasternal fossa; *varices of legs pain*; sacrum feels sore; trembling of the legs.
Expectoration bloody, frothy, pale-red, *rust-colored*; salty, sour, *sweet and purulent.*	Expectoration bloody, tenacious, yellow, sweet, purulent, metallic.
Phthisis pulm. seu abdom., face pale or cheeks red; bowels loose; stools bloody or contain lumps like tallow; flashes of heat with debility, weak knees.	Phthisis pulm. seu abdom. face pewter-like hue; stools contain flakes like epithelium; flashes of heat with intense trembling.

Phos. has a congestive asthma, and then the aggravation is while lying on the back or on falling asleep. The labored breathing indicates its use in threatened paralysis of the lungs. *Zinc.* has a quick, *dry* breathing, with incipient cerebral paralysis, with occipital heat and stiffness of the neck (medulla oblongata).

PHOSPHORUS	ZINCUM
Palpitation with congestion to the heart, cramp between the scapulæ.	Palpitation with an occasional violent jump of the heart.
Pulse full, hard, accelerated; double or small, weak and irregular.	Pulse small and frequent, evening; slow during the day; intermittent.
Back, Limbs	
Burning in *spots* along the spine.	Burning with *crampy* pains along the spine.
Backache, as if broken; impedes motion; *sacrum pains after confinement.*	Backache, worse at the *last lumbar vertebra*; *worse sitting, less walking.*

(4) *Phos.* seems to affect the genitals more interiorly; *Zinc.* exteriorly; the former, therefore, gives us obscenity; the latter, desire for onanism. *Zinc.* seems to exhibit many complaints from checked eruptions, ulcers, exanthema or discharges. Thus we have delirium from undeveloped scarlatina; maddening pain in the brain, when uterine ulceration is locally treated; and here nymphomania from suppressed discharge.

PHOSPHORUS	Back, Limbs	ZINCUM
Paralysis with anæsthesia and heat in the parts ; caused by *sexual excesses ; softening* ; after confinement.		Paralysis with anæsthesia, general sense of trembling caused by *wine*, suppressed foot-sweat ; softening of the brain.

Phosph. has also a paralysis from myelitis, inflammation of the vertebræ (burning in spots) and from chronic softening (with *Calc. C.*). *Zinc.* gives paralysis of the arms with colic ; later, nausea, tremor, paralyzed sphincters ; abdomen retracted. Here it resembles *lead*.

PHOSPHORUS	ZINCUM
Legs so weak, she makes mis-steps; face hot.	Legs weak, worse when hungry ; face pale.
Hands and arms cold with diarrhœa.	Hands bluish, from stagnation of blood.
Soles pain, as if bruised after a journey.	Blisters and soreness, as if *corroded*, after a journey.
Lower limbs covered with fetid sweat.	Foot-sweat, *corrosive*, fetid.

Sleep

PHOSPHORUS	ZINCUM
Usually better after sleep ; except after siesta or when aroused.	Usually worse after sleep ; look haggard.
Awakened by *heat* or chilliness, *hunger* or bad dreams.	Awakened by cold feet, *fidgety feet* or bad dreams.
Coma ; coma vigil.	Deep, fatiguing sleep.

Both have unconsciousness with typhoid symptoms, especially with incipient cerebral paralysis ; but sopor belongs chiefly to *Phos.*

PHOSPHORUS	ZINCUM
Starts in sleep, awakens anxious.	Starts in sleep, awakens terrified.

Fever

PHOSPHORUS	ZINCUM
Chill, evening until 12 P. M.	Chill lasts after eating in the night.
Chill more internal ; worse near warm stove, in a warm room ; better after eating.	Chill more external ; worse in the open air, from touching anything cold, after eating.
Heat afternoon, evening, night ; ascends ; breath anxious ; mammæ swollen ; red cheeks.	Heat forenoon, night ; descends ; breath hot ; milk suppressed ; red face.
Circulation altered when at rest, from tobacco smoke, afternoons.	Circulation altered when ascending, from drinking, evenings.
Sweat clammy, upper part of body; morning, night ; prostration ; milk increased.	Sweat too easily excited ; lower parts ; night ; trembling ; milk diminished.
Typhoid states : Typhus stupida ; exanthematic, enteric, pectoral, cerebral, petechial forms.	*Typhoid States :* Typhus versatilis ; cerebral, enteric forms.

PHOSPHORUS — Fever — ZINCUM

In the Apoplectic forms, with impending paralysis of the brain, both are indicated.

PHOSPHORUS	ZINCUM
Delirum generally mild.	Delirum violent ; tries to esrape.
Senses acute yet indifferent, apathetic ; answers "yes", "no".	Senses dull ; repeats all questions before answering them.
Hot vertex.	Hot occiput.
Lids half covering the dull sunken eyes.	Staring ; cannot or will not open the eye-lids.
Sick, hollow, sunken look ; blue circles around the eyes ; face ashy-pale, dingy or earthy.	Sick, sunken look ; facial muscles relaxed ; face red, cracked or pale, waxy or yellow.
Restless all nlght ; puts hands out, tosses hands.	Trembling, automatic motion of the hands ; picks the bed-clothes.
Lies on the back, sudden spells of weakness, sinking of all the forces ; lips covered with black slime.	Lies on the back ; so weak that he slides down in bed ; lips black, brown, cracked.
Cries out in sleep ; awakens hot, dizzy.	Cries out, as if terrified ; knows no one on waking.
Part laid on feels, as if the bed had been too hard.	Decubitus on the sacrum or trochanters.
Stool unnoticed ; looks like flesh-water or black from decomposed blood.	Stool and urine involuntary with pieces of epithelium.
Roseola spots ; ecchymosis.	Ecchymosis ; petechiæ.
Pulse weak, intermitting, quick, or full and accelerated.	Pulse weak, intermitting, scarcely perceptible, frequent.
Trembling in the morning with jerking of the limbs.	Trembling hands with convulsions, cold extremities.
Hæmorrhages from nose, gums, chest, bowels ; blood black from bowels.	Hæmorrhages with pale blood at the approach of cerebral paralysis.
Small pox with hæmorrhagic diathesis ; eruption fills with blood ; bronchial symptoms.	*Small pox* when the eruption is slow, with convulsions ; no fever but cold feet and pale urine.
Scarlatina, retrocession of the eruption ; typhoid symptoms ; threatened cerebral or pulmonary paralysis ; rattling on the	*Scarlatina*, eruption is slow, imperfect ; threatened cerebral paralysis of cerebral irritation ; breathing short but dry, with

PHOSPHORUS	Fever	ZINCUM
chest, with sweat on the face; sopor with dry tongue, loss of speech and hearing; difficult deglutition; urine involuntary; mouth open; burning in various parts compels a change of position.		cold sweat on forehead, occiput hot; unconscious; loss of speech, difficult deglutition; urine and stool involuntary; mouth open; *eye-lids paralyzed*; a fidgety condition compels the moving of the feet.

Tissues

PHOSPHORUS	ZINCUM
Herpes, vesicular around the joints.	Herpes in the bends of the joints.

Anæmia appears in both. They meet in that disease of exhaustion, known as *Hydrocephaloid*. Compare Head, Stools, Typhus.

PHOSPHORUS	ZINCUM
Sensation of festering of internal parts.	Sensations (pains) occur between skin and flesh.

Small wounds bleed much, although found in both, has proved clinically, characteristic of *Phos.*

PHOSPHORUS	ZINCUM
Cancer, *medullary*; fungus hæm.; *pale, earthy* face; cancer of the stomach with coffee-grounds vomit.	Hard, *scirrhous* lumps in various parts; *pewter-like hue of the face; pressure like a finger in the tumors* (5).
Glands inflamed, swollen, ulcerated; fatty degeneration, atrophy, cancer, &c.	Not many symptoms of the glands; swelling, ulceration, *pressure,* cancer.
Caries, necrosis inflammation and curvature of bones, especially lower jaw and tibia.	Drawing, coldness, tightness in the bones; especially the long bones—they refuse support.
Ulcers, discharge copiously, bloody or yellow.	Ulcers, discharge thin, bloody, acrid.
Tetter, dry, scaly.	Tetter, dry, like rhagades.
Pricking and burning in the skin.	Pricking in the muscles.
Gnawing in outer parts; complaints mostly internal.	*Pungent-biting* in outer parts, (6); complaints mostly external.
Itching; after scratching; vesiculæ; burning; erysipelas; spots.	Itching, after scratching efflorescence, pimples; pricking; rhagades.

(5) That *Phos.* is adapted to bleeding, and hence to open cancers, is certain; it is partly inferential that *Zinc.* is suited to scirrhus, but the symptoms point to it, and it was thought not unwise to insert the comparison.

(6) This sensation is characteristic of ulcers, skin eruptions and erosions in *Zinc.* It is a corrosive feeling, something like that felt when the bare plates of a galvanic battery are allowed to press on the skin.

PHOSPHORUS	ZINCUM
Tissues	
Remission after midnight.	Remission night, noon and forenoon.
Ailments from *Iod.*, table salt (7,8).	Ailments from *Baryta.*

PODOPHYLLUM	CHELIDONIUM
Mind, Head	
Forgetful during the chill.	Difficult thought ; forgets easily.
Low-spirited ; imagines he will die or be very sick ; liver affected.	Troubled, weeps, must move from place to place ; liver affected.
Dull headache, with pain behind the eyes (liver affected).	*Neuralgic pains from occiput to left ear* ; *occiput heavy,* (liver affected).
Face	
Eyes inflamed in the *morning* ; scrofulous ophthalmia.	*Lachrymation* with fistula, with neuralgia ; when looking fixedly.
Complexion sallow as in jaundice.	Sallow or sunken, gray, blue around the eyes.
Not yet given in neuralgia of the face.	*Right supra-orbital neuralgia* ; *eyes water.*
Mouth, Throat	
Tongue white furred or yellow.	Tongue *narrow, pointed* or thickly furred.
Throat sore ; worse right side ; in the morning ; swallowing liquids.	Constricted feeling above the larynx ; sensation, as after swallowing too large a morsel.
Stomach, Abdomen	
Taste *foul* ; *breath foul.*	Taste *bitter.*
Dyspeptic symptoms from *abuse of Mercury* ; *liver torpid,* with soreness, fulness in the right hypochondrium, *better from*	Dyspeptic symptoms, with liver complications indicated by *pain under angle of right shoulder-blade* ; congestion of

(7) *Phos.* has ailments from table salt ; *Zinc.* has herpes in the mouth from salt bathing.

(8) *Phos.* has a tired, drowsy feeling after wine, but generally wine improves.

PODOPHYLLUM	Stomach, Abdomen	CHELIDONIUM
rubbing ; *costive, clay colored stools* ; *sallow complexion, putrid breath, furred tongue* ; dull headache ; aching behind the eyes ; *loathing or regurgitation of food* ; *worse after eating.*		the liver, with *sharp, stitching pains, throbbing* ; *costive,* clayey stools ; jaundice ; *pain from occiput to left ear* ; *longing for milk, coffee, they agree* ; *better* (pains) *after eating.*
Diarrhœa from acid fruit and milk ; *during dentition* ; *discharges yellow, green, slimy.*		*Diarrhœa better from milk* ; *during pneumonia, capillary bronchitis* ; *discharges bright-yellow.*
	Chest	
Loose cough, rattling in the chest during dentition. Whooping cough, with constipation and loss of appetite. Cough associated with remittent fever, lessening during the remissions.		*Rattling cough with capillary bronchitis* ; *bright yellow diarrhœa.* Whooping cough, with forcible expectoration of lumps of mucus. Pneumonia with one cold ear and foot, one warm ; great oppression ; fanlike motion of the alæ nasi ; pain under right scapula.
Palpitation of the heart from physical exertion ; as if the heart were ascending into the throat ; *rumbling in the right abdomen* ; *morning drowsiness.*		Palpitation *so violent as to shake the bed* ; stitches in the heart ; great anxiety ; often associated with congestion of the liver and portal system.
	Back	
Lumbar backache after washing ; *with prolapsus uteri* ; *diarrhœa.*		*Pinching, spasmodic pain on the inner edge of the right scapula.*
	Sleep	
Whining, moaning in sleep ; *rolling the head* (teething).		Sleepy, yet cannot sleep (1).
Sleepy in the forenoon, with flatus in the ascending colon.		Heavy sleep all day in patients suffering from portal congestion.

PODOPHYLLUM	Mind	MERCURIUS
Low-spirited ; fears he is going to die ; hypochondriacal.		Fears loss of reason, fears he will become insane ; anxious.
	Head	
Throbbing temples, eyes ache, hot head, *morning.*		Splitting frontal fulness, head hot ; *evening, night.*

(1) All the *Papaveraceae* have this symptom.

PODOPHYLLUM	MERCURIUS
Head	
Rolling head; grinding teeth; whining at night; head sweaty in sleep, flesh cold. Dentition difficult.	*Fontanelles open*; *restless sleep, moaning, groaning*; sweat all over, *clammy*, cold, sour. Dentition difficult.
Eyes	
Ophthalmia scrofulosa, even perforation of the cornea; *worse in the morning* (1).	Ophthalmia scrofulosa, pustules on the cornea; lids crusty; *worse evening and night*.
Mouth, Throat	
Breath smells foul.	Breath smells fetid (2).
Tongue *white*, dry.	Tongue *yellow, moist, flabby*.
Saliva copious.	Saliva copious, fetid.
Throat sore; worse right side; swallowing liquids; *in the morning*.	Throat sore; worse left side; swallowing saliva and liquids; *in evening air*.
Stomach, Abdomen	
Nausea, *gagging*; vomit of blood, bitter; or, painful retching.	Nausea; vomit bile, bitter or *sweetish* (as from worms).
Flatus in the right abdomen; palpitation, sleepy mornings (*3*).	Flatus not so marked as in *Podophyl.*; *fulness in stomach and hypochondria*.
Liver feels hot, sore; twisting pains; better from rubbing that region; costive; stools hard, dry, difficult.	Liver so sensitive he cannot lie on the right side or bear the least touch; costive, with ineffectual straining.
Colic (as from lead), with *retraction of the abdominal walls*.	Colic as from worms; sweet taste; *hard, tender, distended abdomen*.
Stool *chalk-like, offensive with gagging*; *clay-colored*; black; *watery, profuse, painless, gushing, exhausting*; mealy sediment; bloody, green yellow, mucous, *smelling like carrion*; worse towards morning; *in the morning*.	Stool tenacious, crumbling, small in shape; grayish-white; black, pitch like; not gushing, but burning, *watery, corrosive*; *bloody mucus, slimy, with much tenesmus*; *odorless* or simply sour; worse usually in *evening and night*.

(1) In compounding *Mandrake* pills, the dust causes inflamed eyes, perforating ulcer; itching eruption, worse about the genitals. The morning aggravation is marked, *Merc.* is worse from the glare and heat of the fire.

(2) This fetor comes from ulcerative processes, the foulness in *Podophyl.* is indescribable.

(3) A group many times confirmed by Dr. Jeanes

PODOPHYLLUM	MERCURIUS
Stomach, Abdomen	
After stool exhaustion ; cutting pains ; weak even after natural stool.	After stool cutting and great tenesmus ; sweat ; trembling ; burning in anus.
Prolapsus recti from any exertion ; with diarrhœa.	Prolapsus recti ; inflamed black ; when straining.
Urine, Genitals	
Urine scanty, frequent at night (pregnancy).	Urine scanty with constant, violent urging.
Dragging pains in the ovarian regions.	Shooting from ovaries to hips ; suppuration.
Prolapsus uteri, with backache at sacrum ; *after confinement* ; *from washing* ; *with prolapsus ani* ; with amenorrhœa ; stool frequent, though natural.	Prolapsus uteri et vaginæ with soreness *of the genitals externally and internally* (4) ; much urging in the rectum ; stools crumble or slimy, bloody.
Pregnancy : Can lie comfortably only on the abdomen (early months) ; frequent urination ; prolapsus uteri after.	Pregnancy : Stomach very sensitive to touch or pressure ; scorbutic symptoms, sore gums, etc. ; lochia, with *sore genitals* (4).
Chest	
Cough in remittent fever ; loose during dentition ; whooping cough with constipation and loss of appetite.	Cough with burning and rawness, moist but phlegm does not loosen ; so convulsive, cannot speak ; whooping cough in two paroxysms.
Palpitation from any exertion *with flatulence* ; heart, as if it came into the throat.	Palpitation on *awaking*, *thumping*, *agitation* ; trembling or feeling, as if life were ebbing away.
Fever	
Pulse slow ; scarcely perceptible ; pulseless, collapse, chill 7 A.M., forgets the words.	Pulse usually full, strong ; pulseless with hot body. Chill A.M. (5), but more in *evening*.
Heat with delirium and loquacity ; afterwards forgetful of what has passed.	Heat with ebullitions, constriction of the chest ; anxiety

(4) This soreness is very characteristic, and indicates *Mercury* in scarlet fever, etc.

(5) The morning chill is after rising from bed ; but the evening attack is most important. This collection of symptoms is invaluable in bilious fevers.

PODOPHYLLUM	MERCURIUS
Fever	
Sweat *warm* on the legs ; feet cold; head sweat with coldness of the skin ; sleep during sweat.	Sweat *cold,* clammy on the legs ; cold sweat on the forehead ; skin burns ; *sweat never relieves.*
Flashes up the back and abdominal pains during stool.	*Chilliness between* or *after stool.*
Generalities	
Worse from walking on uneven ground ; mis-step.	Worse from any form of motion.
Worse in the *morning.*	Worse *evening and night.*
Worse from *acid fruit with milk* (6).	Worse from sweets, from *sugar.*

PODOPHYLLUM	NUX VOMICA
Head	
More depression of spirits.	More irritability, anger.
Morning headache ; *hot vertex.*	Morning headache ; *heat in the forehead.*
Eyes	
Ophthalmia worse in the morning; perforation of the cornea.	Ophthalmia worse evening and morning ; ecchymosis of sclerotica.
Face	
Complexion sallow, dingy.	Complexion yellow *with a red flush.*
Nose, Mouth, Throat	
Breath *foul* (night).	Breath offensive, *morning.*
Tongue white or yellow coated.	Tongue red, sore and coated yellow at the base.
Throat sore ; worse from swallowing liquids.	Throat sore, as if rough, scraped ; worse after eating, from solids.
Stomach, Abdomen	
Dyspepsia from abuse of calomel.	Dyspepsia from absue of drastic medicines.
Vomit *hot, sour,* bilious, bloody.	Vomit *sour* or bitter, of dark blood.
Flatus in the ascending colon ; *palpitation* ; *drowsy forenoons.*	Flatus in the hypochondria, *pressing upwards* or *down on to the bladder or rectum.*

(6) *Podophyllum* has received the name of *Vegetable Mercury.* It helps promptly in dyspepsia caused by *Calomel.*

PODOPHYLLUM	NUX VOMICA
Stomach, Abdomen	
Region of the liver sore; *relief from rubbing the right side*; stools black or clay-colored; jaundice; stool difficult.	Region of the liver worse from pressure; *must loosen the clothing*; stools black, large, *ineffectual urging*; jaundice.
Stool difficult from inactive bowels; *prolapsus ani even with loose stool.*	Stool difficult from spasmodic action; *hence ineffectual urging*; prolapsus ani.
Stool *watery, gushing, profuse,* green; *with sudden urging,* often painless; offensive; worse in hot weather.	Stool thin, brown, dark water, small, frequent, offensive; ineffectual urging, worse in cold changes.
Urine, Genitals	
Urine scanty, frequent; or frequent urination during pregmancy.	Painful, ineffectual urging to urinate; even in pregnancy frequent urging.

Prolapsus uteri after washing; after parturition; has frequently yielded to either.

PODOPHYLLUM	NUX VOMICA
Prolapsus; *with falling of the rectum*; stools are *naturally formed, but too frequent and weakening*; sacral pains; aching in ovarian region.	Prolapsus with urging to stool; stools large; *backache worse turning in bed;* tightness in the hypochondria; cough dry, teasing.
After pains with much bearing down, flatulency.	After pains too long lasting; pressure on the rectum.
In pregnancy (early months), must lie on the abdomen; (later) pains above the right groin.	In pregnancy (especially later months) *difficulty of breathing from upward pressure.*
Larynx, Chest	
Whooping cough with costiveness, loss of appetite; cough in remittent fever; cough during dentition.	Whooping cough from costiveness, nose-bleed; stomach-cough; cough of students.
Palpitation of the heart from physical exertion; flatulence; drowsy forenoons.	Palpitation of the heart, the heart feels tired; palpitation lying; wind from the stomach.
Sleep	
Whining in sleep (teething children); languid on awaking in the morning.	Awakens 3 A. M., ideas crowd upon him; if he falls asleep, he re-awakens much fatigued (1).

(1) *Nux Vomica* has a whimpering and moaning in sleep; waking from troubled, busy dreams, frightened, as if some one were in the room (typhus, mania-a-potu).

Fevers

PODOPHYLLUM	NUX VOMICA
Chill 7 A. M.; forgets words he wishes to use.	Chill 1 P. M., goes to sleep between chill and heat.
Heat with delirium and *excessive loquacity*, thirst, headache; forgetful afterwards.	Heat with *over-excited senses*, worse from external impressions.
Sweat warm on the head, with cold face (dentition); sleep in sweat.	Sweat clammy, sour or offensive; one-sided sweat.

Constitution

PODOPHYLLUM	NUX VOMICA
Debility, (especially with bowel disturbances).	Debility, *with over-sensitive nerves*.
Complaints of teething children.	Complaints of "high-livers"
Abuse of calomel; eating acid fruit with milk; poisoning with *lead*.	Abuse of purgatives; indulging in liquids; poisoning with *lead, copper*.

PODOPHYLLUM — SULPHUR

PODOPHYLLUM	SULPHUR
Anxiety; fears he is going to die.	Anxiety, despairs of salvation.
DENTITION: *Rolls the head, grinds the teeth*; child whines at night, restless sleep, half open eyes; head sweats, legs cold, face cold; vomiting frothy mucus, green; or food; or only *gagging*; stools profuse, gushing, green, watery, or white; offensive; *from midnight, but worse in the morning.*	DENTITION: *Child lies in a stupor, eyes half open*; or sleeps in *cat-naps*; jerks the limbs; fontanelles open, pale face, cold sweat on face, cold extremities; vomiting *sour-smelling;* stools watery, green, involuntary, white, sour or offensive; *irresistible, sudden urging in the morning.*

Stomach, Abdomen

PODOPHYLLUM	SULPHUR
Eructations *hot*, sour; smell like rotten eggs.	Eructations sour; taste like rotten eggs.
Worse from acid fruits *with milk.*	Worse in every form from *milk.*
Tongue white or brown.	Tongue white, *red tip.*
Flatus in the right abdomen; *palpitation*; *sleepy forenoon.*	Flatus mostly in the region of the sigmoid flexure.
Bowels move after being washed.	Aversion to washing; generally worse therefrom.
Colic with cramp-like knots or retraction of the abdominal walls.	A similar cramping, as if the intestines were in knots; pains go to chest, to groins.

PODOPHYLLUM	Stomach, Abdomen	SULPHUR

The stools are very similar: changeable, watery, green, mucous, white, undigested; with colic, cramps in the thighs; vomiting, purging; with prolapsus ani (more marked in *Podoph.*). They meet, hence, in cholera infantum, cholera, summer diarrhœas. *Sulph.* has with *Podophyllum* the profuse, gushing, painless stools, but has more marked the *excoriation and redness of the anus*. It pictures, according to Hering, the *whole course of Asiatic cholera*: hence becomes a prophylactic; *Podophyl.* may apply in painless cholera morbus and in cholera when cramps, profuse discharges, prostration, etc., are present. In cholera infantum *Sulph.* shows its supremacy as a nutritive remedy.

PODOPHYLLUM	SULPHUR
Drowsiness or restless sleep, rolling the head; flesh is soft, flabby; sallowness.	*Stupor, suppressed urine* (hydrocephaloid impending); *flesh wrinkled, yellow, dry*; *child looks like an old man.*

Fever

PODOPHYLLUM	SULPHUR
Remittent or intermittent type; forgetful during the chill; loquacious delirium in the heat, violent headache.	More a *continuous remittent* type; between chill and heat delirium sets in; prostration increasing with the congestion and heat; headache.
Tongue coated uniformly white, yellow or brown; jaundice.	Tongue dry, if coated, more yellow-brown centre; jaundice.
After the hot stage forgets all that has passed.	Fever if continuous, causes *slowness in responding* (1).

PTELIA—ARNICA—BRYONIA—NUX VOMICA

PTELIA TRIFOLIATA has many symptoms in common with *Bry.* and *Nux V.* All have weak mind with bodily languor; peevish, irritable; senses too easily impressed by external objects; hence, worse from noise, light, smells, conversation, smell of food, &c. Gastric headache; stomacace; pharyngitis; disgust for meat; hepatic congestion and hepatitis; ascites, (except perhaps *Nux*); dysenteric stool; constipation with hard, dry stool; jaundice; catamenia too soon; urine red, high-colored; red sediment (exccpt *Bry.*); stitches in various parts, worse moving, speaking, breathing; headache with cough; rheumatism, wandering pains; nettle-rash with gastric disorder; languor, must lie down; limbs weak with nausea, &c.

Ptelia stands between *Bry.* and *Nux V.*, and *Arn.*, in gastro-bilious diseases. Like *Bry.*, it has hcpatitis better lying on *right* side but the stitch pains do not appear with the least attempt to breathe,

(1) The latter is an observation of Dr. C. Wesselhœft.

PTELIA—ARNICA—BRYONIA—NUX VOMICA

only in *deep* inspiration and the stool is dry, hard, small, while *Bry.* has stools *large*, dry. *Nux V.* is worse lying on painful side and has large stool.

With *Arnica*, it has eructations like rotten eggs ; aversion to meat and longing for acid ; but eating causes epigastric pain and sensation of goneness ; not fulness, as in *Arn.*

Nux Vomica has a similar periodic aggravation of gastric symptoms (3—4 A.M.) ; but *Ptelia* has aversion to fat ; *Nux* a longing. *Ptelia*, predominating bitter taste ; *Nux*, more sour taste ; *Ptelia* feels the effects of food at once ; *Nux*, an hour or two after a meal. (Duodenal Digestion.)

Ptelia causes dysenteric tenesmus appearing before and *after* stool ; in *Nux* tenesmus ceases after stool.

Ptelia, stool small, hard balls ; *Nux and Bry.*, stools too large.

Ptelia causes dry mouth, cracked lips ; but the saliva is increased and saltish. Tongue shows red papillæ and feels scalded with prickling. Drooling at night. *Bryonia* has dry mouth, thirst ; saliva frothy, soapy ; mouth better when moistened (because "child does not like to take hold of the breast; but when once its mouth is moistened it nurses well."). *Nux V.* has the drooling, but saliva is then bloody ; voice is altered, as if something were being held in the mouth.

In fevers with bilious symptoms : *Ptelia*, hot sweat on *forehead* ; sweat relieves ; (pulse quick, weak or irregular). *Nux*, cold, clammy sweat on face ; sweat aggravates ; worse in open, cold air ; (*Ptelia*, better : pulse full, hard). *Bryon.*, nausea better lying ; (*Ptelia*, worse) : less chilly in open air ; pulse regular.

Ptelia is *worse* : Warmth, mental work, fat-food, meat, lying down, early morning ; and *better* : Open air (except chest), acids, rising from bed, during continued motion.

Bryon. and *Nux* are *better* : Warmth, lying ; and *worse* : Continued motion, open, cold air, acids.

PULSATILLA—LILIUM TIG.

Pulsatilla and *Lilium*, although unlike in their general indications, bear the closest resemblance in their action on the veins. They have the same fulness of veins, chest and heart; worse in the evening and better in the open air. Heart feels too full of blood, with weak, feeble pulse, faintness, inclination to take a deep breath. Such symptoms often occur in enlargement, involving the right heart.

PULSATILLA—LILIUM TIG.

Pulsatilla, though feeling chilly, finds relief in the open air and from walking ; *Lilium* finds relief in the open air (except headache) ; but the cold air makes the heart feel icy-cold ; motion aggravates. If the urine is retained, the congestion seems aggravated.

Lilium like *Pulsatilla*, causes scanty menses ; but the former has irritable mood ; wants to die and yet knows not why ; solicitude about health ; absence of feeling in the head with amenia ; longs for meat; diarrhœa hurries her out of bed in the morning. *Pulsatilla* has gentle, tearful mood; wants to die, but fears it; solicitude about health and salvation ; mania with amenia ; averse to meat ; diarrhœa after midnight. Remission, in *Lilium*, *forenoon* ; in *Pulsatilla*, *midnight*, *until noon* (except diarrhœa).

COMPARISONS OF REMEDIES
OF THE SAME STOCK

THE HALOGENS

In the Affections of Larynx and Chest.

BROMINE	IODINE	SPONGIA
Inspiration difficult ; child starts from sleep ; *relieved by a drink of water.*	Inspiration difficult, *constriction of the throat* prevents swallowing (1).	Inspiration difficult, as *though breathing through a sponge.*
Throat sore ; dry, smooth ; *raw spots* ; *air feels cold.*	Throat sore ; *child grasps it with the hands.*	Throat sore ; *sensation of a plug.*
Hoarse ; *child cries with hoarse voice, evening aphonia.*	Hoarse ; *voice deep or husky ; morning aggravation.*	Hoarse ; deep, harsh voice ; or voice fails in speaking.
Goitre. *Blue eyes,* light complexion ; young.	Goitre. *Black eyes, dark complexion* ; *protruding eyes.*	Goitre. (Living in valleys.) Light complexion.
Cough dry, rough as from vapors of sulphur ; *whistling, hoarse, croupy, spasmodic* ; *no sputa, gasping for breath* ; worse wet weather ; evening, night ; better in warmth.	Cough *moist but harsh* as from tickling all over the chest ; *wheezing, metallic cough* ; *tough or slimy sputa* ; *constriction of the larynx,* worse in wet weather ; morning part of the day.	Cough *barking* ; *with suffocative spells* ; slow, sawing respiration ; scanty sputa; worse before midnight ; *worse from dry cold west winds,* seldom in damp or wet weather.
Croup in children with BLUE EYES.	*Croup in children with* BLACK EYES.	Croup (before exudation) *blue eyes.*
Deep breathing provokes gasping ; asthma better in the sea-air. Eyes AFFECTED ; better in WARMTH.	Breath comes in wave like expansions (2) ; asthma ; *warm air or a warm room always aggravates.*	Breathe *slowly* ; strong action of the abdominal muscles ; always better in wet weather.

(1) *Iodine* has constriction stronger than the rest, *Bromine* has the most marked ptyalism.

(2) This wave-like motion is characteristic of the presence of a membrane. When using the Halogens in croup, a sponge wrung out in hot water and applied externally over the larynx, aids materially.

BROMINE	IODINE	SPONGIA
Rattling as if the chest were full; face puffed, body cold.	Rattling on the chest, yet nothing seems to loosen (3).	Loud rattling on the chest; sonorous ronchi.
Chest weak; EYES AFFECTED.	Chest *so weuk can hardly walk upstairs.*	Sudden weakness of the chest; tottering.
Membrane comes up from the larynx; after *Spongia*; local symptoms very intense; spasm of the glottis.	*Membrane extensive*; *torpid cases*; *jerking breathing*; after *Hepar*, more fever, thirst; more pulmonary congestion.	*Beginning of croupous inflammation*, after *Aconite*; *sawing* respiration.
Phthisis : Cutting up into the axilla; worse in the right lung, *congestion to the head better from nose-bleed*; EYES AFFECTED.	Phthisis : Tickling all over the chest; *tough, stringy*, blood streaked sputa; *hunger, yet emaciation*; *can not bear a warm room.*	Phthisis : Dyspnœa on lying down; *dry, hard, barking cough* on least motion; weak spells; tottering.
Heart : Cutting from heart to axilla; asthma; cannot lie down; pressure referred to the pit of the stomach. Hypertrophy.	Heart : Purring in the region of the heart; heart feels as if being squeezed or very weak; palpitation better lying quietly on the back.	Heart : Deposit on the valves; blowing sound; must sit up; suddenly starting up anxious, choking coughing.
Hepatization of the lower lobes.	Pneumonia when the disease localizes.	Bronchitis.

BROMINE, suffocating spells, *gasping*; excoriation in the larynx; struma.

IODINE, spasm of glottis; rachitic children; *cannot bear warmth.*

FLUORINE, spasm of glottis; *can withstand both heat and cold.*

CHLORINE, *inspiration crowing, expiration impossible.*

---

(3) *Iodine*, here resembles *Hepar* and *Ant. Tart.* If the laryngeal obstruction continues, and if the rattling seems symptomatic of tracheal catarrh, *Iodine* is indicated. If paralysis of the lungs is imminent—blue face, cold sweat, frequent pulse, drowsiness, stupor—*Ant. Tart.* is indicated.

THE KALIS

THE PRINCIPAL SALTS OF POTASSA*

Mind

A state of apprehension, timidity, anxiety is quite general. The patient is easily startled.

In the CARB. the *least touch,* or supposed *"vision of flying birds" makes him start.* In the BROM. this timidity is so intensified we have, *night-terrors* (children) *followed* by *squinting,* cerebral erethism ; in adults this state is coupled with a feeling, as if they would lose their mind. The chemically similar HYDRIOD. shows a symptomatic resemblance ; but the *talkativeness and excitement are a part of the "Iodine-drunkenness."* The third, CHLOR., claims precedence in alternate states of sadness and cheerfulness, associated with congestion ; hence, *nose-bleed relieves.* The NITRAT. produces more than the others, *profuse sweat with the anxiety.*

Dullness of intellect is predominant in all. Associated with this is melancholy, indifference or apathy.

Weak memory, *aphasia,* diminished reflex excitability and profound melancholy, characterize the BROM. Thus it proves curative in cerebral softening.

Vertigo is not marked. More characteristic is a stupid, intoxicated state of mind.

The CHLOR., because of its power to disturb the circulation, determining blood to central organs, gives the best type of congestive vertigo, *especially after violent exercise.* When of gastric origin, we may choose between the BICHR. and the CARB. In the former, *nausea and sour, watery vomit concur,* in the latter, *anaemia, weakness of the legs, pale face.*

Head

In headaches, the BICHR. causes *blindness before the attack, sight returning with the onset of pain.* The HYDRIOD. cures *swellings of the scalp, hard and intensely painful, after abuse of Mercury.* In chronic headaches, there is *coldness of the painful part, relieved by external warmth.*† Under the CARB. the sharp pains are worse from carriage-riding; under the NITRAT. *better.* The latter remedy is indicated when a feeling of constriction ends in *a tightness at the tip of the nose.*

---

*The salts here compared are : *Kali Carbonicum, Kali Bichromicum, Kali Chloricum, Kali Hydriodicum* (otherwise written *Kali Hydroiodicum*), *Kali Nitricun, Kali Bromatum.* The *Nitricum* is usually written *Nitrum.* Schussler's *Kali Phosph.* is omitted. For brevity *Kali* is sometimes anglicized and written in the plural, *Kalis,* when referring to the whole group.

†See Raue's Record, 1872. This coldness, etc., has been confirmed by Dr. J. B. Bell.

THE KALIS—(*contd.*)

Special Senses

Only rarely are the senses too acute. Like its analogue, *Phosphorus,* the CARB sometimes has acuteness of hearing ; but even then, it wavers between acute and dull.

The *sight* suffers in the BICHR. from bile in the blood, *yellow-sight* ; in the CARB. from *loss of semen* ; *anaemia* ; in the CHLOR., from *irritable retina,* in the HYDRIOD., more from *retinal infiltration, scrofulous ophthalmia,* etc. ; while the NITRAT. brings us back again to nervous causes and produces *blackness before the eyes.*

In the KALIS, *dullness of smell is usually traceable to catarrhs, which tend towards ulcerations, thickening and, of course, anosmia. Inflammations of Eyes, Nose, etc., frequently find a cure in the* KALI SALTS.

The BICHR. and the HYDRIOD. answer where *syphilis or scrofula* is at the foundation ; the CHLOR. and the HYDRIOD. when *Mercury* has been abused ; the CARB. for *psora* uncontaminated with syphilis.

Earache finds a remedy in the BICHR., when there are *pulsating pains at night, purulent otorrhœa* ; *stitches extending into the mouth, or down the neck, enlarged parotid.* The CARB. adds an *otorrhœa of liquid cerumen* and pus.

Fetor from the mouth belongs to all ; thus may we expect stomatitis, scurvy, decayed teeth, etc., diminished *taste.* In the BICHR. the ulcers are *deep and yellow,* in the BROM., by reason of its nervous action, infantile stomatitis appears, *with hot, dry mouth, mouth so numb the examining finger can touch the fauces, causing no contraction.* Very similar is the CARB., with mouth feeling *numb, as if burned with caustic,* but the ulcers emit *a smell as of old cheese.* More like *scurvy* is the CHLOR. sore mouth, with spongy, bleeding gums, *patches in the fauces and on the pharynx, like diphtheria* or *follicular disease* ; *fetor unbearable.* Changing to the HYDRIOD. the gums ulcerate as *after Mercury ; the saliva is bloody, smells like onions.*

Scurvy is again pictured in the antiseptic NITRAT., but here *the blood is thin, acrid, like vinegar.*

Saliva increased : Viscid, saltish, BICHR. ; bloody, HYDRIOD. ; tasting brassy, CHLOR.

Toothache : *Throbbing while eating,* CARB. ; reaching the periosteum, the HYDRIOD. gives us a sensation, as though *a worm were crawling at the root of a tooth* ; the NITRAT. infringes on the *Carb., pulsating toothache,* stitches when the teeth are touched, *gums bleed easily.*

Face

All have a bloated face, sickly expression ; *face swells suddenly, parts become œdematous or livid.*

THE KALIS—(*contd.*)

Face

There is commingling of *yellow* in the BICHR. pallor ; the anæmic CARB. adds an *alternately red and pale face, sacs over the upper eye-lids* (1). The expressionless face of the BROM. portrays *incipient softening of the brain.*

Swelling of the cheeks during the menses characterizes the CARB. ; extending to the *tongue after Mercury, the* HYDRIOD.

Catarrhs

Mucus, muco-purulent discharges. The BICHR. develops coryza worse in the open air, flow acrid, sensation of *a feather in the nose or on the tongue,* fauces and bronchi attacked, swollen tonsils, *ropy expectoration* ; *deep-eating* ulcers in the fauces, *syphilitic* ; discharge from the nose of large *clinkers or greenish plugs* ; worse in *warm weather* ; *catarrh alternating with rheumatic pains.* The BROM. has relieved torpid cases of bronchitis with copious purulent expectoration. The CARB. cures coryza, rough voice, *crawling in the throat and difficult detachment of phlegm* ; sensation of a *plug* in the throat ; it belongs principally to the mucous stage with obstructed nostrils, relieved in the open air, discharge of green, bloody or fetid purulent mucus, mostly *from one side* ; *nose scurfy, bloody,* the cough is so difficult and spasmodic that it often causes *retching and vomiting* in the effort to dislodge small, gray lumps of mucus ; like the BICHR. it suits rheumatic patients, but its principal characteristic is the *lassitude and backache* ; even swallowing causes pain in the *cervical spine.* The CHLOR. comes into use when *Mercury is abused*, has developed a tendency to catarrhs with profuse coryza, *twitchings of the masseter muscles,* luminous vibrations before the eyes when sneezing ; *gums bleed* ; *scorbutic* or *aphthous symptoms,* brassy taste, *fetid odor* from the mouth ; the CHLOR. differs from the HYDRIOD. in causing aphthous or diphtheritic states after *Mercury,* rather than croupous and glandular diseases. (This is in keeping to a scorbutic state, the second to a scrofulous.) The HYDRIOD. involves with the differences between *Chlorine* and *Iodine* ; the first corresponding *the frontal sinuses, Highmorian cavities,* etc., the nasal secretion excoriates, *eye-lids are bloated* ; the least cold aggravates ; chilliness alternates with feverishness ; speech nasal ; urine hot, red ; like the others it has rheumatic pains, but worse in *the evening, preceded by chilliness.* The NITRAT. discharges through the posterior nares like the combining Nitric Acid ; *the tip of the nose is red* ; tendency to *nasal polypus.*

Lungs, Heart

RESPIRATION.—*Potash salts are proverbially useful in oppressed breathing, asthma.* The BICHR. breathing awakens the patient at 2 A. M. ; palpitation; orthopnœa, sits bent forward; caused by *mucus, croup, croupous diphtheria, chronic bronchitis, membranous bronchitis,* or, from disturbed

(1) Although Potash Salts readily develop œdema, it is most marked in the HYDRIOD., both internally and superficially.

THE KALIS—(*contd.*)

Lungs, Heart

circulation, cold sensation and tightness about the heart, lower portions of the lungs oppressed ; pressure on the heart after eating. The BROM. dyspnœa is oppressed ; pressure on the heart after eating. The BROM, dyspnœa is more from spasmodic asthma ; breathless with the headache ; also in *chorea, hysteria*, etc. ; *croup, suppuration of the lungs*, etc. The CARB., like its relative BICHR., awakens after midnight with dyspnœa, characteristically *at 2 or 3 o'clock in the morning* ; the patient is *compelled to sit bent forward, the head on the knees* ; worse walking ; in *phthisis, suppuration of the lungs, mucous phthisis, pneumonia, pleuritis, heart disease*. During the cold stages of fevers, the breathing is *loud, dry* ; during the heat *less* marked, then only short ; the difficult respiration comes from *spasmodic pain in the chest.*

The CHLOR. owns a cardiac asthma with a sensation, as if the *heart and lungs were constricted* (*Cadimum*) as from vapors of Sulphur ; congestion of the chest with cold feet.

The HYDRIOD. develops few symptoms of dyspnœa. Like the preceding remedies it has oppression of breathing, which *awakens the patient at* 5 P.M., or at least in the morning hours ; it appears in conjunction with *pneumonia*, specially if *œdema sets in*, catarrhs (especially after *abuse of Mercury*), Bright's disease, when the *lungs become engorged*, and in *membranous croup*

The NITRAT. presents as strong a picture of nervous asthma as any medicine in the Materia Medica, tightness in the larynx during inspiration ; awakens about 3 A. M. ; *so out of breath cannot drink but in sips* ; *child seizes the cup* with *avidity but can only drink in sips* ; throat feels, as if it were about closing up; Camphor aggravates ; also in pneumonia when the *dyspnœa is greater than the extent of disease would warrant*, in *the distressing paroxysms of dyspnœa in Bright's disease.*

LUNGS.—*The* KALIS *seem to attack the lungs, congesting, inflaming and organically altering them.*

The BICHR. causes a bronchitis with thickened or dilated bronchial tubes; *ropy mucus*; purulent mucus, fetid breath; torpidity; *plastic exudation, croup,* the membrane forming even in the trachea and bronchi* ; the head is thrown back ; mouth open ; voice coarse ; tonsils red, swollen ; if parts are detached, they are *tough*, fibrous ; insidious approach of the disease ; *fat, chubby children.* In diphtheria we have similar symptoms, the deposit being *yellowish*, and the bare spots very red *and sensitive* (the *Brom.* is opposite) ; *diphtheric invading the larynx and trachea.* The

---

*I have made six or seven provings of this salt. Generally the cough seems to descend into the chest until there is an annoying *oppression referred to the epigastrium*, the cough seems to start thence. If persisted in, the remedy then causes *a horrible smothering sensation* ; *breathing sounds, as if the tubes were very narrow and lined with metal.* Does this not simulate croup ?

THE KALIS—(*contd.*)

Lungs, Heart

cough is worse undressing, better warm in bed ; *worse* 2 A. M. or on awaking ; cough from every inhalation ; cough from tickling in the larynx or *at the bifurcation of the trachea* ; the least food or drink brings cough ; cough dry, titillating *with smooth or follicular redness of the pharynx and fauces* ; *wheezing and panting precede the cough* ; the BICHR. has it as a characteristic, that *rheumatism co-exists or alternates with gastric or pulmonary troubles.* The BROM. develops a spasmodic cough and may appear in capillary bronchitis, when the child with severe dyspnœa *throws its arms about wildly, spasmodic movements of the muscles,* even opis thotonos ; thus again showing its peculiar combination of the *nervous element with inflammatory processes* ; suppuration of the lungs. Diphtheria *especially with anaesthesia of the mouth.* The CARB. becomes of paramount importance in *pneumonia and capillary bronchitis of children.* It gives us cough with *difficult* expectoration, worse after eating or drinking, vomiting and sour phlegm ; *face pale but red during cough,* pains *referred to the abdomen because the lower lobes of the lungs are infiltrated* ; *œdema of the limbs* ; *livid face with puffed eye-lids.* The difficult expectoration differs from that of the BICHR. Instead of arising only from its tenacity, there is added a muscular weakness, *the sputa must be swallowed again.* The CARB. is the first remedy to be thought of when symptoms of phthisis show themselves after *abortion, confinement, pneumonia.* The pains *are stitching,* worse in *the lower part of the right lung* ; *stitches through right lung to the back* : (the BICHR. also offers stitches, but they are from the sternum to the infra-scapular region ; in similar cases the HYDRIOD. claims attention ; but the stitches are like the BICHR. from mid-sternum to back). The cough is *choking, with so difficult sputa,* that even when loosened *must be swallowed* ; later the sputa is purulent, bloody (especially after pleuro-pneumonia) ; accompanying symptoms are sensation of *a lump in the stomach* ; *empty feeling, goneness before eating, fulness after eating* (thus differing from *Sepia*) ; *coffee or soup produces fulness* ; pulse is *weak,* small, *irregular.* Symptoms *better after breakfast.* In females we add profuse menses. In keeping with the goneness, inability to expectorate, and general languor, is the condition of the chest ; *sensation of hollowness, weakness from talking.* The HYDRIOD. more than the preceding, tends to *inflammations with œdema.* In pneumonia it is preferable to other remedies when the hepatization is so extensive as to develop symptoms of cerebral congestion with *effusion, dilated pupils, dropped jaw, coma, limbs paralyzed* (*Bell.* would be useless here because the congestion is mechanical) ; *the sputa are either frothy, like soapsuds,* showing œdema pul., or copious, *purulent, green* ; stitches through from sternum to back (2) ; pain in the chest, as if cut to pieces. Membranous croup in *scrofulous children* with swollen glands, loss of voice, *awakened choking at* 5 A.M. The CARB. cough is *worse from motion* ; the HYDRIOD., though dry, irritating, is *worse at rest.*

---

(2) It is a remarkable coincidence that all the *Mercuries* have this symptom and *Kali-Hyd.* is one of the best antidotes.

THE KALIS—(*contd.*)

Lungs, Heart

The CHLOR., modified by the combining acid, gives us a constitution tending toward aphthæ, *diphtheritic deposits* ; the cough is associated with *luminous vibrations before the eyes* and a preponderance of congestive symptoms ; *tightness across chest and heart*, palpitation. The CARB. has these luminous vibrations, but less marked than are dark spots. If hoarseness, cough, *fetid breath, diphtheritic patches concur after abuse of Mercury*, the CHLOR. is the only remedy.

The NITRAT. has pneumonia with stitch pains, anxiety. The *dyspnœa is very marked*, as it is in the CARB. ; but in the latter it arises from obstruction of the bronchioles, in the former it is all out of *proportion to the severity of the disease*, appearing even when congestion or hepatization is slight. There is also a troublesome feeling of *heaviness on the chest, as though from a great load* (3). Suppuration of the lungs with profuse colliquative sweat, anxiety, *hot face and forehead* (4). Owing probably to the combining acid, the sweat is more profuse than with any other KALI. In phthisis the cough is violent enough to take away the breath and cause *palpitation* ; *sputa scanty*, with coagulated blood.

HEART, CIRCULATION.—*It is characteristic of the* KALIS *to produce a paretic state of the heart muscle*, qualified, of course, by the combining acid. The BICHR disturbs the circulation but slightly ; pulse accelerated ; especially *awaking at* 2 A. M. ; with nausea, palpitation ; cold sensation in the cardiac region ; pressure on the heart lying, better after rising. The BROM. (5) ? The CARB. better adapted to females than the BICH., cures *throbbing of the blood-vessels felt like a pulse all over* ; pulse more rapid in the morning ; the BICHR., on the other hand, proves curative in local *flushes of heat in the face during the climacteric years* ; a weak, irregular action of the heart with cramp-pains and a faint, empty feeling in the left chest belong to the CARB. The CHLOR. has right pulse full ; soft, sluggish, intermitting every 25 beats, not synchronous with the heart ; the *left*, small, soft, easily compressible. Like the BICHR., it causes a cold sensation about the heart ; but instead of the heaviness, we have *a constriction as from a cord* (the CARB., a cramp) ; congestions to heart and chest, with cold feet and arms. The HYDRIOD. introduces an *Iodine* symptom ; *palpitation while walking*. In cardiac inflammation, we look to the CARB. where with sharp, stitching pains, we find *a blowing noise in place of the first tick and a louder second tick*, showing a stagnation in the pulmonary circulation. However the darting pains might suggest the CARB., we select the HYDRIOD. after repeated attacks (see Raue's Pathology), and if it is a sequel of Morbus Brightii. The NITRAT. must be consulted when palpitation is worse lying on the back ; pulse *slower than the beating of the heart*.

---

(3) This is comparable with the sensation in the limbs, as if they were made of wood.

(4) This feverishness of the forehead is just the state in which the allopaths most successfully use a lotion of nitre.

(5) Lacking potentized provings, we only know the paretic symptoms of KALI BROM.

THE KALIS—(*contd.*)

Stomach

The BICHR. has earned some reputation in dyspepsia when meat disagrees ; longing for *lager beer*, yet worse therefrom ; weight *immediately* after eating ; face red, blotchy, skin thick ; tongue looks flat, broad, with raised, scalloped edges. The CARB. offers a red face made worse by cold washing ; fulness in the stomach *after* eating, emptiness *before* eating ; *soup* causes fulness ; pulsations in the epigastrium ; *pulse weak, irregular* ; pains go *into the back*. The CHLOR. comes to the rescue when portal congestion and enlarged liver are present ; emptiness in the stomach. The HYDRIOD. should be preferred when symptoms common to the KALIS, *weak digestion*, etc., are complicated with frequent belching (like *Iodine*) ; emptiness, unlike CARB., because eating does not relieve it ; food tastes like straw. The BROM. would manifest a curative action when the stomach is so weakened that a heavy pressure follows every attempt at eating. The NITRAT. may, though rarely, counteract a dyspeptic tendency with *crampy pains and colic following veal.*

Stool

Common to all is hard, difficult stool ; *chronic constipation.*

We may distinguish the BICHR. by the painful retraction of the anus (6). The CARB. has *large*, difficult stool, arising from *inactivity of the rectum*. The CHLOR., like the *muriates* causes so decided a dryness that *the stool almost crumble.*

Loose evacuations also appear ; *sudden, forcible urging* ; *watery stool, mucous.* The BICHR. hurries out of bed ; *jelly-like stool*, tongue *dry, red, cracked.* The CARB. and the BROM. develop paretic states, *involuntary stool while passiug flatus* in the former ; in the latter, when *bowels seem as if they would pass with the stool.* Although milk aggravates the CARB. patient, it is more characteristic of the HYDRIOD. In the latter remedy, there is co-existing pain as though the back were being *screwed in a vise.*

Kidneys, Urine

The Potash Salts play a not unimportant part in the treatment of Morbus Brightii.

Buchner recommends the BICHR. in syphilitic cases. The CARB. deserves attention when dropsy of one foot occurs, *with œdematous sacs over each upper eye-lid* ; urine *blackish* ; exciting cause, *getting wet, standing in wet clothes.* The CHLOR. has no clinical confirmation ; but it may appear, because it answers for diphtheritic disease ; afibrinous, pale blood ; congestion to the heart, slow pulse, twitching of the face, dirty yellow, urinal sediment (7). The HYDRIOD. corresponds to the secondary changes ; *pleurisy with exudation*, malaise, chilliness, bruised pain in the lumbar region, *darting* pains ; urine dark, scanty ; *œdema of the lungs.* The

---

(6) Very likely this retraction belongs to the acid, as it comes from a group of which *lead* and *zinc* are isomorphic members.

(7) Also nephritis crouposa with dirty, yellow sediment.

THE KALIS—(*contd.*)

Kidneys, Urine

NITRAT., in sudden œdematous (8) swellings ; pulse *slower than the heart*, painless jerkings here and there ; spasms of the throat, as if choking ; especially *in the distressing dyspnœa* (9).

Pale, watery urine, indicating nervousness, is more characterized under the NITRAT. ; the BROM. also gives us pale urine with *chorea, epilepsy*, etc. In a less marked degree, we find under the HYDRIOD., associated with such an unquenchable thirst, that we are warranted in thinking of *diabetes mellitus*. Here, as elsewhere, the paretic effects of the KALIS. are best known in the CARB., for we note : *Urine discharges slowly*. Such a state may also belong to prostatic enlargement in old people, with prostatorrhœa, nightly micturition. It differs from the same state under the BICHR. In the latter the urine passes readily enough, but *leaves a sensation, as if a drop of urine remained behind.* This may occur in gonorrhœa involving the prostate when the BICHR. rivals *Thuja*. The HYDRIOD. from its powerful action on all glands, so interstitially enlarges the prostate, that the urine is *completely retained.*

Genitals

The KALIS *tend to bring about weakness of the sexual powers*. The BROM. is extolled in *impotence* with *melancholy, loss of memory, nervous prostration and epilepsy* ; or increased irritability with priapismic erections at night, backache and *incontrollable fidgetiness*. The CARB. which always suffers from loss of vital fluids, adds weakness of the body after an embrace, especially *weakness of sight* ; and showing the atony of the ejaculatory muscles we note, *pollutions after an embrace*. The CHLOR. should be thought of when *Nat. Mur.* does not exactly fit and there are present chilliness and apathy. The HYDRIOD. borrows from the *Iodine* its power to *atrophy glands* and with *shrivelling of the testes* comes loss of power. The NITRAT. induces an erethism, which, if not gratified, results in violent testicular *tension* (10).

The CARB. is justly extolled in the *sequelae of abortion and confinement : Backache, night-sweats, dry cough, emaciation or menorrhagia.*

When, however, the uterus refuses to return to its normal size (subinvolution) or when a fibrous tumor forms, the BROM. must be studied.

The KALIS. *alter the time and character of the menses.*

The CARB. as well as the HYDRIOD. own the rare symptom : Menses too profuse *and too late*. The BROM. develops *epilepsy* ; itching, burning

---

(8) *Sudden* hydropical swelling belongs to the KALIS. and often points preferably to their use.

(9) According to Buchner, croupous nephritis as synonymous with Morbus Brightii, is a misnomer ; because the blood in the latter disease is afibrinous, and hence unfavourable to the croupous exudation. However, when gout or rheumatism is at the bottom of the trouble, the croup-forming KALIS must come into use. The symptoms will never deceive if properly characterized.

(10) Tension seems to be produced by fulness of the capillaries combined with nervous constriction.

THE KALIS—(*contd.*)

Genitals

and excitement about the vulva. The local itching under the CARB. is not a pruritus as in the BROM., but comes from the *excoriating flow.* The NITRAT. makes the flow *as black as ink.* The BICHR. adds *suppressed urine or urine with red sediment.*

While the BICHR. has an accumulation of tenacious mucus about the genitals ; the CARB. and the HYDRIOD. develop an acrid corrosive leucorrhœa ; the NITRAT. a thin white leucorrhœa.

Tissues

Stitching or shooting pains are lhe common property of the KALIS. In differentiating we find the localities varying. See Chest, &c.

Rheumatism (11) *is cured by all.* In the BICHR. pains come *periodically and wander from part to part* ; better in warmth (the analogue, *Puls.* opposite); pains come and go gradually or appear and disappear suddenly; rheumatism *alternates with gastric* or pulmonary affections. The BROM. answers more for paralytic pains ; weakness of the muscles of the arms ; the BICHR. has sensation of lameness in the right arm, as if had gone to sleep and suggests itself in rheumatoid paralysis ; the BROM. suggests at once increased reflex action and may serve in the spasmodic jerkings in rheumatism, if other symptoms concur. The CARB. is the best proved in muscular paresis ; thus, arms numb after cxercise, want of strength in the arms, limbs go to sleep, even after a meal ; faint, weak, after a walk, &c. Rheumatism with swelling, worse at rest. The lumbago is *worse* 3 A.M. ; *pains shoot into the buttocks and thighs* (12), pains cause the patient to *jerk* ; *jerks the limb if the foot is touched.* The HYDRIOD., like the BICHR., appears in *syphilitic and mercurial rheumatism* ; it is more closely allied to gout ; pains *worse at night, tearing* (periosteal) ; *rheumatic nodes* ; *contractions of the joints from gouty deposit.* The CHLOR. is adapted to mercurial rheumatism with *facial twitchings.* The NITRAT. cures rheumatism with the usual *stitch pains*, but the parts feel, as if *they were growing large* ; *feet feel, as if made of wood.* Rheumatic paralysis when numbness and creeping alternate with articular pains.

SPASMS.—*We can sometimes look to the* KALIS *to relieve spasms. Just as they are better serviceable in paresis than in paralysis* ; *so analogously, they are oftener indicated in muscular twitchings*, &c., *than in general convulsions.*

The BICHR., so far as proved, gives us only spasmodic contraction of the hands and this in connection with rheumatism. The BROM., however, is one of the greatest "*reflex*" *medicines we have* ; hence, twitchings, *chorea*, and from the same cause, *mental disturbances* ; as *spasms from emotions, delusions, night-terrors* ; characteristic here is *the hands constantly busy tying his shoes, picking threads from his clothes* ;

---

(11) Potash in different combinations is a physiological necessity to muscular tissue. Its deficiency develops a paretic state. The KALIS become nutritive remedies in muscular rheumatism, paralysis, especially in old people. Compare Heart.

(12) Several cases were promptly cured with *Kali-Carb., 2c.*

THE KALIS—(*contd.*)

Tissues

busily working ; *always worse when trying to sit quietly.* The CARB. is recommended in epilepsy and puerperal eclampsia when *eructations relieve.* The spasms co-exist with spinal irritation in the cervical region and involve the pneumo-gastric nerve. A similar increased reflex excitability to that noticed in the BROM. is also observed here : *Starts when touched, especially on the feet* ; *head jerked forward, unconsciousness, blindness* ; *a drink relieves but she remains weak, nauseated.* Epilepsy selects the *morning hours of the night* and as with the BROM. there is always a debility bordering on paralysis. The CHLOR. should be given when *twitchings occur in the facial muscles after Mercury* ; also, jactitations in the inner canthi, lower forehead. There always concurs a congestion of nervous centres; for we note as concomitants, heat in the head, vertigo after exercise, face hot, better from nose-bleed ; delirium after convulsions. The HYDRIOD. obedient to its contained *Iodine*, is curative when *subsultus tendinum* is very marked ; contraction of the tendons ; distortion of the limbs, with gout, with chronic spinal meningitis. The NITRAT. gives us tension in the cheeks and *tip of nose* (the BICHR. pains in the cheeks, as if bruised ; the CARB., pressure ; the CHLOR., twitchings and the HYDRIOD., tearing). Like the CARB. the NITRAT. produces spasms of the stomach ; the former after food or drink ; the latter after veal.

Hips

SCIATICA—The BICHR. promises well when the left nerve is the seat of disease ; tendons feel, as if stretched.

In pains referable to hip disease, we may be called upon to select between the CARB. and the HYDRIOD. The former, though acting but slightly on bone and periosteum, prominently affects joints ; gout, paralytic weakness, *tubercularization* (coxarthrocace). The latter adds periosteal and osseous inflammation with interstitial infiltration. From the CARB. then, we would expect only *crampy, tearing pains from hip to knee* ; *the limb goes to sleep, twitchings in sleep and when lightly touched.* From the HYDRIOD., *gnawing, boring pains, worse at night* ; *fluctuation over the hip with a doughy surface around* : darting in the hip at every step, must limp ; abscesses discharging a *curdy or thin ichor.*

Skin, Bones

The KALIS *arrest profuse and abnormal secretions, whether they appear as haemorrhages or purulent or serous secretions.* Goullon.

The CARB. has dryness of the skin, deficient perspiration ; hence, scaly, dry eruptions ; occasionally an exudate under the epdermis develops herpes of the scrotum, perineum or edges of the labia ; only exceptionally do phagedenic blisters develop. The skin is *painfully sore*, with *stitches in the liver* ; long, lasting, *gastric weakness, empty feeling. Urticaria* with uterine disease. *Ulcers* with *livid edges, bleeding at night.* Glands swollen after contusions. *Erysipelas.* Bones and periosteum escape.

To always discriminate between the BICHR. and the HYDRIOD. is not easy. The former develops *a measle-like eruption* on a hot, dry skin ; yet

THE KALIS—(*contd.*)

Skin, Bones

its tendency is always towards *pustulation* ; *the pustules resemble small-pox.* If blisters form (as in the CARB. and NITRAT.), they tend to *deepen* and form thick scabs after breaking. Just such a picture is seen under the HYDRIOD., but the choice falls here upon the *abuse of Mercury*. The blisters form thick, lamellated scabs, with continuous suppuration beneath ; that is, a complete picture of rupia appears. Although both (BICHR. and HYDRIOD.) cure ulcers which grow *deep*, yet in the former, they are usually *dry*, *oval*, contain *a dry*, *black scab* ; in the latter the discharges are *thin*, *corroding*, *ichorous*. In osseous affections, the BICHR. cures caries, *syphilitic caries of the septum narium* ; the HYDRIOD. develops also *exostoses*, *tophi*, *necroses* ; abscesses with a *curdy* discharge ; *nightly mercurio-syphilitic bone-pains*. The BROM., the CHLOR. and the HYDRIOD., when taken in excess, bring out a *papular eruption*. In scrofulous enlargement of the tonsils with enlarged glands elsewhere, similar to *Merc.*, *Hep.*, etc., I suggest the subsitution of the HYDRIOD., when *dryness of the throat and papulae on the face concur*. The BROM. is excellent for acne.

Equally difficult is it to differentiate the *tuberculous tumors* produced by the BROM., BICHR. and HYDRIOD. In the first two, the centres present *a navel-like depression* and, on disappearing, leave thick crusts or scars. The BICHR. develops them more in *summer*, and they degenerate into *deep*, *solitary ulcers*). The BROM. selects *winter* ; and if ulceration ensues, we note *a flat*, atonic ulcer, which, healing, leaves a yellow, scaly surface.

The KALIS *appear in the treatment of boils*, *boils that are small* (*furuncles*). Of these the HYDRIOD. comes nearest to the character of *carbuncle*, both from its action on the nape of the neck (a common locality for this disease) and because of its destructive inflammation of cellular tissues.

Skin of the Hands. For *the fingers* the KALIS *have an especial affinity*. The BICHR. develops pustules at the roots of the nails, the inflammatory process involving the lymphatics up the arm, engorging the axillary glands. The CARB. selects the thumb and gives us superficial subcutaneous inflammation about the nail (run around) in *rheumatic patients* ; sensation of *subcutaneous ulceration*. The HYDRIOD. dips deeper to the *periosteum* (felon) ; *drawing*, *as if the thumb would come off* or *the nail be torn out*. The NITRAT., true to its character, affects the *tip* of the thumb, but the inflammation is furuncular.

Generalities

So general is the aggravation (especially of chest symptoms) in the *morning hours* that this may be denominated *a family characteristic* : BICHR., 2 A.M. ; CARB., 3 A.M. ; HYDRIOD., 5 A.M. ; NITRAT., 3 A.M.

Weakness of the lower limbs. When concomitant symptoms agree, the KALIS, may serve in spinal irritation, passive congestion, (as in CARB., BICHR. and NITRAT. at the menstrual epoch) and in paralysis. The BROM.

THE KALIS—(*contd.*)

Generalities

has cured backache with anæsthesia, phosphatic urine ; *loss of memory* ; *impotence* ; *after venery*, The CARB. restores the spine *after abortion.* So general is *backache* in diseases cured by the CARB. that it must be considered an *essential "key-note"*. In sore throat (*cervical spine stiff*) ; in pharyngeal and œsophageal diseases (*food swallowed hurts the spine*) ; in dyspepsia (*pains in back and legs after eating*) ; in genital troubles ; in spasms ; in constipation ; in erysipelas ; in tuberculosis. The HYDRIOD. used by the old school comes into play in chronic myelitis and meningitis ; *back feels, as if in a vise* ; limbs contracted.

Constitutions

The BICHR. suits *fat, chubby children.* The CARB. corresponds to *dtseases of old people, females, fat and flabby.* The HYDRIOD. suits the mercurialized in whom there is a tendency to glandular diseases, *atrophy of glands,* who have had *syphilis.* It absorbs *normal fat.* It develops inflammations which tend toward *infiltration, œdema, necrosis.* The BROM. absorbs *pathological fat* ; so-called *nervous diseases* The CHLOR. may be used in the mercurialized in whom *a scorbutic state has been created.* The NITRAT. pre-figures the *asthmatic.*

Analogues

Although possessing many points of resemblance, the respective *salts* diverge greatly when their individual characteristics are compared with analogous remedies. The BICHR. bears an intimate relation to *Puls., Lach., Ars., Thuja.* The BROM. mostly resembles *Nat. Mur.* (mind) (C. Wesselhoeft). The CARB. is allied to *Phos., Carbo Veg., Nitric Acid, Lycop., Nat. Mur.* The CHLOR. finds a counterpart for its symptoms, in *Cadmium.* The NITRAT. encroaches on *Lycopod.* in pneumonia, and is very similar to *Canth.* in bladder diseases. The HYDRIOD. holds a wonderful relation to *Mercury*, and finds an all-sufficient antidote in *Hepar.*

THE MERCURIES

THE PRINCIPAL COMPOUNDS OF MERCURY

Head

MERCURY has long been known to the Arabs, from whom, it is said, the Moors brought it into Spain. Paracelsus had the honor, however, of introducing it as an official medicine.

Its history is but a sad repetition of many other powerful and valuable medicaments, which have been abused greatly to the detriment of humanity. Its poisonous effects are destructive to health and even to life. A long and painful train of symptoms follows its excessive administration.

The several preparations with which we have to do are :

1. **Mercurius Vivus** (Quicksilver).

THE MERCURIES—(*contd.*)

1. (*a*) **Mercurius Solubilis** (a Black Oxide with some Nitric Acid and Ammonia).
2. **Mercurius Dulcis** (Calomel).
3. **Mercurius Corrosivus.**
4. **Mercurius Aceticus.**
5. **Mercurius Cyanatus.**
6. **Mercurius Proto-Iodatus** (Yellow Iodide of Mercury).
7. **Mercurius Bin-Iodatus** (Red Iodide of Mercury).
8. **Mercurius Præcipitatus Ruber** (Red Precipitate of Mercury).
9. **Mercurius Sulphuricus** (Sulphate of Mercury).
10. **Cinnabaris** (Sulphide of Mercury).

Generally stated, there is metallic taste, gums swollen, tender, dark red ; tongue swells, breath fetid, increased saliva, which is rich at first but becomes watery and contains fat. Salivary glands become swollen and painful and later stomacace sets in, progressing even to sloughing and caries of the jaw. Individual susceptibility and certain diseased states modify the mercurial symptoms. Thus, children are not easily salivated, neither are those who are suffering from some inflammation ; but if scrofulous, symptoms will soon develop. Body wastes, blood becomes impoverished, less fibrin, albumen, etc., and has a fatty material ; fever sometimes with pustular eruption ; tremor worse in upper extremities extending all over ; sleeplessness ; loss of memory, delirium, headache, even convulsions ; ulcers form on legs. Skin all over is brownish. The tremor of *Mercury* at first looks like chorea, later like delirium tremens, or like paralysis agitans.

Mercury attacks the entire organism, but its primary action is in the vegetative sphere. Here it increases absorption and also the secretion of the glands everywhere. Both the quantity and quality of these secretions are changed. They become increased, thinner and more fluid, acrid and excoriating, oily, as is the sweat ; thus differing from *Hepar* and *Conium* with their thickened secretions. And, also, from *Euphrasia* in ophthalmia, which gives a very similar picture to *Mercury*, but with thick, acrid pus instead of thin, acrid pus.

These changes are wrought by a lessening of the plasticity of the secretions and by the actual substitution of minute particles of *Mercury* in the place of the displaced plastic materials, It is, therefore, more than a poetical license to speak of the *Mercury* in one's bones. The albumen of the blood escapes through the kidneys, and thus we have albuminuria. *Mercury* has been found in the blood, urine, saliva, and in every tissue, even in the fœtus, and urine of infants whose nurse took the *Mercury*.

Mercury at first, according to Kaspar, causes by its stimulating action an excitation amounting even to inflammation and suppuration. This is followed by torpidity and weakness even to exhaustion. These various

THE MERCURIES – (*contd.*)

remarks show just where *Mercury* stands in inflammations. It follows *Belladonna*, and stands parallel with *Hepar*, *Arsenic*, *Lachesis*, *Silicea* and *Sulphur*.

In erethism it resembles *Belladonna*, and *Arsenic*, and thus far is opposite to *Lachesis* and *Silicea*. It differs from *Belladonna* and *Hepar* in that it is only applicable after pus has formed. And it differs further from *Belladonna* because it acts on the sensorium secondarily to its changes in the vegetative sphere. So it may follow *Belladonna* in a cerebral affection, but never precede it. And, we must also have decisive symptoms of the glands, nutrition, state of gums, etc., hence, the general value of the *Mercury* symptom so often quoted as a key-note "scorbutic gums".

Silicea is its substitute when pus discharges and refuses to cease.

Sulphur may be needed whenever *Silicea* fails.

Arsenic resembles *Mercury* because it causes erethism with destruction of tissue (opposite to *Lochesis*, *Carbo Veg.*, etc.), formation of pus, etc.

Mercury and **Arsenic** are excellent in Pyæmia.

The changes wrought in absorption and secretion necessarily lead to a retarding of nutrition, emaciation and laxity. Skin and mucous membranes become earthy or pale. Tissues turn spongy, especially the gums. Tendency to hæmorrhage. Bone diseases. The blood loses its plasma and the tone of the vessels themselves is depressed. Hence the pulse is frequent but feeble, or slow and soft. These forms of pulse are very characteristic.

The congestions and inflammations give place later to hyperæmia and stases, exudations. These venous stases, owing to the impoverished fluid blood, readily lead to cellular infiltration or dropsies. Associated with these nutritive changes is an erethism, which sometimes seems to mask the depression and produce an appearance of increased strength.

Secondary to these phenomena are the nerves : Depression, restlessness ; lack of motor power, the motions are tremulous like paralysis agitans. Loss of speech, dysphagia, etc. The mind suffers from irritability, mania, and finally, imbecility. The neurilemma (as a parallelism with the periosteum) may be inflamed, giving rise to neuralgiæ, notably aggravated by changes in the temperature and atmospheric humidity. So, similarly, the spinal membranes may be attacked, and we have thus a valuable remedy in spinal meningitis, myelitis, etc. (If syphilitico-mercurial, consult symptoms of *Kali Iod.* ; also, *Sulphur.*)

Upon serous and fibrous tissues, *Mercury* acts so as to cause secretions; as in the joints, serous cavities, sheaths of muscles, under the periosteum, etc. Hence, its utility in articular rheumatism, pleuritis, peritonitis, periostitis, etc.

The liver is enlarged by *Mercury*, and often, from incomplete reproduction, fatty liver results. (Compare : *Picric Acid*, *Aurum*, *Nitric Acid*,

THE MERCURIES—(*contd.*)

Phos., *etc.*). Many of its hepatic symptoms are due to a catarrh of the duodenum, extending into the hepatic duct.

Mercurius, then, is to be thought of for patients who have a tendency to mucous and bloody discharges ; to suppuration ; to enlarged lymphatic glands ; who are erethistic, who are anxious, restless, especially in evenings, with fear of loss of reason ; irritable ; desire to flee, with nightly anxiety, and whose manner and speech is hurried. Ebullitions with trembling on the least exertion.

Dyscrasiæ : Syphilis ; soft chancres with lardaceous bases and increasing rapidly in breadth and depth, tending to become indolent, spongy and to bleed. Circumference red and edges puffed. Pustular syphiliderma.

Mercurius Cor. is to be substituted when the local inflammation is very severe, with serpiginous ulcers, threatening the destruction of the penis ; pus stains linen looking like melted tallow.

Arsenic comes in here when the phagedenic inflammation persists with danger of gangrene. (See also *Lachesis.*)

Nitric Acid also develops phagedenic chancres, but with irregular edges, exuberant granulations and bleeding from least touch. It is far superior to *Merc. Sol.* in syphilis of mouth and throat, hence to sccondary syphilis.

Merc. Iod. and **Bin. Iod.** are to be preferred for the genuine Hunterian chancre.

Cinnabaris is the form of *Mercnry* needed for sycotic excrescences ; small, shining red points on glands ; small ulcer on roof of mouth, tip of tongue, etc.

Coral. Rub. for chancres, which are very red and sensitive, with offensive discharge.

Jacaranda, prepuce inflamed, raw, bleeding, yellow pus from the inner surface of prepuce ; chancres.

Nux Vomica, according to Dunham, for chancroids, shallow, flat, spreading irregularly without lardaceous base, exuding thin, serous fluid,

In bone-pains, etc. :

Mercurius, Nitric Acid, Hepar (after *abuse of Mercury*).

Stillingia—great torture from bone-pains and nodes.

Kali Iod. and **Aurum**—caries of bones of skull, nose and palate.

Asafœtida—caries with much soreness to touch.

Kali Bich.—nose and throat.

Hecla Lava and **Corydalis**—nodes on skull.

THE MERCURIES—(*contd*).

Phytolacca—long bones.

Nasal catarrh : *Mercury*, *Nitric Acid*, *Kali Iod.*, *Kali Bich.*, *Hydrastis* (blood ; also salivation) ; *Aurum.*

Exanthemata : Vesicular and pustular eruptions; hence in pustular itch. Variola with suppuration or pyæmia. It follows *Ant. Tart.* in variola, especially when suppuration progresses, and the secondary fever develops. (Compare also *Thuja* here, which, according to Bœnninghausen, prevents pitting) Herpes Zoster ; boils with pus—to make them "break". Impetigo, etc. Measles, etc. Discharges are acrid ; pimples around the main eruption. Itching aggravated evening and night. Inflammations localized and advanced to exudation of pus or plastic matter.

Puerperal fever, symptoms agreeing.

Hectic fever and other irritative forms with thirst, tendency to sweat without relief ; anxiety, restlessness ; cannot bear the warmth of the bed, the pains become much worse; moist tongue, taking the print of the teeth; tongue dirty yellow.

Gastric and bilious fevers, with the addition of gastric symptoms presently to be mentioned.

Scrofula ; child has large head, open fontanelles, oily or sour sweat on scalp.

Silicea very similar in scrofula, etc. ; but head-sweat is sour, not oily, and face is pale, waxen.

Veratrum has cold sweat on forehead.

Mercurius cold skin of forehead with sweat. Teeth imperfect ; limbs cold and damp ; slimy diarrhœa with straining ; gums spongy ; glands swollen. Face of a dirty colour.

SYMPTOMS IN DETAIL WITH OTHER COMPARISONS

Head

Faintings follow sweetish rising, followed by sleep (often with worms). (Compare *Stannum.*) Vertigo with nausea, momentary blindness or things turn black ; lying on back. Semilateral nightly tearing in head ; nape of neck weary, sore and tired ; head aches, as if it would split, increased by heat of bed. Head feels, as if bound with a hoop (also *Gelsemium*, *Carbolic Acid*, *Sulphur*, *Iodine*, *Nitric Acid*, etc.) Dullness in forehead, stitches though temples. (This and above often accompany gastric symptoms, q.v.) Headache with cold forehead.

Scalp : Exostoses ; yellow eruptions, fetid, stinging burning. Sweat oily, sour, forehead icy-cold.

Silicea very similar in scrofula, etc. ; but head-sweat is sour, not oily, and face is pale and waxen.

THE MERCURIES—(*contd.*)

Head

Veratrum has cold sweat on forehead.

Mercurius cold skin of forehead with sweat. Painful to touch (*Mezereum*, *Natrum Mur.*, *Nitric Acid*).

Eyes

Eyes and lids inflamed ; tarsi ulcerated, scabby, suppurating; discharge thin, acrid pus. Eyes aggravated by heat or glare of fire. Profuse excoriating lachrymation increased at night ; head sore. Increased with syphilis. Iritis : *Mercurius Corr.* (generally the best) ; *Kali Iod.*, *Nitric Acid*, *Asafœtida* (after abuse of Mercury—burning, throbbing, ameliorated from pressure, thus opposite to *Aurum*).

Thuja : Iritis with thin blue film over contracted pupil.

Euphrasia, profuse acrid lachrymation; pus thick and acrid ; blurred vision aggravated by winking.

Arsenic also has thin, excoriating burning discharges ; but warm applications relieve with spasmodic closure of lids and all aggravated after 12 P.M.

Hepar similar but better from warmth (*Mercury* is aggravated) and is very sore to least touch. Pains throbbing.

Mercurius Corrosivus has inflammation but more violent ; pustules and ulcers tend to perforate cornea ; discharge excessively ichorous. Iritis syphilitica. This is the best form of *Mercury* in retinitis albuminurica.

Mercurius Dulcis in scrofulous condition ; in pale, flabby children.

Mercurius Proto-Iod. is distinguished by its ever present thick yellow coating at the base of the tongue (corneal ulcers not deep).

Ears

EARS : Tearing aggravated at night : boils in ear ; otorrhœa, thick yellow. Parotid large, hard, pale. (In catarrhal otorrhœa compare *Cham.*, *Puls.* and better *Hepar*, *Silicea*, *Sulphur* when deeper parts are inflamed. It follows *Belladonna* very well).

Nose

NOSE : Red, shining. (Like *Aurum*, *Pulsatilla* and *Hamamelis*.) Catarrh with thick yellow, green discharge, or coryza excoriating with sneezing, watering eyes and sore, raw burning throat aggravated by damp weather. (Don't give it unless the cold is 'ripe'. It retards cure. But if they have coryza made worse in damp weather it may be given. It compares with *Nux*, but the latter remedy has rough throat and is aggravated by dry cold weather. *Pulsatilla* is bland. *Arsenic* has throbbing in forehead and is very weak. *Mercury* alone has heavy aching.)

Mouth

MOUTH : Salivation, sore, spongy gums aggravated at night, by touch and by eating ; teeth loose. Ulcers on gums, cheeks and tongue with acrid, discharges ; irregular circumference ; have white dirty look and bleed easily,

THE MERCURIES—(*contd.*)

Mouth

and are surrounded by dark halo. Opening of Steno's duct affected. Profuse bloody fetid saliva. (A common form of stomatitis. Compare, *Nitric Acid* which, according to Dunham, is more alike the syphilitic form.)

Hydrastis : Mucus long, shreddy ; mucous membrane raw, dark ; very weak ; empty at pit of stomach.

Carbo Veg. : Gums white and bleeding.

Staphysagria : Gums pale ; whole system run down ; face sunken, sickly, blue around eyes.

Mercurius Corr. is very like the *Solubilis*, only more intense.

Toothache

Toothache, teeth hollow or dentine inflamed, aggravated by warmth of bed, damp air and at night.

Stomach

STOMACH : Dragging feeling about stomach after a meal ; qualmish ; epigastrium very sensitive and weak. Upper abdomen bloated, worse from touch and from lying on right side. Canine hunger. Insatiable burning thirst. Nausea and sweet taste. Liver enlarged, painful to least contact or lying on right side. Stinging pains. Jaundice. Sweat stains yellow.

Stools

Stools slimy, bloody, or green, bilious, sour and acrid, making anus-sore. Prolapsus ani when straining; it looks dark red and bloody. Tenes, mus continues after stool ; a never-get-done feeling. Cutting, griping stabbing pains in abdomen, worse at night and in cool evening air ; but better while lying down. It is often useful in enteritis, peritonitis, typhlitis and metritis, after pus has formed.

Staphysagria also has the feeling of relaxation.

Mercurius Corr. has, says Dudley, often cured dyspepsia from chronic gastric catarrh ; distension, sore epigastrium (like *Arsenicum*). It is certainly excellent in enteritis and peritonitis when there are sharp pains (like *Bryonia*), griping, colicky pains, forcing double (like *Colocynth*), burning ; distension, anguish, excessive tenesmus vesicæ and recti, with burning, worse than *Mercurius Sol.*

Mercurius Dulcis is useful in children who have pale, clayey, pasty, stinking stools. The liver symptoms of *Mercurius Sol.* are excellent.

Cinchona stands near it in jaundice.

So does **Leptandra**, but here the soreness of posterior of liver, black, tarry stools and cessation of tenesmus after stool, distinguish.

In dysentery, compare also **Thrombidium** ; brown, morning stools, bloody or not ; violent colic ; mucous fæces, much drawing, which is ameliorated after stool. Very sore pains in abdomen.

THE MERCURIES—(*contd.*)

Stools

Nux, also, is useful when the tenesmus is ameliorated after stool.

In typhlitis : Compare *Belladonna, Lachesis* and *Ginseng* ; in prolapsus ani : *Podo., Thrombidium, Nux, Ignatia*, etc.

Urine

Urine : Frequent and scanty; often followed by mucus; dark, offensive or pale and abundant. *Mercurius Corr.* causes Morbus Brightii, albuminous urine, uriniferous casts, backache, dropsy, cough with blood-tinged mucus and tightness of chest, as in *Phos.* Dyspnœa in catarrh, etc. *Mercurius Aceticus* has cutting with last part of urine. Desire sudden, irresistible.

Sexual Organs

SEXUAL ORGANS : Genitalia, either sex is inflamed (excellent during measles, scarlatina, etc.). Gonorrhœa ; discharge yellow, green, worse at night, has more burning, tenesmus, paraphimosis, etc.

Mercurius Corr. has thick and yellow discharge. Orchitis, often from checked gonorrhœa (useful after *Gels., Tussilago, Puls., Hamamelis, Nux Vomica*, if checked discharge was green). Penis is swollen, with phimosis; bubo. Sweat on genitals, parts raw. Phimosis. . Ill-effects of masturbation with usual *Mercury* symptoms (like *Staphys.*). Bloody semen.

Bubo : *Mercury, Merc. Iod.* and *Bin-Iod., Mercurius Corr., Ars. Iod.* (tends to ulcerate or discharge ichorous, burning). *Badiaga* (indurated bubo, spoiled by opening.). *Carbo Animalis* (indurated bubo).

Menses : *Copious*, with anxiety and cramps. Congestion to uterus. Labia swollen, red, shining. Leucorrhœa acrid and contains lumps or pus.

Respiratory Organs

Coughs, so that cannot utter a word. Cough, as if head and chest would burst. Cough worse from night air ; burning in chest. Pains through lower part of right lung, (Useful in pneumonia with erethism). Stitches in left chest (*Lachesis* and *Lycopodium*). Stitches in chest, sneezing or coughing, as in catarrh. Difficult breathing as from copper vapors.

Mercurius Sulph. is a remedy in hydro-thorax, when a copious watery, burning diarrhœa relieved. Great dyspnœa ; must sit up. Legs œdematous. Burning in chest.

Mercurius Præcip. Ruber has cured suffocative fits at night, on lying down, while falling asleep, must jump up suddenly. (See also *Kali Iod., Lachesis, Grindelia, Lactuca, Kali Bich., Sulph.* and *Sepia.*)

Peculiarities : Symptoms aggravated after getting warm in bed; in wet, damp weather ; in the damp evening air, especially catarrh. Thus the dysentery is frequently caused by cold nights following hot days. (Like *Aconite*, which it follows well.) Sweats on least exercise. Pains never improved by sweat. In typhus fever with this symptom look rather to *Stramonium* (children) and *Phos.* ***Mercury* is often useful as an intercurrent to 'spur up' *Sulphur*.**

THE MERCURIES—*(contd.)*

Throat

I wish now to revert to the throat symptoms, that I may pass under review that *Mercurial salts* in their application to diphtheria, scarlatina, etc.

Mercurius Sol. is not often indicated in true diphtheria. Indeed, it generally aggravates. It may be given in scarlatinal angina, general symptoms agreeing. Dr. Raue lays great stress, and justly too, on the soreness and inflammation of the genitals as a complication. (See *Cantharis.*)

Mercurius Iod. is said to follow *Lachesis* when fauces are blue-red, ulcerated, glands enormously swollen, voice lost.

As already hinted, the *Solubilis* cures tonsilitis after pus has formed. Also dry throat, mouth full of saliva, must swallow continually. Stitches into ears on swallowing (*Phytolacca*). Liquids return through the nose. Much mucus in the throat, necessitating hawking. Throat worse on swallowing drinks and saliva.

Mercurius Corr. has swelling of the throat to suffocation, heat as from a glowing coal. Soft palate and throat ulcerated ; raises clots and membranous pieces. Membrane over throat and into nose. Constriction and burning. Uvula elongated. Pillars of velum dark red. Swallowing causes violent spasmus glottidis and even spasm of œsophagus and stomach (like *Cantharis*). Externally, throat enormously swollen and glands are large. Breath fetid ; adynamia ; face expressing great weakness and suffering.

Mercurius Cyan. has won deserved laurels in diphtheria ; fauces red with difficult swallowing ; a white coating on velum palati and tonsils. Glands swollen. Posterior nares and larynx were found, in a case of fatal poisoning, coated with mucus. In diphtheritic croup, general symptoms agreeing, it is a good remedy. In addition to above we have : Great weakness, fainting, heart beat and pulse weak. Fever, skin hot or blue and cold ; tongue coated yellow at base. See *Merc. Proto-Iod.*, but in *Merc. Cyan.* we have in addition edges red, and later, gray membrane ; later still it becomes dark, almost black-coated. Profuse epistaxis (a dangerous symptom, suggesting also, *Crotalus, Lachesis, Carbo Veg., Merc. Iod., Arsenic, Sulphuric Acid, Nitric Acid, Muriatic Acid*). Ulcers covered grayish-white ; with thin, fetid, excoriating discharge (like *Arum Tri.*). Gangrene. Paralysis following diphtheria (like *Gels., Ars.*, etc.).

Mercurius Proto-Iodatus is useful when the membrane is worse on right side. Throat very red reminding one of *Belladonna*, but with constant secretion of mucus and thick, tenacious saliva, which he must constantly hawk ; amelioration from warm drinks, Cervical glands swollen. The tongue is always coated on its base, thick, dirty, yellow. Faintness. Tired all over ; hence, weakened by the poison. Pulse weak, irregular. Dr. C. Neidhard and others declare it and the *Bin-Iod.* useless in true diphtheria. If the above symptoms are present, it is certainly the remedy for the time. If it fails to relieve in sixteen to eighteen hours, select another. It is often serviceable in scarlatinal angina. It differs in affecting more the left side

THE MERCURIES—(*contd.*)

Throat

and in not having so well-defined yellow base to the tongue. Feels worse on empty swallowing.

Cinnabaris causes dry throat at night, must moisten it every time he *awakes*. Much dirty, yellow mucus in the posterior nares. Dr. Williamson used it in scarlatina.

Nearly related to the *Mercuries* is *Phytolacca*; throat dark-red, swollen, feels full if he would choke; much mucus in throat and posterior nares, causing hawking. Pain and aching in neck, back and limbs. Weak. Faint on rising (like *Bryonia*). Shooting into ears when swallowing. Cannot drink hot fluids. Feeling, as of a hot ball in throat. Also *Lachesis* and *Lycopodium*.

COMPARISONS OF ALLIED REMEDIES

APIS
&
OTHER ALLIED REMEDIES

Apis Mellifica.—The virus of the *honey-bee* acts with great intensity, causing a rapid swelling of the part stung, soreness, heat, redness, and burning stinging, with itching and prickling. When administered internally, in trituration or in alcohol, it readily develops a similar train of symptoms ; hence they are characteristic.

The redness of the APIS inflammation is either a rosy pink, or in advanced cases, a livid, bluish red.

The swelling is the result of a rapid serous effusion into the cellular tissues. It is a universal symptom. Akin to this effect are the wale-like lumps which appear on the skin, presenting often a paler appearance than the surrounding parts. They are often sore to touch, with burning stinging, or, less frequently, painless.

In addition to the pains mentioned, APIS relieves also when there are lancinating-stabbing pains, which cause, by their keenness, sudden crying out and starts.

The mucous membranes are irritated and inflamed everywhere. And here, too, the tendency to œdema is to be observed.

Apis patient is exceedingly nervous and restless. This state must not be confounded with the excitement of **Belladonna**, nor with the restless moving of **Rhus Tox**.

As with many other animal poisons, there is a marked periodicity of the symptoms.

Mental Symptoms

Anxiety, premonition of death. He feels so strangely.

Irritable, fidgety, and restless.

Is himself conscious of an extremely disagreeable, violent, and sensitive mood ; he would like to kill a dog, which barked at him ; nothing pleases him.

Jealousy (in women).

Excitable, dances with excessive joyousness. Laughs at the greatest misfortune, as he would at a comedy.

She feels like crying about everything.

Mental restlessness.

APIS & OTHER ALLIED REMEDIES—(*contd.*)

Mental Symptoms.

Inclination to change the occupation; will not keep steadily at anything, with dulness of the head.

Confused ; cannot think clearly.

Complete loss of consciousness.

Moaning, unconscious.

Sopor, with sudden piercing shrieks.

Head

Confusion of the head, dizziness, a constant pressive pain above and around the eyes, which is sometimes relieved by pressure with the hands.

Vertigo ; worse sitting than walking ; extreme when lying down and closing the eyes. Dizzy and faint.

Head feels big and confused. Bursting, expansive feeling.

Dulness of the head, with restlessness.

Rush of blood to the head, which feels too full ; worse in a warm room. Irritable, prostrated.

Throbbing in the head.

Pressure generally relieves the headache. Photophobia during headache.

Violent shooting pains over the right eye, extending down to the eye-ball.

Stinging, prickling, or stabbing pains.

Inflammation of the meninges wiih effusion; bores the head in the pillow ; gives sudden shrill shrieks; tongue sore ; big toe turned up ; one side twitching, the other paralyzed ; much fever. *Especially indicated when caused by suppressed eruptions.*

Hydrocephaloid, with the same shrill cries, with open, sunken fontanelle ; great prostration and restlessness.

Scalp sensitive to touch. Stinging, prickling-itching.

Special Senses

In **Apis** the eyes are irritable and weak. One prover had starting from sleep at any noise. Though not confirmed, this last sympton is in keeping with the irritating effect of the drug and is doubtless genuine.

Sensitive to light. Eyes pain and water when looking at any light or when using the eyes, Smarting and sensation of burning in the eyes, with bright redness of the conjunctiva.

Eyes easily fatigued, with redness and stinging pains when used ; worse evenings; feeling as of a small foreign body in the eye, with burning and lachrymation.

Blindness with the vertigo.

APIS & OTHER ALLIED REMEDIES—(*contd.*)

Special Senses

Intense pains shooting through the eye. Piercing pains. Burning and stinging. Photophobia. Swollen lids and dark-red, chemosed conjunctiva. Hot gushing tears. Relief from cold applications—indicating the remedy in keratitis, ulcerative or scrofulous conjunctivitis, etc.

Dim vascular cornea, hot lachrymation ; scrofulous ophthalmia. Staphyloma. Opacity of the cornea.

Swelling of the eye-lids and adjacent cellular tissue. Margins of the lids smart, burn, sting, or itch ; lachrymation.

Eye-lids œdematous, rosy red, much swollen, even everted.

Eye-lids erysipelatous, dark, bluish-red. (See FACE.)

Piercing, itching around the eyes, in the brows and lids; desire to rub them.

RELATED REMEDIES

The essentials of **Apis** are severe pains, photophobia, hot lachrymations, and above all, œdematous swelling and erysipelas. Similar remedies, therefore, are : RHUS, ARSENIC and BELLAD.

Rhus Tox. is very similar, especially in œdematous swelling of lids ; chemosis, hot, gushing lachrymation ; erysipelas. But APIS has less tendency to the formation of pus—a symptom highly characteristic of RHUS. In the former the pains are stinging, the time of exacerbation is evening, and cold water relieves the inflamed lids. If erysipelatous, the lids are blue-red, looking watery—as if semi-transparent. In the latter, the pains are worse at night, particularly after midnight ; warmth relieves. The erysipelatous lids are of a dusky-red colour and together with the cheeks are studded with small watery vesicles. The pains are usually drawing, tearing, though in erysipelas they may be burning stinging, but with more itching than the *bee-poison*. The eye-lids often feel heavy and stiff.

Arsenic compares with APIS in hot tears, violent pains, œdematous lids. But the lachrymation is more acrid. The œdematous lids are pale, not blue-red. The palpebral conjunctiva and edges of lids are very red. The restlessness is more pronounced. Relief is usually obtained from warm applications, though the scrofulous patient can open his eyes in the open cool air, but not in the room, even if dark. Worse at and after 12 P.M.

Belladonna, in erysipelas, usually lacks the œdematous puffiness of APIS. The pains are more throbbing, and the parts are bright-red, shining; or from intensity of congestion, deep-red.

Face, Nose and Lips

Pale, sickly face ; pallid, deathlike, waxen.

Face red and hot, swollen, with burning, piercing pains. Burning, with feeling of fulness, as if the vessels were overfilled with blood.

APIS & OTHER ALLIED REMEDIES—(*contd.*)

Face, Nose and Lips

Burning, which leaves a long-lasting, livid or bluish-red colour.

Erysipelas : Skin red. swollen, especially under the eyes ; or, bluish-red. Parts feel sore ; or, burning, stinging pains, with occasional sharp stabbing pains; fever, thirst.

Red stripes on the face.

Nose swollen, red, œdematous. Inflamed at point.

Dry nasal catarrh, with a sensation of swelling and obstruction ; sneezing.

Nettle rash. Bold hives, the swelling being large and white.

Pimples on the face, painfully sore and sensitive to touch.

Burning of the lips, which are red, swollen, cracked and finally desquamate.

Lips œdematous. Prickling, with swollen and contused feeling. Sensation, as if swollen.

Dark stripe on the vermillion of the lips, which are dry, rough, cracked.

RELATED REMEDIES

Apis is a valuable remedy when erysipelas assumes an œdematous form, and there is exquisite soreness; or burning and stinging. The sensation of swelling is marked here as well as under "Head" Pimples and nettle rash are very characteristic. The pallor and waxen appearance are present in general dropsy, renal affections, and cachectic conditions. Similar remedies are BELLAD., RHUS, LACHESIS, ARSENIC, *Canthar.*, *Acetic Acid.*

The first two form with **Apis** an interesting group, frequently indicated in erysipelas.

Belladonna is required when the face is smooth, swollen, bright-red, streaked-red, or, from intensity, deep dark-red.

Rhus Tox. when the color is dusky red, and there are vesicles and œdema or even pustules.

Apis stands between the two in nervousness, partaking something of the *Rhus*-restlessness with the *Belladonna* cerebral excitement.

Neither produces exactly the livid or blue-red hue noticed in severe APIS cases. Here LACHESIS is the nearest.

When the nose is mainly attacked, APIS compares with **Canthar.** ; but the latter has larger blisters and more burning. When the nose reddens and the alæ become sore from every cold, we have found **Hepar** serviceable.

APIS & OTHER ALLIED REMEDIES—(*contd.*)

Face, Mouth and Lips

Those who are subject to facial erysipelas are sometimes troubled with pimples, which become intensely sore, red and threaten to develop into the full-fledged disease. BELLAD., APIS and RHUS have helped us here. The first when they are very painful and form rapidly ; the second when they are of a rosy hue and sting and itch. When the face, after a spell of erysipelas, is sensitive to the cold air : RHUS, Bellad., *Hepar*, *Silicea*, Sulph.

In dropsy, compare ARSENIC, Acetic Ac. The first has thirst, which is generally absent in the APIS dropsy. The second has anæmia, waxen face, feeble, soft pulse, diarrhœa.

Mouth and Throat

Buccal cavity is fiery red and swollen ; feels dry, raw and scalded, with prickling heat or burning and stinging.

Similar sensations on the tongue, which is swollen. Edges covered with blisters, which feel sore, raw, and burn and sting ; can neither speak, move his tongue, nor swallow.

Tongue dry, trembling ; it catches in the teeth when he tries to protrude it. Typhoid fever.

Saliva viscid, tough or soapy.

Throat dry, without thirst.

Sensation of constriction and erosion.

Throat swells inwardly and outwardly ; hoarse voice, breathing and swallowing difficult from irritation of the epiglottis ; every drop of fluid which touches his tongue nearly suffocates him. Regurgitation on attempting to swallow.

Throat intensely red, dry, glazed and puffy ; uvula elongated and looking like a sack of water; grayish patches of diphtheritic membrane; tonsils swollen ; mucous membrane of mouth and throat rosy red ; or later, livid. Early and disproportionately severe debility, drowsiness and serious swelling of the subcutaneous tissue about the neck, which is of an erysipelatous color. Fever and drowsiness worse 5 P.M.

Sore-throat, with a hoarse, hard, spasmodic and somewhat hollow cough, from a sensation of filling up in the throat.

RELATED REMEDIES

Apis produces glossitis. This with the red, swollen throat, suggests the remedy in scalds, extension of erysipelas faciei, scarlatina.

The swelling, difficult swallowing and suffocation indicate the remedy in œdema glottidis, and in that puffy, infiltrated state of the pharynx and cellular tissue so frequent and so alarming in diphtheria.

APIS & OTHER ALLIED REMEDIES—(*contd.*)

Mouth and Throat

Similar remedies are : LACHESIS, *Lac Caninum*, MERC. SOL., *Merc. Corr.*, *Kali Bich.*, BELLAD., RHUS TOX., ARSENICUM, *Canthar.*

In glossitis compare : Acon., Bellad., MERCUR., Laches.; none of which, however, cover the ground so completely as the APIS. If a burn or scald is the cause, compare also : *Canthar.*, *Caust.*, SAPO SODA, Arsenic.

In œdema glottidis compare : *China*, *Stramon.*, *Laches.*, ARSENIC.

In diphtheria compare : LACHESIS, *Lac Can.*, *Canthar.*, *Rhus Tox.*

Lac Caninum has served us well when the throat was swollen externally and internally, with difficulty of breathing, similar to APIS and to LACHESIS. In each case the hands were burning hot, and there was great bodily restlessness, must move or be carried from place to place.* This restlessness resembles that of ARSENIC and of RHUS. It is different from the nervous fidgetiness of APIS. The first has more mental anxiety.

In one case the restlessness and hot hands were present, and the pharynx was puffed and covered with a membrane,† which looked like unvarnished silver. So great was the swelling, the child could not lie down. Snoring breathing. On dropping off to sleep, it would awake grasping for breath. So near was the disease to the larynx, that a suspicious croupy cough was occasionally given. Lachesis failed, but *Lac Can.* 2c cured.

Apis, Canthar., and **Lac Can.** ‡ have scanty urine and strangury, a symptom sometimes present in diphtheria. The CANTHARIS, like the *bee-poison*, induces great weakness, death-like turns ; but the local inflammation is more violent, with burning-like fire, and tough, stringy mucus in the throat and posterior nares. And the debility is rather a sequel to a violent disease than an early manifestation as in APIS.

Stomach, Abdomen and Rectum

No thirst, with heat, with dryness of the throat ; burning thirst.

Nausea to vomiting, with fainting; nausea and must lie down.

Vomiting of bile, of ingesta ; or, with profuse diarrhœa.

Burning heat in the stomach ; soreness ; pressure.

Soreness of stomach and abdomen. Bowels feel sore when he sneezes. Abdominal walls sensitive to touch or pressure.

Fulness and sensation of bloatedness in the abdomen.

Pains in the abdomen, worse mornings, with urging to stool.

Violent cutting pains in the abdomen.

Ascites, with vomiting and diarrhœa, can breathe only when sitting erect ; even leaning back causes suffocation.

---

* See Dr. H. W. Taylor's excellent provings in the *Organon*, July and October, 1880.

† See Dr. A. Lippe's symptom in the *Organon*, July, p. 404.

‡ Taylor's provings, ibid, October, 1880, pp. 530, 531.

APIS & OTHER ALLIED REMEDIES—(*contd.*)

Stomach, Abdomen and Rectum

Burning-stinging or stabbing pains coming suddenly and making him cry out.

Loose, yellow stools, with griping and urging in the morning. Passage of flatus.

Greenish-yellow mucous diarrhœa, without pain.

Thin yellew stools, great prostration, coming with every motion of the body, as if the anus was constantly open.

Tenesmus, bowels feel bruised or crushed ; bloody, slimy stools.

Diarrhœa contained small bright lumps, like chopped beets.

Sensation of rawness in the anus, with diarrhœa.

Varices burn and sting, making him fidgety and irritable.

RELATED REMEDIES

Thirstlessness is characteristic, though burning thirst may be present. The nausea is like that which is often noticed in erysipelas, diphtheria, with great prostration. Vomiting and diarrhœa suggest the remedy in cholera infantum, ascites, gastro-enteritis. Pains, tenesmus and stool indicate it in dysentery. Soreness and sensitiveness of the abdominal walls, with stabbing pains, show its applicability in peritonitis. The anal symptoms are very important.

Compare with ARSENIC, *Merc. Corr.*, SULPHUR, PULS., Phos., LACHESIS, *Rumex*, Nuphar Luteum.

Arsenic causes more violent gastro-intestinal inflammation ; and though restless change of place is found in both, it is a fidgety nervous state in APIS and an anxious inconsolable state of mind in ARSENIC. In ascites the latter has thirst, the stomach rejects fluids at once ; the former, thirstlessness.

Merc. Corr. causes peritoneal exudation and enteritis ; but the pains are atrocious and the tenesmus violent, with intense burning.

Sulphur aids APIS in ascites and in effusion from peritonitis.

Lachesis causes abdominal tenderness, bus it is more a hyperæsthesia than a bruised, exquisitely sensitive condition.

Phos., **Pulsatilla,** and **Secale C.** resemble the *bee-poison* in open anus. The first causes "involuntary movements the moment anything enters the rectum", and, clinically, discharge of mucus from the wide-open anus. The second has, precisely like APIS, sensation, as if the anus is open. The last has "anus stood wide open." The color of the discharges will distinguish APIS.

Coloc. has a relaxed state of the anus, but only after diarrhœa. Yellow morning diarrhœa, often painless, and so characteristic of APIS, is also in *Rumex* and *Nuphar Luteum.*

Some years ago APIS helped in cholera infantum, when the stools were small, mucous, and contained little specks of blood. Then, as now, it was especially useful when the anterior fontanelle was open and sunken.

APIS & OTHER ALLIED REMEDIES—(*contd.*)

Urinary Organs

Sharp stinging pains and tenderness over the kindneys ; soreness, worse on stooping.

Frequent sudden attacks of pain along the ureters.

Irritable bladder, with frequent desire to urinate, and strangury.

Prostatitis, with incessant desire to urinate, bearing down, pricking in the urethra ; scanty or suppressed urine.

Urine bloody, with casts and albumen.

Urine scanty, dark, albuminous ; generally with thirstlessness.

Urine scanty, with frequent desire. Bearing down in the region of the sphincter vesicæ.

Anuria.

Frequent and excessively profuse discharge of natural urine.

Burning before and after urinating. Soreness, as if scalded ; burning when urinating, as if scalded.

Urine high-colored, scanty.

RELATED REMEDIES

Apis cause an irritation of the kidneys and the bladder very similar to the early stages of Morbus Brightii. It has been found useful in post-exanthematic desquamative nephritis with the above symptoms and with dropsy. The swelling may be general, but is usually worse under the eyes and in the upper half of the body, with thirstlessness and absence of sweat.

It is also serviceable in cystic irritation, and also strangury, particularly when accompanying other diseases (scarlatina, erysipelas, etc.).

Compare with ARSENIC., *Merc. Corr.*, LACHESIS, *Terebinth.*, Phos., *Helleb.*, *Sulph.*, CANTHAR.

Arsenic here has a more extended range than APIS. It also causes more thirst and restlessness ; cannot sleep after 12 P.M. Sharp stitching pains in the renal region ; tubal nephritis. All forms of casts.

Mercurius Corr. suits when the face is pale, puffed, doughy ; thirst, swollen tongue ; renal region painful ; scanty, bloody urine ; profuse sweat, while APIS has little or none.

Helleborus has dark, coffee-grounds urine ; dropsy after scarlatina, like APIS. There is more dulness of mind, with slowness in responding ; jelly-like stools.

Terebinthina, dark, scanty urine, presenting a smoky appearance ; bronchial catarrh, with rales over the chest.

OTHER ALLIED REMEDIES—(*contd.*)

Genital Organs

Lachesis also causes dark urine and dropsy, post-scarlatinal ; the urine is black, foaming ; and the oppression is worse when he goes to sleep, arousing him.

Cantharis in cystic symptoms is similar, but acts more violently.

Female : Sexual desire increased, with stinging in the ovaries ; jealousy.

Coition causes stinging in the ovarian organs.

OVARIES : Acts especially on the right ; stinging-burning pains ; extreme sensitiveness; pain in right ovary, with pain in the left pectoral region, and cough ; lancinating ; extending down the thighs, on right side, sometimes with numbness ; feeling of weight or of bearing down; drawing.

In the region of the left ovary, pain as if strained, more when walking, evenings at 6 o'clock; after several hours, also a bearing down on the right side and a lame feeling in the shoulder-blade ; toward 11o'clock, when walking, she is compelled to bend forward, on account of a contractive, painful sensation in the abdomen ; still felt in the following morning, somewhat to the left.

When stretching in bed, fine cutting pain in the left ovarian region across to the right.

Ovaries (right) swollen, indurated, with soreness, tenderness, and burning heat.

UTERUS : Bearing-down pains, as if the menses were coming on with aching and pressure in the hypogastrium, or as in early stages of parturition. Feeling of weight or heaviness.

Plunging, stabbing pains in the uterine region.

MENSES : Pressure in the abdomen, back and sacrum, as if the periods were coming on. Bearing down. Period flows two to three days, then stops one day, and returns, and so on for ten days. Menses profuse and early.

Metrorrhagia at the second month ; flow profuse, heaviness of the abdomen, uneasiness, restlessness and yearning. Abortion in the early months. (Skin symptoms usually present.)

Amenorrhœa in young girls who are awkward, silly; feels, as if menses would come, but they do not.

Mucous leucorrhœa with sensation of internal burning in the abdomen.

Pruritus vulvæ, with erysipelatous inflammation or with exquisite soreness, stinging and burning.

APIS & OTHER ALLIED REMEDIES—(*contd.*)

Genital Organs

Inflammation of the labia. Œdema.

Mastitis ; high fever, but little or no sweat ; breast hard, swollen, erysipelatous ; relieved by cold application.

RELATED REMEDIES

Apis acts on the ovaries (right). It would seem from the concatenation of symptoms that ovarian irritation underlies all its "genital" effects. Thus we note abortion, with ovarian pains and bearing down ; weight and bearing down in the ovarian region, preceding the menses. Ovarian sensitiveness, worse during coitus, etc. It has cured ovaritis, ovarian cysts, neuralgia and induration.

Compare with ARSENIC, LACHESIS, *Belladonna*, *Sepia*, Graph., Lilium Tig., VIBURN. OPULUS, Iodine, Coloc., Nat. Mur., Bromine, *Podophyl.*, *Conium*, Kali Carb., Sabina, Secale.

Arsenic cures ovarian induration, swelling, and inflammation ; but with restlessness, some relief from constantly moving the feet ; burning pains.

Lilium Tig., like APIS, causes dragging, heaviness, swelling, pain shooting from ilium to ilium, stinging. But it affects more the left ovary ; the accompanying bearing down is funnelled towards the vulva, with consequent relief from external support. The neuralgic pains are intense, shooting burning, *grasping* ; better from rubbing with the warm hand ; APIS is worse from touch and from warmth.

Sepia causes ovarian congestion, stinging, pressure and weight. But pains come around from the back over each hip ; the bearing down is more purely uterine than ovarian.

Natrum Mur., Amm. Mur., and **Arnica** somewhat resemble APIS, by causing sprained, tense sensation in the ovarian region.

Belladonna causes a more violent condition of congestion or inflammation than the *bee-poison*. The ovarian dysmenorrhœa is intensely painful, with exquisite soreness in the right groin and bearing down.

Podophyllum compares with APIS in the side affected, and in what we may term abortion from ovarian irritation. Co-existing hepatic affections or prolapsus ani will distinguish.

Iodine, *Coloc.*, *Arsenic*, *Graph.*, *Laches.*, with APIS, have cured ovarian tumors.

Conium has more lancinating pains in the indurated ovary.

Viburnum Opulus is much superior in threatened abortion. It has produced and cured pains beginning in the back and coming around either side to the hypogastrium, and there culminating in intense squeezing, cramping, and bearing down.

APIS & OTHER ALLIED REMEDIES—(*contd.*)

Genitals

In early abortion, **Secale** is distinguished by the strong contractions and the hæmorrhage, which is dark, passive, fluid ; from **Sabina** by the profuse bright and clotted flow and pain from sacrum to pubes ; from **Kali C.** by the weak back, with pains which pass from the lumbar region down into the buttocks.

In mastitis compare **Bryonia,** which, however, has more tense, stretched feeling ; dull headache ; white tongue ; useful in beginning with soreness from caking, induced by imperfect emptying of the ducts ; **Rhus Tox.** ; which has phlegmonous form, suppuration, and discharge of clots of milk ; pains in the limbs producing restlessness ; breast deep red ; **Belladonna,** which has bright-red radiating inflammation ; the pains are shooting, tearing, often with throbbing, while those of **Apis** are stinging or stabbing.

Larynx, Chest and Heart

Hoarseness, with difficulty of breathing ; also with dry throat and soreness in supra-sternal fossa.

Feeling of rawness, with inclination to hawk.

Cough caused by a crawling irritation in the supra-sternal fossa ; cough from tickling in a spot deep down on posterior wall of windpipe ; worse on lying down, often arousing him from his first sleep ; it ceases as soon as a small lump of mucus is loosened.

Great dyspnœa ; it seems impossible to breathe ; it seems, as if he could not long survive for want of air.

Intcnse sense of suffocation ; he throws the collar open ; can bear nothing about the throat ; face dusky, lips blue.

Hurried and difficult breathing, with fever and headache ; difficult breathing from swelling of tongue, fauces, pharynx, or larynx, as from œdema ; also from constriction, as in croup.

Sensation, as of rapid swelling of the lining membrane of the air-passages.

Asthmatic breathing from checked hives.

In the chest fulness, pressure, tension ; sensation of soreness, bruised feeling.

Stitches through the chest ; lancinating pains come suddenly.

Pain above the clavicle, and thence down through the chest, when coughing.

Pains just below the heart, arresting the breath ; sudden, stabbing.

Acute pain, sudden, just below the heart, extending diagonally towards right chest.

APIS & OTHER ALLIED REMEDIES—(*contd.*)

Larynx, Chest and Heart

Dull, aching pains in the left side of the chest, near the middle of the sternum, with sensation of fulness and short breath.

Violent, audible palpitation ; beats are rapid but feeble.

Pulse accelerated, full and strong; or feeble, scarcely discernible at the wrist ; pulseless at the wrist ; intermittent pulse.

Faintness, with feeble pulse, and other symptoms of cardiac weakness.

Sulphur has been found clinically to act well after APIS in pleuritic effusions.

Back and Limbs

Pressure, heaviness, and fulness in the occiput (diphtheria).

Glands of neck swollen. Vascular goitre.

Sense of stiffness in neck and back (diphtheria, etc.)

Back feels bruised, as if muscles were internally sore ; region of last ribs.

Spine feels weak, as if she could not lie on it.

Hyperæsthesia of the spinal region.

Burning pressing in the coccygeal region, worse trying to sit.

Arms and hands are sensitive ; burning, pricking, stinging, with redness and swelling.

Spots on the arms or hands, red or bluish-red, with burning, stinging, itching, and extreme soreness.

Œdema of limbs ; parts red, tense ; erysipelatous ; feel bruised, or are pale, waxy.

Œdema of hands and feet.

Limbs feel weak, as if paralyzed, with numbness, heaviness, and stiffness, or with crawling.

Numbness of the fingers, especially of their tips.

Coxitis, when the inflammation is sudden and the fever high, with violent, lancinating pains.

Synovitis, with stinging, lancinating pains, tense, exquisitely sensitive swelling from exudation.

Gouty concretions.

Dull pains, as if in the bones.

APIS & OTHER ALLIED REMEDIES (*contd.*)

Back and Limbs

Jactitation of the muscles ; paralysis of one side, with twitching of the other (hydrocephalus).

Excessively irritated ; restless change of place.

Surface of the body exceedingly sensitive to touch.

Great prostration, with trembling ; deathly faintness ; tired, bruised, as after exertion.

RELATED REMEDIES

Apis is needed in erysipelas, dropsies, effusions into serous membranes rheumatism, etc., when its characteristic pains, swelling, and skin eruptions are present.

The swelling and pain have led to its employment in boils, carbuncles, and, above all, in panaritium. The peculiar pains also indicate it in rheumatism, muscular and articular, while its inflammatory effects with serous effusion have led to its efficient use in coxitis and synovitis.

The pale and painful tumefaction suggested its trial in phlegmasia alba dolens, in which it acts well, symptoms agreeing.

The stiff back, hyperæsthesia, bruised feeling, and the paralytic weakness ought to suggest the remedy in spinal meningeal affections ; but, in such cases, the general characteristics should be present for the sake of necessary definiteness.

Rhus is said to be inimical. It is so similar in prostration, erysipelas, hives, coxitis, restlessness, etc., that great attention must be paid to such distinctive symptoms as the momentary relief from change of position, darker or deeper hue of skin eruptions, form of weakness, etc.

Sulphur follows APIS well, and, conversely, the latter antidotes the abuse of the former in panaritium.

Pulsatilla bears some resemblance in urticaria, tension, and stinging about the joints ; and, above all, in milk leg, with aggravation from warmth and in fever, without thirst. But the pains are erratic, or are located with tension, jerking, and a feeling as of subcutaneous ulceration.

The paralytic weakness of APIS is that form which is so common a result of animal poisons, and compares with the sudden and violent effects of certain vegetables and minerals.

Sleep

Anxious starting in sleep. Awakes with a shrill shriek (cephalic cry).

Sleepless from being fidgety ; restlessness.

Tormenting dreams, of journeys, of care and toil, etc.

Sleepy, yet so nervous he cannot sleep.

Very sleepy, also with prostration (with many ailments).

APIS & OTHER ALLIED REMEDIES—(*contd.*)

Sleep

Sleeps long in the morning. On awaking, head confused, as if brain had not rested ; feels bruised ; the symptoms of the sting, however, may be better.

Yawning in uterine hæmorrhages.

RELATED REMEDIES

Apis induces a state of nervous excitement, eoupled with weakness, even to prostration. The extreme of this is stupor and apathy.

It compares with BELLAD., LACHESIS, RHUS TOX., *Baptisia*, *Zinc.*, *Opium.*

It is distinguished from the apparent agreement with the first by its greater prostrotion, asthenia, and tendency to torpidity. In both there is sleeplessness from cerebral excitation ; in APIS, however, there is a condition of more restlessness and less violent excitement. Therefore, it stands between *Bellad.* and *Rhus Tox.* Its dreams of toil, etc., are yet to be confirmed, while the tiring, hard-working dreams of RHUS are well attested.

Apis again, somewhat like the latter drug, has bruised paralytic feeling in the morning, as after over-exertion ; must stretch. But RHUS adds aching in fibrous tissues, stiffness and soreness, better from continuing to move.

Zincum agrees in several points bearing on cerebral irritation with weakness.

Chill, Fever and Sweat

Chilly at 3 P.M., shoulders, worse in warmth ; chills run down the back ; hands feel, as if dead. Nettle rash. Thirst. Oppression of the chest, as if smothering.

Cold feet ; burning cheeks, also with burning toes.

Heat, with oppression of the chest and *drowsiness* ; rarely thirst. Skin burning hot oll over, especially on chest and stomach. Nettle rash. Heat of the room is intolerable.

Sweat occasionally ; often alternating with dry skin. (This stage may be absent.)

Sweat after trembling and fainting, then nettle rash.

RELATED REMEDIES

Apis induces, as several times mentioned, a continuous high heat with accelerated pulse and nervous excitement or increasing drowsiness. It, therefore, becomes eminently useful in such affections as scarlatina, when the temperature remains up, breathing rapid, etc. Here it excels *Belladonna*, and compares with ARSENIC, Rhus, Sulph.

APIS & OTHER ALLIED REMEDIES—(*contd.*)

Chill, Fever and Sweat

In intermittent fevers, it suits chronic, spoiled cases, where it compares with NATRUM MUR.—its complement, and also with ARSENIC, RHUS TOX. (especially with nettle rash), Carbo Veg., *Opium*.

Arsenic is relieved by external heat. **Rhus** has a dry cough before and during chill, and less oppression. **Opium** compares in heat with deep sleep, but there is more stertor and hot, *profuse* sweat. **Carbo Veg.** has cold knees and oppression like APIS and is called for in the weak ; but the skin is apt to be icy-cold, and the breath cool. During heat wishes to be constantly fanned.

In typhoid, APIS compares with LACHESIS, *Hyosc.*, *Rhus Tox.*, *Baptisia*, *Zinc.*

Skin and Cellular Tissue

Rapid swelling of the whole body.

Skin sensitive to the least touch.

Diffuse cellulitis, followed by destruction of the tissue ; parts intensely sore, then burning and stinging, with rosy redness of the skin, then purple.

White miliary eruption.

Erysipelas (see FACE).

Elevated spots and wales, either red or unnaturally white, with prickling, itching, soreness, burning and stinging.

Œdema ; also indurations of cellular tissue.

Carbuncles, boils, abscesses, cancers, with burning-stinging, erysipelatous inflammation ; restlessness, anxiety, and often scanty urine and strangury. Pains lancinating.

Small pustules burn and sting ; hence in variola.

RELATED REMEDIES

Apis, as must have appeared from the preceding pages, has many and important skin symptoms. Its various forms of dropsy have been sufficiently dwelt upon. In nettle rash it suits in acute cases, while CALC. OSTR. is more frequently needed in chronic forms. For the consequences of suppressed hives APIS is useful and compares with ARSENIC and SULPHUR.

Urtica Urens also develops vesicles and bullæ.

In diffuse cellulitis, with destructive tendency, compare APIS with LACHESIS, RHUS, *Tarent. Cubensis*, ARSENIC, etc. In cellular induration compare SILICEA, HEPAR, SULPH., etc.

Modalities

Apis has general relief from cold applications. Sitting erect is the most favourable position with dyspnœa.

APIS & OTHER ALLIED REMEDIES—(*contd.*)

Modalities

Many complaints are worse evenings and night, though diarrhœa increases in the morning (see also Fever).

Wine relieves ; sour things aggravate (diarrhœa, etc.).

Motion generally aggravates.

APIS antidotes—ailments from Anthrax, Quinine, Iodine, Cantharis, Sulphur. Stings of bees require heat, *salt*, *earth* and LEDUM.

CANTHARIS
&
OTHER ALLIED REMEDIES

The most important of the Coleoptera is the Spanish fly, **Cantharis Vesicatoria.** This insect has long been known to the profession, both as a medicine and as an ingredient in many philter-powders.

There are several species of this fly, all of which blister. Among these are : *C. Vittata*, potato fly ; *C. Cinerea* ; *C. Marginata* ; *C. Atrata* ; *C. Nuttalli* ; *C. Strigosa* ; *Mylabris Cichorii et Phalerata,* two insects imported from China.

The vesicatory properties of the Spanish fly are also shared by Formica, Atherix Maculatus, Mezereum, Juglans Cinerea, Arum Mac., Ran. Scel., Urtica, Clematis Crispa et Vitalva, Euphorbious plants, especially Croton Tig., Thapsia Garganica, Plantago Alisina, Rhue, Oleum Cajuputi, etc.

Cantharis contains, as its active ingredient, a principle called *Cantharidin.* Its effects on the human system are quite easily comprehended ; hence, as a drug, it is among the plainest studies in the Materia Medica.

When applied topically it quickly develops an inflammation which soon results in blistering. This removed, there may be observed a deposit of lymph, constituting a sort of false membrane. In some cases the blister dries rapidly, without any plastic exudate ; in others free suppuration ensues The process has been known to extend even to diphtheritic, ulcerative. or gangrenous degeneration.

Among the characteristic peculiarities of the drug is its marked affinity for the urinary tract. Not unfrequently its topical application, quite distantly removed from the kidneys or bladder, is followed by an absorption of *Cantharidin*, with consequent renal symptoms, and notably, strangury.

In studying this unique remedy, we may readily follow its symptoms, if we keep in mind its evident effects Highly irritant to all tissues, it

CANTHARIS & OTHER ALLIED REMEDIES—(*contd.*)

creates extreme irritation and inflammation, with fever. The results of this violent action are suppuration, plastic exudation, gangrene, or delirium and convulsions. And, moreover, as a necessary sequel, we must add excessive prostration, even collapse.

The aphrodisiac properties of this drug are so uncertain that their validity has been questioned.

Experience has demonstrated that nearly always when CANTHARIS is indicated, cystic or renal symptoms are present.

The pains are violent, cutting, stitching, tearing, or burning, with anguish, tenesmus, and constriction of the sphincters.

Nervous System and Vitality

Furious delirium—also, with sexual excitement, priapism—convulsions and priapism. Howls frightfully like the barking of a dog, and then is seized with spasms; eyes sparkling and rolling in their sockets; constriction of the throat, worse from even the sight of water; attacks renewed by pressure or touch. (See under Stomach.) Coma follows.

Restlessness, particularly when sitting or lying; must move constantly. Uneasiness with change of place.

Insolent, contradictory.

Anxious restlessness, ending in rage.

Face expressive of extreme suffering.

Face pale, suffering, death-like during the pains; also, hippocratic.

Face glowing red, anxious.

Body feels raw and sore internally and externally; or as if crushed to pieces, with great weakness.

Faintness; extreme sinking of strength.

Collapse, sunken features, distressed face, coldness; or, lies unconscious, arms stretched along the sides, sudden starts, with screaming and throwing about of the arms; results of intense inflammation, with suppuration, effusion, internal ulceration, or uræmia.

RELATED REMEDIES

Cantharis may be required in meningitis, cerebral or cerebro-spinal; also, possibly, in hydrophobia, sexual mania, uræmic delirium, etc. In any case, however, we have safe guides in the characteristic constriction of sphincters; furious excitement or, conversely, coma; sexual excitement and the well-marked facial expression.

Its value in effusions will appear as we go on.

Compapre with: BELLAD., STRAMON., HYOSC., ARSENIC, *Cannab. Indica*, CAMPH.

CANTHARIS & OTHER ALLIED REMEDIES—(*contd.*)

Nervous System

The first three agree in furious delirium, constriction of the throat ; the second and third have sexual excitement (STRAM. especially during delirium), though neither causes priapism. But these remedies lack the intense suffering look and anguish of CANTHARIS. Though HYOSC. and STRAM. cause great weakness, manifested between paroxysms, neither they nor BELLAD. induce collapse. The restlessness and distress belonging to these solanaceous plants arise from direct cerebral disturbance, while in CANTH. it is associated with or reflex from abdominal or genito-urinary affections.

Much more nearly related to CANTHARIS are CAMPHOR and ARSENIC. In all, the anxiety, restlessness and suffering face indicate severity of disease or sinking of vital forces. **Arsenic** closely resembles CANTH. in violent inflammations, with intense burning, agony, thirst, subsequent collapse. The two may also meet in uræmia.

Arsenic lacks the sexual erethism, and its delirium is associated with a tendency to self-mutilation,* or to suicide. Fear of death. Restlessness alternating with stupor.

Camphor acts as an antidote to the *Spanish fly*, hence, probably, in an opposite dirction. Both cause delirium, convulsions, sexual mania, priapism ; strangury ; internal burning, with external coldness ; hyperæmia or inflammation of internal parts, as brain, stomach, bladder, etc. Toe coldness and sinking of vital forces in CAMPHOR are usually regarded as its most characteristic effect, the symptoms of excitemnt being reactionary. In CANTHARIS, on the contrary, the principal effects are those of excitement, coldness expressing the result of its continued or prolonged action.

Practically, we may decide for CAMPHOR when delirium, mania, or convulsions exist with coldness and extreme prostration ; especially if caused by suppressed eruptions.

Cannabis Indica compares in uræmia. But it is readily distinguished by its headache, as if the vertex was opening and closing, and by its peculiar mental state, extraordinary over-estimation of time and space.

In collapse with exudation, as in peritonitis and meritis, compar ARSENIC, APIS, MERC. COR., *Terebinth.*, Bufo.

Arsenic as observed above, closely resembles CANTHARIS in expression, alternate convulsion and coma, etc., but lacks the presistent urging to urinate, so essentially present when the latter remedy is needed.

Apis has a similar strangury, though less severe ; and its pains are more stinging and lancinating. Serous effusion.

---

*Confirmed in the Middletown Insane Asylum.

CANTHARIS & OTHER ALLIED REMEDIES—(*contd.*)

Nervous System

Merc. Corr. has almost identical indications ; as, burning, strangury, cutting-burning pains, exudation into the peritoneal cavity, coldness, suffering face etc. But the *Mercury* tongue and sweat without relief, distinguish.

Terebinthina may be compared in metritis with strangury, much burning in the uterus, and excessive prostration. The urine is scanty and beclouded with blood. The tongue, however, is dry and smooth, and there is much tympany. So far as we know, the alternation of coma and spasm, in such cases, has been cured only with *Ars.* and *Canth.*

Head

Confusion in the morning, with pulsating in the forehead. Vertigo, with attacks of unconsciousness. Pains deep in the brain, with expression of anguish on the face. Heaviness, confusion. Pressure, especially as if everything was being pressed out of the forehead. Stitches, tearing. Gnawing, as if in the bones. Burning in the sides of the head, ascending from the neck, with soreness and giddiness ; worse in the morning and afternoon, standing or sitting ; better walking or lying down, semilateral right-sided headaches. Stitches, tearing deep in from left occiput towards forehead. Pains in the head, with spasms or coma.

RELATED REMEDIES

Cantharis has frequently cured right-sided headaches. Poisoning with this drug induces hyperæmia and inflammation of the cerebrum, but especially of the cerebellum, which has been found covered with lymph. These phenomena, however, appear late, and may, therefore, serve as well in affections which secondarily involve the brain and spine.

The characteristic pains are heavy, pressive, with the congestion ; tearing, stitching often deep-seated, with stiff neck and other symptoms of brain and spine, as well as with facial anguish ; or convulsions, and, lastly, pains, with sexual erethism.

Compare : *Bellad.*, *Hyosc.*, *Stram.*, *Cann. Ind.*, *Camph.*, Bufo *Cannabis Ind.* has marked cerebellar symptoms such as throbbing, fulness, pressure preceding the convulsions, surging from posterior head toward forehead ; stunning pains with vertigo, on rising. As these may be associated with renal symptoms, or with satyriasis, the remedy should be compared with CANTH.

Camphor has marked occipital pulsation.

Bufo causes lancinating pain from interior of head to the eyes, loss of consciousness and convulsions ; but sexual and urinary symptoms materially differ.

Belladonna, like CANTHARIS, is useful in hyperæmia and inflammations ; both, too, cause pressure, heaviness, pushing out of the forehead, but the former has throbbing carotids, red face, rolling of the head, CANTHARIS more an expression of deep suffering, with pale, sallow, or sunken face.

CANTHARIS & OTHER ALLIED REMEDIES—(*contd.*)

Eyes, Ears and Face

Dimness of vision. Dilated pupils. Eyes protrude. Gaze fixed, eyes flashing. Eyes sunken, surrounded with blue rings. Inflammation of the eyes. Glowing heat, as from coals. Eyes red, suffused with tears. Smarting in the eyes, as from salt. Tearing in the ears and mastoid. Nose-bleed only in the morning. Erysipelas begins on the nose, with burning and itching. Blisters form. Face swollen, puffy. Prosopalgia, terrible burning pains, twitching of the facial muscles; dilated pupils : frowning ; face expressive of severe suffering.

RELATED REMEDIES

Clinically, the Spanish fly has been successfully exhibited for inflamed eyes from steam, or burns from other causes. In erysipelas it seems to act best when blisters form, or when the inflammation is intense, and there is accompanying strangury.

Compare with ARSENIC, KREOSOTE, *Graph.*, RHUS TOX. *Apis*, *Bellad.*

The first two resemble the Spanish fly in neuralgia, with burning ; the last four, in erysipelas of the nose,

Kreosote, like CANTHARIS, causes tearing and burning ; but if urinary symptoms concur, there is more urging and haste, with profuse urine —symptoms which belong more to the female genital affections than to idiopathic cystic disease. The pains affect more over the teeth, too ; teeth dark, decayed. The pains are worse from motion, and the patient is nervous and irritable.

Rhus has followed well after the Spanish fly in erysipelas. If there is any possible confusion with *Apis*, the less intensity of the pains and smallness of the blisters compared with the blebs of CANTHARIS will decide.

Belladonna compares here only in the severity of the symptoms. Blisters are not apt to form, nor is there the same co-existing strangury in the latter remedy. They follow each other well, however. In one instance *Bella.* promptly relieved when CANTHARIS helped but for a short time. In this case there were no blisters.

Mouth, Throat, Larynx and Chest

Tearing in the teeth and gums. Gums red, swollen. Fistula dentalis following a red-pointed blister, with swelling of the upper lip. Tongue furred, red at the edges,—swollen and thickly coated,—excoriated and covered with blisters. Lining membrane of the mouth and throat red and covered with blisters, excoriated, with burning and smarting. Profuse salivation, margin of tongue and gums covered with aphthæ, teeth loose. Early in the morning a clot of blood comes into the mouth. Tongue and lips denuded ; dysentery. Throat inflamed, coated with plastic lymph. Tough mucus is drawn from the posterior nares. Burning from mouth to stomach ; throat feels as if on fire. Burning in the throat, scraping sensation, brings up blood with hawking. Constriction and intense pain at the

CANTHARIS & OTHER ALLIED REMEDIES—(*contd.*)

Mouth, Throat, Larynx and Chest.

back of the throat. Aphthous ulcers at back part of fauces, and on right tonsil, covered with a white adherent crust. Swallowing very difficult. Burning thirst, but liquids are vomited, or cannot be swallowed. Even the sight of water chokes him and brings on strangury. Burning and constriction of pharynx and œsophagus, craves drinking. Burning in the larynx, especially when attempting to hawk up tough mucus. Voice hoarse, rough. Speech low, with sensation of weakness of the vocal organs. Cough, with frothy, bloody sputum. Sticking in the chest from one side to the other. Stitch from right axilla into the chest – from forepart of right chest downwards to lower ribs – from lower right towards middle of sternum,—Burning in the chest, as from fire. Pressure on the sternum. Sense of weakness in the respiratory organs. Respiration difficult and oppressed. Precordial anxiety. Palpitation. Pulse hard, full, accelerated, at times intermittent. Less frequently, weak, slow, almost imperceptible. Pulsation through the trembling limbs.

RELATED REMEDIES

Cantharis causes an intense inflammation of mucous membranes, with plastic exudation, extreme congestion, burning, blisters or ulceration; marked constriction of sphincters. The intensity of this process accounts for the syncope, weak voice. The pains are a combination of stitching and sticking. As marked as are the symptoms just given, they are not always conclusive unless the inevitable urinary symptoms are present. These latter agreeing, CANTHARIS has cured aphthæ, diphtheria, pleurisy, pneumonia. In diphtheria, it is suggested especially when the resulting debility is marked.

In pleurisy, the drug has won favour in the relief of effusion, especially when anxious dyspnœa, distressed face, threatening syncope, and moderate fever, are present.

In scarlatina it is used when there are hawking of tough mucus from throat and posterior nares, albuminuria.

Compare : *Bellad.*, *Capsicum* MERC. CORROS. *Arum Tri.*, ARSENIC, *Apis*, *Cinnabar*

The mucous membrane in the former is rosy, puffed, or, in bad cases, bluish. The inflammation is less violent.

In fistula dentalis, compare Fluoric Acid.

In pleurisy, compare BRYONIA. Dr. Jousset claims that CANTHARIS is very useful here when the fever is not marked. If it only palliates, he at once resorts to BRYONIA. It is important to observe how similar the two are. Both cause stitches, dyspnœa, fever and pressure on the sternum and the heart (so characteristic of BRYONIA). CANTHARIS causes more syncope, weakness, sunken face. The expression of BRYONIA is merely that of oppressed breathing ; so the patient wishes to be quiet, though at the same time he is irritable and anxious.

CANTHARIS & OTHER ALLIED REMEDIES—*(contd.)*

Stomach and Abdomen

Mouth dry.

Burning in mouth, pharynx, and stomach.

Nausea and vomiting. Vomiting of blood and frothy mucus ; membrane-like shreds.

Acute pain in the region of the stomach and bladder ; such exquisite sensibility that pressure produces convulsions.

Violent epigastric pains, causing agonized tossing. Inflammation of stomach, liver, and intestines, with erosions (see collapse under Nervous System).

Abdomen swollen, tympanitic and tender.

Incarceration of flatus under the short ribs.

Cutting, griping, burning, abdominal pains, wandering about ; but worse in the lower abdomen.

Burning along the bowels to the anus.

With the stools, cutting in the abdomen ; after stool burning like fire in the anus, shivering.

Very severe tenesmus, with cutting and tormina.

Stools of blood and mucus ; of white tough mucus, like scrapings from the intestines, with streaks of blood ; of pure blood ; of red mucus, fecal masses. Cold hands and feet, small pulse ; dysentery.

RELATED REMEDIES

Cantharis inflames all of the abdominal viscera, though its most characteristic attack is on the lower bowels and rectum. The pains and stool are well defined. Urinary symptoms are usually present.

Compare : MERC. CORROS., CAPSIC., *Colchicum, Colocynth,* MERC. SOL., *Arsenic, Zincum Sul., Sulphur* and *Kali Bich.*

Relatively these drugs stand as follows :

Distended abdomen (tympany) : Canth., Colch., Merc. Corros., Merc. Sol., Coloc., and Sulph., each *3.*

Cutting pains, with agony : Canth. 4 ; Coloc. 4 ; the others much less.

Griping : Coloc. 5 ; Merc. Corros. and Merc. Sol., each 3.

Tenesmus : Canth. the least ; Colch., Capsic., Merc. Corros., Merc.Sol., and Sulph., each 4 ; Coloc. 3.

Burning in the abdomen : Arsenic most.

Burning at the anus : Arsenic, Capsic.. Merc. Corros., and Merc. Sol., each 4 ; Sulph., Canth. and Coloc. each 3.

CANTHARIS & OTHER ALLIED REMEDIES—(*contd.*)

Stomach and Abdomen

Cantharis, then, is indicated by the locality of the pains, lower abdomen ; cutting pains, worse from pressure ; and by the stools.

The Mercuries are indicated by their tenesmus and griping, especially by tenesmus continuing after stool.

Colocynth has most griping ; this is worse after the least food, and better from external pressure.

Colchicum has stools with shreddy pieces, and chilliness up the back ; but this latter follows spasms of the sphincter ani.

Capsicum has thirst, and yet drinking excites the urging, and causes shuddering. There is co-existing tenesmus of the bladder ; but not so marked as CANTHARIS, which even causes blood from anus and bladder. The distended abdomen in CAPSICUM, causes suffocative arrest of breathing.

Pain in the region of the stomach, worse from pressure, is found under CANTHARIS, ARSENIC, and *Cuprum.*

Only the first and last have pressure causing convulsions. Confirmed in the first, it is quite probably a genuine symptom also of *Cuprum*, and so should be remembered. Copper has relieved death-like feeling behind the ensiform cartilage.

Camphor has in the provings, pains in the epigastrium, loins, and bowels, with strangury and vomiting. Burning. Suffocative dyspnœa, as if from pressure in the pit of the stomach. The latter is not a gastric symptom, but may be present in the general state, which would call for the remedy ; gastric inflammation, great sinking of strength, icy coldness.

Urinary Organs

Inflammation and ulceration of the uro-poetic organs.

Kidneys : Dull pressing pains, with urging to urinate ; sensitive to least touch ; with paroxysms of cutting and burning. These latter often alternate with pain at the end of the penis. Post-scarlatinal nephritis, with impending uræmia.

Aching pains across the loins, tearing into testicles. Cutting and contracting pains from the ureters down towards the penis ; at times passing from without inwards ; pressure on the glans relieves.

Bladder : *so* irritable can not bear but a spoonful or so of urine in the bladder without urging to urinate.

Violent cystic pains, with intolerable tenesmus and urging, extorting screams.

Cystitis with vomiting, fever, anguish, restlessness, etc. Burning and cutting in the neck of the bladder, extending to the fossa navicularis.

Excessive tenesmus of bladder and rectum.

CANTHARIS & OTHER ALLIED REMEDIES—(*contd.*)

Urinary Organs

Pain in the perineum, seemingly from the neck of the bladder, Gangrene of the lining membrane of the bladder. Continued urging to urinate, the urine passing only in drops, with unbearable burning, sticking, and tenesmus.

On urinating, cutting as with knives.

Before, during, and after urinating, cutting pains, forcing him to scream out and to bend double. Urging, with passage only of hot, scalding drops, or of drops of blood ; sometimes with dribbling of urine or urine and blood.

Urging, with strangury and ischuria.

Urging, less sitting, more standing, most walking.

Frequent, painful urination, preceded by pain in the glans.

Urine : bloody ; blood-mixed ; bloody and mucous ; turbid, scanty ; cloudy, meal-like, with white sediment, which adheres to the vessel.

Urine contains albumen, membranous pieces, which are rolled up, organized lymph, epithelial cells, etc.

Urinary sediment looking like old mortar.

Urine frequent and more copious than usual.

Urine retained or suppressed.

Atony of the bladder from too long retention of urine. Paralysis of the bladder, with frequent desire but inability to urinate.

RELATED REMEDIES

No remedy is more frequently called for in irritation of the urinary organs than CANTHARIS. Its characteristics here are, briefly, painful or violent strangury, urine in drops and vesical tenesmus ; nephritis with strangury ; and tubal nephritis. Paralytic weakness rarely calls for it, though it not infrequently relieves dribbling with strangury - a defective control, spasmodic rather than paralytic. Sometimes, however, atony and paralysis may require it.

Uræmic symptoms have been considered under the Nervous System.

The following may be compared, since they cause severe irritation, inflammation, or violent pains, and hence more or less resemble the main drug under consideration.

Kidneys : ACONITE, *Terebinth.*, Cann. Ind., CANN., SAT., *Bellad.* ; BERBERIS and Chimaphila.

Renal Colic : *Ocimum*, *Pareira*, *Berberis*., Bellad., *Lycopod.*,Uric Acid and *Ipomœa.*

CANTHARIS & OTHER ALLIED REMEDIES—(*contd.*)

Urinary Organs

Cystitis : *Capsic.*, Berberis, *Cann. Sat.*, *Coloc.*, *Copaiva*, *Cubebs*, *Senega* and *Zinc.*

Dysuria : ACONITE, CANN. SAT., Cann. Ind., CAMPH., BELLAD., *Equisetum*, *Doryphora*, MERC. CORROS., *Merc. Viv.*, FERRUM PHOS., Poland Water, *Linaria*, PETROSEL., *Capsicum*, *Digitalis*, *Nux Vom.*, *Apis*, *Kali Nitricum*, Thuja, Rhus Aromatica, *Chimpah.*, Epigea Repens, *Pulsat.*, Populus, Sassaf., *Merc. Aceticus*, Oniscus, *Clematis*, *Conium*, Colchic., *Copaiva*, *Erigeron*, *Sarsap.*, Mitchella, Hedeoma, *Terebinth.*, Benzoic Acid and Ant. Tart.

Bloody urine, with much pain : *Aconite*, TEREBINTH., ERIGERON, Capsic., UVA URSI, Epigea, Merc. Sol., MERC. CORROS., *Colchic.*, Erechthites, *Mezer.*

Camphor and **Kali Nitricum** are approved antidotes of CANTHARIS in urinary affections. *Apis* too is stated to relieve the cystitis caused by the Spanish fly.

Aconite frequently suits the incipiency of renal and cystic affections, which, unmodified, progress into a CANTHARIS-condition. The urging to urinate, dysuria and hæmaturia, are accompanied with an anxious restlessness and high fever, altogether different from the expression of Cantharis.

Belladonna induces violent renal congestion, with copious urination, or with retention of urine, intense urging and strangury. The urine may be fiery red or yellow. It may also contain albumen.

In renal colic it is sometimes of use for its well-known spasmodic pains.

It has caused irritation at the neck of the bladder very similar to CANTHARIS, though mostly as a symptom of some exanthem.

In cystitis, violent fever, co-existing brain symptoms, hot fiery-red urine and local sensitiveness, so marked as to render touch or jarring unbearable, are its indications.

Cannabis Sativa may supplant the drug under study in simple nephritis ; but it has no record in Morbus Brightii. Drawing pain in the region of the kidneys extending into the inguinal glands, with anxious nauseous sensation in the pit of the stomach. (Compare Genital Organs.)

Cannabis Indica has burning, stitching, aching in the kidneys ; pains when laughing. But its greatest use here is in what may be termed 'renal debility', with frequent urination, pains in the kidneys and restlessness.

Berberis develops a great variety of pains in the renal region, and hence may be confounded with the Spanish fly. **Indeed** it is too often forgotten for more commonly employed drugs.

CANTHARIS & OTHER ALLIED REMEDIES – (*contd.*)

Urinary Organs

Tension, pressure ; sticking pains from kidneys to bladder or to hips and groins. Burning stitches. Tearing, sticking in region of the loins and the kidneys, as if parts were crushed or bruised, with a feeling of stiffness ; numb sensation. Pains radiate from the kidneys in all directions. Sticking in the abdomen just over the front of the kidneys. Cutting from the kidneys to the urethra. Burning along the length of the urethra ; cutting.

This is an excellent remedy in broken-down patients. The face is sickly, pale or dirty-gray, sunken, with blue circles around the eyes ; tendency to gall-stones and to gravel ; liver congested, torpid ; urging to stool ; long-lasting sensation after an evacuation, as if one had just been to stool. It may be distinguished from CANTHARIS by the hip-pains, and also by the urine, which though mealy in both, deposits a thick reddish or yellowish meal-like sediment characteristically in BERBERIS.

In renal colic and gravel CANTHARIS is recommended when the pains are cutting, burning and constrictive, with strangury. *Pareira* differs here from the spanish fly, as well as from BERBERIS, by the direction of the pains which extend to thighs and feet (rarely below hips in BERBERIS). The urine deposits a copious red sediment. The strangury compels the patient to get on all-fours. *Ocimum* has the same sediment after the attack ; but the pains cause vomiting. *Ipomœa* is needed when the pains are worse in the back, causing nausea. *Uric Acid* relieved a case of gravel promptly. We know of no provings.

Terebinthina produces congestion of the kidneys, progressing to inflammation It also inflames the bladder and the urethra. Heaviness and pain in the region of the kidneys ; pressure in the morning, while sitting. Violent burning and drawing pains. Strangury, with bloody urine. Urine cloudy, dark, albuminous ; contains blood-casts of the renal tubes. Dropsy.

As with CANTHARIS, so here, many ailments yield to the drug, provided only the urinary symptoms agree. But such accompanying affections are quite different in the two remedies.

Equisetum causes dull pain in the renal region, with urging to urinate. The bladder is tender, sore, with severe dull pain which does not lessen after urination. There is constant desire to urinate, sometimes with a feeling of distension, and with profuse urination. But it likewise causes high-colored, scanty urine, containing mucus ; burning in the urethra during urination ; cutting pains. Passes a small quantity of urine, but feels as though he had not urinated for hours—a symptom akin to the distended sensation.

The remedy has won most favour in enuresis. But even when the vesical irritation increases, with scanty urine, it has proved curative, especially with women ; urine blood-mixed, albuminous ; pain worse just after urinating. (*Marsden's Prac. Midwifery*).

CANTHARIS & OTHER ALLIED REMEDIES—(*contd.*)

In the latter respect it compares with CANTHARIS ; but still more with *Linaria* and *Eup. pur.* The former of these two has produced and cured frequeut painful urging to urinate ; must rise at night. Also enuresis. The latter irritates the kidneys and the bladder, causing frequent and painful urging; excess of urine, or scanty, high-coloured mucous urine. Dr. Hughes used it in vesical irritability in women. Its symptom "feeling as though it had retained the urine a long time," is somewhat similar to *Equisetum*.

In catarrh of the bladder, caused by stone, UVA URSI is superior to CANTHARIS. There are frequent painful attempts to urinate, with burning ; slimy or bloody mucous urine. It often palliates.

Sassafras, which has caused burning urine, presents skinny particles in it. **Nux Vom**. with ineffectual urging. **Merc. Sol.** and **Merc. Aceticus,** the latter with cutting just at the close of urinating (like *Natrum Mur.*). **Cochlearia Armoracia** has produced burning, cutting at glans during and after urination, strangury and jelly-like urine.

In Morbus Brightii, CANTHARIS stands near ARSENIC and MERC. CORROS., though not in far-advanced cases. **Merc. Corros.** is needed when the urine is scanty and bloody, containing casts ; face pale, puffy and doughy.

Colocynth, like the Spanish fly, causes cramp of the bladder, forcing the patient to bend double; but only the former has a urinal deposit of stringy mucus. It is adapted to cases, which have been modified by CANTHARIS but not cured.

Bloody urine, with irritation or inflammation, suggests, in addition to CANTHARIS : *Erigeron*, an excellent remedy ; **Erechthites,** a promising remedy in bright hæmorrhages. **Epigea**, bloody sediment and vesical tenesmus, with burning. **Merc. Corros**., bloody urine in drops ; terrible strangury with burning ; **Colchicum**, during strangury writhing in the renal region ; TEREBINTH. ; UVA URSI, etc.

In the course of colds, fevers, pneumonia etc. , bladder symptoms are not uncommon. They may suggest CANTHARIS. If so, the case should be readily distinguished by local and concomitant symptoms from cases calling for the following : Ant. Crud., *Ant. Tart.*, *Scilla,* MERC. SOL., *Merc. Aceticus*, CEPA, *Apis*, etc.

The first suits in cystic catarrh, with frequent, burning urination ; but more often with gastric ailments. Thus, for instance, it is needed for a child who cries on urinating, has a white tongue, and the urine deposits red crystals, more abundant the more he has colic.

The second causes frequent urging, spasm of the bladder, scanty urine, passing dark, or even in drops, and bloody. This looks like CANTHARIS but clinically, *Ant. Tart.* has removed these symptoms when they accompanied its rattling cough, sneezing, dyspnœa, etc.—all foreign to the Spanish fly.

CANTHARIS & OTHER ALLIED REMEDIES—(*contd.*)

Merc. Aceticus has cured colds, when an accompanying symptom is cutting with the last drops of urine ; and CEPA is readily distinguished by its coryza.

Urethra and Genital Organs.

Urethra contracted, urine passes in a thin stream.

Inflammation of urethra, even gangrene.

Glans swollen, painful. Meatus very red.

Prepuce hot, red, tumefied, with phimosis.

Pruritus glandis penis ; ardor urinæ.

White watery urethral discharge, as in gonorrhœa ; particularly when there is violent inflammation, terribly painful erections, and involvement of the neck of the bladder.

Strong and persistent erections, painless, and without voluptuous sensation. Erections at night, with contractions and sore pain in the whole urethra.

Satyriasis.

Burning in the excretory ducts of the vesiculæ seminales, during and after coition.

Drawing pain in the spermatic cord while urinating.

Seminal emissions caused by irritation of prepuce, urethra, or seminal vesicles.

Self-abuse ; partially blind after emissions, shivering, cannot sleep. Genitals cold, relaxed. Ringing in the ears, palpitation, cold sweat ; despondent, stupid ; suddenly dizzy and faint, various colored objects float before him.

Prostatitis following gonorrhœa, other symptoms agreeing.

Blood is discharged in stead of semen.

Sterility.

Abortion, especially with bladder symptoms. Retained after-birth.

Menses early, profuse, black ; nausea and colic.

Membranous dysmenorrhœa, especially in the sterile.

Tenderness and burning in the ovary ; stitches, which arrest the breathing; pinching, or bearing towards genitals, also after suppressed gonorrhœa.

Burning in the uterine region ; co-existing peritonitis over uterus and bladder. Ulceration, with coldness, patient lies unconscious, with arms stretched out along the body, interrupted by sudden screams and convulsions.

CANTHARIS & OTHER ALLIED REMEDIES – (*contd.*)

Urethra and Genital Organs

Purulent discharge from the womb, burning and soreness; gums spongy.

Swelling of the neck of the uterus; burning in the bladder; abdominal pains; vomiting, hot fever.

Bloody mucus from the vagina after urinating.

Burning in the vulva, itching; swelling

Pruritus vaginæ, exciting strong sexual desire; rubbing causes little tumors.

RELATED REMEDIES

Cantharis is not a remedy for gonorrhœa. unless the violence of the symptoms demands it; or the bladder or ovaries are involved.

Its sexual excitement we have already discussed. We have found this remedy eminently serviceable in seminal emissions, when the vesiculæ or the urethral tract is irritated, whether from self-abuse or not. It suits some of the cases which Lallemand so graphically describes, and for which he cauterizes the prostatic urethra. It ought to be a valuable preventive of neurasthenia, reflex from genital irritation.

Dr. O. B. Gause finds Cantharis 6 frequently useful in aiding the expulsion of the placenta. Others have failed with it. It has, however, an undoubted power to contract the uterus, and must be the remedy in some cases. This same property renders the drug of use in impending abortion, especially if depending upon inflammatory irritation of the pelvic viscera.

Cantharis is far preferable to the vaunted *Caladium* in pruritus vulvæ—so potent a cause of masturbation.

In affections of the urethra, compare the following:

Cann. Sat., more important in gonorrhœa, with thin discharge, smarting and burning on urinating; glans dark-red and swollen; chordee; biting at the orifice of the urethra. Less cutting.

Capsicum is required when the discharge is thick and creamy; stitches between micturitions and fine stinging in the meatus urinarius.

Sulphur helps to remove the remnants. In chordee, CANTHARIS compares with: CANN. SAT., CANN. IND., and *Mygale*. The latter has several times removed the symptom.

Petroselinum is similar to the Spanish fly, since it attacks the neck of the bladder and urethra. It is an excellent intercurrent when the patient is frequently and suddenly seized with an irresistible desire to urinate. "First cases" of gonorrhœa, when the inflammation develops.

CANTHARIS & OTHER ALLIED REMEDIES—(*contd.*)

Urethra and Genital Organs

Clematis has to wait for urine to come ; interrupted stream ; urine bites and burns ; worse on beginning to urinate ; contracted urethra—all similar to CANTHARIS. The latter, however, has more symptoms just after urinating.

Conium may be needed. Its characteristic here is, flow of urine suddenly stops and continues again after a short interruption.

Copaiva and **Cubeba** are so abused that we are too apt to neglect them ; or are called upon to antidote their misuse. The former causes urethritis ; burning in the neck of the bladder and in the urethra ; milky, corrossive discharge ; orifice of urethra tumid, inflamed, sore as if wounded; nettle-rash. The latter causes cutting and constriction after micturition ; mucous secretion. Both are useful in the irritation attending thickening of the lining membrane of the bladder (Senega).

Neither acts as violently as CANTHARIS.

Thuja has continued desire to urinate ; wants to pass water, but feels as if a tape was hindering. Violent urging, passes only a few bloody drops ; if these do not pass, there is intense itching. Burning in the urethra ; dark-red itching pimples. Stitches from rectum to bladder. Stitches in the urethra with urging to urinate. Feels as if drops were trickling down the urethra after micturition.

Thin, green, urethral discharge. Warty excrescences.

Nightly painful erections, preventing sleep.

In CANTHARIS, the erections prevent urination ; not so in THUJA. Moreover, the symptoms of the latter are those of continued or oft-repeated gonorrhœa.

The essential symptoms of gonorrhœal prostatitis are rectal tenesmus, deep perineal pains, dysuria, retained urine ; cutting at beginning of urination, the pain descending the urethra to a point just above the external meatus ; urine spurts out, or slowly drops ; scalding and cutting at the close of urination.

CANTHARIS is needed, as are also THUJA, Chimaphila, *Digitalis*, PULSAT. and CAUSTICUM. The latter has perineal pulsation ; after a few drops pass, pain in urethra, bladder, and spasms in the rectum, with renewed desire.

Merc. Corros. is similar to CANTH., with intense burning ; urine full of mucus.

Pulsatilla causes spasmodic pains after micturition, extending from bladder to pelvis and thighs ; flattened stools.

Thuja is often the remedy ; stitches from rectum to bladder.

Cannabis. S. urine is filled with thready mucus,

CANTHARIS & OTHER ALLIED REMEDIES—(*contd.*)

Urethra and Genital Organs

In frequent seminal emissions, compare CANTHARIS with *Camphor, Nux Vom., Sulph., Merc., Cann. Sat., Ledum* (the last three with bloody emissions).

Staphisagria is somewhat similar in prostatic and urethral irritation, as is also CANNABIS SAT.

If a child continually pulls at the penis, it may be caused by local irritation, for which CANTHARIS and *Merc. Sol.* are both useful.

Petroleum and **Sulphur** suit when the skin about the genitals is pimply ; though if the itching is intense (especially with painful urination), CANTHARIS is needed ; or, CROTON TIG. (worse at night) ; MEZEREUM, Clematis, Cinnab. (red spots) ; *Mercur-Sol., Cann. Sat.* (red spots) ; RHUS TOX. (eczema) ; *Thuja* (alternating with stinging at anus).

Chest and Heart.

Voice hoarse, rough, or weak and low, as from weakness of vocal organs.

Hawks a tenacious mucus from the larynx, with burning and stinging.

Cough dry and hacking.

Sputa forthy and bleeding.

Breathing difficult and oppressed, partly from contracted larynx and trachea, but also from dry nose.

Stitches from right axilla into chest, shooting from front to back ; fore-part of right chest, downwards into right lower ribs ; lower right chest extending towards middle of sternum. (A similar stiching on left side, but confirmed on right.)

Burning, with stitches.

Pressure on the sternum ; also from the heart towards the sternum.

Anxiety in the precordium.

Stitch in the heart, followed by a crawling sensation.

Pulsation of the heart intermits.

Pulse : hard, full, as in inflammatory fevers ; thready, weak and imperceptible. Slow and full.

Pulsations through the trembling limbs.

Neck, Back and Limbs.

Stiff neck, with tensive pain on stooping.

Tearing in the muscles of the neck and the back.

Tearing extending upwards, towards the vertex.

CANTHARIS & OTHER ALLIED REMEDIES—(*contd.*)

Neck, Back and Limbs.

Cutting in both loins, extending to the scapulæ, where it becomes stitching.

Pains in the loins, with incessant desire to urinate.

Dragging in the back, as if about to be "unwell."

Stitching and tearing in coccyx.

Tearing in the anus.

Coxagra, with spasmodic pains in the bladder.

Limbs weak, tremble. Also numb.

Convulsions in all the limbs.

Pains are tearing and stitching, with dysuria

Fearful pains in the soles, like an ulcer.

Pains more right-sided, and abate when lying down, and from warmth.

Skin.

Erythema from exposure to the sun.

Burns ; many cases.

Exfoliation of the skin of the penis and the scrotum, with strangury and hæmaturia.

Burning, itching, and tearing, here aad there.

Pimples burn when touched.

Skin pains when touched, as from an ulcer.

Eruptions : Pimples. Vesicles, with surrounding redness ; violent burning and itching ; smarting as from salt. Bullæ, herpes zoster.

Eczema rubrum ; surrounding skin raw ; watery and scalding discharge. Erysipelas. (See Face.)

Ulcers on the legs.

Ulcers, with itching, tearing, and lacerating, or burning, smarting and stinging. Pus copious, inodorous, slightly yellow, sometimes blood-tinged ; worse from rubbing and scratching ; better lying down.

Psoriasis, especially in women.

Dandruff ; the scales copious and large.

Carbuncular and gangrenous inflammation.

Alopecia areata.

The skin symptoms of CANTHARIS, while they are limited, are neverthe-less, equalled in importance by no other of its effects except the urinary symptoms. In burns its topical application has proved very soothing and

CANTHARIS & OTHER ALLIED REMEDIES– (*contd.*)

Skin

effective, especially in blistered skin from exposure to the sun's rays. In eczema rubrum it compares favorably with Rhus Tox. In gangrene its clinical record is not large, and its selection, as in so many affections, would seem to demand that urinary complications be present.

Exfoliation of the genitals has also been observed in Arsenic, Rhus Ven., and Crot. Tig. ; but in CANTHARIS we read in addition, "with strangury and hæmaturia."

There are many substances which applied topically or taken internally produce vesication.

Cantharis locally has, in some instances, caused a plastic exudation. It stands here almost alone. Compare *Arg. Nitric.*

Lymph in the vesicles is attributed to Rhus Ven., Calc., Caust., Ran. Bulb., Bellad., Croton Tig., but it is doubtful if it would organize into a false membrane in these cases.

ANT. TART., *Hydrastis*, Ant. Crud., and Copaiva produce vesicles, which soon pustulate and resemble the variola eruptions.

In burns, compare CANTHARIS lotion with Sapo Soda, Sodi. Bicarb., Ars., and Carbol. Ac.—the later when the parts ulcerate.

Chill, Fever and Sweat

Skin icy cold and clammy. Temperature reduced.

Coldness without subsequent heat, and coming a little later each day. Thirst afterwards.

Chill, with violent pains in knees and calves.

Chill, afternoon or evening ; generally not relieved by warmth.

Chill, with frequent micturition, in nursing children.

Icy-cold hands and feet, with fearful pains in the urethra.

Feeling of coldness in the vertebral column.

Heat, anxious and burning, with thirst. Burning heat, not felt by the patient himself. Averse to uncovering.

Sweat profuse ; smells like urine ; increased at every movement.

Cold sweat. Averse to uncovering.

Sweat with painful urination.

According to Bœnninghausen, painful urination is most marked as a concomitant of the sweat.

In the provings we find the following produced in a patient by a blister applied over a swollen cervical gland : "Fever ; scanty, painful and blackish urine, followed by micturition four-fold more copious than the water drunk, with great thirst, and much desire for meat."

CANTHARIS & OTHER ALLIED REMEDIES—*(contd.)*

Chill, Fever and Sweat

And again, a girl anointed her whole body with Unguent Canth. for scabies. Of her it is reeorded that she had "general fever, with the usual urinary symptoms."

Still another observation is, "fever during pain in the renal region." (See Allen, vol. iii.)

The only urinary symptom with sweat is straining and cold sweat with extreme prostration. This observation is subsequent to Bœnninghausen's time.

We have not sufficient facts, therefore, upon which to judge of the case. We presume that Bœnninghausen based his conclusions upon clinical experience.

Certain it is, however, that we are often called upon to prescribe CANTHARIS in renal and cystic affections when fever is a prominent symptom.

In collapse, **Cantharis** is not one of the most important remedies. It is less frequently needed than its analogue, **Camphor**. As before observed, the prostration is a result of intense inflammatory action ; hence we find it most needed in peritonitic sero-purulent effusions and internal suppuration. It is also given in post-diphtheritic prostration, symptoms agreeing. It is further needed at times when coldness or cold sweat characterize the renal and the cystic affections, in which it is indicated.

Nenning's provings furnish a group of symptoms suggestive of cerebro-spinal meningitis : "Tearing in left servical muscles ; tearing from the neck towards the vertex ; tearing in the limbs ; squeezing and contraction in the fore-part of the chest, with impeded respiration, better on lying down ; whole body as if crushed to pieces". These with amorous frenzy and the urinary symptoms may make it of use.

Doryphora Decemlineata contains Cantharidin, and so presents some similarities with the Spanish fly. But there are numerous points of differences too. The delirium resembles more that of certain of the Solanaceæ. The blood is disorganized very much, as it is under the influence of the snake-poisons. Inflammations are not plastic, nor are they vesicular. They present a dark-purplish hue, with infiltration of pus. The tendency of the fever is typhoid-ward : Delirium, muttering, dark-brown coating on the tongue, dark vomit and utter exhaustion.

There are over ten thousand species of the Radiata, and yet but two or three are represented in our materia medica. We have provings of Asterias, Physalia, Medusa, Corallium, Spongia and Badiaga. But since these low forms of life link, as it were, of the animals with the other kingdoms, no doubt a more extended acquaintance with their medicinal effects would be of great value.

CANTHARIS & OTHER ALLIED REMEDIES—(*contd.*)

Chill, Fever and Sweat

The SPONGES, so far as known, exhibit similarities with the animal medicines, and with the minerals which enter into their composition. Thus, SPONGIA TOSTA contains and is similar to IODINE, BROMINE, *Carbonate* and *Phosphate of Lime*, Sulphur, Alumina, Chloride of Sodium, Peroxide of Iron, Magnesia, and Silica. Badiaga differs in the absence of the first two salts and Sulphur.

It is quite probable that these mineral substances are rendered more active by what may be termed "animalization". Hering refers to a patent medicine which gained considerable reputation ; but after a while the market supply seemed to have lost its efficacy. A wealthy nobleman, failing to be cured by it, brought a suit against the proprietors. The chief ingredient of the medicine was Phosphate of lime. At first it was prepared from bones, but afterwards a less expensive manufacture in the laboratory was substituted, with corresponding decrease in the power of the medicine.

Of the Sponges two species have been proved. The BADIAGA, or *Spongia Flaviatilis*, is an inhabitant of fresh waters ; it therefore lacks, as has been mentioned, the chemical substances which belong to the sea-sponges.

The **Badiaga** has long been a popular drug in Russia, from which source we derive several clinical effects. The more common variety of sponge from salt-water came into common use through the doctrine of *signatura rerum*. "Old women" fancied they traced a resemblance between the sponge and the goitre, and so strapped the former about the neck as a "signature". Cures occasionally resulted, confirming the popular notion. It was not until Chemistry revealed the constituents of the sponge that the real reason of its curative value became evident.

Sponges cause some nervous excitement, with disturbed circulation and palpitation of the heart ; glandular inflammations, catarrh, and muscular soreness with weariness.

If it is true that Iodine does not exist in the Badiaga, it is a mistake to attribute the glandular symptoms solely to that substance, since the Badiaga has often relieved indurated glandular swellings.

Spongia Tosta, however, has some symptoms which are evidently intensified by the iodine, if not wholly caused thereby. (See below.—croup, heart disease, anæmia, with tuberculosis, etc.)

Badiaga,— Severe headache, still the mind is clear.

Frontal headache, with pain extending into the posterior portion of the eye-balls ; worse moving them.

Dandruff increased.

Scrofulous inflammation of the eyes, with hardening of the Meibomian glands.

Sneezing, with coryza ; cough causes sneezing.

CANTHARIS & OTHER ALLIED REMEDIES—(*contd.*)

Chill, Fever and Sweat

Hawks a viscid, solid lump of bloody mucus in the morning. Tonsils red, swollen, worse on swallowing, especially solids.

Severe spasmodic cough, ejecting a viscid mucus from the bronchial tubes, which at times comes flying out of the mouth ; caused by a tickling in the larynx, as from sugar dissolving in the throat.

Vibrating, tremulous palpitation of the heart upon the least elating or other emotion of the mind. While lying ln bed, forcible pulsations up into neck, from slightest emotion or thought.

Stitches on both sides of chest, worse from motion and touch.

Soreness and lameness, with stitches in nape of neck ; stitches in posterior right side below the scapula, both worse from bending backwards.

Flesh and muscles feel sore to touch, even of the clothes ; sore feeling as if beaten. Contusions. Soreness and numbness of the muscles of the leg.

Glands indurated. Cellular infiltration and hardness. Buboes. Sore cicatrices remaining after maltreated syphilitic buboes.

RELATED REMEDIES.

Spongia Tosta of course bears many relations to its congener ; but the headaches are associated with morose humor, and are worse from thinking there-on. The sore-throat is worse from sweets.

The laryngeal symptoms are those which accompany goitre, or which indicate valvular deposit. The patient starts up from sleep as if suffocating; livid lips, bellows murmur ; cough. In BADIAGA the exciting cause of palpitation is some elating thought.

The chest pains in both the remedies are chiefly muscular. Only SPONGIA, thus far, has gained a reputation in tuberculosis pulmonum. It is indicated by the charaeteristic hard, ringing cough, and also by rush of blood to the ehest, with palpitation and sudden weakness while walking ; flushes of heat, which return when thinking of them.

Both the drugs cause sore muscles, with weakness and numbness. This is so marked in BADIAGA that the Russians employ it in contusions. SPONGIA has also burning feeling all over, though the thighs are cold and numb, with cold neck.

The former causes fever and thirst, hot breath, etc., as from catarrhal fever ; the latter, attacks of anxious heat, weeping, inconsolable mood.

In glandular affections BADIAGA has helped in scrofulous and syphilitic indurations. It removes the stony hardness, acting like BARYTA C., GRAPHITES, CONIUM and *Carbo An.* SPONGIA has cured goitre, orchitis, indurated mamma, etc.

Compare BADIAGA also with Phosph., Coffea and Convallaria Majalis, in heart affections.

CANTHARIS & OTHER ALLIED REMEDIES—(*contd.*)

Chill, Fever and Sweat.

Sneezing is a sort of nasal cough and not uncommonly alternates with cough, It may aid in the selection of a proper drug for a cold.

Sneezing causes cough : *Senega*, *Bellad.*, *Cupr.* and NUX VOM.

Sneezing causes irritation in the throat, and then comes cough : Petrol., Sep., Sul. and Sul. Ac.

Cough followed by sneezing : Badiaga, *Bellad.*, HEPAR and Bry.

Sneezing and cough intermixed : Bellad., Hep., Sep., Sil., Cina, Ant. Tart., Alumin. and Bry.

In dandruff, compare BADIAGA with CALC. OSTR., ARS., *Graph* , PHOS. and *Staphis.*

The first has white and yellow scales, scalp sensitive ; hair comes out on one side; scalp feels cold. The second, ARSENIC, causes bran-like scales. The third causes itching like fine needles ; hair turns gray ; worse on top and sides of head. The fourth induces copious dandruff ; hair comes out in bundles ; scratching relieves the itching, but is worse afterwards, with burning ; skin over fore-head feels tight. The last is useful when vexation seemed to disturb nutrition. Itching as from needles ; dandruff over nape of neck, behind ears, etc. (C. Hering and others.)

In **Badiaga** it is described as tetter-like.

Spongia.— In addition to the symptoms already referred to as belonging to this drug, we may allude to the following :

Chronic hoarseness ; voice gives out when singing or talking.

Voice cracked : can speak only with difficulty.

Croup, with harsh, barking cough, worse in the first part of the night ; sawing respiration ; child arises from sleep startled, suffocating, with long-drawn breaths and barking cough ; better by holding the head back. Caused by exposure to dry, cold winds.

Dry cough, with burning in the chest ; better from eating or drinking.

Difficult respiration, as if a plug was sticking in the larynx, and the breath could not get through on account of constriction of the larynx ; glands enlarged.

Pain in the chest and bronchi, with rawness in the throat when coughing.

Dyspnœa ; great weakness in the chest ; she can hardly talk after exercise.

Spermatic cords swollen, painful ; pinching, bruised, squeezing pain in the testicles ; pressive, painful swelling of the testicles.

CANTHARIS & OTHER ALLIED REMEDIES—(*contd.*)

Chill, Fever and Sweat.

Strangulating pain in testis and cord, the former being hard, smooth, and swollen ; any motion of the body or clothing causes a throbbing pain.

Menses too early and profuse, preceded by colic, soreness in the sacrum and craving in the stomach ; violent drawing in the limbs during menses.

Ailments are worse from dry, cold wind ; from lying in a horizontal position (except the headache).

RELATED REMEDIES.

In grandular affections the toasted sponge has gained some reputation in goitre, and still more in orchitis, especially in mismanaged cases of gonorrhœal origin.

In croup the drug is often the only remedy needed for the spasmodic forms without much fever. It also frequently follows Aconite, the latter failing to prevent a recurrence of the paroxysms in the succeeding night. In true membranous croup relief must be prompt, and if not, resort must be had to such analogously acting remedies as Hepar, Iodine or Bromine. The cough, rawness, and dyspnœa have led to the successful use of SPONGIA in laryngitis, especially after dry cold winds, Aconite failing.

The symptoms of tuberculosis pulmonum are invaluable. They represent this dread disease in the stage of solidification. One or the other apex is invaded ; the cough is dry, hard and ringing, while the faintness and rush of blood to the chest from exercise are not of uncommon attendance, particularly in young patients.

Compare in glandular affections : Pulsat., Rhodod., Iodine.

In croup : ACONITE, HEPAR, BROMINE, IODINE, *Causticum*, Kali Brom., etc.

Aconite is preferable in croup, when the child arises with suffocation and the cough is harsh and barking ; face expressive of anxious fear ; skin hot or bathed in sweat. Caused by exposure to cold winds. If the anxiety or the heat continues or returns the next night, persist with the same remedy ; but if the respiration becomes more sawing or labored, as if forced through a sponge, the anxiety present but less marked, the fever somewhat diminished, sputum still absent or scant, change to SPONGIA.

Hepar often follows SPONGIA when the cough is accompained with a mucous sound, though it preserves its barking tone. This frequently occurs after 12 P. M., towards morning. Hence HEPAR is generally required later than the sponge. It must be remembered, however, that HEPAR also develops a tedious, dry, barking cough, coming on so soon as the child lies down at night. This cough, common in croupy children, is relieved by HEPAR promptly. *Causticum* is a good substitute in some cases of catarrhal or spasmodic croup. Child while inspiring chokes as if suddenly clutched by the throat ; raw, burning feeling, in a streak down the course of the trachea.

CANTHARIS & OTHER ALLIED REMEDIES—(*contd.*)

Chill, Fever and Throat.

Kali Bromatum is not to be forgotten in weak, nervous children, who arise with a dry, spasmodic cough, which greatly frightens them, causing them to cry out in terror.

It has several times happened in our experience that DROSERA was needed for a barking, evening cough, simulating that of SPONGIA. The coughs were frequent and persistent, combining the spasmodic with the croupy sound. SPONGIA failed.

Bromine and **Iodine** may follow. The first suits in membranous croup, whether diptheritic or not ; the larynx seems to be full of loose mucus. Child is aroused suddenly choking ; a drink of water relieves temporarily. IODINE causes a dry cough, with noisy respiration and fever. Child tears at the throat ; raises large flakes of tough, but not stringy exudation.

Phosphorus resembles SPONGIA in tuberculosis. Both are indicated in youth, with weakness and rush of blood to the chest ; but the cough and the laryngeal symptoms are different. Much more nearley related here are SPONGIA and HEPAR. They suit in cases which cannot tolerate dry, cold air ; beginning solidification. The former is needed when the cough is dry, hard, worse before 12 P.M. ; the latter when the cough sounds hard, but there is phlegm in the larynx and bronchi ; in the morning, on going into the open air, his throat fills with mucus, making his voice husky.

In the selection of SPONGIA for goitre the choice must depend upon general as well as local symptoms. Among the latter the provings include: Region of the thyroid seems indurated ; on breathing feels as if air was forced in and out of the thyroid ; pressive pain in the region of the larynx while singing ; drawing towards the larynx with contraction.

Symptoms of a more general character, which may possibly be associated with goitre, are : Sensation of a plug in the larynx ; catching of the breath after dancing ; rapid, sobbing respiration ; weak after exertion, chest so weak can scarcely talk ; hot in the face ; nauseated. After moderate motion in the open air, weak ; anxiety, nausea, pale face; short, sighing respiration, with surging of the heart, as if it would force out upwards ; orgasm, face hot, body aglow, blood-vessels hard, distended. These symptoms suggest Morbus Basedowii.

Among similar remedies IODINE stands foremost. Here, too, the heart symptoms are prominent. The bronchocele itself may be painless, or sensitive to touch, with feeling of oppression. The heart, when this remedy is needed, is exeessively active ; exercise causes throbbing, which with a weary, weak feeling of the heart, akin to muscular fatigue, lasts after exercise.

Natrum Phos. has been used to cure goitre. The guiding indication was a feeling of pressure in the swelling. Twice in our experience the symptom was removed, but the goitre remained undiminished in size.

CANTHARIS & OTHER ALLIED REMEDIES—(*contd.*)

Chill, Fever and Sweat.

In cardiac affections SPONGIA resembles ACONITE, *Spigelia*, *Naja*, *Laches.*, Arsenic, Lycopus Virg., *Kali Iod.*, *Aurum* and Cactus.

Aconite has awakening with congestion to the chest, oppressed breathing, anxiety, etc. ; but in SPONGIA there is added valvular deposit, the real cause of the suffocation ; while in the former remedy there exists only cardiac irritation or simple hypertrophy.

Naja and **Lachesis** have arousing from sleep, smothering. The first is indicated in valvular lesions, the heart acting tumultuously, with fronto-temporal headache. Like SPONGIA it has removed the murmurs. The second is preferable in the incipiency of heart disease, when threatened during acute rheumatism ; on going to sleep, aroused smothering ; must sit up in bed and loosen the clothing ; heart feels enormously expanded.

Spigelia precedes SPONGIA. It is indicated by purring over the heart (pericarditis) ; dyspnœa from any motion ; tumultuous action of the heart, sharp pains, etc. It may prevent valvular lesion.

Aurum resembles the sponge in causing thoracic congestion during exercise. But the bursting, full, sub-sternal sensation indicates cardiac hypertrophy.

Kali Iod. is a remedy for valvular deposits ; it produced in a prover, fluttering about the heart on awakening ; must jump up or smother.

LACHESIS
&
OTHER ALLIED FEMEDIES.

Medicines derived from the animal kingdom act energetically and rapidly. They vary in intensity from the fatal snake-bite to corals, sponges, etc., which are more or less modified by their mineral constituents.

Lachesis has been most frequently used, and consequently more fully confirmed clinically. It may be distinguished from the others with a degree of certainty ; but the latter need further proving and testing.

Mental Symptoms.

Lachesis has loquacity, with a constant shifting from subject to subject ; vivid imagination ; jealousy ; frightful images ; proud ; sadness and anxiety, worse on awaking.

Mental activity ; he sits up late at night at mental work.

Memory weak ; makes mistakes in writing and reading ; has to stop to think how to spell.

LACHESIS & OTHER ALLIED REMEDIES—(*contd.*)

Mental Symptoms.

Loss of consciousness, with cold feet ; cold, clammy sweat.

Muttering delirium ; tendency of lower jaw **to drop** ; eyes sunken ; tongue protruded with difficulty ; it trembles and catches behind the teeth ; tongue dry, red, or cracked ; stupor, with anxious expression ; debauched look.

COMPARISONS.

Lachesis and **Crotalus.**—*Crotalus* is almost identical with *Lachesis* in its action on the brain and in its effects on the sensorium and vital forces. Both may meet in the treatment of scarlatina, yellow fever, erysipelas, especially with meningitis, diphtheria, and typhoid. Clinical experience with *Crotalus* has been chiefly in yellow fever, erysipelas, and diphtheria. Both have mental excitability, ecstasy. *Lachesis* only seems to have the peculiar loquacity, though simple garrulity may belong to both. In the epistaxis of diphtheria—thin, persistent, dark red—the rattle-snake has acted best, other things being equal. In erysipelas *Crotalus* affects the right, *Lachesis* the left side, with dark-red puffiness, delirium, stupor and suspicious coolness of the extremities. Yellow skin is most marked under *Crotalus.*

Lachesis and **Naja Trip.**—*Naja Trip.* also excites the mind, and conversely causes depression and forgetfulness. Like *Lachesis* there is a state of moral persuasion. In the former this is expressed as a consciousness of some duty to be performed, but attended with an unacountable inclination *not* to do it. In *Lachesis* it is described as a feeling as if the patient was under the control of some super-human power. *Naja* develops sadness, which is characteristically connected with an intense frontal headache, fluttering of the heart and spinal pains—a group more marked than in *Lachesis.* And, besides, the latter remedy causes pains down to the root of the nose, or over the left eye.

In delirium compare *Lachesis* with *Hyoscyamus, Lycopodium, Rhus Tox.* , *Belladonna, Opium, Apis, Baptisia, Muriatic Acid* and *Arnica.*

Hyoscyamus and **Lycopodium** resemble *Lachesis* in severe cases where the vital powers are waning, and paralysis of the brain seems imminent, as in stupor, dropping of the lower jaw, involuntary stool and urine.

Lachesis, Hyoscyamus and **Lycopodium** together with *Opium, Arnica, Muriatic Acid, Apis* and *Rhus Tox* have trembling or prarlysis of the tongue.

Opium has, in distinction, dark brown-red face, cheeks flap in breathing, more stertor ; body hot and sweaty.

Arnica pictures apathy, stupid expression, sugillations ; even in stuper, restless as if bed was too hot and hard, and seems momentarily relieved when the position is changed.

LACHESIS & OTHER ALLIED REMEDIES—(*contd.*)

Mental Symptoms.

Muriatic Acid displays a sunken face, tongue smooth, as if deprived of papillæ, or brown, shrunken, and hard ; slides down in bed from muscular weakness.

Apis has sensitiveness of a bruised feeling, differing from the hyperæsthesia of *Lachesis ;* and this fact may be elicited from the patient while he is unconscious, for in *Apis* he resists pressure as well as touch, while in *Lachesis* slight touch is more annoying than more firm pressure or friction.

Lycopodium is a drug which induces depression of function from a slight *ennui* to complete stupor. This quality often demands the fern, and happily frequently yields to it. If we examine Hahnemann's masterly provings we shall see numerous illustrations of this property. Thus, talks rationally on exalted subjects, but is confused when conversing on every-day things. Prostration and paralysis of the arms, he must let them fall ; but while at work they are strong. Thus we see, that by an exertion of will, the functional activity is somewhat aroused. Now carry this effect further, and we see the patient becoming drowsy ; he is worse from 4 to 8 P.M. (which is the time of *minimum* tension of electricity of air) ; he is worse after sleep or arises cross, frightened, and very irritable ; his muscles refuse their support, his face looks sunken, lower jaw drops, breathing becomes rattling, eyes filled with mucus ; rumbling in the bowels and constipation—all picturing just such a giving out of the vital forces as may suddenly or insidiously follow some poison, as that of scarlatina, or diphtheria, or typhus. And experience teaches that *Lycopodium* acts well after *Lachesis.*

Hyoscyamus.—*Hyoscyamus* bears strong symptomatic resemblances to *Lachesis,* but it does not act so profoundly. It causes, at first, perverted sensorial action, strange hallucinations ; he grows suspicious and fears of being poisoned ; he talks in a rambling manner ; jumping in a meaningless way from subject to subject ; he seems more *agitated* than violent ; he talks with imaginary persons. Now such illusions are not foreign to the snake-poisons, but *Hyoscyamus* has, as very characteristic, the following group ; suddenly sits up in bed, looks inquiringly around, and then lies down ; talks of his business ; answers correctly, but immediately becomes delirious again ; scolds, raves ; stares, pupils dilated ; starts in terror and tries to escape. Lascivious, throws off the clothes and uncovers the genitals. Muscular twitchings in single groups ; plays with his fingers. Now, this picture may change, for underneath all these maniacal manifestations is a systematic weakness, which existed from the beginning. The patient is weak, ataxic ; his mucles fail him, and he may fall into a typhoid state. Then he grows stupid, lies with eyes closed, distorted features, dropped jaw, twitchings of muscles ; tongue trembles, black sordes on the teeth ; tympany, stool and urine involuntary; respiration stertorous, with suffocation and rattling ; pulse weak, irregular, etc. If now

LACHESIS & OTHER ALLIED REMEDIES—(*contd.*)

Mental Symptoms.

the case grows worse, with cracked bleeding lips, horribly offensive stools, and cold extremities, *Hyoscyamus* will be of no further service, while *Lachesis* may yet save.

Rhus Tox.—*Rhus Tox* has its well-known restlessness. Loquacity is not prominent, the patient remaining silent or answering abruptly, as if nettled and too weak to waste words ; later his answers grow more and more incoherent. The tongue has a red triangular tip, while in *Lachesis* the point is often cracked and bleeding. The stools are watery, often greenish-brown and flocculent, and are passed involuntarily at night ; but they are never so offensive as those of *Lachesis*. Its cellular infiltration usually partakes of the erysipelatous inflammation ; thus, if about the neck, as in scarlatina, the surface looks red—a sort of dusky red. The patient is also very drowsy and at the same time restless ; worse after 12 P. M. The left parotid swells and threatens to suppurate, and the uvula is dark-red and œdematous. Under *Lachesis* the engorged throat present, a dark-bluish cast ; patient arises from sleep as if smothering ; the least touch upon the throat induces suffocating spells ; sleep always aggravates, while in *Rhus Tox* this is not so uniformly so. The latter has much restless tossing in sleep ; nose-bleed or some other symptom becomes aggravated or appears about 3 A. M., arousing the patient ; after a while he falls asleep, and upon again awaking feels heavy and sore, as if he had not slept ; these sensations pass away after he has stirred about his bed. In *Lachesis* the torpor is supposed to be farther advanced, the adynamia more marked, the swollen throat is hard and dark and the fever is low, with cool extremities and weak pulse. In threatening suppuration the snake-poison is preferable when the swelling softens here and there, presenting ash-colored or livid points, which "break" very tardily or degenerate into sloughing, as if vitality is wholly inadequate for the work imposed.

In jealousy, compare *Lachesis* with *Apis* and *Hyoscyamus*.

In pride, *Lachesis* with *Lycopodium* (imperious, commanding), *Hyoscyamus*, *Stramonium* and *Veratrum Album*.

In ecstasy, *Lachesis* with *Crotalus*, *Tarentula*, *Cuprum*, *Opium*, *Antim. Crud.* and *Anacardium*, the last having—soul feels as if freed from the body.

Anxiety and apprehensiveness are symptoms of many animal poisons, especially of the ophidians. In the latter, exciting reading may be a cause. It is also precordial in *Lachesis*, *Crotalus* and *Naja*.

Lachesis is attended with sensitiveness of the brain ; it returns when riding in the open air. We may likewise note an anxiety when mixing with the world, seeing many people, suggesting *Lachesis* in uterine affections. Dreads going to bed from fear of apoplexy.

Naja.—*Naja* brings about a depression of spirits, during which any little imaginary trouble brings about mental agony.

LACHESIS & OTHER ALLIED REMEDIES - (*contd.*)

Mental Symptoms.

Elaps.—In *Elaps* it is developed as a fear of rain. It has a fear of being alone, lest rowdies break in ; apprehensive of some fatal disease, with faint feeling in the pit of the stomach.

Hydrophobinum.—*Hydrophobinum* has strongly marked apprehensiveness.

Actæa Racemosa.—Like *Lachesis*, it is indicated in the distressing fore-bodings of women.

Aconite.—*Aconite* is anxious in crowded streets.

Phosphorus.—*Phosphorus* fears being run over.

Weak memory is a natural result of a poison which so powerfully depresses the mind. After the intellectual excitement, which is especially noticed in *Lachesis* and *Naja*, the mind grows confused, speech and writing are performed imperfectly and incorrectly. This is common to all the ophidians. It is profitable to compare the snake-poisons in defective memory as a symptom of senility, idiocy and apoplexy. *Lachesis*, as quite thoroughly known, may be useful in the impaired memory of drunkards ; also after partial recovery from an apoplectic stroke with paralysis of the left side ; or, again, the stroke may have been preceded by absence of mind, vertigo. As exciting causes, violent or protracted emotional disturbances and intemperance have been noted. Over-study, entailing severe taxation of the mind, may also lead to loss of memory, and *caeteris paribus*, *Lachesis* be needed.

RELATED REMEDIES

In apoplexy, compare *Lachesis* with *Nux Vomica* and *Arnica*. Here there will be also left-sided paralysis, but it is rather suited to stout persons, and suggillations are also present ; the patient remains indifferent for weeks. *Nux Vomica* precedes *Lachesis*.

For inebriates, compare *Opium*, *Apis*.

From over-study, compare *Nux Vomica*, *Sulphur*, *Picric Acid*, *Phosphorus*, *Cocculus*, *Sepia*, *Anacardium*, *Lycopodium*, *Calcarea Ostrearum*.

For mistakes in spelling, compare *Nux Vomica*, *Fluoric Acid*, *Lycopodium* and *Sulphur*.

Lasciviousness, amativeness, is a part of the ophidian excitation. The provings of *Elaps* do not mention it ; but it is present in the remaining members of the group under consideration. Indeed it is related that some of the *Lachesis* provers were thus urged into hasty marriage. The latter drug is useful for epilepsy from onanism. Emissions at first relieve, leaving the mind clearer and more active ; later they weaken and are followed by profuse exhaustive sweats. Lasciviousness attends the feeling as if the patient (female) was in the hands of some stronger power.

Naja.—*Naja* has palpitation, spinal pains, and mental gloom from sexual irregularities.

LACHESIS & OTHER ALLIED REMEDIES—(*contd.*)

Mental Symptoms.

Compare *Lachesis* with *Platina*, in nymphomania and epilepsy from onanism.

Lachesis with *Bufo*, in onanism and spasms.

Lachesis with *Hyoscyamus* and *Phosphorus*, for lasciviousness.

Lachesis with *Picric Acid*, in headache and excessive erections.

Lachesis with *Agnus Castus*, in which excesses cause impotence, but lascivious thoughts remain.

All the ophidians cause vertigo, congestion to the head, frontal pains, mental confusion and general weakness. Fainting from cardiac weakness.

Head Symptoms.

Lachesis has vertigo after rising, on awaking, mornings, with feeling as if he would have a fit ; worse on closing the eyes ; on awaking occiput feels heavy, with sick, weak feeling and dizziness ; the joints feel as if sprained ; with pale face and fainting ; with staggering to the left ; in forehead, with misty vision.

Headaches, generally worse on the left side ; caused by heat of the sun, menstrual irregularities, climacteric disturbances, abuse of alcohol, rheumatism, catarrh etc. ; throbbing in head from the least movement ; whizzing ; congestion, with bright-red nose-bleed.

Forehead : bursting, throbbing, undulating pain in the forehead, worse after sleep and on stooping, with vertigo, nausea, weak mind and weak, numb limbs ; sore aching above the eyes, extending to the root of the nose ; sore pain in left frontal protuberance, worse early in the morning ; frontal headache ; faint on rising.

Temples and sides : Pulsating headache, usually in left temple and over the eyes, with mental confusion, before the development of a coryza ; pains from right side of head to neck ; muscles tense ; rheumatic headache.

Vertex : Burning, as at climaxis ; boring.

Crotalus.—*Crotalus* is provokingly similar in character. Clinically, *Lachesis* has cured more headaches on the left side ; *Crotalus*, on the right. Both have congestive headaches with abdominal ailments : *Crotalus* having relieved when constipation seemed to be the cause ; *Lachesis*, with hæmorrhoids. Although both have an attendant bilious vomit, it seems strongest in the rattle-snake poison.

Elaps.—In *Elaps* the vertigo is accompanied with inclination to fall forwards, rather than to the left. The headaches increase and decrease gradually—a useful symptom, if confirmed.

Naja.—*Naja* simulates *Lachesis* very closely, with headache on waking, fluttering at the heart, and melancholy. But the former has relief

LACHESIS & OTHER ALLIED REMEDIES—(*contd.*)

Head Symptoms.

from alcohol ; the depression of spirit is very marked, and there are more spinal pains. *Naja* also has weight and pressure on the vertex, with cold feet and flushes in the face.

Catarrhal and rheumatic headaches :—In catarrhal and rheumatic headaches, compare *Mercurius*, *Cinchona*, *Pulsatilla*, *Bryonia* and *Gelsemium*. Undeveloped or suppressed coryza, especially in the debilitated, is serious, because so distressing. Pains over the eyes, languor, and mental confusion combine to make the sufferer miserable. *Lachesis* often relieves, as does also *Cinchona*, when the head is worse from the least draft of air. Apropos of nerve pains, *Pulsatilla* relieves when they go into face and teeth, *Lachesis* as well into neck.

Special Senses.

The special senses are usually depressed or perverted by the snake-poisons.

Lachesis.—*Lachesis* cures the following : Dim vision, worse on awaking ; mistiness and flickering.

Blue ring about the light, filled with fiery rays. Flickering, as from sun-rays. Zigzag figures.

Pains above the eyes (left), shooting to the temples, top of head, and occiput.

Obstructed feeling in the ears, with roaring, hammering, or chirping; better when inserting finger in external meatus and shaking it.

Tearing from zygoma to ear. Stinging, piercing deep in the left ear, with a disagreeable sensation between ear and throat.

Soreness of the mastoid ; swelling between mastoid and ear, with stiffness, pain, and throbbing.

Ear-wax pale, pap-like ; or dryness, want of wax, and hardness of hearing.

Nose-bleed, bright red or *dark*, persistent ; with the headache ; before the menses, at climaxis, from blowing the nose ; all worse mornings. In diphtheria it is very useful, other symptoms agreeing.

Coryza (see Headache), preceded by obstinate sneezing ; becomes dry and suddenly *breaks* out again ; nose sore, remaining long after the discharge ceases ; nostrils red ; accompanied with stiff neck and sore-throat ; worse in weak persons, and especially in the spring.

Ozœna, syphilitic or not, with discharge of blood and pus ; and headache.

Redness of the point of the nose.

LACHESIS & OTHER ALLIED REMEDIES – (*contd.*)

Special Senses.

Crotalus.—*Crotalus* and *Elaps* are most similar. *Crotalus* cures, though less frequently than *Lachesis*, an apoplexy of the retina. Like *Elaps*, it also relieves keratitis, when there are cutting pains around the eye, lids swollen in the morning ; ciliary neuralgia with these cuttings, worse at menses. Similar too, is its amblyopia, with coloured flames before the vision ; the eyes are apt to be yellowish ; blood exudes from the eyes.

In the ears *Crotalus* causes a stuffed feeling, worse in right ear, with feeling as if hot ear-wax was trickling out.

Elaps.—Elaps also causes blue appearances in field of vision ; large, red, fiery points, becoming violet, then black, with congestion as in *Lachesis* ; blood oozes from eyes.

The ears are subject to catarrh as in *Lachesis*. In *Crotalus* and *Elaps* there are black cerumen and buzzing in ears and otorrhœa.

Compare *Lachesis* with—

Belladonna, *Lycopodium*, *Strontium* and *Stramanium* in blue ocular illusions.

Causticum, *Lycopodium*, *Belladonna*, *Hyoscyamus* and *Phosphorus* in misty vision.

Actaea Racemosa, *Spigelia*, *Cedron* (over left eye) in ciliary pains.

Cinnabaris has pains that go round the eye-ball ; hence compare with *Crotalus*.

Phosphorus, *Belladonna*, *Glonoin*, *Arnica* and *Hamamelis* in retinitis apoplectica.

Nux Vomica and *Carbo Veg*. when blood oozes from eyes.

Crotalus, *Conium*, *Iodium*, *Kali Bichromicum*, *Phosphoric Acid*, *Vipera*, *Curare* and *Arsenic* in yellow color of the whites.

Nitric Acid, *Aurum*, *Hepar*, *Mercurius*, *Capsicum* and *Silicea* in affection of the mastoid process.

Compare *Elaps* with *Mercurius*, *Nitric Acid*, *Thuja*, *Pulsatilla* in otorrhœa and with *Cinchona* (bleeding).

Compare *Pulsatilla*, *Selenium*, *Muriatic Acid*, *Elaps* and *Lachesis* in affection of ear-wax, hard.

In *Lachesis* the ear-wax is pale and pap-like.

In *Conium* the ear-wax is like mouldy paper.

Compare *Lachesis* with *Carbo Veg*. and *Calcarea Ostrearum* in want of wax.

LACHESIS & OTHER ALLIED REMEDIES—(*contd.*)

Special Senses.

Lachesis with *Mercurius Cyanatus, Nitric Acid, Carbo Veg., Cinchona* and *Arsenic* in nose-bleed (in diphtheria).

Compare *Pulsatilla, Phosphorus, Hamamelis, Secale Corutum, Sepia* and *Bryonia* in nose-bleed with menses.

Compare *Sambucus* with *Elaps* in "snuffles".

In *Sambucus* the child arises smothering.

In *Sticta* the child cannot breathe through the nose ; dry hard cough.

In *Nux Vomica* and *Chamomilla* the nose is stuffed up and yet water drops (*Lycopodium* and *Ammon. Carb.*).

Compare *Lachesis* with *Gelsemium* and *Quillaya Saponaria* in coryza.

Gelsemium and *Quillaya Saponaria* both cause cattarh in the spring ; are preceded and followed well by *Mercurius*. It is marked by thick green catarrh ; raw, sore throat, worse from exposure to damp evening air, after a warm day; or thin, excoriating coryza, sneezing, bone-pains and sweat (*Hepar*).

Lachesis with *Aurum* and *Phosphorus* in red tip of nose

In *Phosphorus*, the tip of nose is shining, the nostrils being dry.

Compare *Lachesis* with—

Rhus Tox, Belladonna and *Hepar* in erysipelas.

Nitrum, Rhus Tox and *Ruta* in drunkards.

Nitric Acid, Hepar Sulphur, Carbo Animalis—all of which are sensitive to touch.

Compare *Lachesis* with *Causticum* in misty vision. *Causticum* is unlike *Lachesis* in misty vision; the melancholy, weak memory, yellow face, blue lips, paralytic weakness, make it a not improbable choice after the snake-poison in cases of debility. As an evidence of heart disease and syncope, in dim sight, *Lachesis* leads the list of remedies and may save in apparently hopeless cases.

Carbo Veg.—*Carbo Veg.* necessarily compares with *Lachesis* and *Crotalus*, since it suits in cases of torpor, loss of vitality, etc. The charcoal may be aptly termed "a torpid Arsenic," and so stands with *Arsenic* as related to the snake-poisions. Its points of resemblance are : cold surface, weak pulse, persistent hæmorrhages—as for instance, nose-bleed and bleeding from the eyes—gangrenous inflammations, collapse, etc. Both *Lachesis* and *Carbo Veg.* have burning of external parts; but the latter, like *Arsenic*, has it more in inner parts. Mentally they differ widely, the latter not causing marked delirium, excitement, etc. It is, therefore, as observed, in torpidity that they meet, especially in typhoid of drunkards. *Lachesis*

LACHESIS & OTHER ALLIED REMEDIES—(*contd.*)

Special Senses.

has hot head and cool feet ; *Carbo Veg.* has, very characteristically, feet and legs cold to the knees, oppression of breathing, desire for fanning. In severe cases : tongue moist, face hippocratic, breathing rattling, constipation, or at least, absence of defecation ; while in *Lachesis* there is usually diarrhœa. In epistaxis, as in diphtheria, metrorrhagia, etc., some of the above will be present as a result of the loss of blood, and then *Carbo Veg.* is decidedly preferable.

Face Symptom.

The face expresses how seriously the snake-poisons affect the system. Change of complexion shows that the contents of the blood-vessels are altered, while the look of anxiety and the distorted and sunken features complete the picture of suffering and exhaustion.

Lachesis has : Expression anxious, painful, with stupor ; face disfigured ; puffy ; looks as after a debauch ; hot, red, swollen ; sunken features ; blue circles around the eyes ; earthy gray, with abdominal troubles or ague.

Rush of blood to the face.

Cheeks of a circumscribed yellow-red ; also the nose. Convulsions of the face ; lock-jaw; distortion. Stretching of the body backwards ; screaming ; feet cold and itching.

Sudden swelling of the face.

Erysipelas ; bursting headache on stooping. Face bloated, red, with cerebral symptoms, drowsiness, etc., or parts bluish-red, gangrenous, pustular. Worse left-side. Itches so that it can hardly be endured.

Throbbing in the face ; full, slow throbbing of carotids.

Tearing in the zygoma extending into the ear.

Screwing and digging in the malar bone.

Swelling of the lips : they crack and bleed.

Crotalus and **Naja.**—*Crotalus* and *Naja* claim the same expression and changes in color, as well as the trismic symptoms. *Crotalus* causes the same erysipelatous inflammation and sudden facial puffing.

Elaps.—*Elaps* develops a similar train of effects, though clinically *Crotalus* and *Lachesis* have the greatest repute.

Compare *Apis, Belladonna, Pulsatilla, Hepar Sulphur, Anacardium, Euphorbium, Rhus Tox, Ammon. Carb., Hyoscyamus, Sulphur, Mercurius* and *Carbo Animalis* in erysipelatous appearance.

Mouth Symptoms.

The Ophidians affect the mouth and throat, causing stomatitis, copious saliva, loosened or decayed teeth, swollen gums, swelling of the tongue, constriction and burning in the throat. Swollen tongue is very marked under *Crotalus* and *Lachesis*.

LACHESIS & OTHER ALLIED REMEDIES—(*contd.*)

Mouth Symptoms.

Lachesis has teeth crawling, feel too long ; hollow, crumbling ; jerking, tearing in the roots of lower teeth through upper jaw to the ear ; periodic, always after waking from sleep, soon after eating, also from warm and cold drinks ; gum about a hollow tooth swollen, relieved by a discharge of pus.

Gums swollen, spongy, white, bleeding.

Tongue mapped ; red, dry, glistening, cracked, especially at the tip ; trembles, catches in the teeth when he tries to put it out; inflamed, swollen, ulcerated ; gangrenous ; paralyzed.

Talks as one drunk, unintelligibly, after an apoplectic fit.

Aphthous, denuded spots, preceded by burning pain and rawness.

Mouth dry, parched, cracks in various places, which bleed ; blisters on the sides of the tongue, burning, with the roof sore ; mucous membrane feels as if peeling off ; offensive odor ; saliva abundant, tenacious ; also with the sore-throat.

Compare : ANTIM. CRUD., *Staphysagria*, MERCUR., *Kreosotum*, HEPAR, SILICEA, RHODODENDRON and *Thuja* in decayed teeth.

Fluor. Acid, *Petrolcum*, LYCOPODIUM, NATRUM MUR., THUJA, MERCUR., HEPAR and SILICEA in ulceration at roots.

MERCUR., CARBO VEG., NUX VOMICA, *Natrum Mur.*, STAPHYSAGRIA and *Sarsaparilla* in spongy gums.

HYOSCYAMUS, *Baptisia*, RHUS TOX, NUX VOMICA and *Belladonna* in red tongue.

Kali Bichromicum and BAPTISIA (edges) in glistening tongue.

APIS, CARBO VEG., ARSENIC, BRYONIA, STRAMONIUM, *Muriatic Acid*, RHUS TOX, *Mercur.*, KALI BICHROMICUM, *Phosphorus*, *Nitric Acid*, *Baptisia* and *Sulphur* in cracked tongue.

Apis, GELESEMIUM, BELLADONNA, ARSENIC, *Lycopodium*, SECALE, *Stramonium* and *Hyoscyamus* in trembling tongue.

APIS, ARSENIC, *Conium*, MERCUR. and BELLADONNA in inflamed tongue.

ARSENIC, NATRUM MURIATICUM, LYCOPODIUM, *Ran. Scel.*, *Tarax.*, *Niiric Acid* in mapped tongue.

Baryta Carb., BAPTISIA, BELLADONNA, DULCAMARA, *Laurocerasus*, HYOSCYAMUS, *Opium*, MURIATIC ACID, STRAMONIUM and LYCOPODIUM in paralyzed tongue.

Baptisia, BELLADONNA, STRAMONIUM, OPIUM, HYOSCYAMUS, *Rhus Tox*, *Laurocerasus* and *Lycopodium* when the patient talks as one drunk.

LACHESIS & OTHER ALLIED REMEDIES—(*contd.*)

Mouth.

Apis, Arsenic, Carbo Veg., Baptisia, Conium, Kali Chlor., MERCUR., *Muriaiic Acid*, NITRIC ACID, *Hepar, Lycopodium*, NATRUM MUR., *Staphysagria, Sulphur, Sul. Acid, Salicylic Acid, Helleborus* and PYTOLACCA in sore-mouth.

Arsenic, Belladonna, Carbo Veg., Lycopodium, MERCUR., *Rhus Tox.*, STAPHYSAGRIA, OPIUM, *Sulphur*, HEPAR, *Cinchona*, HYOSCYAMUS, LAUROCERASUS, *Nitric Acid*, SUL. ACID and STRAMONIUM when saliva is increased or altered.

Arnica, Arsenic, Baptisia, Belladonna, CARBO ANIMALIS, *Cinchona, Helleborus, Hyoscyamus, Kali Bichromicum, Lycopodium*, MERCUR., *Nitric Acid*, RHUS TOX., SUL. ACID, SILICEA and SULPHUR in bad smell from mouth.

Throat, Lungs and Heart.

In **Lachesis** there is dryness of the mouth and throat ; he awakens choking ; can hardly breathe until the dry, shining throat is moistened.

Throat and larynx painful to touch, when the head is moved.

Pains : Left side of throat to tongue, jaw and ear ; rawness and swelling, feels ulcerated, burning ; feeling as of crumb of bread sticking ; as from a plug ; throat sensitive as if sore, from taking cold, with pain in the left side in the evening.

Swallowing : Eating relieves the pain in the throat ; liquids cause more difficulty than solids ; drinks return through the nose ; empty swallowing causes constant pain, food does not. After chewing his food he cannot get it down, because it rests on the back part of the tongue, causing a thrilling there. Deglutition causes pressure, as if a lump was sticking in the throat ; causes sharp pain extending into the ear ; throat feels ulcerated ; throat feels swollen, as if two lumps as large as the first came together ; only on empty swallowing.

Sore-throat, with deafness ; typhoid fever.

Hawking of mucus with rawness, after a nap in the day-time.

Feeling of hollowness, as if the pharynx had disappeared.

Throat inflamed, tonsils enlarged ; disease travels from left to right. Velum and pharynx inflamed. Mucous membrane looks dark red or purplish, and often has a dull dry appearance. Diphtheritic deposits, spreading from left to right ; fetid odor from the mouth. Great debility, especially noticed in cardiac symptoms, such as feeble pulse, cool limbs, fainting ; inflammation assumes a malignant type ; glands enlarge ; cellular tissue of the neck swells and looks blue, with burning ; tongue coated thinly white, shading into thick yellow towards the root.

LACHESIS & OTHER ALLIED REMEDIES—(*contd.*)

Throat, Lungs and Heart.

Tonsils enlarged ; he hawks up oily whitish lumps.

Ulcers in the throat, extending up to the posterior nares.

They often cause a teasing, tickling cough.

Uvula elongated ; parts look purplish.

With all the throat and laryngeal symptoms there are intolerance of the least touch or pressure upon the neck ; must loosen the clothing ; spasmodic contractions, which arouse from sleep or develop as he awakes. Touch provokes them anew. Spasms of the glottis ; suddenly something runs from neck to larynx, awakening him and stopping the breathing. Disposition to frequent return of angina of throat.

Feels as if a piece of dry skin was in the pharynx.

Audible beating of the carotids ; sometimes they beat slowly.

Larynx: Swollen, sore, raw, scraping ; somewhat also when pressing on it ; obliged to swallow. Throbbing, narrow sensation, very painful to touch ; sensation of a plug, which moves up and down, with short cough ; sensation as of something fluttering.

Pain in the pit of the throat, extending to the root of the tongue and into the 'hyoid' and to the left 'tragus', behind which it shoots out, painful to touch.

Hoarseness, worse evenings ; something in the larynx prevents speech, which cannot be hawked up, though mucus is brought up.

Cough : Dry, spasmodic, hacking, tickling. Caused by pressure on the larynx, throwing the head back, eating, drinking, smoke, as from tobacco ; ulcers in throat ; a tickling in the throat, under sternum or in stomach ; heart diseases. Worse after sleep, during sleep without awakening him, from change of temperature, alcoholic drinks, mental emotions, getting wet through riding in the wind (tickling in the left side of the larynx caused cough). At every cough, stitch in the hæmorrhodal tumours.

Expectoration : Mucus and blood, as in heart disease ; blood-streaked, thick, yellow, as in phthisis pulmonalis ; grayish lumps, dislodged with difficulty ; a watery, scanty sputum, mixed with mucous lumps ; the effort causes vomiting and pain, compelling him to hold the stomach, worse after sleep, after talking.

Breathing : Loud rattling, dyspnœic upon any exertion, in suffocative attacks, arousing from sleep ; suffocative feeling during the heat, must loosen clothes about the neck, feels as if they hindered circulation ; fits of suffocation, must sit up in bed ; constantly obliged to take a deep breath, especially while sittng; shortness of breath, with many affections ; breathing difficult and feels so weak that he faints, worse moving around.

LACHESIS & OTHER ALLIED REMEDIES—(*contd.*)

Throat, Lungs and Heart.

Chest so tight in the evening, after lying down, almost suffocated.

Oppression of the chest, with cold feet ; also during sleep. Pressure on the chest as if full of wind ; this seems to rise up into the chest ; better from eructation.

Constriction of the chest ; it feels stuffed.

Stitches in the left chest, with difficult breathing, worse when coughing or on perspiration.

Soreness in the chest and of sternum.

Burning in the chest at night, with pains in the sternum or deep in the chest.

Hepatization, especially of the left lung ; great dyspnœa on waking, heart weak.

Deposit of tubercle after pneumonia, symptoms agreeing.

Purulent dissolution of hepatized lung.

Threatened gangrene of the lungs.

Œdema pulmonum, hydrothorax, etc., when the characteristic respiratory and laryngeal symptoms are present. Better lying on the left side.

Heart : Feels constricted, cramp-like pain in the praecordia, causing palpitation with anxiety.

Feels the beating of the heart, with weakness even to sinking down.

Palpitation : Causing anxiety, fluttering, with weakness to fainting, with nausea and weakness at the stomach with choking, caused by suppressing old ulcers.

Pressure as if from the stomach or during fever.

Irregular beat of the heart, every intermission accompanied by a strange feeling ; sensation as if the circulation were restored by crying a little.

Spasmodic affections of the heart, with a feeling as if the ear-drums would burst.

Cyanosis, with suffocating fits when moving.

Heart feels as if too large ; can bear nothing to touch throat or chest ; must sit up, slightly bent forwards ; aroused suddenly, during acute rheumatism, with a smothering and oppression at the heart and palpitation ; great anguish ; left arm numb ; stiff shoulders on taking a deep breath or upon turning to the right side.

LACHESIS & OTHER ALLIED REMEDIES—(*contd.*)

Throat, Lungs and Heart.

Spasmodic pain about the heart.

All the Ophidians affect the throat and cause constriction, dryness, impeded deglutition, hoarseness, sensitive larynx, dyspnœa, cough, blood-spitting, oppression of the chest and palpitation ot the heart, with anxiety.

Vipera Torva causes violent chest pains, with chilliness ; chest swells, with difficulty of breathing ; violent congestion to the chest ; he tears his clothes open, with sick sensation in the abdomen ; cardiac anguish ; upper extremities numb and lame.

In heart affections *Lachesis* suits more accurately the incipiency of rheumatic carditis.

Naja suits more accurately to the after-effects of rheumatic carditis. *Naja* causes a tumultuous fluttering action of the heart ; cannot lie on the left side, but great relief from lying on right side ; nervousness, pain at the heart ; sensation as if a hot iron had been run into the chest ; temporo-frontal headache, with great depression of spirits. Cardiac weakness is prominent in both. *Naja* also has palpitation, with crampy pains in the left ovary.

Elaps causes a constriction of pharynx and œsophagus ; liquids are suddenly arrested, and then fall heavily into the stomach, as does also food. It seems as if the spasm suddenly gives way, leaving an opposite paretic condition. Spasmodic stricture of the œsophagus is found also in *Lachesis* and *Naja,* if not in *Crotalus* ; but if the paretic effect is confirmed, it will help to differentiate ; for although not contrary to the genius of the others, it has not yet been recorded for them. It also causes a sensation as if the heart was being squeezed. Rush of blood to chest and throat.

RELATED REMEDIES.

Mouth and throat dry : Alumina, *Arsenic,*—BELLADONNA, with moist tongue, or with feeling of a skin on tongue ; Bryonia, Hyoscyamus, burning and dryness of tongue and lips ; they look like singed leather ; *Cinnabar*, mouth and throat must be moistened every time he awakes ; much mucus comes down from the posterior nares ; bridge of nose feels as if pressed by a metallic substance. Causticum ; Hepar ; Kali Bich. ; Kali Carb., evenings without thirst ; Lauroc., *Lycopod.*, *Mercur.*, palate dry as from heat. *Nux. M.*, *Natr. Mur.*, *Nux Vom ,* Opium, PHOSPH., Phos. Ac., Plumb., Rhus Tox., Secale C., Silicea, *Stram.*, Sulph., Verat. Alb., *Wyethia.*

Hoarseness with those who talk much : Lachesis, PHOSPH., Calc. Ost., CARBO VEG,

Larynx painful to touch : PHOSPH., *Bellad.*, *Apis, Spongia, Hepar,* Chin. Sulph., Bromine, Baryta C. (throat), Bryonia (throat , Iod. (pressure on larynx).

LACHESIS & OTHER ALLIED REMEDIES—(*contd.*)

Throat, Lungs and Heart.

Feeling of rawness in throat : Alumina, CARBO VEG., CAUST., Ignat., *Lycopod.*, MERCUR., *Nitric Acid*, Nux Vom., Phosph.

Feeling of a crumb, splinter : Alumina, Argent. Nit., Canth., HEPAR, Ignat., Kali C., *Merc.*, NIT. ACID, Rhus Tox.

Feeling of a lump or plug : Alumina, Apis, Arsenic, Baryta C., *Bellad.*, Caust., Carbo Veg., *Hep.*, Hyosc., *Ignat.*, Kali Bich., Kreos., Lycopod., Mercur., Nitric Acid, *Nux Vom.*, Phos. Acid., Phytolac., Sepia, Sulph., etc.

Feeling of something rising up like globus hystericus : ASAF., Con., IGNAT., Lycopod., Mercur., *Mosch.*, Nitric Acid, Nux Mosch., Plumbum, Spig., Sulph., etc.

Worse empty swallowing or swallowing saliva : Baryta C., Bellad., *Bryon.*, *Cocc.*, *Hep.*, Lycopod., *Mercur.*, Mercur. Corros., *Pulsat.*, *Rhus Tox.*

Fluids return through the nose : BELLAD., *Lycopodium*, Aurum, Canth., Cupr., Ignat., Mercur., Phosph., Silica.

Better from swallowing food : Mangan., Ignat.

Pharynx feels hollow : *Phytolac.*, Cinchona.

Ulcers in the throat : Alumina, *Apis*, *Arg. Nit.*, *Arsenic*, Baptis., Carbo Veg., Hepar, Ignat., Iod., KALI BICH., LYCOPOD., MERCUR., *Merc. Corros.*, MERC. CYAN., *Mur. Acid.*, NITRIC ACID, Phos. Acid, Sanguin.

Tonsils suppurate : *Ammon. Mur.*, BARYTA C., Bellad., Canth., HEPAR, *Ignat.*, *Lycopod.*, MERCUR., *Merc. Corros.*, *Phytolac.*, Sabad., SILICA, SULPH.

Diphtheritic deposit : Ailanthus, *Apis*, *Arsenic*, BAPTISIA, Ignat., *Kali Bich.*, LYCOPOD., LAC CAN., MERC. CAYN., *Merc. Bin. Iod.*, *Merc. Proto. Iod.*, Mur. Acid, *Nitric Acid*, *Phytolac.*, Rhus Tox., Sul. Acid.

Spasmodic stricture of the œsophagus : Alum., Arsenic, Arg. Nitric., Baptis., BELLAD., Bryon., *Carbo Veg.*, Cicuta, Coccul., Hydrophob., Hydroc. Acid, Hyosc., Ignat., Kali Bich., Kali Carb., *Naja*, Natr. Mur., Nit. Acid, PHOS., Plumb., Verat. Vir.

Throbbing of the carotids : BELLAD., Phosph.

Spasmus glottidis : CHLORINE, *Cupr.*, *Iod.*, Mephitis, *Bromide of Camphor*, PLUMB., *Bellad.*

Dyspnœa on going to sleep or arousing from sleep : *Arsenic*, *Sepia*, *Sulph.*, *Grindelia*, SAMBUC., *Carbo Veg.* Cough until phlegm is raised, especially *Apis*.

Cardiac cough, especially LAUROC.

LACHESIS & OTHER ALLIED REMEDIES—(*contd.*)

Throat, Lungs and Heart.

Oppression of chest, as if full of wind : Carbo Veg., Cinchon., Lycopod., Sulph., Zinc.

Neglected or badly-treated pneumonia, especially Sulph., LYCOPOD.

Œdema pulmonum ; hydrothorax : Ant. Tart., Ammon. Carb., Apoc. Cann., APIS, ARSENIC, Asparagus, Carbo Veg., *Digital.*, *Kali Carb.*, Kali Hyd., Lactuca, LYC., Merc. Sul., *Phos.*, Sulph.

Gangrene of lungs : *Arsenic*, *Carbo A.*, *Carbo Veg.*, *Cinchon.*, *Kreos.*, Osmium, Secale C.

Heart feels constricted : Arnica, Bufo, Justitia, Kali C., Kali Chlor., Lycopus, Cadmium.

Left arm numb, in heart affections, especially RHUS TOX.

Awakes smothering, with heart-disease, organic or not : ARS., *Digital.*, Grindelia, Kali Hyd., Lactuca, Merc. Præc. Rub.

Cyanosis : Ant. Tart., LAUROC., Aconite, *Secale Cor.*, *Digital.*, *Camph.*, *Op.*, *Cupr.*, Verat. Alb.

Heart feels too large : Sulph.

Rheumatism attacks the heart : Apis, ARSENIC, *Bryonia*, *Digital.*, *Kali C.*, *Phos.*, SPIG., Kalmia, Sanguin., Rhus Tox.

AMONG the Related Remedies referred to the following are the most important.

Both **Phosph.** and **Lachesis** have nervous cough, constriction and sensitiveness of the larynx, hoarseness evenings ; cough from tickling in the larynx or trachea. The former has the burning rawness most marked ; talking causes severe pain, for the larynx is inflamed, not merely irritated. And further, the tendency of the inflammation is to extend down the trachea and even to the bronchioles. Tightness across the chest is a prominent symptom and it is accompained with a sense of weight and oppression, as if the air-vesicles did not fill. Hoarseness is more prominent ; but both may meet in membranous croup and require careful discrimination. The hoarseness in LACHESIS is attended by a feeling as if something in the larynx prevented clear speech, it cannot be hawked up. This may be the membrane or more likely, a closure of the rima glottids. It is accompained with suffocating spells in sleep ; the child arises in agony, as if choking. Now PHOSPH. is needed in croup rather when hoarseness or aphonia remains as a sequel ; or when the nervous system is prostrated and the child lies cold, sweaty, with rattling breathing. It has the distinctive aggravations after sleep.

LACHESIS & OTHER ALLIED REMEDIES – (*contd.*)

Throat, Lungs and Heart.

Both cause præcordial anxiety, palpitation, feeble pulse and rush of blood to the heart. Only PHOSPH. has the violent beat on the least motion. If it be true that both affect the pneumogastrics, the resulting symptoms are not at all alike. In PHOSPH. there is created a feeling of hunger, demanding food, which relieves ; in LACHESIS, the nervous symptoms are choking and constriction of the throat.

The former remedy is not all comparable with the latter in its many forms of nervous palpitations.

In the after treatment of pneumonia, great care is necessary in the selection of PHOSPH., if there is a deposit of tubercles. LACHESIS, in such an emergency, is often indicated. By thus qualifying the former it is not intended to teach that this remedy can never be used ; but as its imperfect application will result disastrously, we must be sure of its appropriateness before venturing. No one is so skilful in the selection of the similimum that cautionary advice is useless.

Phytolacca depresses the vital powers and causes vomiting and purging. These latter effects are accompained with coldness and extreme weakness. They are slow in their development, and so resemble the gastro-enteric symptoms attendant on just such blood-poisioning as marks the development of diphtheria. Consequently, we find as characteristic, dizzy and faint when rising in bed, nausea and vomiting. The heart's action is not much weakened at first, though later its beat is feeble. Fatal poisonings do not seem to depend upon paralysis of the heart, but upon that of respiration. Therefore, the cardiac weakness cannot be so important a symptom as it is in LACHESIS. And further, it is a more acrid drug. The patient complains of chills, followed by fever. The body aches all ever as if pounded, with violent pains in forehead, occiput, back and limbs. LACHESIS has a hard aching all over, necessitating change of position. Both may affect the left side of the throat, with much constriction, swelling, purple color, and with putridity. Only the pokeberry has the feeling as if a hot ball was lodged in the fauces and sensation as after swallowing chokepears.

In **Mercurius Cyanatus** the corrosive effects of the mercury are manifest in the rapid ulceration of mucous surfaces ; while the no less rapidly developed prostration and gangrenous degeneration mark the added effects of the Prussic Acid. Other mercurial symptoms are the swollen glands and tenesmus with bloody stools. To the acid are chiefly due the cyanotic face and cold surface, the weakened heart, which post-mortem shows is attended with heart-clot, and the diphtheritic form of inflammation. This remedy holds out some hope when the diphtheritic deposit is also about the anus and in the bowels, with shreddy, bloody, and horribly offensive stools. The systematic poison causes that dangerous symptom, aversion to all food. If the child will not eat and cannot be

LACHESIS & OTHER ALLIED REMEDIES—(*contd.*)

Throat, Lungs and Heart.

compelled to, his situation is very critical. In such an emergency the remedy under consideration stands with Mur. Acid, Nitric Acid, and Liq. Calcis Chlor. as among the best. The heart is of course weak, so weak that the patient should not be raised to a sitting pasture, lest fatal syncope results. Even in the beginning of the disease the fever is adynamic and the strength sinks before the local deposit in the throat is sufficient to account for the sudden giving way of vital power—a strong indication.

The mouth and fauces are swollen and red, varying from a bright to a dark purple. The deposit is white, opalescent, or grayish ; and later, gangrenous and putrid. The tongue has a yellow base ; but soon becomes coated with a diphtheritic gray coat, the edges remaining red. As the disease advances, the tongue is dark, probably from changes in its coating. The disease spreads into the posterior and anterior nares and also downwards to the larynx. Profuse epistaxis.

Lac Caninum has won long-disputed laurels in true diphtheria. It bears many resemblances to LACHESIS, but may be distinguished by the following. The symptoms tend to affect the two sides alternately; Membrane is yellowish-gray or ulcers shine like silver. Mucous membrane red, glistening. Corners of the mouth sore (as in Arum. Triph).

Merc. Proto. Iod. and **Merc, Bin. Iod.** affect characteristically opposite sides of the throat. The former has most effect upon the right and is distinguished by the thick dirty-yellow coating far back on the tongue. In the latter, the patches are numerous on the left tonsil. Both have engorged glands and great prostration. Nose-bleed may be a symptom, though it is never so constant as in the snake-poisons, rather indicating congestion than dissolution of the blood.

Lycopodium is an acknowledged complement of LACHESIS. Its symptoms in the sick, move from right to left, shift about or remain stubbornly fixed in the right side of the throat. Upon swallowing, the throat feels tight ; food and drink regurgitate through the nose. Constant inclination to swallow. Fauces deep red, with burning and soreness. Cervical glands swollen and sensitive. The nose is generally involved, with stuffing of the nostrils, compelling the child to breathe with the mouth partly open and the tongue protruded. The child has a silly expression, which is a result of this method of getting breath ; but also, we believe, dependent upon the relaxed features caused from mental and physical weakness. Early in the case the child awakens as if frightened ; he strikes and kicks any one who attempts to console him. Stupor. If, in addition, the urine, whether passed involuutarily or not, deposits a red, sandy sediment, the choice is certain.

Like **Phosph.** this remedy may be needed for hoarseness remaining after croup ; and like LACHESIS, there may be suffocating spells at night ; cough as from tickling in the larynx, constriction of the chest, etc. In the

LACHESIS & OTHER ALLIED REMEDIES—(*contd.*)

Throat, Lungs and Heart.

Fern the hoarseness and cough are accompained with rattling of mucus, worse during sleep, making the breathing difficult and short. The tickling is as if form sulphur-fumes.

The chest symptoms are plainly those of catarrh. Rales are heard on both sides, though more on the right. The difficult breathing is in part due to accumulated mucus and is better when the latter is raised. Flatulent distension of the abdomen also contributes to the discomfiture by its upward pressure. But there are two other causes to be observed. One is the already mentioned alternation of contraction and expansion universal in this remedy. The other is the tendency to produce paralytic weakness of organs (see under Mental Symptoms). The relaxation tends to render the catarrhal and other chest symptoms persistent, permits the accumulation of mucus and muco-pus and gives rise to the rattling breathing, which is noticed along with the dropped jaw and stupor. Several forms of disease, then, frequently call for the remedy, viz.—phthisis pulmonalis, neglected pneumonia, typhoid pneumonia, catarrh of weakly children etc. And it is in the first three that the remedy compares with LACHESIS. The latter, however, has alternate chills and flushes, afternoons ; spasmodic, gagging cough, compelling patient to sit up and hold his stomach. Finally, he half expectorates and half vomits a purulent, offensive sputum, with some relief. So soon as he sleeps, he sweats, especially about the neck. LYCOPOD. develops a loose, deep cough, as if he were about to expectorate the whole pulmonary parenchyma. Fever worse from 4 to 8 P.M. Sputa are mucous, purulent, lemon-colored or gray, salt-tasting.

In hydrothorax, the latter is useful when the patient can lie only upon the right side ; the former, when only upon the left. Both have accompanying œdema of the limbs. In the Fern the urine deposits a red sediment ; in the other the urine is dark, almost black.

Kali Bichromicum has choking on lying down, wheezing-panting on awaking ; dyspnœa in sleep; oppression of the chest, which arouses him suddenly. Oppression at the bifurcation of the trachea into the bronchial tubes. The asthmatic symptoms are worse in early mornings, and seem to be associated with, if not caused by, a swelling of the bronchial mucus membrane and an accumulation of tough or stringy mucus. The removal of the latter greatly relieves. These sorts of difficult breathing make the bichromate useful as a successor to LACHESIS in diphtheria and croup, especially when the disease is spreading downwards. Experience proves that they follow each other well and profitably.

Baptisia has already been differentiated. All that need be added here is its use in malignant diphtheria. Typhoid symptoms are prominent, and the stupor is decided. The patient can only swallow liquids. Mouth and hroat look dark, the membrane is gangrenous, and the breath is horribly

LACHESIS & OTHER ALLIED REMEDIES.—(*contd.*)

Throat, Lungs and Heart.

putrid. There is great oppression of breathing, which is caused by pulmonary congestion and is relieved when air is freely admitted into the room. Compare *Ailanthus* which has also drowsiness ; livid throat. There is a thin acrid coryza, and the ulcers in the throat discharge an acrid fluid. Of the mineral acids, ARSENIC, *Mur. Ac.*, and *Nitric Ac.* present the greatest similarities. The first is distinguished by its general symptoms. The second has developed a gray-white membrane on the fauces, with choking on swallowing ; the parts appear dark bluish; rawness and smarting. Dark fetid nasal discharge. Weak, empty feeling at the stomach, with significant loss cf appetite ; nose-bleed ; weak, drowsy ; pulse weak, intermits every third beat ; hoarseness. The third is more acrid than the second ; the disease involves the nasal cavities, with excoriation of the lips. This is present in the second also, though less severe. The pulse intermits every fourth beat. Sometimes the child complains that a stick or splinter is in his throat.

Nux Vomica, like LACHESIS, has a morning aggravation ; but in the former remedy, it is the time of the day when many of the Nux symptoms appear ; in the latter, it is because of the aggravation from sleep. In the former sleep helps, unless the patient is suddenly awakened ; the throat feels scraped and rough, and though there are fetid ulcers, constriction and sensation of a plug during empty deglutition, yet the throat feels worse during and after solids ; while LACHESIS may have relief from solids.

Ignatia, according to the toxic symptoms noticed in India, corresponds very closely to the symptoms of diphtheria. Like LACHESIS, swallowing food relieves, and there are ulcers on the tonsils, etc. But in the former the patient has more marked aggravation between the acts of deglutition, and the ulcers are small, flat and open, on the indurated tonsils. The temperament, too, is important ; the patient is irritable, whining, nervous.

Spasmodic œsophageal stricture often calls for PHOSPH. The cardiac end is especially affected like LACHESIS, ARG. NITRIC., *Arsenic*. **But** LACHESIS has also spasms of the upper portion, when it more resembles BELLAD., *Hyosc.*, *Stram.*, *Carbo Veg.*, Canth., *Alumina,* Ignat., *Lycopod.*, Cicuta, etc. ARSENIC, *Rhus Tox.*, and Verat. Viride, have the spasm as a symptom of œsophegitis. LACHESIS, *Ignat.*, *Asaf.*, *Coccul.* etc. suit in hysterical, nervous patients, when there is also a reverse peristalsis. (See Globus Hystericus.)

To distinguish from H*yosc.*, remember that the latter is worse from cold liquids; solids and warm things give the least trouble; and hiccough is an accompaniment.

Carbo Veg. causes a sensation as if the pharynx was contracted or drawn together; food cannot be easily swallowed; throat seems contracted, with spasm, but no pain.

LACHSIS & OTHER ALLIED REMEDIES.—(*Contd.*).

Throat, Lungs and Heart.

Alumina causes constriction of throat ; soreness and constriction of the whole length of the œsophagus from swallowing a morsel of food ; but warm drinks relieve, as does the saliva.

Bellad. is closely related to LACHESIS, though its faucial and œsophageal spasms are more severe. It causes constriction, frequently recurring, particularly during efforts at swallowing ; the whole canal feels narrowed. It may likewise be employed when a large morsel of food or a bone obstructs the œsophagus and incites violent spasmodic contractions. (Compare also Cicuta, Ignat.) LACHESIS has rather a sensation of a crumb or button lodged in the œsophagus ; or the attempt at deglutition produces a gagging and smothering, as if food had gone down "the wrong way"

In sore-throat involving the tonsils, Bellad., Mercur., Hepar and Lachesis form a very interesting group, to which may be added Amygdala Persica, Apis, Vespa and Phosph.

Bellad. has dryness, scraping, burning, stinging ; violent and painful constrictions, worse when attempting to swallow fluids. Throat bright red, or, when inflammation is intense, deep crimson. Attacks come suddenly and develop rapidly, with throbbing pains, frontal headache, red face. Tonsils rapidly enlarge and threaten to suppurate ; cervical glands swollen, Sometimes there is a ropy mucus in the throat. According to the provings, the left side is most affected ; clinically, in agreement with the law of direction of symptoms (Hering), they are mostly right-sided.

Even if pus should form the remedy need not be changed, if the general characteristics of intensity, rapidity etc. remain. But if, with chills and local throbbing, the faucial color becomes livid, with pains as from splinters sticking and the external throat is very sensitive, HEPAR is the substitute. Or, again, if pus has formed but will not break forth, much badly-smelling phlegm collect and is hawked out with great pain, throat dark red, sweat aggravates rather than relieves, stitches extend into the ears, drinks regurgitate, then MERCUR. is needed. Now LACHESIS goes farther—the throat is purplish, and the patient very nervous ; the least touch is intolerable, more from hyperæsthesia than from inflammatory soreness, as in the others ; pus from tonsils is unhealthy and they tend to degenerate into ulcers. (Compare *Silicea, Sulph.*).

Amygdala Persica causes a dark-red throat and severe pains shooting through the tonsils. The pulse is not as strong as in Bellad. It has been employed when the latter, though seemingly indicated, does not relieve the pains ; and also when diphtheritic membrane forms. (Here compare *Merc. Proto Iod.* and *Merc. Bin. Iod.*).

Phosphorus affects tonsils and uvula ; the latter is elongated and sometimes œdematous ; the pharyngeal wall also looks swollen and glistening ; stinging pains, worse in the evening ; rawness, worse from talking ;

LACHESIS & OTHER ALLIED REMEDIES—(*contd.*)

Throat, Lungs and Heart.

hawks mucus, mornings, which has a nasty taste. Worse swallowing fluids, and during and after solids.

Apis Mel. induces a swelling of the mucous lining of the throat, which is rosy, with stinging and a constricted feeling, as if choking ; feeling of erosion. The main feature is the tendency of the mucous membrane to puff up or swell, causing the sense of choking and smothering. If ulcers form, they present œdematous borders. VESPA is nearly identical. It may, however, be needed when the symptoms recur periodically.

Among the new aspirants for distinction in throat affections is *Wyethia Helenoides*. As this remedy is said to cause nervousness, apprehensiveness, weakness, slow pulse, pain in left ovary etc., it may be that its throat symptoms will occasionally need differentiation from LACHESIS. The throat feels dry, with burning ; swallows with difficulty ; constant desire to swallow, but without relief of the dryness. Hemming to clear the throat, though unsuccessful. Similar dryness, with pricking, in the posterior nares.

Awaking smothering is deservedly considered as an excellent indication for LACHESIS. But in asthma, œdema of lungs, hydrothorax, heart disease etc., we may be compelled to decide between it and several others.

Arsenic awakens at 12 P.M. or later, with anxiety and smothering. **Kali Carb.** and **Kali Bich.**, towards 3 or 4 A.M.

Lactuca has tightness of lower part of chest ; he awakens at night and springs up for breath.

Graphites has a similar symptom, but it is relieved by eating.

Sambucus has starting from sleep with suffocation ; head and hands bluish, puffy. So soon as he awakens he begins to sweat, while during sleep he has hot face.

Belladonna arises choking and frightened ; face is red ; cries out in sleep.

Sepia and **Sulphur** awake smothering : the latter has markedly a sudden jerking of the legs as he drops off to sleep.

Phosph. induces suffocation just as the patient drops off to sleep. He is tall, slim, and predisposed to bronchitis. Palpitation and smothering from growing too fast.

Kali Hyd. awakens choking. This indicates it in heart disease, and also in œdema pulmonum. In the latter case, the sputum looks like greenish soap-suds.

Merc. Praec. Rub. has suffocative fits on the point of falling asleep ; he must spring up. It has cured this symptom in cases of simple debility, without any organic disease.

LACHESIS & OTHER ALLIED REMEDIES—(*contd.*)

Throat, Lungs and Heart.

Grindelia Robusta : Oppressed breathing ; heart feels too weak to take care of the blood sent to it ; on dropping off to sleep, the respiration ceases—he awakens smothering.

Baptisia has relieved the following : Awakes with difficult breathing ; better when the window is opened.

Asparagus should be thought of for dyspnœa of hydrothorax in the aged, with weak heart and pain at the left acromion.

Compare :- *Lachesis*, *Apoc. Cann.*, DIGITAL., ARSEN., *Phosph.*, *Gelsem.* All have weak heart, and the second, like the first, has many symptoms worse on awaking ; it also has goneness in the epigastrium, and the heart feels prostrated, flutters now and then, is very feeble, then slow—all common in hydropericardium. The *Gelsem.* may be distinguished by a feeling as if he must move or his heart will stop.

Rhus Tox., like LACHESIS, causes numbness of the left arm, and indeed, more characteristically. If there is any doubt, decide by the restlessness and by the lame and weak feeling about the cardiac walls.

Spigelia and **Lachesis** have suffocation provoked by moving the arms and by anxiety. But in cardiac rheumatism, the latter is called for when the invasion is announced by a sudden arousing from sleep, with anxiety, oppression and intolerance of pressure. The former is adapted to undulatory motion of the heart, purring feeling. sharp stitching pains etc., with anxiety. The intermittent pulse, which both cause, is very characteristic of SPIGELIA. In advanced heart-affection with dropsy, *Spigelia* has aggravation from sitting bent forwards ; LACHESIS, amelioration.

The Digestive Organs

THE Snake poisons weaken digestion, cause bitter or sour taste ; sour or acrid eructations, bilious or bloody vomit ; colic, flatulency ; swollen abdomen ; diarrhœa—bilious, slimy, bloody.

MOUTH—Taste : salty ; sourish and saltish taste of mucus and saliva ; bitter, also early in the morning and at night ; food tastes bitter ; metallic, with dry mouth.

STOMACH—Thirst.

APPETITE—lost in many complaints. At one time good, at another, absent. Hunger, cannot wait for food ; face pale, he feels faint. Aversion to warm food ; to warm things. Craves oysters, which agree ; wine, but it disagrees ; coffee, which agrees ; milk, but it causss nausea.

WORSE FROM : brandy ; fruits ; tobacco. Acids cause diarrhœa, feverishness, or retard the case.

LACHESIS & OTHER ALLIED REMEDIES—(*contd.*)

The Digestive Organs.

Before eating : languid, can scarcely move ; drowsy.

After eating : drowsy, with repletion ; indolenee, desires to lie down ; heaviness after every copious meal ; nausea and vomiting ; pressure in the stomach, with weak feeling in the knees ; raises a sour water ; regurgitation of ingesta. Eating relieves gnawing in stomach for a while.

Eructations : sour ; feels very ill until he eructates.

Nausea with faintness ; must loosen the clothing.

Nausea in paroxysms. Nausea after drinking.

Inclination to vomit, with sensation of illness, rousing him from a sound sleep—also in the morning in bed, as with drunkards or during pregnancy.

Vomits ingesta, bile, especially mornings, with mucus.

Spasmodic vomitting, with diarrhœa.

Vomits blood.

Vomitting renewed by the slightest motion ; nausea with great flow of saliva.

Pressure as from a load after eating, feels relieved by eructations of wind ; worse after siesta.

Feeling as if something was gnawing, though without pain ; the same in both sides and across ribs, deep in abdomen.

Pit of stomach very painful to touch.

Great discomfort from having the clothes tight around the waist.

Stitches extending from stomaeh to chest.

Great weakness of digestion ; with many eructations ; scarcely any sort of food agrees. Accompanying symptoms are : pale, sunken face vertigo. Causes are : abuse of Cinchona, Mercury, Alcohol etc. Feels bad immediately after eating. Very costive.

Digestive derangements, with hypochondriasis ; thinks he is an object of dislike, suspicion or hatred to his friends.

LIVER—Violent pains in the hepatic region ; clothing annoys.

Pain as if something had lodged in the right side, with stinging, and a sensation as if forming into a lump, moving towards the stomach.

Ulcerative pain in the liver, especially when coughing.

Suppuration of the liver. Burning pains.

LACHESIS & OTHER ALLIED REMEDIES—(*contd.*)

The Digestive Organs.

ABDOMEN, RECTUM and STOOLS.—Pain across the abdomen, after walking.

Sensation of a ball rolling in the abdomen.

Tearing in the abdomen. Cutting, lacerating and burning pains.

Enteritis, peritonitis, when gencral symptoms agree ; especially during suppuration.

Burning in the abdomen, mounting towards the chest and descending to the thighs. Burning and sensitiveness. Burning with pressure extending to throat, with scanty menses. Burning about the navel.

Cramp-like pain in the abdomen which is hot and very sensitive.

Incarcerated flatus. Eructations relieve ; pit of stomach painful to touch.

Abdomen distended and hard. Distended, must loosen clothing and remove all pressure, however slight.

Cutting pain in right side of abdomen, throwing her into fainting attacks.

Hernia, with strangulation ; skin mottled, bluish.

Griping pains, left to right ; feels as if diarrhœa would set in.

Painful stiffness from thc loins down the thighs.

Drawing from the anus to the navel.

Typhlitis—must lie on the back with kness drawn up.

Burning in the anus during and after stool.

Prolapsus ani, followed by painful constriction of anus,

Spasmodic pains in the anus, internally, shortly before and after stool.

Beating in the anus as from little hammers, as in piles ; and also after the evening diarrhœa.

Piles protruding and strangulatcd ; every cough or sneeze causes stitches in it. Worse in drunkards ; at climaxis ; with scanty menses, etc.

Tormenting constant urging in the rectum, but it increases the pain ; so he must desist without a stool.

Stools hard, like the sheep's dung. Unsuccessful urging, the anus feels closed.

Constipation of years' standing, with hard, distended abdomen.

The stool lies in the rectum, down to the anus, without any urging.

After great straining, discharges offensive, croupous masses.

LACHESIS & OTHER ALLIED REMEDIES—(*contd.*)

The Disgestive Organs.

Soft, bright-yellow stools.

The desire continues after thc evacuation of a pap-like, offensive stool.

Sudden diarrhœa, with great urging about 12 P.M.; movements excessively offensive.

Even formed stools are horribly offensive.

Watery stools, with burning in the anus, in the evening.

Bloody, purulent discharges. Dark, chocolate-coloured or looking like charred straw and very offensive,

Diarrhœa : in the spring ; from acid ; of drunkards ; at the climaxis ; evening or night ; during typhoid ; after sleep.

Alternate diarrhœa and constipation.

Hæmorrhage from the bowels ; blood decomposed.

Of the remaining Ophidians, **Elaps** is the best confirmed here. It may be distinguished by the fact that cold drinks feel like ice in the stomach. There are also :—a sinking feeling at the pit of the stomach, relieved by lying on the abdomen ; burning in thc stomach ; desire for sweetened butter-milk. The stools resemble the others, but it is particularly called for when the diarrhœa consists of black, forthy blood, with twisting in the bowels. Useful for consumptives.

Crotalus has burning thirst ; violent, greenish or bloody vomit ; black vomit. Stomach so irritable that it can retain nothing but brandy or gelatin. Cannot bear the clothing to touch the epigastrium. Irregular stools with pimples on the face, headache and nausea, worse in spring weather. Colic, after dinner and early in the morning. Hæmorrhages from the anus, as from every other orifice. Fetid diarrhœa. Sore pain from pit of stomach to hepatic region, with qualmishness, nausea and greenish vomit. Mouldy smell from the mouth.

Naja has similar symytoms, but as yet they ase not confirmed.

RELATED REMEDIES

Carves oysters : Lycopod., Brom., Rhus Tox.

Longs for wine or brandy : STAPHIS., *Sulphur, Selen., Hepar,* SUL. ACID, etc.

Coffee agrees : Angustura, Arsenic.

Complaints of drunkards : ARSENIC, Actæa Rac. (see Mind), *Carbo Veg., Nux Mosch., Cinchon., Hyosc., Opium, Stram., Cannab. Indica.*

Must loosen clothing : *Nux Vomica,* LYCOPOD., *Carbo Veg.,* Kreos., Sulph., Amm. Carb., *Graphites,* Kali Bich., Phos. Ac., Stram., Aurum, *Cinchon.,* Bovista.

LACHESIS & OTHER ALLIED REMEDIES—(*contd.*)

Stomach.

Vomiting bile, black vomit : ARSENIC, Curare, CONIUM, *Phosph.*, *Plumb.*, Opium, *Verat. Alb.*

Eating relieves stomach : *Petrol., Chelid* , ANAC. (while eating), Mezer., *Graph.*

Acids cause diarrhœa ; *Ant. Crud., Arsenic*, Phos. Acid, Apis.

Digestion weak : HEPAR, CINCHON., LYCOP., Arg. Nitric., *Mercur.*, SUL. ACID, PULSAT., KREOS., NUX VOM., *Digital.*, CARBO VEG., *Arnica*, *Nat. Mur.*, *Nat. Carb.*, Graph.

Before eating face pale, lassitude : Kali Carb.; Zinc. has weakness, trembling, legs weak. SULPH., Phosph., Natr. Carb.,—have gone, hungry feeling, 10 to 11 A.M. Pale, sunken countenance : ARSENIC, VERAT. ALB., *Nux Vom.*

Nausea with faintness : Alumin., ARSENIC, Cinchon., *Hepar, Phosph.*, *Tabac.*, *Verat. Alb.*, Kali Carb., Kali Bich.

Pressure as from a load, after eating : NUX VOM., *Abies Nigra*, *Lobelia* (like a plug), BRYON., ARSENIG, *Calc. Ostr., Kali Carb.*, LYCOP., *Mercur.*, *Pulsat.*, *Plumb.*, *Phosph.*, (cardialgia), Sepia (before and after eating), Opium (as from too hard food).

Cold sensation in the stomach : Lachesis less than ELAPS. Compare :- *Arsenic*, Camph., Cinchon,, *Colchic.*, Kali Bich., Nat. Mur., Phos. Ac., Sabad., Sulph., Sul. Ac., Verat. Alb.

Stomach worse on awaking : *Arg. Nitric.*, Kali Bich., Kali Carb., *Lycopod.,* Natr. Mur., Pulsat., Oxalic Acid., *Staphis.*, *Sulph.*, *Nux Vom.*

Hypochondriasis : NUX VOM., *Cinchon., Sepia, Aurum,* SULPH., *Silica*, *Nat. Carb.*, *Nitric Acid.*

Pit of stomach sensitive, with weak digestion : *Arnica*, *Nux Vom.*, CALC. OSTR., *Pulsat.*, *Cinchon*, *Arsenic*, *Sulph.*, *Phosph.*, Secale C., *Mercur.*, *Bryon.*, *Carbo. Veg.*, Graph., *Sepia.*

Liver sensitive : *Phosph.*, MERCUR., *Bellad.*, Lycopod., *Arsenic*, *Rhus Tox.*, *Carbo Veg.*

Burning pains in liver : *Mercur.*, ARSENIC, Bryonia, Anac., Kali Carb., Phos. Acid, Sulph., Phosph.

Abdomen sensitive to touch : APIS, NITRIC ACID, *Phosph.*, Phos. Acid.

Pains across upper abdomen chiefly : LYCOPOD., IPECAC., Carbo Veg., Sepia, Stannum, Arnica.

Inflammatory conditions, especially with exudation, suppuration, or with typhoid symptoms : MERCUR., *Bryonia*, RHUS TOX. *Merc. Corros.*, *Lycopod.*, *Plumb.*, ARSENIC, BAPTISIA, *Apis*, *Hyosc.*, *Canthar.*, *Oxalic Acid.*

LACHESIS & OTHER ALLIED REMEDIES—(*contd.*)

Stomach.

Typhlitis : Bellad., Mercur., Ginseng., Opium, Plumb., *Rhus Tox.*

Burning in the abdomen : Apis, Arsenic, Bellad., Carbo Veg., *Colchic.*, *Kali Bich* , Mercur., Phosph., Arnica, Phos. Acid, Secale C., Silica.

Incarcerated flatus : *Arnica*, Carbo Veg., Coccul., Graph., Lycopod., Plumb., Staphis., Anilin Sulph., Sulph., Phosph.

Faint, with pains in abdomen : Alumin., Ammon. Carb., Calc. Ostr., *Cinchon.*, Sepia, Sul. Acid.

Strangulated hernia and gangrene : Arsenic, *Carbo Veg.*, Plumb..

Prolapsus Ani, with painful constriction : *Mezer.*, *Nitric Acid*, Sepia. Spasmodic pains in the anus : Lauroc.

Beating at the anus : Berberis, Caustic., Apis, Alumin., *Natr. Mur.*

Constriction of the anus : Bellad., *Alumin.*, Caust., *Colchic.*, *Kali Bich.*, *Lycopod.*, Natr. Mur., *Nitric Acid*, Nux Vom., Plumb., Sepia, Silica, Ignat., Staphis., Coccul., *Mezer.*, Sarsap., Secale C.

Constriction after stool : Ignat., Sepia, Sulph., Kali Bich., *Nitric Acid*, *Colchic.*

Constipation, abdomen distended : Bellad., *Graph.*, Hyosc., *Sulph.*, Phosph., *Lycopod.*

Costive, urine retained : Laches.. Hyosc., Lauroc., Opium, Morphia Acet.

Stool lies in rectum, no urging : Opium, Alumin., *Lycop.*, Hyosc., Carbo Veg., Sepia, Kali Carb., Nux Mosch., Silica, Verat. Alb., *Cinchona*, *Graph.*

Piles, with stitches at every cough : *Ignat.*

Piles protrude and become strangulated : Silica, Nux Vom., Ignat.

Varices hinder stool : Lachesis, Caustic., Sul. Acid.

Hæmorrhages from the bowels, blood dark : *Alumen*, Alumin., Hamam., Mercur , Ant. Crud., *Pulsat.*, Secale C., Mur. Acid, *Carbo Veg.*, Nitric Acid (black, offensive, or bright), Terebinth.

Diarrhœa sudden : Apis, Kali Bich., Croton Tig., Podoph.

Stool invulantary : Opium, *Mur. Acid*, Rhus Tox., Colchic., *Hyosc.*, Baptis., Carbo Veg., *Arnica*, Phos. Acid, *Apis.*

Offensive : Baptis., Cinchon,. Arsenic, Graph., *Colchic.*, Lycopod., Kreos., Nitric Acid, *Opium*, Podoph., Rhus tox., Secale C., *Arg. Nitric.*, Carbo Veg., *Stram.*, Silica, *Sulph.*, Arnica.

LACHESIS & OTHER ALLIED REMEDIES—(*contd.*)

Stomach.

Bright yellow, papescent : CHELIDON., Apis, (orange), *Podoph.*, *Gelsem.*, Nuphar, Yucca, GAMBOGE, *Hepar*. Rhus Tox., *Natr. Sulph.*, *Aloes, Sul. Ac.*, *Colchic.*

Watery : APIS, Apoc., Cann., ARSENIC, *Arnica*, CINCHON., CROTON TIG., *Colchic.*, *Chelidon.*, *Elatcrium*, *Gamboge*, *Hyosc.*, *Kali Bich.*, *Magn. Carb.*, Mur. Ac., PODOPH., PHOSPH., PHOS. AC., *Secale C.* SULPH. AC., VERAT ALB., *Rhus Tox.*

Purulent : *Arnica*, ARSENIC, Bellad., Apis, Calc. Ost., *Carbo Veg.*, *Calc. Phos.*, CANTH., Cinchon., Kali Carb., *Lycopod*, MERCUR., *Pulsat.*, SULPH., SILICA.

Croupous : MERC. CYAN., *Arg. Nitric.*

Of the drugs enumerated above, only a very few bear more than a partial similarity to the special remedies under study. A succinct account of the action of LACHESIS here shows that it relieves when digestion is weakened from want of vitality. And with this, there are always hypersensitiveness to touch, aggravation after sleep, and either obstinate constipation or offensive stools. Contractions and constrictions are here, as everywhere, predominant. So can we explain the difficult stool and colic. The sphincter ani tends to this constriction ; and, in the one case, holds back the faeces, despite the urging ; in the other, threatens the protruding piles with strangulation. Inflammations in the abdomen or in its pareties partake of the low grade, so characteristic of the snake-poison.

Examining now the analogous remedies in the light of these essentials, we find the following, amongst others, of special interest :

Lycopod. requires that food have its natural flavor. There may, however, be sour taste, and in the morning, bitter taste. Eructations relieve the sense of repletion, but not the feeling of illness. The smallest quantity of food fills to bursting, and then the clothing must be loosened. There are water-brash, oppression of the chest, heat in the abdomen, cold face, and oppressed breathing from flatulency, not from constriction of the throat. Distended abdomen, with rumbling, worse in region of splenic flexure, and pains in consequence. Constipation predominates ; urging is frequent enough, but the anus constricts and thus retards defecation ; but the rectal urging is less painful.

In hepatie abscess the one often follows the other. LACHESIS has a contractive feeling; LYCOPOD , a feeling as of a cord constricting the hypochondria. In the former the urine is black, frothy, or rarely turbid, with red sediment ; in the latter, it deposits a red sand. Though both have gastralgia, it is far more marked in LYCOPOD., and only the snake-poison has temporary relief from eating.

* For details of other remedies consult Farrington's "Clinical Materia Medica."

LACHESIS & OTHER ALLIED REMEDIES—(*contd.*)

Stomach.

Nux Vom. materially alters the taste ; it is, particularly in the morning, sour, putrid or bitter, after raising mucus from the throat. Hunger is usually wanting, except sometimes as a precursor of gastric disorder. Worse generally after meals, especially after dinner. Very marked is an aggravation, one to two hours after eating (duodenal digestion). Nausea is attended with a faintness and illness as in LACHESIS, and the pressure of clothing is annoying. When these symptoms result from abuse of alcohol, the choice from merely local symptoms is difficult. Usually NUX suits when there are mental and bodily over-impressibility ; LACHESIS, when the sufferer if greatly weakened by repeated debauchery. If constipation obtains, the urging in the former is spasmodic, fitful and ineffectual ; in the latter, painful and fruitless from constriction of the anus ; and this, with large purplish piles, increases with the amount of alcoholic abuse.

The abdomen is distended by the action of NUX, but the principal sensation, as we understand it, is a tense feeling out of proportion to the objective swelling ; and the characteristic irritability of the remedy is displayed in the griping colic, feeling of a load in the abdomen, sensitiveness to touch, and' withal, irregular urging to stool. Constipation prevails ; but diarrhoea may be present, when it is usually scanty, with straining ; bloody, slimy, with tenesmus.

In typhoid conditions, when the abdominal symptoms are severe, with involuntary stools, sopor, dropping of the jaw, compare **Lachesis** with **Opium** when the stertor is marked.

Hyoscyamus, if the apathe is complete, with mucus rales in the chest, stools watery, sphincters paralyzed.

Apis, when the watery, yellow stool escapes from the open anus at every movement of the body.

Muriatic Acid, when the patient slides down in bed and the involuntary stool is fetid and often accompanied with profuse hæmorrhages.

Urinary Organs.

Lachesis : Sticking pains shoot from place te place, from the small of the back to the liver (perhaps also to the kidneys), and thence downward to the urethra.

Renal affections : Albuminuria, Morbus Brightii, after scarlatina, after excessive use of alcohol, etc In such cases the urine is dark, turbid, and there may be dropsy, with suffocating spells, and pale, puffy, yellow face ; uriue black in spots, after scarlatina.

Feeling, when turning over, as if a ball rolled over in the bladder. Dull pain in the bladder when constipated.

Peculiar unpleasant sensation in the bladder, desire to urinate, and slimy sediment in the urine. Offensive mucus in the urine ; cystic catarrh.

LACHESIS & OTHER ALLIED REMEDIES—(*contd.*)

Urinary Organs.

Urging to urinate is violent, with copious escape of a dark, foaming urine.

Frequent micturition.

Burning during urination.

Urine suppressed.

Of the remaining ophidians but little can be said in this connection, as their clinical use is almost *nil*. *Crotalus* causes hæmaturia and stains the urine, as in jaundice, just like LACHESIS. Elaps causes a constriction of the spincter vesicæ ; but although this symptom is not so exprsssed in the provings of Lachesis, it is by no means contrary to the genius of the latter.

RELATED REMEDIES.

Albuminuria after abuse of alcohol :ARSENIC, CINCHON., Ledum, Sulph., Aurum, Bellad., Calc. Ars., Cuprum.

Albuninuria after scarlatina : APIS, ARSENIC, DIGITALIS, HELLEB., Canth., Kali Carb., Lycopod., Hepar, Terebinth., Helon.

Urine black : *Colchic.*, Natrum Mur., *Helleb.*, *Carbolic Acid, Digital.*

Urine dark, turbid : *Apis*, Ammon. Benz., *Arsenic*, *Benz. Acid, Digital.*, Arnica, Opium, Carb. Veg., Kali Carb., *Terebinth.*

Strong odor from mucus : Dulca., Phos. Acid, Pareira Brava, Lycopod., Uva Ursi, Coloc., Petrol.

Urine foaming : Lauroc., Copaiva, Cubebs, Lycopod., Thuja.

Urine suppressed : *Apis*, *Apoc. Cann.*, Elaps, Vipera, Crotalus, *Helleb.*, PULSAT., LYCOPOD., SULPH., STRAM., Bellad., *Arnica*, *Hyosc.*, *Lauroc.*, *Arsen.*, *Camph.*, Plumbum, Rhus Tox., Kali Bich., *Cuprum*, Tabacum, Canthar., Carbolic Acid, Merc. Corros., Digital., Terebinth., Colchic., Secale.

Carbolic Acid is eliminated by the kidneys, causing a black urine, black and usually clear. We may infer, then, that the drug acts on the kidneys, but whether the black urine is to be regarded as a symptom remains to be seen. It should be tried when renal disease, albuminuria, etc., accompany other affections in which the acid has been successfully employed, such as diptheria, scarlatina, with the charateristics of Carbolic Acid. When urinating, involuntary discharge of mucus from the anus. Suppression of urine and simple retention should be carefully distinguished, for though both are serious symptoms, the farmer is speedily fatal. Our text books are inexcusably careless in including, as they often do, both conditions under the one heading of "retained urine" (see Boenninghausen's

LACHESIS & OTHER ALLIED REMEDIES—(*contd.*)

Urinary Organs.

Therapeutical pocket-book, et al) ; or, which is still worse, denominating as suppression that which is merely a retention.

Of the list of remedies for suppressed urine which we give above we feel quite positive, though from the defective wording of provings and from the neglect of catheterization, we cannot speak with the certainty we could wish. Agaricus Phal., Arsenic, Camph., Bellad., Canthar., *Cupr. Acet.*, Digit., *Plumb.*, *Secale C.*, *Stramon.*, Tabac., Hyosc., Elaps, Vipera, Ailanthus, Merc. Cor., Merc. Cyan., Phosph., Sul. Ac., Conium and Causticum are stated by provers to have caused suppression of urine. Traumatic cases require Arnica. Renal hyperæmia, with suppression of urine, has been produced by large doses of *Cantharides*. And any remedy causing scanty urine as a symptom of renal congestion or inflammation, as Bellad., *Cannab.*, may be indicated when the disease is severe enough to entirely suppress secretion.

The cases in which we may suppose LACHESIS indicated—typhoid conditions—may also demand *Apis, Arseuic. Apoc. Cannab.*, *Helleb.*, *Arnica*, Hyos., Stram. Lycopod., or Sulph.

Apoc. Cannab. causes a tropidity of the kidneys. Indeed, the general effect of the drag is functional torpidity of many organs ; as, drowsy and heavy, bewildered sensorium ; pulse 50 ; muscular ennui, etc. It may, therefore, be called for when the ischuria attends weak heart, dropsy, etc.

Helleborus operates more deeply ; the sensorium is so depressed that the patient is stupid, cannot comprehend, or answers slowly, the senses act sluggishly, the muscles fail and the heart beats slowly. The pupils are dilated ; the nose is dry and the nostrils look as if smoked. In severe cases the mouth is partly open and the forehead drawn into wrinkles Compare Lycopod., which we have shown to cause functional torpidity.

Sulphur has relieved suppression in cholera infantum, when the child lies semi-conscious, with cold sweaty face, starting of the limbs, etc. In puerperal fever, compare also, *Secale C.* (Baptisia), Arsenic.

In Cholera Asiatica, ischuria may yield to CAMPH., *Verat. Alb.*, Lauroc , *Secale C.* (Carbo Veg.), *Cuprum*, *Arsenic* or *Kali Bich.*

Genital Organs.

GENITAL ORGANS.—The ophidians, so far as proved, weaken the virile powers of man, and this often with lascivious imaginings. Several of them also affect the uterus and ovaries.

Lachesis.—*Males* : Lascivious thoughts and dreams ; either with erections and sexual desire, or with physical weakness.

Emissions make him more cheerful and increase his mental activity ; or, cause profuse sweat.

Epilepsy from onanism.

LACHESIS & OTHER ALLIED REMEDIES – (*contd.*)

Genital Organs.

Prepuce inflamed, indurated.

Phagedenic chancre. Gangrene from para-phimosis.

Red pimples and spots on the glans penis.

Syphilis with above symptoms and also flat ulcers on the legs, with blue surroundings ; caries of the tibia, the parts are sensitive and livid ; ulcers iu the throat ; bone-pains at night ; all after abuse of Mercury.

Buboes after abuse of Mercury, with sore-throat and violent headche, either in back or front of head.

Females : Nymphomania, lascivious dreams ; tickling jerking from thighs to sexual organs ; sad on awaking ; labia swollen with much mucous discharge ; the menstrual flow relieves.

Menses scanty, feeble ; flow acrid, or lumpy, black, intermittent.

Before menses : Leucorrhœa ; nose bleeds a few drops ; tendency to faint ; wants fresh air ; bruised pain in the hips ; cutting in the abdomen ; vertigo ; headache. During menses : Many symptoms ease with the flow and return when it lessens or ceases ; there may be blood or mucus from the anus, throbbing in the head, labor-like bearing down. The latter seems to follow a slight menstrual flow. Menstrual colic beginning in the left ovary.

Uterus prolapsed, especially at climaxis. Cutting, like knife-thrusts in the abdomen. Very weak from any exercise. Pains in left ovarian region and left side.

Shooting across from left ovary to right.

Ulcers on the cervix, syphilitic, with condylomata.

Affects more the left ovary, with tendency to the right. Induration, swelling, or suppuration, with burning-boring pains, relieved by a discharge of blood from the vagina. Moral emotions or exertion aggravate.

Pains in the right groin, extending towards the uterus, or upwards to liver and chest.

In uterine and ovarian affections the following are some of the concomitants : Flushes of heat during day, chills at night. Cannot bear the pressure of the clothing. Faints easily. Hysterical, with globus hystericus, smothering spells on dropping off to sleep, awakes mornings distressed and unhappy ; is jealous and lascivious ; apprehensive ; mistrust of everything; pride; suspicious mood; ecstasy ; great mental excitement; talkative, with rapid flow of ideas, or frequently, mental inactivity. Restless as if hurried. Emotions aggravate pains in the right ovarian region. Very sad during menses ; sighing relieves.

LACHESIS & OTHER ALLIED REMEDIES—(*contd.*)

Genital Oagans.

Gulping of a sour fluid ofter meals, during pregnancy.

Faints during labour ; lies as if dead from cardiac syncope.

Puerperal convulsions commence on the left side, and are worse about the throat and neck, with trismus and blue face : body bent backwards ; extremities cold.

Mastitis, suppuration ; the skin around is bluish.

Milk blue, thin ; especially if the mother has long suffered from some mental trouble.

Puerperal fever ; abdomen distended ; she says that the pains seem to ascend to the chest; urine suppressed; fetid ichorous lochia; skin alternately burning hot and cold. See also peritonitis, under "Abdomen".

In complaints at the climaxis, often indicated, especially for : Flushes of heat ; vertigo ; fainting ; spells of blindness ; weakness, trembling, desire to lie down, worse before breakfast; palpitation, cold sweats, etc.

Of the remaining ophidians, *Naja Trip.* has gloomy headache, spinal pains, and palpitation from sexual irregularities. Strong sexual desire with physical powerlessness.

In females its most characteristic effect is a crampy pain in the left ovarian region. The secretion of milk is lessened.

Crotalus induces the same sexual excitement with lax organs. "The milk poisoned the baby, 5 months old". The Crotal. Casca. caused : Lancinating in the uterus when washing with cold water. Mania alternating with a bright-red metrorrhagia.

Elaps : Prepuce inflamed, as in Lachesis. Weight in the uterus, worse rising and walking ; lancinating up to the epigastrium. Weight on the vagina after a hysterical colic. White leucorrhœa. Secretion of milk lessened.

RELATED REMEDIES.

Lascivious thoughts : CANTH., HYOSC., LYCOP., *Calc. Ostr.*, PHOSPH., PLAT., STRAM., Origanum, *Lilium Ttg.*, *Verat. Alb.*

Lascivious thoughts, with weakness of the sexual organs, or without much local irritation (which seems characteristic of the ophidians); Ambra, Calc. Ostr., Agnus, Staphis., Ignat., Calad., Sepia, Aurum, Graph., Selen., Sulph., Agaric.

Emissions relieve : Agnus, Calc. Phos., Zinc.

Epilepsy from onanism : *Bafo*, *Platin.*, CALC. OSTR., Kali Brom,, Silica, *Sulph.*

LACHESIS & OTHER ALLIED REMEDIES—(*contd.*)

Genital Organs.

Syphilis after abuse of Mercury : KALI IOD., NITRIC AC., HEPAR, *Aurum*, *Staphis.*, *Carbo Veg.*, Arsenic, *Phytolac.*

Prepuce inflamed and indurated : Sulph., Sepia.

Para-phimosis, with gangrene : Ars., Merc. Corros., Canth.

Phagedenic chancre : *Arsenic, Merc. Corros.*, *Nitric Ac.*

Buboes maltreated with Mercury, and which are accompanied with violent headache : KALI IOD., *Carbo An.* (back of head), *Hepar* (forehead), Phytolac. (forehead).

Nightly pains in the limbs, syphilis : MERC., NITRIC AC., *Lycopod.*, Mezer., KALI IOD., HEPAR, Stillingia, Syphilin. *Asafœt.*

Pains cease after a flow of blood from the uterus : Zinc (better during menses).

Pains in the left ovarian region : Apis, *Arg. Met.*, Eup. Purp., Bromine, Coloc., *Lilium*, Graph., ZINC, THUJA, Ustilago, Podophyl., Psorinum, Silica, Capsic., Merc. Viv., Ambra, Bovista, Nat. Mur., Rhus Tox., Carbolic Acid.

Syphilitic ulceration of the os uteri, with condylomata : NITRIC AC., THUJA, *Nux Vom.*

Prolapsus uteri, with pains in the left ovarian region : *Arg. Met.*, *Lilium*, Podophyl.

Pains from uterine or ovarion regions upwards : GELSEM., Calc. Ostr., *Apis*, Hydrophobin, *Sepia*, Podophyl.

Ovary inflamed : APIS, BELLAD., *Hamam.*, *Lilium*, *Pallad.*, Canth.

Suppuration of the ovaries : Mercur., Hepar, Platin.

Induration of ovary : Apis, Arsenic, Baryta Iod., Baryta Mur., Couium Bellad., Graph., Iodine, Psorin., Pallad., Platin.

Ovarian pains are boring : *Coloc.*, *Lycopod.*, *Zinc.*, Lilium.

Ovarian pains are lancinating : *Conium*, *Apis*, Curare, *Lilium*, *Lycopod.*

Ovarian pains are stitching : Ambra, Bryon., Bufo, Canth., Carbo Anim., *Conium*, Curare, Graph., *Kali Carb.*, Mercur., Lycopod., Coloc., Picric Ac., Plat., Sepia.

Complaints at the climaxis : *Sepia*, Sul. Ac., Sulph., Amyl-Nitrite, Glonoin, Pulsat., Sang. and Kali Bich.

Back, Limbs and organs.

Lachesis.— Creeping sensation slowly down the back from the neck in epilepsy.

LACHESIS & OTHER ALLIED REMEDIES.– *contd.*)

Back, Limbs and Nerves.

Neck painful to least touch.

Neck stiff, with rheumatism or catarrh.

Neck swollen.

Ulcers on the neck.

Pain in the small of the back, with constipation, palpitation, dyspnœa, etc.

Tearing, with bruised sore pains, sore throat ; cold in spring weather.

Drawing in small of back and into legs, worse in the ischia ; worse in the evening.

Coccyx pains ; when sitting he feels as if sitting on something sharp.

Rheumatic pains and heaviness in the shoulders ; drawing and stiffness in back and limbs ; tearing. Tension and shortening of the hamstrings, with swelling of the soft parts and intolerable pain on touch. Joints and back feel sprained. Pains hinder sleep. Chronic rheumatism, worse in changes of weather. Bluish-red swellings. Curvatures of the joints. Profuse sweat, but it does not relieve. Pains go (in the sick) from right to left, or alternate. Aching in the bones.

Nervous exhaustion with nearly all complaints. Langour, weariness ; trembling (as in drunkards). Sinks down from exhaustion. Feels as if body is disintegrating, with sinking of the vital forces.

Left-sided paralysis, especially from apoplexy.

Gait stumbling, awkward, with numbness of hands and feet, and mental and physical weakness. Helpless mornings ; occiput heavy as lead ; weak, faint ; feels stiff until two or three hours after rising. Feet ice cold. Flushes of heat.

Gressus gallinaceus.

Swelling of hands and feet.

Legs swell, worst left ; dropsy : elephantiasis.

Swelling of the feet, worse after walking (pregnancy).

Cracked skin between and on the toes ; deep rhagades across the toes. Sometimes syphilitic.

Panaritium, with stinging, pricking pains ; violent pains at night, especially if the bone is affected ; surrounding parts dark, bluish. Suppuration slow, insufficient. Lymphatics inflamed. Proud flesh. After abuse of mercury : or if Hepar is insufficient.

Gangrene of the toes ; bluish-black vesicles ; tingling, with heat and numbness ; parts feel as if touched with ice : itching ; rubbing causes painful spots to appear.

Ulcers on the legs.

LACHESIS & OTHER ALLIED REMEDIES—(*contd.*)

RELATED REMEDIES

Lachesis, it will be observed, causes tearing pains, sprained feeling about the joints, and shortening of the tendons. Hence it may be required in rheumatism, especially if chronic. The history of the case will usually reveal abuse of mercury, syphilitic taint; or, quite commonly, accompanying nervous weakness, bordering on paralysis. In acute rheumatism, it is needed when the heart becomes invaded.

This state of rheumatism, with nervous weakness, suggests a comparison of LACHESIS with LYCOPOD., COLCHIC., RHUS TOX., *Silica, Caustic., Arsenic*, Rhodod., Ledum, Kalmia etc.

Lycopodium suits chronic forms ; the affected parts are numb ; there are tearing in the limbs at night, and stiffness on beginning to move in the morning ; sweat without relief—thus far very similar to LACHESIS. But the former always has, in addition, flatulent distension of stomach and abdomen. Worse on alternate days. Rheumatism of the dorsa of the feet. Lithic Acid deposit in the urine more marked than with LACHESIS.

Colchicum induces great sensitiveness of the parts, numbness, prickling and tearing pains in feeble, debilitated persons. The inflammatory swellings are pale red and the accompanying pains unbearably severe in the evening. The disease travels crosswise, or goes from left to right.

Rhus Tox. compares with the snake-poison in the morning stiffness, weakness, with numbness and formication ; sweat, and no relief etc. Both have stiff neck, but only the latter has it with little annoyance when moving the head. In RHUS the patient moves conveniently after the parts are "limbered up" but on beginning to move, pains and tension force him to cry out. The pains go from left to right, and there is relief from continued motion, with aggravation again *after* moving. While in LACHESIS there is also increased suffering on begnning to move, yet the relief from its contiunance is not marked. So only RHUS has the following : pains annoy him until he changes position, then they are better for a short time, but soon he is again compelled to change. Indeed LACHESIS is usually worse from such change of position.

Both, as was said, cause numbness ; but this is most prominent in RHUS, while in LACHESIS, oversensitiveness exists exclusively. Worse from straining is found only in the former.

Causticum, like LACHESIS causes trembling. weakness, paralysis, contractions of tendons, curvature of joints ; nightly pains. Both may be employed in arthritis deformans of women. But the exciting cause of rheumatism is different. In the former it is dry, cold weather or snowy air ; in the latter it is damp, warm air, as in spring or before a thunder-storm. In acute cases there is no resemblance whatever.

In rheumatism with prominent affection of fibrous structures, LACHESIS compares also with RHODOD., *Ledum, Kalmia, Manganese;* Mezer.

LACHESIS & OTHER ALLIED REMEDIES—(*contd.*)

Back, Limbs and Nerves.

Phytolac. The first three also cause nervous weakness, but are readily distinguished from LACHESIS. **Rhodod.** has tearing pains, tingling and weakness, better from motion ; and worse in rough, windy weather. Both have aggravation before a thunder-storm. **Kalmia** affects the heart, but the pains in the limbs are characterized by their severity, with notable absence of swelling. **Ledum** causes pains which ascend ; and there is aggravation from warmth in general. Both have aggravation from warmth of bed.

Weakness of the nervous system, paralysis etc. are among the evident effects of LACHESIS. They are the direct results of the blood-poisoning, and so suggest this remedy when they are produced by such diseases as typhoid fever, diphtheria, scarlatina etc. But they may result from other causes, such as apoplexy, alcoholism, especially apoplexy of drunkards, or from organic cerebral or spinal changes.

The paralysis is usually left-sided, with tingling, prickling, numbness and trembling.

There is, however, a condition developed by the snake-poison which is suggestive of the early stages of spinal disease, and which may also arise from extension of rheumatism to the fibrous sheaths. This condition is expressed in the following : Always after sleep, so stiff, he can scarcely stir ; rubbing relieves. Helpless stumbling gait which disappears an hour or two after rising ; caused by a pain as from a sprain in the small of the back that prevents every motion. Joints feels sprained.

In paralysis of toxic origin, compare : BAPTISIA, GELSEM., ARSENIC, *Rhus Tox.*, MUR. AC., *Apis*.

In paralysis from apoplexy, compare : *Apis*, *Arnica*, BELLAD., BARYTA C., OPIUM, Gelsem., Lauroc., Hyosc., *Nux Vom.*

In paralytic weakness, with stiffness : RHUS TOX., *Lycopod.*, *Contum*, *Silica*, *Causticum*, Rhodod., *Natr. Mur.* (tendons, hamstrings shortened). See also CAUST., Am. Mur.

Awkward : *Apis*, *Bovista*, *Natr. Mur.*, Silica, Agaricus.

Compare here typhoid symptoms mentioned in the preceding pages. MUR. AC., GELSEM. and ARSENIC have, with LACHESIS, great weakness of the musular system.

Gelsemium has only motor paralysis. Ptosis is often present and the blood-vessels are enlarged from defective vaso-motor control ; henee the face is suffused and the pulse full but not hard. There are never the evidences of putrescence etc. of the snake-poison.

Apis is said to suit in profound coma, even more pronounced than that of Opium. Paralysis of one and convulsions of the other side.

Belladonna suits when the face is bloated, red ; there are convulsive movements ; right-sided paralysis. LACHESIS follows.

LACHESIS & OTHER ALLIED REMEDIES—(*contd.*)

Back, Limbs and Nerves.

Baryta suits the aged, and childishness is marked.

Opium : face more brown red ; hot sweat ; drunkards.

Nux Vom. in drunkards. Incomplete paralysis, with vertigo, weak memory ; gastric ailments ; costive.

Rhus Tox. is distinguished by the fact that the stiffness is not especially after sleep, but on beginning to move or after exertion.

Conium : but it is principally motor ; sluggish accommodation of vision ; vertigo, worse when turning the head.

Causticum : also chiefly motor. Partial paralysis ; as ptosis, one-sided paralysis of the face. Central irritation as shown in contractions of limbs. Staggering gait ; the brain is weak ; ankles give way and he falls, thus differing from the "cock-walk" of LACHESIS.

Panaritium, compare : APIS, HEPAR, *Rhus*, *Silica,* Bufo, Arsenic, Lycopod., Asafœt.

Apis produces similar stinging, but the inflammation is more superficial and the parts are tense, red, and exquisitely sore and sensitive ; after abuse of Sulphur.

Hepar presents a livid, throbbing swelling, intolerant of touch or pressure ; pus has formed. If this remedy fails to evacuate the pus, or, if after breaking, the abscess continues to discharge, retaining its bluish surrounding, LACHESIS must be substituted.

Asafœtida compares with the snake-poison when the bone is affected, threatening necrosis, with violent pains at night.

Rhuu Tox., the swelling is dark red, dusky ; slow development.

Skin.

The Ophidians act almost identically upon the skin and cellular tissues, causing : Itching ; vesication, the surrounding parts being dark-red or bluish ; peeling of the skin ; pustules ; ulcers ; erysipelas. Yellow skin. Swellings of the limbs, with œdema. Dark-red or purplish swellings. Malignant pustules (LACHESIS). Gangrene. Capillaries enlarged and dark-colored. Symptoms return periodically.

Vipera T. cures tumefactions with marked "bagging."

Lachesis.—Sore spots become fungoid, dark-red to brown, with whitish spots and burning on wiping. Fungus hæmatodes. Burning and itching preventing sleep ; scabies, especially if with large purplish blisters.

Herpetic eruptions ; the vesicles are large, yellow, soon turning dark. These break and leave an excoriated surface, which burns when touched ; worse periodically every spring.

LACHESIS & OTHER ALLIED REMEDIES—(*contd.*)

Skin.

Erythema worse from exposure to the sun or to damp air. Different parts of the surface feel as if burned by the sun. When rubbed, sensitive spots appear, with dark, blue-red margins and dry scurf.

Pemphigus.

Scarlet-red spots.

Rash, which turns livid or black or is scanty ; scarlatina.

Small flat warts on the hands or fingers.

Erysipelas.

Miliary eruption.

Old cicatrices become painful and re-open or bleed.

Small ulcers or pustules around the large.

Chimney-sweeper's cancer.

Open cancer with bleeding and with bluish base.

Ulcers burn at night or when touched.

Boils (or carbuncles) near the spine, with burning, throbbing pain.

Bed-sores with black edges.

Ulcers, flat, spread rapidly.

Small wounds bleed profusely and for a long time.

Varicose veins of the legs, especially with blueness and threatening ulceration.

Gangrene of an ashy-gray color and offensive.

Traumatic gangrene.

Malignant pustule.

Dropsy from liver, spleen or heart affections ; also after scarlatina ; urine black ; legs œdematous, first left, then right.

Severe symptoms follow stings of insects.

Poisoned wounds : parts look blue, are swollen and burn, with a purple line along the lymphatics, and great general prostration, stupor etc. Septicæmia.

Skin yellow, as from jaundice, with ecchymoses and hæmorrhages.

Purpura hæmorrhagica during typhus and kindred diseases.

RELATED REMEDIES.

The essentials of LACHESIS are : eruptions of a dark or bluish color ; inflammations which degenerate into ulceration or gangrene ; ulcers which

LACHESIS AND OTHER ALLIED REMEDIES—(*contd.*)

Skin.

are sensitive to touch, bleeding and offensive ; erysipelas which soon assumes a low type. Similar in these respects are : APIS, ARSENIC, CARBO VEG., *Cinchona*, *Secale*, NITRIC AC., LYCOPOD., *Phosph*. *Phosph. Ac.*, *Mur. Ac.*, Silica.

Fungus hæmatodes : PHOSPH., *Silica*, *Carbo A.*, *Carbo Veg.*, *Nitric Acid*.

Malignant pustule : *Bufo*.

Flat warts : Fluor. Acid., Dulc.

Erythema, worse in the sun : *Canthar*.

Pemphigus : *Ran. Scel.*, RHUS TOX., ARSENIC, Causticum, Bufo.

Blackish spots with old people : *Con.*, Arsenic, Opium, Sul. Ac.

Carbuncle near spine : SILICA, HYOSC., Nitric Acid.

Small wounds bleed profusely : PHOSPH., *Sul. Ac.*

Varicose ulcers : SECALE C., *Arsenic*, *Hamam.*, Sulph.

Poisoned wounds : *Crotalus*, CARBO VEG., *Rhus Tox.*

Stings of insects : Apis, Ledum.

Chimney-sweepar's cancer : Arsenic, Rhus Tox., Secale.

PHOSPHORUS is similar in fungus hæmatodes, wounds bleeding, etc. In LACHESIS, however, the escaping blood does not coagulate, while in the former it does. Spots on the skin appear in both, but in PHOSPHORUS they are reddish-brown. Only LACHESIS has marked blueness and tendency to gangrenous ulceration.

Both may be employed in erysipelas with suppuration, as in mastitis. But here again the color distinguishes, for PHOSPHORUS is required when the inflammation is characterized by red spots or streaks.

Sulphuric Acid is of interest, since it offers several resemblances to LACHESIS ih traumatic gangrene, blue spots like suggillations ; bed-sores ; fungus hæmatodes : hæmorrhages from wounds ; dark pustules.

The ACID follows Arnica when bruises remain black and blue, or when wounds bleed profusely. In typhoid states, with petechiæ and dark, persistent hæmorrhages and great exhaustion, the two remedies certainly appear, at least from a superficial view, very similar. But the form of the debility in the two is quite different. In SULPH. ACID there are deathley pale face, subjective sense of trembling : and the tongue is dry, or red and brown. This is the well-known acid debility. In addition there may be aphthæ, or the tongue may be red as if eroded.

In gangrena senilis LACHESIS is certainly more often indicated. In scabies SULPH. ACID is required when in every spring the skin itches and

LACHESIS AND OTHER ALLIED REMEDIES—(*contd.*)

Skin

single pustules develop. Though the periodicity reminds one of LACHESIS, the large, yellow blisters of the latter are sufficiently distinctive. In the former too scartching causes the Itching to change place. In the latter, scartching causes vesicles, burning of the skin, or bleeding.

In carbuncle, Hyosc., SILICA, and CARBO VEG. are similar, as well as ARSENIC and *Anthracinum*. The latter two are distinguished by the dreadful burning.

Hyoscyamus is occasionally needed when the patient is excessively nervous ; coma vigil etc.

Silica, like the snake-poison, suits when the disease progresses very tardily, with want of vitality and scanty, thin, ichorous discharg. But the prostration is greater in the latter, the limbs being cold and clammy and the mind befogged. The parts are bluish and the skin over the diseased part is dead, scaly. Blue swelling of the lymphatics. In the former there is hectic fever, with accompanying prostration and sweats towards morning. The remedy has the effect of hastening the removal of the decayed masses and of promoting healthy granulations.

If suppurating boils threaten to become gangrenous SILICA is useful, but if they look bluish before breaking, LACHESIS is preferable.

The yellow skin of the snake-poison may indicate jaundice or those conditions in which the skin rapidly tinges yellow, as in pyæmia and yellow fever. In the latter affection, however, when in the second stage jaundice and hæmorrhages supervene CROTALUS is advised.

Sleep.

The Ophidians induce two opposite states depending upon cerebral irritation and, conversely, nervous depression and blood-poisoning. In the first, sleeplessness obtains ; in the second, drowsiness and even stupor. As they all affect the heart it is not to be wondered at that they cause anxious, vivid and repeated dreams, with restless sleep.

Lachasis.—Sleepy but cannot sleep.

Wide-awake, talkative; persistent sleeplessness night after night ; sleeplessness from nervous exhaustion, as after excessive mental exertion etc.

Cannot sleep from internal restlessness ; abdomen and chest seem swollen.

Sleepless from crowding of ideas.

Child sleeps restlessly, with tossing, moaning and groaning.

Drowsiness ; sleepy during the day.

Stupid state ; coma : with many ailments.

LACHESIS & OTHER ALLIED REMEDIES—(*contd.*)

Sleep.

Awakes and cannot sleep any more.

Aroused from sleep suddenly, especially with the laryngeal and heart symptoms.

Awakes, *always worse* ; frightened.

Dreams : continual ; they arouse him, but he as often dozes and repeats them. Lascivious ; pleasant ; full of fancy ; merry.

Epilepsy worse after sleep.

Always worse after sleep.

RELATED REMEDIES.

Lachesis is characterized by sleeplessness, with mental excitement. This may attend nervous weakness constituting what is termed "irritable weakness", and may result from fever, loss of blood, the incipient action of blood-poisons etc. Again, it may indicate an over-active brain rendered so by protracted study ; and again, it may accompany heart disease.

Conversely there is drowsiness, which suggests LACHESIS in some of the most alarming forms of fever, as well as in diphtheria etc.

Very important is the aggravation after sleep. Care is needed not to confound the remedy under consideration with BELLADONNA. Although both induces sleepiness, but cannot sleep, restless tossing etc., yet the causes are different. In LACHESIS the cerebral irritation arises from blood-poisioning ; in BELLAD., from a more sthenic congestion or inflammation.

In deep sleep, sopor, compare LACHESIS with OPIUM, BELLAD., *Hyos.*, *Nux. Vom.*, APIS, *Pulsat* , *Stram.*

Opium suits if there are convulsive twitchings, stertor, reddish-brown face.

Belladonna may be employed if the face is red, or if it is pale and cold; the pulse in the latter case being small and quick ; furious look on awaking.

Fever.

The Ophidians induce coldness from want of animal heat, even collapse ; chilliness, with irritable weakness ; heat ; flushes of heat ; cold sweats. Burning heat. Fever with cold feet and legs. Typhoid type of fever. Intermittent or remittent fevers. They are, therefore, called for (especially LACHESIS and *Crotalus*) in low forms of fever.

Lachesis – Pulse : small, weak but accelerated, frequently alternating with full and strong beats ; unequal, intermitting.

Blood-vessels : distended about the neck. Varicose.

Congestions : to the head, face, lower limbs.

LACHESIS & OTHER ALLIED REMEDIES—(*contd.*)

Fever.

Worse from : brandy, wine, emotions and from unpleasant news.

Long-lasting chill, with shaking and something like trismus.

Chill beginning in the small of the back and ascending ; worse on alternate days.

After icy coldness of the calves, shaking chill, with warm sweat ; then strumming through the limbs intermingled with flushes of heat.

Thirst more before than during chill.

Chill and heat alternate and change from place to place.

Cold feet, with oppression of the chest.

Chills at night, flushes of heat by day.

Chills along the back mingled with heat ; blackness before the eyes and failure of thought.

Chilly afternoons, followed by heat and shivering if the bed-clothes are lifted ; then sweat.

Chills worse : afternoon and evening ; every other day, or returning every spring. After abuse of quinine.

Accompanied with : restlessness (begnning of chill) ; glistening eyes, chattering of the teeth. Spasms in nursing children. Oppression of the chest. Headache, red face, and cold hands and feet.

During the chill wants to be near the fire and to lie down ; this makes him feel better, although it does not shorten the paroxysm. Wants to be held down firmly to relieve the shaking and the pains in head and chest.

Heat, with internal chill.

Heat, especially evenings, in hands and feet.

Internal sensation of heat, with cold feet.

Burning in palms and soles at night.

Flushes of heat with great sensitiveness of the neck, evening and night. Orgasm of blood.

Flushes of heat at the change of life.

Burning dry skin ; dry coated tongue, thirst ; small, quick pulse and dull eye.

Catarrhal fever with heat, fulness of the head, drawing in the teeth and facial bones, glistening eyes ; coryza.

Heat ascends.

Heat of various parts ; œsophagus, hands, palms, legs, feet, soles etc. Spreads from the feet.

LACHESIS & OTHER ALLIED REMEDIES—(*contd.*)

Heat worse : evening and night.

Heat accompanied with : loquaciousness. Face red or yellow, ashy. Headache. Pains in the throat. Thirstlessness, usually. Fluent coryza. Diarrhœa. Sleep. External throat sensitive. Burning, rending pains ; bilious fever maltreated with quinine.

Offensive night-sweats.

Sweats too easily.

Sweat : red ; bloody. Stains the linen yellow. Cold. Profuse with many complaints.

Worse : with the pains. At night or after 12 P.M. During rheumatism much sweat, but without relief.

Types of Fever : *Intermittent*. TYPHOID. *Remittent*. Yellow. *Bilious*. Catarrhal, after getting the feet wet. Hectic. *Puerperal*, etc.

Of the remaining Ophidians, *Crotalus* and *Elaps* have been most frequently used.

Crotalus, it is claimed, is needed in yellow fever, when there are hæmorrhages, black vomit, etc. Delirium, with open eyes ; restlessness and pains over body and limbs ; small pulse, with faintaing spells ; bloody sweat ; can retain nothing in the stomach but gelatin or brandy ; skin yellow ; purple spots. Second Stage.

Elaps Coral has been successfully employed in intermittent fever. The symptoms are : Coldness in the back. Chill, no thirst, and followed by heat. A cold drink makes him shiver ; it feels icy cold in the chest and abdomen. Heat at night. He must uncover. Dyspnœa. Flushes of heat at night.

Cyanosis is produced by Lachesis, Crotalus, Bothrops Lanceolatus and Vipera. The former has it during the fever.

RELATED REMEDIES

Chill ascends : *Digitalis*, *Hyosc.*, *Phosph.*, *Sepia*, *Gelsem.*, *Sulph.*

Chill spreads from the back : *Hyosc.*, *Eup. Perf.*, *Eup. Purp.*

Thirst before chill : *Arsenic*, *Capsic.*, *Cinchon.*, *Eup. Perf.*, *Pulsat.*, *Sulph.*

Thirstless during fever : Arsenic, *Carbo Veg.*, *Cinchon.*, *Helleb.*, *Mur. Ac.*, *Nux Vom.*, Phosph. Ac., Pulsat., *Sepia*, Sulph.

Chill returns every spring : Carbo Veg., Sulphur.

With the chill, glistening eyes : *Lachnanthes*, Bellad., Sepia.

With the chill, oppression of the chest : Apis.

With the chill, spasms : Helleb., *Hyosc.*, Arsenic, Camphor, Opium.

LACHESIS & OTHER ALLIED REMEDIES—(*contd.*)

During chill wants to be near the fire : *Arsenic*, CAPSIC., IGNATIA, *Kali Carb.*, *Menyanth.*, Therid., Helleb.

During chill wants to be held down : Gelsem.

Burning in palms and soles : STANN., PHOSPH., *Arsenic*, LYCOPOD., MUR. AC., Sepia, Sulph.

Flushes of heat : SULPH., *Sepia*, SUL. AC., PHOSPH., *Lycopod.*, *Calc. Ostr.*, *CarboVeg.*, Elaps, *Ignat.*, Rhus Tox.

With the heat, loquacity : STRAM., Carbo Veg., Bellad., Verat., Rhus.

With the heat, burning, rending pains : *Arsenic*, CINCHON., Eup. Purp., *Rhus Tox.* (less burning), Lycopod.

With the heat, drowsiness : *Ant. Tart.*, *Apis*, *Arnica*, *Bellad.*, *Capsic.*, *Hepar.*, GELSEM., OPIUM, *Stram.*

Sweat is bloody : Nux Mosch., Crotal., Arnica.

Sweat red : *CarboVeg.*, NUX MOSCH., Arnica.

Sweat stains yellow : *Carbo A.*, GRAPH., *Mercur.*, SELEN., *Verat.*

Sweat cold : ANT., TART., ARSENIC, CAMPH., CARBO VEG., CINCHON., Elaps, *Digital.*, *Helleb.*, *Hepar*, *Hyosc.*, *Ipecac.*, *Stram.*, *Sulph.*, VERAT.

Sweat does not relieve in rheumatism : MERCUR., *Cinchon.*, *Lycopod.*,

Sweat in the axilla, smelling like garlic : Tellur., Osmium, Bryonia, Nux Vom., Sepia.

Sweat offensive-smelling : *Hepar*, Dulcam., *Nitric Ac.*, *Selen.*, *Sepia*, Sulph., PETROL.

Lachesis seems to require that there be desire for warmth, burning heat or flushes, and aggravation in the spring, after the previous abuse of quinine. In severe cases the heat is characterized by sleep with deep breathing, or by talkativeness. In still another class of cases, representing the debilitated, whether such weakness is from drugging or from other causes, the symptoms are : Icy coldness, especially of the feet, of the tip of the nose, the ears etc. The skin looks livid and shrivelled, and the pulse is filiform.

In catarrhal types, there is coryza, general aching and well-defined pains in the throat ; headache precedes the coryza and the patient feels weak, must lie down.

In intermitting types of fever, compare : CARBO VEG., CINCHON., *Capsicum*, *Arsenic*, Menyanthes. If with great debility, bordering on collapse : CAMPH., CARBO VEG., *Arsenic*, *Lauroc.*, or HYDROC. AC., and VERAT. ALB., *Cuprum*, *Helleb.*, *Apis*, *Phosph.*, *Digital.*, *Secale C.*

Ailments from : Cinchona, the Solanaceae, Hepar, Mercury, Mercurial vapours, abuse of Apis, abuse of Alcohol.

LACHESIS & OTHER ALLIED REMEDIES—(*contd.*)

Fever.

Antidotes. The Ophidian poisons are antidoted by Alcohol, heat, Ammonia. And some of the symptoms and chronic effects by Arsenic and Bellad.

PICRIC ACID & OTHER ALLIED REMEDIES.

Picric Acid.—A picture of disintegration forcibly bespeaks the use of *Picric Acid* in spine and brain diseases, in typhoid conditions and in other conditions in which the red blood is impoverished and imperfectly regenerated. When the symptoms are related in detail, it will be seen that this acid is destined to prove invaluable in overworked patients especially if overtaxed mentally ; and how often are we called to treat men whom close study or perplexing business matters have broken down ! We find, when *Picric Acid* is the remedy, that there is headaehe, dull, pressive, with aggravation from using the mind ; dull occipital pains ; heaviness extending down the spine; no desire to study or work ; always tried; heavy feeling; great weakness of legs or back, with soreness of muscles and joints; burning along the spine, worse when studying. In other patients with cerebro-spinal affections we note restless sleep—disturbed by priapismic erections ; severe pains in the neck and occiput to supra-orbital notch, and then down into the eyes ; hot feeling in the lower dorsal and lumbar regions ; heavy dull pains ; aching, dragging in the lower lumbar region and legs, worse from motion ; tired sensation in lumbar region and legs when awaking ; legs heavy and weak ; heavy, numb, with crawling, trembling, pricking as from needles ; lips tingle ; heavy tingling feeling and formication in head. Prostration on least motion or exertion, sexual desire increased, terrible erections—these are common symptoms in spinal diseases.

Phosphorus also resembles *P'cric Acid* in causing fatty changes in the blood, the kidneys, and also in softening of the brain and spine. The sexual symptoms are similar ; both, too, may be useful in brain-fag from study, mental over-exertion etc. Both have hot head, tingling, formication, numbness, weak back and legs, burning in the spine and trembling, congestive vertigo, great general nerve weakness even with organic changes in the nerve centres, especially with softening of the spine, jerking of the muscles with backache, darting pains here and there.

Phosphorus causes more irritable weakness, over-sensitiveness to external impressions ; hence the senses are often acute, or if failing, photopsies are present—loud noises in the ears, sensitiveness to odors, to electric changes etc.

Sadness, followed by anxiety, restlessness ; worse at twilight. Excitable, head weak, cannot think, worse from loud noise. music etc., again displaying the irritable weakness ; the backache is a feeling as if it would break on motion ; burning in spots, better from rubbing; the sexual

PICRIC ACID & OTHER ALLIED REMEDIES—(*contd.*)

excitement is very strong, but the erections are not so intense as under *Picric Acid*; not so much like priapism, although the lasciviousness is more marked in *Phosphorus*. Even in extreme cases when all irritation has ceased the history shows that it once characterized the case.

Nux Vomica sometimes resembles *Picric Acid* in cerebro-spinal affections, but the irritability (akin to that in Phosphorus), the prominence of gastric symptoms etc. distinguish it.

Argentum Nitricum is thought to be similar, especially in blood changes. Its cerebro-spinal symptoms are, however, so unique that they cannot be easily misunderstood; vertigo, dreads passing a projecting object, fears it will fall on him ; nervous, anxious, timid ; backache, worse on first rising ; bones at sacrum give out; limbs tremble. Impotence; sexual organs shrivelled.

Alumina is distinguished by the pains in soles on stepping, as though soft and swollen ; burning in the spine as from a hot iron ; when walking in the dark with eyes closed he staggers ; costive from inert rectum ; nates go to sleep.

Silicea is quite similar to *Picric Acid* ,in nervous exhaustion. Jones, quoting Dunham, remarks that *Silicea* is useful when the patient dreads exertion, mental or physical, but warmes up to it when started. In spinal troubles there is the well known constipation ; legs feel as if they had lost their power ; numbness of fingers and toes, limbs go to sleep easily.

Of the remedies causing violent erections compare :—*Cantharis* (said to be an inconsistent symptom), *Phosphorus, Capsicum, Agaricus, Pulsatilla, Mygale, Platinum, Opium, Hyoscyamus, Stramonium, Ambra Gris., Zinc., Physostigma, Piper Methys., Petroleum, Selenium* (which has priapism without curvature of the penis). Thus *Cantharis. Capsicum, Cannabis Ind., Mygale* and *Pulsatilla* are excellent in erections with gonorrhœa, though *Cantharis, Mygale* and *Pulsatilla* may be used in cases of cerebral or spinal affections.

Silicea has priapism with spinal affections.

Oxalic Acid has erections with dullness in occiput.

Œnanthe Crocata has semi-priapism as in epileptics.

Nux Vomica, Cicuta, Staphysagria, Thuja, Graphites, Fluoric Acid, Lachesis, Kali Carb.—many erections with spasmodic constriction of the cord.

Moschus—a small retracted penis in an octogenarian, suddenly attains its former size; an impotent man becomes natural, with excited desires etc.

Natrum Carb.—a kind of priapism towards morning ; emission and no desire.

PICRIC ACID & OTHER ALLIED REMEDIES – *(contd.)*

Natrum Mur. and **Magnesia Mur.**—erections and burning in penis.

Rhus Tox. – erections even with spinal diseases ; *Sulphur, etc.*

Of these the following may be studied in spinal affections : *Phosphorus, Silicea, Rhus Tox, Oxalic Acid, Staphysagria, Lachesis, Moschus, Natrum Carb., Kali Carb., Natrum Mur., Nux Vomica, Pulsatilla, Mygale, Agaricus, Platinum, Physostigma* and *Zincum.*

In old people—*Fluor. Acid, Ambra,* with numbness.

With sexual excesses – *Phosphorus, Nux Vomica, Staphysagria, Kali Carb., Agaricus* and *Zinc.*

With lasciviousness—*Phosphorus, Cantharis, Lachesis, Platinum, Stramonium, Hyoscyamus, Nux Vomica, Thuja, Natrum Carb.* and *Piper Methys.*

When nervous, better when occuping the mind, etc. - *Sulphur, Staphysagria, Moschus.*

Additional symptoms of Picric Acid.

Head.

Vertigo : congestive, with headache and nausea, worse stooping, rising, walking or going upstairs. Headache : dull, bursting, full, heavy, sharp pains, throbbing ; worse studying, stooping or moving eyes, any motion ; better in open air, from rest or binding head up tightly.

Eyes.

Sight dim, blurred from mucus ; pupils dilated, sparks before the eyes. Inflamed, dry, burning, smarting with feeling of stick in the eyes ; worse working ; lids heavy, thick matter in canthi, worse from lamplight.

Ears.

Burn ; are puffy ; crawling as from worms.

Nose.

Epistaxis with heat and congestion of head. Nose full of mucus ; can breathe only with mouth open, better in open air.

Mouth.

Saliva frothy, stringy ; taste sour, bitter.

Throat.

Rough, scraped, better from eating ; hot, red ; sore on empty deglutition, worse after sleep ; thick, white mucus on tonsils ; on swallowing throat feels as if split ; sensation of a plug when swallowing saliva.

Stomach.

Thirst ; appetite increased or diminished ; eructations sour, with frontal headache ; bitter water-brash ; nausea, 5 A.M. ; death-like, faint, worse rising and moving around, with vertigo, with headache. Pressure and weight in stomach, wants to belch but seemingly powerless to do so.

PICRIC ACID & OTHR ALLIED REMEDIES—(*contd.*)

Rectum.

Destroys epithelium of the intestines.

Diarrhœa thin, yellow, oily, with straining, with burning ; smarting at anus and prostration.

Urging to stool unsuccessful.

Kidneys.

Cortex congested ; urine contains suggar ; Sp. gr. 1030 ; is albuminous, dark-red ; excess of uric acid and phosphates, diminution of sulphates and urates.

Skin.

Yellow ; also eyes and urine. Papules on face becoming small furuncles.

Limbs.

Feet cold ; chilly, cannot get warm, followed by clammy sweat.

General Symptoms.

Chilliness predominates. Heat in head and spine ; throbbing, jerking of the muscles with severe chills ; great pains between the hips ; dull, heavy, dragging, darting pains here and there ; into bones.

SEPIA
&
OTHER ALLIED REMEDIES.

Of the sub-kingdom Mollusca, Sepia is the most important.

As a remedial agent **Sepia** is the peculiar property of Homœopathy. Hippocrates employed it, as did also Dioscorides, Plinius and a few others. But it is so unofficinal now that Stille and Maisch refer to the cuttle-fish *bone*, and recommend it in powder as an ingredient of dentifrices on account of its hardness.

We do not use the bone, but prepare triturations and tinctures from the juice of the Sepia, the SUCCUS SEPIAE.

Sepia acts profoundly and lastingly on the human system. It is chiefly indicated in ailments arising from disturbances in the sexual sphere, especially of women, though it may not-uncommonly suit men also.

Mind and Sensorium.

Sad, weeping mood ; with lassitude ; with concern about the future. Every few minutes inclined to cry without known cause.

Low-spirited, does not care what becomes of her.

Depressed and easily irritated.

Anxiety with ebullitions ; restlessness and irritability.

SEPIA & OTHER ALLIED REMEDIES.—(*contd.*)

Mind and Sensorium.

Passionate, irritable ; fretful from slight causes ; disposed to scold ; becomes heated in discussions.

Indifferent and apathetic. Does not care what happens; indifferent to those dearest to her ; no ambition for work or thinking.

Heavy flow of ideas. Past recollections of unpleasant circumstances make her ill-humored.

Ailments from one-sided mental occupation.

Language comes slowly; cannot fix attention. Forgetful; worse in damp weather. Moody ; depressed.

Stupid feeling, with dizziness, unfitting him for mental work.

Painful confusion of the head, particularly of the forehead.

Vertigo while walking, as if objects were in motion; objects turn in a circle.

Sudden dizziness, as if drunk, while walking.

Vertigo as if the senses would vanish. Stupid and dizzy; he does not know what he is doing.

RELATED REMEDIES.

Sepia induces a state of sadness, anxiety and hopelessness. Mingled therewith is an excitableness, such as is common with women suffering from uterine disease, and also from disturbed circulation.

The mental condition, then, is a part of the general effect already alluded to, namely, erethism. But this is soon followed by depression, and hence, excitement gives place to a condition of indifference and languor, and the flow of ideas is changed to mental sluggishness and forgetfulness.

A commingling of states is observed, as for instance, depression with irritable temper : sad and nervous ; dull, forgetful and moody etc.

The vertigo arises from disturbance of cerebral circulation, as a reflex uterine symptom and also as a result of brain-fag, whether produced by mental strain, loss of animal fluids or other depressing causes.

It may also indicate impending apoplexy, especially in one who has weakened his vital powers and developed venous hyperæmia of the brain by the abuse of alcohol, or who has been guilty of sexual excesses. He is dizzy on walking, feels dull, confused, forgets easily ; drops things from the hands. Or, he is dull, dizzy on awaking. Physical exercise produces numbness. Coitus is followed by weakness of thought, sadness, dejection and numbness.

The state of indifference is very characteristic. It may accompany dyspepsia, uterine disease or hepatic disorders.

SEPIA & OTHER ALLIED REMEDIES—(*Contd.*).

Mind and Sensorium:

Compare with : PULSAT., NATR. MUR., *Phosph.*, *Actæa Race.*, Stannum, Hepar, LILIUM TIGRINUM, *Platina*, GRAPH., SULPH., CAUST., *Nux Vom.*

Pulsatilla is without doubt the nearest analogue. Both develop a state of weeping, anxiety with ebullitions, peevish ill-humor, solicitude about health etc. But only the former has the mild, yielding disposition, clinging, seeking consolation. In this remedy there may be moroseness and peevishness or irresolution. But there is ever lacking the angry irritability of SEPIA. Neither has the former the cool indifference of the latter.

In **Pulsatilla**, too, the vertigo is relieved by walking in the open air, and the drunken dizziness is accompanied with internal heat of the head, the face being pale.

Natrum Muriaticum *is complementary to Sepia.* They agree in causing weeping mood, depression of spirits.

Confusion and vertigo. Hasty manner, nervousness. The former has prominently, worse from consolation. Clinically the same has been recorded for SEPIA. Both, too, have ailments aggravated by vexation or anger.

The former remedy may be called for when the mental state depends upon uterine disease or menstrual irregularity. But it will only be a prolapsus, never the engorged uterus of the latter remedy.

The indifference of NATRUM MUR. is more akin to, though less pronounced than, that of Phosph. The indifference of SEPIA is more like that of Fluor. Acid : indifference, even hatred, towards those loved best.

Head.

Rush of blood to the head, with red and hot face.

Weakness of the head—she can scarcely think ; worse in damp weather.

Head aches as if it would burst.

Heavy pressing pain or fullness in left orbit and left side of head, with occasional darts through the eye-ball and side of the head, or over side of head towards occiput ; worse from mental labor ; better after meals.

Single, violent, undulating jerks of pressing headache quite in forepart of forehead.

Violent stitches outward over the left orbit ; drawing together of the eye.

Tearing in the left frontal eminence. Also in upper part of the right side of the forehead.

Stitches in the forehead with nausea ; better from lying down.

Headache in forehead and on vertex, followed by anxiety in the pit of the stomach, with trembling ; afterwards violent nose-bleed.

SEPIA & OTHER ALLIED REMEDIES.—(*contd.*)

Head.

Fulness in the temples and the forehead and throbbing of the carotids.

Tearing in the left temple to the upper part of the left side of the head.

Beating, painful headache in the vertex, in the morning soon after rising.

Pressure on the vertex, after mental labour. Pressive, contractive pain.

Headache in the right side of the head and face, with a surging like waves of pain rolling up and beating against the frontal bone ; after the sweat.

Headache in the morning with nausea until noon.

Boring headache from within without, forenoon till evenings, worse from motion and stooping ; relieved by rest, when closing the eyes, from sleep and from pressure.

Pulsating headache in the cerebellum, morning till noon or evening ; worse from motion ; better during rest and in the dark.

Heaviness, pressure, in the occiput and down the spine ; passes off after rising.

Hair falls out ; also with chronic headaches.

Scalp pains when touched, as if roots of hair were sore.

Scurf on the head. Eruption on the vertex and back part of head, offensive, with stinging-itching and tingling and cracks ; it extends down behind the ears. Dandruff in patches shaped like ring-worm.

Jerking of the head backwards and forwards ; worse sitting, forenoon.

Coldness of the vertex.

Sepia is a useful remedy in hemicrania, in hysterical females who are ill-nourished, with pale or dirty-yellow skin, delicate frame, and who have scanty menses. Sudor hystericus is stated to be present in many instances. The pains are piercing, boring or throbbing ; they shoot upwards, are severe enough to extort cries and culminate in vomiting. The paroxysms are renewed or aggravated by motion, light, noise or by a thunder-storm, and are relieved by sleep or rest in a dark room.

It is also useful in arthritic headaches, especially when, like NUX VOM., they are worse in the morning, with nausea and vomiting. The liver is, of course, affected and the urine is loaded with urie acid.

Open fontanells have closed under the influence of SEPIA when the peculiar jerking motion of the remedy was present.

In headaches from brain-fag SEPIA is to be selected by its general cachectic condition. It is said to be particularly efficacious when a one-sided occupation has led to brain exhaustion.

SEPIA & OTHER ALLIED REMEDIES.—(*contd.*)

Head.

Heaviness of the eye-lids often accompanies the SEPIA headache.

Nux Vomica is more suitable to men, but it may be needed in some instances in which SEPIA is similar, and, as we shall see, the two drugs are synergistic. NUX cures a drawing-aching feeling, as of a nail driven into the head, or as if the brain was dashed to pieces. The face is pale, sallow or red on a sallow ground. The attacks commence early in the morning and gradually increase to a frantic degree. Like SEPIA, exciting causes may be hæmorrhoids, abdominal plethora or brain fatigue. But in general the two drugs diverge greatly.

Eyes.

Vanishing of sight. Objects suddenly get black before the eyes, with great weakness, passing off when lying ; also during menses.

Fiery sparks before the eyes. Zigzags of colors. Black spots passing in all directions.

Vertical hemiopia.

Eyes readily fatigued, especially in reflected light.

Eyes feel tired and are injected ; feel heavy, lids inclined to close. Lids droop with the headache.

Swelling in the eyes, burning ; flow of tears, which affords relief.

Burning, sore, rough feeling after walking in the cold wind, worse by gaslight and reading.

Cataract, especially in women.

Eyes feel like balls of fire.

Redness of whites of eyes in the morning, with burning, smarting and pressure.

Eye-lids pain on awaking, as if too heavy.

Margins of lids dry and hot; itching; scaliness or small pustules on the ciliary border. "Scratching sensation in the eyes, worse at night than at any time during the day, upon closing the lids ; they feel as if they were too tight and did not cover the eye."

"Acute catarrhal conjunctivitis, with drawing sensation in the external canthus, smarting in the eyes ; better by cold bathing and worse morning and evening." Muco-purulent discharge in the morning and great dryness in the evening.

Follicular conjunctivitis, worse during hot weather.

Trachoma, with or without pannus, especially in tea drinking females.

The eye symptoms of SEPIA we may summarize as follows : Cataract ; conjunctivitis, especially in asthenic cases ; trachoma ; scaly lids,

SEPIA & OTHER ALLIED REMEDIES—(*contd.*)

Eyes.

pustular lids with eruption on the face ; muco-pus in the morning with dryness in the evenlng; eyes irritable to light, lids close in spite of him: eye-lids droop ; aching, sticking pains, worse by rubbing. Causes : uterin or liver diseases, scrofula, tea-drinking. Worse morning and evening, in hot weather ; better from cold washing and in the afternoon.

RELATED REMEDIES.

Pulsatilla : but the muco-pus is bland, worse at night. gluing the eyes in the morning ; fine granulations on the lids ; repeated, highly-inffamed styes.

Graphites : but the canthi crack and bleed, edges of the lids are pale and swollen as well as scaly.

Thuja : especially with tea-drinkers; brown, brank-like scales about the cilia; tarsal tumors like warts.

Staphis. : dry margins of lids, old nodulated styes, abuse of Mercury.

Sulph. : small pustules, like SEPIA, but generally edges very red ; pains worse early morning ; both worse in hot weather.

Nux Vom. : both in liver-diseases ; morning exacerbation and relief of some symptoms from cold bathing.

Natrum Mur. : reflex uterine ; lids droop. But there is more spasmodic elosure of the lids in conjunctivitis etc. ; the discharges are thin, acrid ; there are cracks in the canthi (Graph.), and also in corners of the mouth ; pains over the eye, worse when looking down.

Alumina : both have falling lids, dryness, burning, dim sight ; but Alumina is worse evening and night ; inner canthi affected.

Drooping of the lids marks the Sepia asthenia ; but it is less genuinely paralytic than that of RHUS, CAUST., GELSEM., Conium etc.

In hemiopia, compare : Lycopod., Natr. Mur., Calc. Carb., Bovista, Viola. Od., Mur. Ac., Lobelia Inf., Chin. Sulph., Titanium.

Ears, Nose and Face.

Very sensitive to noise.

Wheezzing and roaring in the ears; they feels as if stopped. Deep-toned roaring when lying on the ear, synchronous with the pulse.

Otalgia, worse walking in the wind, better in a warm room. Pressure from within outwards ; or pain extending to the parotid gland and to the mastoid.

Thin pus flows out of the ear, with itching ; purulent, whitish cerumen.

Sense of smell acute.

Nose dry, fells stuffed. Dry coryza and cough.

SEPIA & OTHER ALLIED REMEDIES—(*contd.*)

Ears, Nose and Face.

Nose-bleed during the menses. Blows blood from the nose, or blood and mucus. Profuse nose-bleed.

Nostrils sore, burning, aching in alæ ; right side feels stuffed, yet there is a slight watery discharge.

Frequent sneezing, almost without coryza. Spasmodic sneezing every morning.

Yellow discharge from the nose. Green plugs are hawked out in the morning. Nose inflamed, swollen, with sore, ulcerated nostrils, which feel raw, with smarting.

Tip of the nose painful, red ; eruption.

Face red, flushed—pale, puffed—yellow, especially about the mouth, and like a yellow saddle across the upper part of the cheeks and nose.

Small red pimples on the forehead ; roughness. Liver spots.

Tearing pains in the facial bones and in the teeth ; worse, or only, at night.

RELATED REMEDIES.

Studying these local effects of SEPIA in conjunction with the universal characteristics we see that erethism, vascular fulness and organic changes qualify the effects of SEPIA on ears, nose and face. The senses are excited as they often are in nervous or hysterical women. Roaring in the ears, nose-bleed and flushed face indicate venous fulness; and the yellow, earthy skin and altered nasal mucus mark organic changes. Even the sensations in the nose are one with the universal symptoms of mucus membranes, as acted upon by SEPIA : rawness, smarting and tingling. And the susceptibility to cold and damp, resulting in otalgia or coryza, is also a universal characteristic. SEPIA compares well with SULPH. in chronic otalgia. It also resembles the following in chronic inflammation of the external auditory canal with itching—SULPH., ARSENIC, GRAPH., *Petroleum*, *Nux Vom.*, *Silic.*, *Tellur.*, *Baryta C.* and *Psorin.*

Sepia has, it is claimed, itching and scratching, and causes a watery oozing.

In **Arsenic** the canal is dry and full of scales.

In **Graph.** there is more gluey discharge.

In Petroleum there is marked dryness, but with humid soreness behind the ear ; occipital throbbing headache.

Scurfy, moist ears also call for *Scpia*, PSORIN., GRAPH., SULPH., CALC. OSTR. and OLEANDER.

In **Sepia** it is tettery, rough, red, with pustular eruption, much scaling and some moisture.

SEPIA & OTHER ALLIED REMEDIES—(*contd.*)

Ears, Nose and Face.

In **Psorinum** there is scabby, offensive eruption on ear and cheek.

In **Oleander** there is intolerable itching of various parts of the body when undressed ; skin chafes from slight friction.

Sepia has relieved nasal catarrh when green plugs were hawked out, especially in the morning. Here it resembles KALI BICH., in which, however, the plugs are firmer, more tough.

Teucrium, according to Dr. Walter Williamson, cures large, irregular "clinkers" (Lycopod., Arum Tri., Natrum Ars. etc.)

SEPIA is distinguished from all by the aggravation during menses.

The color of the SEPIA face suggests SULPH. and NUX VOM. in bilious patients (see further on under Stomach and Bowels), and CAUST. CAUSTICUM has more yellowness about the temples ; Nux and SEPIA about mouth and nose.

For so-called "liver spots" SEPIA compares with *Nux Vom.*, LYCOPOD., *Sulph.* and Woorari, recommended by Dr. Baruch. We have twice relieved with it. Caulophyllum has also been suggested.

Mouth, Stomach and Abdomen.

Lips dry ; they crack readily.

Swelling of the lower lip, with soreness, burning pain, and pricking, as from a splinter of wood.

Mouth and throat dry, rough, in the morning.

Inside of mouth swollen ; small white blisters and ulcers, which are painful.

Tongue feels as if scalded, especially at the tip ; blisters and pains as if burnt ; dry and rough.

Tongue coated white—dirty yellow, with putrid taste mucus-coated.

Salivation : mouth full of a saltish fluid, and yet fauces and throat are so dry that the patient can hardly utter a sound (Dunham).

Gums bleed easily; swollen, dark-red. with very painful throbbing, as if beginning to suppurate; sore, ulcerated. Toothache and throbbing in the gums during menses.

Toothache : drawing, tearing in the left ear; sticking; stitches extending to the ear. Worse at night, from cold air or wind, from hot or cold things in the mouth (the drawing), during pregnancy or at the menstrual period.

Teeth decay quickly. Teeth become loose. All the teeth are painful, especially a hollow molar, which pains as if elongated and swollen, with swelling of gums and cheeks, with which the pain ceases.

SEPIA & OTHER ALLIED REMEDIES—(*contd.*)

Mouth, Stomach and Abdomen.

Taste : Bitter or sour in the morning ; bitterish-sour ; foul as from old catarrh ; foul or putrid ; like bad eggs, with similarly tasting eructations.

Eructations frequent, bitter, sour, or sour and offensive, like rotten eggs. Heart-burn. Hiccough after a meal.

Nausea : Mornings with weakness, better after eating ; things grow black before the eyes, even fainting. Makes her sick to rinse the mouth or clean the teeth.

Nausea at intervals all day, also after a meal ; afflux of watery saliva ; bitterish sour taste ; no appetite, but food has a natural taste. Vomiting during pregnancy; it often follows the morning nausea; bilious, with much retching. During the day attacks of constriction in the hypochondria and nausea. Vomits a milky water.

Hunger, craving ; hungry soon after meals. Desires vinegar, pickles, piquant things.

Loss of appetite; things are tasteless, or there is a positive aversion to food ; nausea when thinking of it.

Thirst ; though generally it is absent.

Stomach : Pressure, burning, distress, with sensitiveness to touch or to pressure of the clothes ; aching and throbbing, relieved by eructations ; distress worse in the afternoon, nearly ceases after supper.

Beating in the pit of the stomach in the morning, then ebullitions in the chest like palpitation of the heart, followed by subjective burning heat of face and body ; no thirst, but some sweat.

Goneness : With weakness and dragging—empty feeling, with nausea at the thought of food ; faint, sinking feeling—with or without pain on pressure.

After eating : Heat and palpitation of the heart ; or the patient is irritable, averse even to those ordinarily loved best ; bloatedness of the abdomen; acid mouth; water-brash ;nausea, vomiting; diarrhœa (after meat or milk) ; pressure in the stomach, as from a stone etc.

Liver : Fulness ; pinching pain ; stitches ; sore pain. Sensitive while riding over rough roads. Sense of fulness and bloating across the epigastric region.

Abdomen : Sensation of emptiness, dragging, heaviness ; distended with flatus, worse after eating even a little food ; loud rumbling.

Cutting pains horizontally across the abdomen, sometimes extending up into the chest (Dunham). (See also Genital Organs.)

Burning, smarting and itching in the anus.

SEPIA & OTHER ALLIED REMEDIES—(*contd.*)

Mouth, Stomach and Abdomen.

Heat, burning and swelling of the anus.

Aching in the anus, better by fast walking.

Weak feeling in the rectum, evening in bed, with restlessness.

Contractive pain in the rectum and thence to the perineum and vagina, or up into the abdomen.

Hæmorrhoidal tumors, painful and bleeding; discharge of mucus, with stinging and tearing, but without stool.

Prolapsus ani during stool.

Sensation of weight in the anus, not relieved by stool.

Stools : Much urging, even with soft stool; insufficient, retarded; like sheep-dung; whitish.

Diarrhœa, green, slimy, sour or fetid.

Small, jelly-like stools, with tenesmus and debility.

Diarrhœa, worse from milk, whether boiled or not.

Ascarides or round worms.

RELATED REMEDIES.

The alimentary canal, with associated organs, is profoundly influenced by SEPIA. Its especial characteristics are here very manifest—as the venous plethora, relaxed tissues, sluggish functions, irritation of mucous membranes, with burning and smarting, yellow skin etc. Dunham has well described the relation of SEPIA to functional derangements of the liver; and Raue refers to its use in abdominal affections, when the whole aspect of the patient indicates a deep-seated disturbance in the digestive functions.

One of the provers had a yellow-coated tongue, with red tip and edges; brown-coated with red edges; dry, cracked lips; nausea; dull, heavy feeling, very weak back.

The peculiar symptom of the lower lip has led to its successful use in epithelioma. The splinter-like feeling suggest a comparison with NITRIC ACID and HEPAR.

In diseased teeth, SEPIA, as an antipsoric, should be compared in scrofulous children with : LYCOPOD., CALC. OSTR., SULPH., *Mercur.*, *Carbo Animulis* etc. According to one author LYCOPOD. follows lime, if there is dull aching in the teeth; worse after eating; little tumors or ulcers on the gums.

Calc, Ostr. acts well, general symptoms agreeing, when the carious teeth are always worse from a draught of cold air.

SEPIA & OTHER ALLIED REMEDIES.—(*Contd.*).

Mouth, Stomach and Abdomen.

Mercurius differs with the tongue taking imprint of the teeth, aggravation from the warmth of the bed, no relief from sweat.

Carbo Animalis relieves when there are rending, tearing pains from salt food : sensitive to the cold.

In toothache during pregnancy, compare *Mag. Carb.*, *Phos.* and *Ratanhia*, all of which have, like SEPIA, nightly aggravation. In *Mag. Carb* and *Ratanhia* the patient is compelled to walk the floor for relief.

In gastro-enteric affections SEPIA is useful particularly in chronic cases. It is characterized by sour and offensive secretions, the two combining often, goneness at the epigastrium, nausea and bilious vomiting in the morning ; awakes with nausea and headache, as from debauchery. After a little food, full to repletion like LYCOPOD. Abdominal plethora like NUX and SULPH., but with more dragging, faint, gone sensation. The accompanying mental indifference to near and dear friends is an important symptom. Defective action of the liver, as shown by yellow eyes and skin, whitish stools, offensive gases from the bowels ; urine deposits a red sediment. Catarrh : as indicated by slimy mouth, rawness in the throat, mucus-coated faeces ; slimy, green, or jelly-like discharges ; proctitis, with mucous or purulent oozing.

In "morning sickness" SEPIA is unsurpassed. One prover referred to nausea with distress in the pelvis, and it is because of the power of the drug to affect the pelvic circulation and to influence the os uteri that it promises so well. Compare here : NUX VOM., PULSAT. and Kreos ; and, when there is aggravation from a morning ride, COCCUL. and PETROLEUM. Only SEPIA has vomiting of a milky water.

In abdominal complaints compare : LYCOPOD., NUX VOM., SULPH., *Pulsat.*

Lycopodium, like Sepia, depresses the functional activity leading to torpidity and chronic disease. There are, in both, repletion from small amount of food, bloatedness ; constipation ; yellow skin, defective action of the liver, with abdominal congestion, piles ; impaired nutrition ; red sand in the urine.

But repletion is more characteristic of LYCOPOD. ; emptiness, goneness, etc.. of SEPIA. Indeed, with the former the repletion overshadows the other symptoms, often existing without marked changes in the appearance of the tongue. Sour taste and sour or burning eructations, however, are very common. The abdomen is in a state of ferment ; disturbed circulation after eating, with irresistible drowsiness. Urinal sediment of free, red sand. Constipation, with urging and constriction of the anus. In SEPIA, on the other hand, there are more foul eructations ; erethism ; anxious faintness after eating ; urinal sediment adheres to the sides of the vessel ; costiveness, with inertia of the rectum.

SEPIA & OTHER ALLIED REMEDIES.—(*Contd.*)

Mouth, Stomach and Abdomen.

Lycopodium (Teste and Hughes confirm it) cures enteritis of infants who are fed on food which they cannot digest.

In **Sepia** we have a remedy for indigestion of children which exacerbates at every change of weather. The breath is sour, tongue white and blistered, anxious dreams, high fever.

Sulphur resembles the drug under consideration in many respects. Both are suited in torpid cases, with defective reaction. There are abdominal plethora, congested liver, piles, constipation ; hunger about II A.M. ; bitter or sour taste ; eructations sour or like bad eggs ; fulness from a little food etc. Subacute lingering inflammations.

In **Sulphur** the face is more blotched, red, spotted at times ; saliva nauseates him ; vomits food, chronic vomiting ; craves brandy or beer ; craves sweets, but they disagree ; hunger at II A.M. While in SEPIA it is more of a gone, faint feeling. The constipation is attended with ineffectual urging, like NUX. There is no inertia as in SEPIA, but congestion, irritation of muscular fibre, with resulting sensitiveness, tenesmus, fitful urging etc. A universal of SULPHUR is : anxiety, ebullitions of blood, irritability with mental despondency. If there is inflammation present, the tongue displays a red tip and there is accompanying fever, with persistent dry heat.

Sepia stands between PULSAT. and NUX VOMICA, favouring in the former, mucous states, chilliness, putrid eructations, and in the latter, yellow skin, abdominal plethora, sour stomach, morning headache as from debauchery, constipation.

For gone, empty feeling in epigastruim, compare : *Calc. Ostr.*, *Ignatia*, *Actaea Rac.*, *Kali Carb.*, Niccolum. *Hydrastis*, *Phosph.*, *Mercur.*, *Sulph.*, *Natr. Carb.*, Natr. Mur., Natr. Phos., Murex, Thea, Podoph., *Stannum*, COCCULUS, *Carbo Animalis* and *Staphysag.*

Sepia usually has associated hunger, though eating may not relieve. It is a part of the general relaxing effect of the drug, as manifested in nearly all the regions of the body.

Ignatia, with sighing.

Carbo Animalis, from loss of vital fluids, as nursing.

Sarsaparilla, with rumbling in the abdomen.

Niccolum, but without desire for food.

Olender, with sensation of distended abdomen ; chest feels empty and cold.

Ipecac, **Thea** and **Staphis.**—all with empty, relaxed feeling of the stomach, which seems to hang down.

SEPIA & OTHER ALLIED REMEDIES—(*contd.*)

Mouth, Stomach and Abdomen.

Hydrastis, Mercury and **Calc. Carb.**, like SEPIA, have a faint-like weakness.

Actæa Rac. is excellent when, with the faint, empty feeling in the epigastrium, there is a trembling, wavy sensation, proceeding from the stomach over the body.

Hydrastis relieves when there is sinking sensation, palpitation of the heart and mucus-coated stools.

Thea produces a gone, faint feeling ; sick headache, radiating from one point ; the left ovary pains, then sick headache.

Throat and Chest.

Throat red, dry, feels rigid and yet mucus collects.

Fauces rough, red, smarting, burning ; cutting in the throat, worse when hawking.

Pressure in the region of the tonsils as from a tight neck-cloth. Feeling as of a plug. Cervical glands swollen.

Larynx, dry ; feels sore, raw, scraped, with cough. Mucus collects. Hoarseness with coryza.

Cough, from tickling in the larynx, from pit of the stomach, abdomen, or seemingly from constipation. Worse from getting wet, cold damp air, sour food, after a meal etc. Sometimes relieved by lying down, though frequently there is hacking cough in the evening after lying down, with or without bitter vomiting ; cannot sleep on account of incessant cough ; dry, whooping, choking cough, which dos not awake her, but is severe when she docs awake.

Sputa are saltish ; purulent, with oppression of the chest ; the least motion takes the breath and causes exhaustion; blood-streaked, coagulated blood ; gray, yellow ; of putrid taste and smell ; profuse. Worse—morning, evening and night.

Cough accompanied with stitches in the epigastrium, liver, chest ; bitter or bilious vomit, then vomiting of food.

Breathing, short when walking; loses breath from least exertion; awakes with dyspnœa and sweat ; asthmatic after mental exertion, with palpitation. Expiration long, difficult and noisy.

Congestion to the chest, with palpitation.

Oppression of the chest, worse morning and evening. Constriction. Contraction.

Feeling of emptiness.

The chest symptoms compel and are relieved by pressure of the hand upon the chest (Bœnninghausen).

SEPIA & OTHER ALLIED REMEDIES—(*contd.*)

Throat and Chest.

Brown spots on the chest.

Violent palpitation of the heart and beating of the arteries ; also with stitches in the left chest. Worse after emotion or exertion, when sweat breaks out. Accompanied with hot flushes, faintness etc. One form is relieved by fast walking.

Ebullitions of blood, with anxiety, faintness, nausea, restlessness ; worse at night. Feels the pulse all over, but worse in the whole left chest.

Pulse, quick at night, slow mornings ; intermittent.

On the mucous membranes, as already observed, SEPIA acts as an irritant, causing dryness, burning, rawness and smarting. Mucus is altered, becoming thick, yellow or yellowish green ; muco-purulent. In the bronchial tubes, pus or putrid expectoration may collect. The symptoms point to chronic catarrh, neglected bronchitis, and also to tubercular deposit.

The drug may be needed for cough caused by abuse of tobacco, especially if following the injurious custom of swallowing the smoke from cigarettes. Compare here Nux Vom. and Atropine. Twice have we verified the symptom of the latter. Sore feeling in the throat ; dry, trickling cough excited by smoking.

The night and evening coughs of SEPIA are very important, for the remedy has been used in phthisis when these coughs were present.

The spasmodic cough, with bitter vomit, has led to its successful use in whooping cough. Compare, in this latter respect, KALI CARB., *Bryon.*, Carbo Veg., Laches., *Sulph.*

For evening cough, worse after lying down, compare also : CALC. CARB., *Kali Carb.*, SULPH., CONIUM, *Phosph.*, *Rhus Tox.*. *Bryon.*, *Pulsat.*, *Hyosc.*, ACTAEA RAC., DROS., HEPAR, *Carbo Veg.* and Nitric Acid.

Cough from stomach or abdomen : *Ant. Crud.*, Verat. Alb., *Bryon.*, *Nitric Acid*, Hepar, Puls. and *Sulph.* (ensiform cartilage).

Relieved by lying down : Mangan. and Calc. Phos.

Purulent sputum : CALC. CARB., CARBO VEG., *Conium*, *Hepar*, KALI CARB., LYCOPOD., PHOSPH., *Phos. Ac.*, *Rhus*, SILICA, SULPH etc.

Foul, putrid taste or smell of sputum : *Carbo Veg.*, *Carbo A.*, Conium, LYCOPOD., Rhus, *Sulph.*, *Silica*, *Phellandrium*, *Sang.*, *Stann.*

But generally when SEPIA is the remedy, the case is chronic, or appears in a patient ill-nourished, prostrated, sallow, whose digestion is imperfect, with torpid liver and abdominal plethora. Perhaps it is a child, which is scrofulous, thin, weak, suffering from diarrhœa after boiled milk. Or she

SEPIA & OTHER ALLIED REMEDIES.—(*contd.*).

Throat and Chest.

is a female who has long endured uterine or ovarian disease. It would seem, too, that the tendency to catarrh of nose, throat or bronchial tubes in this remedy has much to do with its effect on the vascular system ; for passive congestions certainly favour catarrh.

Of all its cough symptoms, however, that is most characteristic which refers to an evening or night paroxysm, with gagging, vomiting loss of breath and exhaustion. Not infrequently, in agreement with what has been already stated, this symptom yields to SEPIA when the case fails to yield to such ordinary remedies as Drosera, Bryonia etc.

Referring again to the analogous remedies, we may have to compare Sulph., Calc. Carb., Silica and Lycopod., when there is an underlying scrofulous constitution ; Stannum, Pulsat., Kali Carb. and Actæa Rac., if uterine diseases qualify the case ; Nux Vom. and Sulph., with abdominal plethora.

Sulphur is very similar, but the cough starts from the throat or from the ensiform cartilage. There is more pain through the left chest, instead of the middle or right lung. Cough may arise from the motion of mucus in the air-tubes, when it is generally a loose cough.

Calcarea agrees with **Sulphur** in evening, tickling cough, though in the lime it may continue into sleep, ceasing, however, as the night advances—common during dentition. Fat, fair children, open fontanelle. Cough as from a feather or from dust in the throat. Chest sensitive to touch, while in SEPIA pressure relieves. Sputum thick, portion of it sinks like a shooting star, leaving a trail behind.

Siliea has cough from tickling in the supra-sternal fossa, or as if from a hair extending from tip of the tongue to the trachea. Fetid foot-sweat, more marked than in SEPIA. Cavities in the lungs, with copious, offensive pus. Children with large, sweaty head ; poorly nourished, rachitic.

Lycopodium has cured dry cough in feeble, emaciated children. Often there is a sensation as if the lungs were full of mucus, and the child has marked rattling breathing while asleep. Dry, tickling evening cough, as from a feather (Calcarea), or as from sulphur-fumes. Loose cough, sounding as if the whole parenchyma of the lungs were softened.

Several of these drugs may be needed in old cases of catarrh of the lungs. **Silica**, in old people ; cough sounds as if lungs were full of mucus ; when sputum is raised it is purulent, offensive ; several small vomicæ – a not uncommon sequel to long-standing cases of fibroid phthisis.

Lycopodium, in neglected pneumonia ; frequent attacks of lobular pneumonia ; loose, rattling cough ; gray, offensive. purulent sputum ; mucous rales, mostly in right chest ; dyspnœa, partly due to the state of the lungs, partly to spasmodic constriction of the chest, with fan-like motion of the **alæ nasi.**

SEPIA & OTHER ALLIED REMEDIES.—(*Contd.*).

Throat and Chest.

Sepia has much purulent sputum, rattling ; least motion takes her breath and exhausts her, etc.

In the beginning of tubercular disease, especially in females, **Sepia** vies with **Actæa Rac.**, which has teasing, hacking cough, worse at night and renewed by every exposure to cold. It often helps.

Drosera : just as soon as she lies down, she is harassed with a constant cough ; or it comes on in paroxysms ; spasmodic contractions of the diaphragm, she must press the stomach or hypochondria—not the chest, as in SEPIA.

Hepar : if the teasing cough in the evening follows exposure to dry, cold wind, rather than damp, wet atmosphere. The cough may be a combination of harshness with rattling.

Conium : cough at night, or whenever she lies down.

Since **Sepia** causes dyspnœa on awaking and is of use in chronic cases of bronchitis, it has also been employed in bronchiectasis and emphysema—sequels of bronchitis.

It compares with SULPHUR and LACHESIS, both of which have dyspnœa on awking. Consult also : ANTIM. ARSENITE—**a** very valuable drug for the dyspnœa, *Chinin. Ars.*, Naphthalln, *Carbo Veg.* ARSENIC etc.

Clinically, **Sepia** has relieved asthma with long, difficult, noisy expiration. This is a symptom of emphysema, and finds a parallel in ARSENIC. We always relived with the latter remedy a lady, who suffered for years from asthma. Sitting up in bed, she breathed heavily. Auscultation revealed difficult, labored inspiration, followed by long-drawn, very difficult expiration. The chest was distended, as in emphysema. After Arsenlc, the spells were less frequent, and now seldom return.

The Urinary Organs.

Dull aching in the region of the kidneys. Stinging.

Bladder feels full and as if its contents would fall out over the pubis ; constant desire to press them back.

Pressure ; urging to urinate : burning after micturition.

Sensation of drops from the bladder, which however, do not come.

Burning in the bladder. Spasms.

Urethra : moisture oozes after micturition. Gleet.

Burning in forepart of the urethra : smarting ; tingling at the meatus.

Urine frequent, with urging and bearing down in the pelvis ; urging referred to the neck of the bladder. Frequent micturition at night, with itching in the region of the bladder.

SEPIA & OTHER ALLIED REMEDIES—(*Contd.*).

The Urinary Organs.

Has to wait for some time before the urine will start.

Urine : Turbid, offensive, thick, slimy. Pale and copious. Contains bile-acid etc. Discharge of mucus periodically in small lumps, after urination ; it ls admixed with dark pigment.

Sediment yellow, pasty, or reddish, sandy, adherent : white. Cuticle on the surface.

Involuntary urination at night, especially in the first sleep (lIttle girls).

RELATED REMEDIES.

The peculiar sensations in the urethra, together with a milky or yellowish mucus discharge, have led to the employment of SEPIA in gonorrhœa or gleet. Dr. Franklin, probably following Jahr, uses this remedy at the beginning of gonorrhœal inflammation. The tingling, smarting, burning etc. certainly point definitely in this direction. So we have no doubt of the validity of his claim that the disease is ehecked or modified by the early exhibition of a dose or two of SEPIA. It acts well, too, in gleet.

The peculiar pressure recorded under SEPIA, as well as the delayed micturition, designate precisely when to use the drug in cystic irritation associated with uterine disesses (*q. v.*).

The sediment and odor of the urine are highly characteristic. Compare: LYCOPOD., *Nat. Mur.*, PULSAT., *Dulcam.*, *Benz. Ac.*, *Calc. Carb.*, LILIUM TIG., *Hepar Sulph.*, Nux Vom. and *Kreos.*

As regards odor or sediment, SEPIA may be confounded with LYCOPOD., *Calc. Carb.*, *Benz. Ac.* and *Kreosote*. From the first, it is distinguished by the adhesiveness of the sediment ; from the second, by a preponderance of red sediment and by a fetid rather than a pungent odor ; and, besides, the *Calcarea* urine is more apt to be clear. Confusion with *Benzoic Acid* is not likely, owing to many differences in the actions of the acid and SEPIA. The odor of Benzoic Acid urine is not so much fetid, as it is like the horses', from the presence of an undue amount of Hippuric Acid.

The odor of the SEPIA-urine seems to be due to decomposing mucus etc. Pathologically lt here resembles Dulcam., Senega, Lycopod., Pareira, Pulsat., Laches., Salicyl. Ac., Carbolic Ac., Nitric Ac., Phos. Ac. etc.

In cystic catarrh, the nearest relative of SEPIA is undoubtedly PULSAT. The former is better adapted to chronic cases, the latter to either the acute or the chronic. PULSAT. has more sensitiveness over the region of the bladder and uneasiness in the abdomen. After micturition, spasmodic pain in the neck of the bladder, extending to pelvis and thighs.

Incontinence of urine suggests CAUSTICUM (also in first sleep ; but better than SEPIA in children who are annoyed especially during cold weather, day or night), SULPH., GRAPH., PLANTAG. Maj., *Equisetum*, *Kreos.*, Silic., *Puls.* and Chloral (latter part of night).

SEPIA & OTHER ALLIED REMEDIES.—(*contd.*).

The Urinary Organs.

Delayed micturition from atony rather than spasm or inflammation, is under SEPIA, HEPAR, MAGNES. MUR. (must use abdominal muscles), Ammon. Mur.. Selen., Stramon., Natrum Phos., Lauroc. and Alumina (can only pass water while at stool).

Male Sexual Organs.

Inclination for coitus, with weakness of the organs. The act is followed by weakness of thought, relaxed tissues, lowness of spirits,vertigo, or anxiety and restlessness. Emissions may be weak and watery. Erections weak, or strong with too quick emission.

Involuntary emissions during sleep.

Loss of prostatic fluid or semen at stool, also of the former after micturition.

RELATED REMEDIES.

Sepia, as already stated, applies to men whose sexual powers are weakened by abuse or by general nervous weakness. Coitus weakens, even if seldom indulged in.

It compares with : SULPH., LYCOPOD., GRAPH. (the latter is excellent when desire remains but thc organs fail), PETROLEUM, SELEN., PHOS. AC., *Nux Vom.*, SILICA (the latter with sensation on right side of the head as if paralyzed ; bruised feeling all over).

Female Sexual Organs.

Sexual desire diminished. Coitus is painful and followed by blood from the vagina.

Menses scanty, dark, clotted—scanty, pale, acrid—too late ; less often early and profuse or scanty. Delay of first menses.

Before menses a few drops of blood (fifteen days before the time) ; colic, aching in abdomen, shuddering over body; faintness, bearing down ; mania (profuse menses); acrid leucorrhœa ; vulva excoriated, swollen ; perinæum feels enlarged and sore. Aggravation of all complaints.

During menses, bearing down with spasmodic contractions in the abdomen ; must cross the limbs for relief; restlessness, drawing pains in limbs, tearing in the tibia ; tootache ; obscured vision ; faint spells ; palpitation, dyspnœa ; headache, epistaxis; great mental depression, weeping. Tearing in the back, chills and heat, thirst and painful contraction of the chest, preventing sleep. Sensation of a heavy lump in the rectum. Dragging and weak feeling in the back. Pains passing around the pelvis from sacrum to groin (with scanty flow).

Menorrhagia or metrorrhagia ; flow only or mostly mornings ; change of life etc. Ebullitions, flushes of heat, faint spells.

Uterus : Lancinating from the womb to the navel.

Painful feeling of stiffness in the uterine region.

Shooting feeling of stiffness in the uterine region.

SEPIA & OTHER ALLIED REMEDIES.—(*contd.*).

Female Sexual Organs.

Shooting stitches, generally upwards, in the cervix, with burning.

Womb feels as if clutched and then suddenly released : nausea.

Uterus congested, enlarged, indurated, especially the neck. Dropsy.

Malpositions ; either versions, prolapsus or flexions.

Bearing down (and kindred sensations) : weight in the abdomen; heaviness; bearing down, dragging from the chest, abdomen, pelvic region or back, with oppression of breathing or with empty "gone" feeling in the abdomen and chest. Crowding and pressing downward in the pelvis ; feeling as if everything would push out of the vulva. Relieved by sitting with the legs crossed ; worse while standing. Bearing down with a peculiar intra-pelvic distressed feeling. Pressure on the bladder as if it would fall out over the os pubis, partially relieved by hard pressure. Bearing down on the pelvis, with slight dragging from the sacrum. Burning pain in the small of the back with dragging. Sensation of a weight in the anus.

Ovaries : Pressure and weight and pressure to urinate. Stinging. Congestion. Sharp, darting pain (right). Like a thread from right ovary to uterus, drawn tightly ; soreness on pressure. Stitching through the left ovary.

Vagina (similar pains etc. to uterus) : Burning, sharp shooting pains, worse sitting quietly. Jerking pain from below upwards, worse in the morning on awaking. Contractive pain.

Vulva : Labia sore, red, also between the thighs and on the perinæum. Offensive sweat.

Leucorrhœa like milk, with burning excoriation between the thighs—profuse after urinating—of lumpy mucus, fetid, acrid—with soreness of the pudendum - looking like pus—yellow, greenish—brownish, acrid, watery and offensive.

Nipples crack across the crown ; bleed ; itch and sting.

Labour pains retarded by indurated os uteri, with spasmodic contraction of the cervix and pains shooting upwards. Shuddering with the pains.

Abortion at the fifth or seventh month ; abdominal plethora, sensation of weight in the anus.

RELATED REMEDIES.

The anatomical relation of the uterine and ovarian blood-vessles wlth the portal system on the one hand and the hæmorrhoidal veins on the other, favours the extension of vascular derangements from one of these parts to the rest.. Hence, we observe, SEPIA causes portal stasis, uterine stasis, and piles. So, too, piles associate with vaginal catarrh, because the internal iliac supplies the vaginal and the hæmorrhoidal vessles.

Sepia will seldom be needed if there is no increase in the amount of pelvic blood.

This remedy, we think causes its well-known bearing-down pains, by relaxing the tissues, from the diaphragm even to the perinæum. It thus favour gravitation of the abdominal viscera ; hence comes the dragging. By increasing the amount of blood this effect is intensified, and the overcharged vessels irritate the muscular fibres and make them contract. There is also some ovarian irritability, which is not violent so as to favour, by reflex action, severe hysterical spasms, wild excitement etc. It is rather subdued, but nevertheless rersistent, because made chronic by long-lasting congestion, with want of reaction. The resulting symptoms are, therefore, a combination of erethism, nervousness and anxiety, with depressed spirits, faintness and excessive languor.

Organic diseases of the uterus, that is to say, enlargement, induration, ulceration etc. may follow long-lasting congestion. Continued irritation favours the growth of fibrous tissue; and post-partum return of the uterus to its unimpregnated proportions may, under such conditions as SEPIA favours, be only partial ; hence results sub-involution.

In estimating the relation of this remedy to others we should regard it as entering into several groups of similar drugs, but most intimately with those which cause abdominal congestion. From another and equally important point of view it holds a relation of chronicity with other drugs. It is, as Hering said, "a finishing remedy." And, therefore, unless symptoms emphatically declare to the contrary, it should be viewed as a remedy to follow others, rather than one with which to begin treatment. It is, of course, distinctly understood that the "totality" always decides conclusively. But in uncertain cases the rule mentioned has served us well, and thus explained we do not hesitate to suggest its use.

We may then compare SEPIA with MUREX, NUX VOM., SULPH., *Alocs, Aurum*, BELLAD., *Pulsat.*, LYCOPOD., *Podophyl.*, Æsculus, Collinsonia (all with congestion). STANNUM, *Ant. Crud., Asterias Rub.*, Alumina, *Apis*, Agaricus, LILIUM, *Platina*, ACTAEA RAC., Aletris, *Calc., Calc. Phos., Conium, Kreos., Inula,* NATR. CARB., NATR. MUR., Kalı Ferrocyan,, Phytolac., Ferrum, *Ferrum Iod.* (bearing down, pushing etc.). AUR., *Aur. Mur. Natro.*, PLATINA, CARBO AN., BELLAD., Alumen, Am. Mur., NATR. CARB., Iodine (induration). LILIUM, BLLAD., APIS, *Graph., Arg. Met., Conium, Carbo An., Podophyl.*, Phytolac., *Plat.. Pallad.* and *Kali Carb.*

Lilium has bearing-down, funnelling at the vulva ; hence manual pressure there relieves. Ovarian pains, as well as uterine, are more intense than in SEPIA ; boring, drawing, shooting, cutting, in the (left) ovary ; stinging, darting. Ovarian region sore, sensitive to touch. Sharp pains across thc pubes ; better from rubbing with a warm hand. Crampy pains. Burning, like coals of fire. Uterus so sensitive she cannot bear the least jar or walking on uneven ground. (In pains it resembles more Actæa Rac.) Burning all around the pubes and genitals.

Lilium,, further, has a nervousness similar to SEPIA, but more marked ; she is excited, her sexual desire is increased, and she is forced to exercise for relief ; her manner is bustling and hurried.

Female Sexual Organs.

Sepia, per contra, has lack of sexual erethism. The former has diarrhœa and urination, followed by smarting in the passages ; bilious stools. The latter has not the smarting, but merely burning. The former, like the latter, causes disturbed circulation ; but it appears as oppression, fluttering of the heart, congestion to the head and chest ; better in the open air (hence much like PULSAT.) ; faint in a warm room. Fluttering papitation after walking ; better when busy ; SEPIA—better from walking fast. Pain through the left mammary region to the back is characteristic of LILIUM.

As to time of exacerbation, LILIUM is worse in the afternoon ; SEPIA in the forenoon.

Lilium may so excite as to lead to hysterical paroxysms. Here it departs from SEPIA and draws near to PLATINA, with which it also agrees in sexual desire.*

RELATED REMEDIES.

Aloes, Helonias, Platinum, Graphites, Cimicifuga, Ustilago, Viburnum, Murex and Kreosote.

Back and Limbs.

Stiffness of the neck and of the back.

Backache, worse sitting ; pressure usually relieves. Heaviness on awaking, mornings, as if she could not turn or rise ; or as if she had lain in a wrong position. Backache, better from belching.

Aching between the shoulders and under the left scapula, extending into the left lung ; worse on expiration. Constant pain between the shoulders and down the back. Aching across the loins.

Drawing pressure and burning pain across the dorsal region, as from sewing (Dunham).

Pain in the small of the back; weakness; tired pain. Pain as if sprained.

When stooping, pain as if struck ; relieved by pressing the back against something hard.

Stitches posteriorly over the right hip ; could not lie on that side ; when touched, the part pained as from subcutaneous ulceration.

Pressing, dragging pain over the sacrum and hips ; burning pressure in the spine.

Aching in the sacrum, relieved by pressure ; pain in the sacrum through the hips and thighs to the kness, with weakness and lassitude when moving, especially when going upstairs, as if the limbs would refuse to act.

Limbs.—Go to sleep ; feel heavy ; sore, bruised, as if beaten.

Uneasiness, especially at night.

Joints stiff, or feel weak, as if they would easily become dislocated. Shoulders, after exertion, feel as if out of joints. Arthritis.

---

*For further details, consult Farrington's Clinical Materia Medica.

Back and Limbs.

Cramps in the thighs when walking ; cramps in the buttocks when stretching, at night.

Swelling of the feet ; also of the limbs ; worse standing, better walking.

Tension in the tendo-achilis ; swelling.

RELATED REMEDIES

Sepia is not one of the best remedies for spinal irritation with hyperæsthesia. It is preferable when there are aching, stiffness, and weakness. There is some irritability still existing, shown in uneasiness of the limbs, fidgetiness, sense of subcutaneous ulceration etc. But exhaustion predominates, the back aches and is passively congested ; there is weakness of the back and legs, with fatigue of the muscles and joints and numbness of the limbs after exertion. This last symptom is very characteristic. The joints are weak ; it seems as if exercise would cause their dislocation. This effect is a part of a universal property of SEPIA—relaxation of tissues.

The remedy, therefore, is useful after long abuse of the sexual organs ; also for women who have suffered from uterine and ovarian affections, or who have been weakened by loss of vital fluids. In all cases, when SEPIA is needed, the symptoms are substantially those already referred to as universals of the remedy.

Among the modalities of the spinal symptoms, the following are very characteristic : Sacro-lumbar pains ; worse standing ; she feels faint and sick. Backache, pressure and burning, with congestion ; relieved by pressure ; *worse from sitting*. Backache worse at night. On awaking, stiff, tired ; headache ; great weakness.

Among the allied remedies are : Natr. Mur., Puls , Helon., Murex, Sulph., Lilium, Actæa Rac., Lycopod., Picric Ac., Nux Vom., Coccul., Kali Carb., Kreos., Graph., Calc Carb., Mitchella.

Pulsatilla has more of the sensation of sub-cutaneous ulceration ; it has also heaviness, as from a stone ; and above all, a sensation in the small of the back as from a tight band ; back feels as stiff as a board. This latter symptom we have relieved in both men and women.

Natrum Muriaticum, like SEPIA, has paralytic weakness of the back, stiffness, bruised feeling ; pain in the joints as from luxation ; legs weak, "go to sleep" ; cramps ; sweaty feet, etc. ; uneasiness of the legs. But the salt causes more irritation, with sensitive vertebræ and contraction of the tendons (ham-strings). The small of the back feels as if broken. Only SEPIA, causes pains from the sacro-lumbar region down the legs, or around to the groins. The concomitants differ. In NATRUM MUR there are flutterng of the heart, trembling, faintness ; constriction. In SEPIA there are more marked ebullitions, violent heart-beat, cardiac fulness, faintness.

Weakness of the back is also caused by COCCULUS, CONIUM, HELONIAS, PICRIC ACID, ZINC, Lilium, *Alumina*, Actæa Rac., ÆSCULUS HIP., GRAPH. , SULPHUR, PHOSPH., *Arg. Nitric.*, *Gelsem. etc.*

Back and limbs.

Cocculus depresses the vital powers, causing muscular paralysis, often associated with twitchings and even spasms—a form of irritable weakness not unlike the effect of Ignatia and Nux Vomica. The patient is intolerant of external impressions ; thus, noises disturb, she is over-susceptible to odors, to tobacco smoke, to cool air etc. There are paralytic pains over the hips, the loins feel stiff; spasmodic constriction—the whole length of the spine. Paresis of the eye-lids, tongue, pharynx, limbs, with trembling ; at one time one hand and foot and at another time the other hand and foot are asleep ; depression of spirits—all, however, transient.

Such symptoms are common in weak, nervous women. And consistently, with the tendency in such persons to spasmodic symptoms and excitement—symptoms depending upon the irritation of weakened nerves—we find the drug called for in eonvulsions after loss of sleep ; in menstrual colic, sharp cutting in the uterus, which feels distended ; in sleeplessness from mental activity, etc. But generally torpor of the animal nerves obtains ; the patient is dizzy and feels faint if she rises from a recumbent position ; sea-sick feeling ; back feels weak, as if paralyzed, with or without twitching of the muscles. Empty, hollow feeling in any one or in all of the splanchnic cavities ; hence her head feels light, empty ; the occiput feels as if opening and shutting ; talking exhausts and causes or intensifies a weak, empty sensation in the chest.

Conium paralyzes the spine from below upward (Hughes, but see symptom 991, Allen). It has caused and removed the following : "Leucorrhœa, with weakness and paralyzed sensation in the small of the back before the discharge and followed by weakness." In this respect it resembles SEPIA (back weak when walking ; aches after sitting a while) ; GRAPH. (leucorrhœa more profuse and watery) ; ÆSCULUS H. (sacro-iliac symphyses give out when she walks) ; *Natrum Mur.* (back feels lame. bruised) ; and, of course, COCCULUS.

Argentum Nitricum, like SEPIA, has backaehe ; worse while the patient is sitting. But with the former it is a paralytic heaviness and rigidity ; the legs are weak and trembling ; sacro-iliac symphyses weak, as with Æsculus. There are not the pulsation and other evidences of congestion which eharacterize SEPIA.

Picric Acid in one of its aspects, resembles SEPIA. We refer to tiredness and backache. Not infrequently women complain of being so tired ; their muscles ache and feel sore ; walking is very laborious, if not impossible and their hands and feet are numb and pithy.

Helonias often affords at least temporary relief ; back weak, aches, burns ; she becomes tired from the least exertion.

Actæa Rac, too, helps, especially in rheumatic patients ; weight and trembling of the muscles of the back and legs ; lame, tired feeling ; pulse weak ; general soreness and stiffness as after exertion.

SEPIA & OTHER ALLIED REMEDIES.—(*contd.*).

Back and Limbs.

Gelsemium has relieved, "I feel so tired", and her face shows it; the eye-lids are only half opened, the speech is heavy or thick and she can scarcely lift her arms. She is weak, sore, and drowsy. But in another class of cases PICRIC ACID is the remedy : muscles feel sore, *heavy*, weak; *heaviness* and dragging in the back, with heat. Tired all over; lack of will-power to undertake anything.

With both **Sepia** and **Picric Acid** there is spinal exhaustion. With the latter, exhaustion predominates, the fully developed symtoms closely simulating spinal softening. Of course, the classes of cases to which we refer above, do not include so serious a lesion as softening. Still they include cases of exhaustion, in which functional action is so impaired that symptoms arise closely resembling the more persistent effects of organic changes.

Skin and Glands.

Eruptions red with roughness of the skin. The epidermis peels off, especially on the hands. Psoriasis.

Yellow-brown spots; they scale when rubbed. Scaly and moist eruptions.

Fine rash all over, but worse in the bends of the elbows and knees : in the cold air it disappears, when it is followed with rheumatic pains in the elbow and knee joints.

Itching in various places, relieved by scratching; afterwards there is a pinkish color of the skin. Itching and acridity on the posterior part of each elbow. Pricking skin, worse when he is warm in bed. Rhagades.

Skin sensitive to knocks. Scratches heal slowly. Ulcers painless; or itching, stinging and burning : situated most frequently on or near the small joints—also on the heels, following blisters.

Small, itching pustules. Boils. Vesicles becoming pustules; scabies. Ecthyma.

Nails yellow; crippled. Warts hard, horny, or long and rough; especially if on hands and fingers.

RELATED REMEDIES.

Sepia causes yellow-brown spots, itching, redness, vesicles, humidity and rawness, scaling, pustules. The warm room makes the urticaria-patient feel comfortable; but the warmth of the bed aggravates pricking of the skin.

Ring-worm, it is asserted, is frequently cured with SEPIA. We have been so unfortunate as to have failed with it several times.

Dr. Dunham, guided by the tendency to scaling, recommends SEPIA as an antidote to Rhus-poisoning.

Jahr, after curing ecthyma with SEPIA, which remedy he employed because it produces isolated pustules, used it in scabies when some of the vesicles were filled with matter.

SEPIA & OTHER ALLIED REMEDIES.—(*contd.*).

Skin and Glands.

The nearest relatives of SEPIA in skin-affections are Natr. Mur., Natr. Phos., Sulph., Rhus Tox., Thuja, Tellurium, Calc. Carb., Calc. Acetica, Lycopod., Woorari etc.

Soda salts are similar in itching, herpetic, scaly skin, worse about small joints, especially about the ankle.

Thuja, like **Sepia**, causes white scaly eruptions ; but in the latter case the parts are humid ; in the former, dry.

Tellurium, Calc. Carb. and Calc. Acetica are, according to Dunham, useful for ring-worm—the first named, when the eruptions cover a great portion of the body in intersecting rings. Sulphur may be needed in ring-worm ; and if the itching is severe, Croton Tig. and Arsenicum.

Yellow-brown spots have been removed by Lycopod., Nux Vom. and Sulph. Dr. Baruch uses Woorari. We think the latter modified one case for us, and we know it cured another.

Sepia stands well in the treatment of psoriasis, though inferior to *Ars.* and ARS. IOD. Compare Hepar, Copaiva (hands), Sulph., Teucrium (skin of finger scaly), Iris Vers. (shining scales), Graph., Lycop. Kafka gives first Sulph. and then SEPIA, in a descending scale of potencies.

In rhagades SEPIA is inferior to PETROL., SARSAP. and CALC. CARB.

Crippled nails is a symptom more characteristic of GRAPH., CAUST. and *Silica.* But yellowness of the nails is more marked in SEPIA than in any of the above. CONIUM, SULPH., MERC., NITRIC ACID and *Nux Vom.* are about equal with SEPIA in this discoloration.

Herpetic eruption is very characteristic of SEPIA. Thus, we find blisters about the mouth (like RHUS, Natr. Mur.); also on the nape of the neck, behind the ears, in the bends of joints and on the genitals. The glans penis is hot, the prepuce sore, itching and smarting. Labia sore, red, as is also the perinæum—the characteristic in most cases being humidity, rawness, smarting and itching.

For warts on hands, compare : THUJA, *Sulph.*, *Dulc.* etc.

A valuable concomitant of SEPIA in skin symptoms, especially in moist eruptions about the head, face and behind the ears, is frequent jerks of the head to and fro. This qualification is a good distinction from Graph., Petrol. and Oleander in eczema aurium.

The eczema marginatum of SEPIA finds a counterpart in *Natrum Mur.* Compare also *Arsenic*, Hydrastis and Arg. Nitricum.

Sleep.

Sleepiness, during the day, especially during the forenoon.

Restless sleep from heat and ebullitionss of blood, or from a sense of weight on the body. Talks in sleep ; awakes screaming, as in affright. Limbs jerk on dropping off to sleep. Awakes about 3 A.M., and cannot again go to sleep ; sometimes with rush of ideas.

SEPIA & OTHER ALLIED REMEDIES.—(*contd.*).

Sleep.

On awaking, mornings, is tired, stiff ; can hardly move ; headache and nausea, as after "a spree".

RELATED REMEDIES.

The sleep symptoms of **Sepia** are all in keeping with the general action of the drug. Sleepiness and sluggishness, restlessness and sleeplessness caused by ebullitions, and ennui on awaking, all depend upon a disturbed circulation and a depressed condition of the nervous system. The time of aggravation, about 3 A. M., places SEPIA with remedies which act upon the liver and bowels ; hence with NUX VOM., SULPH., *Arsenic* etc.

The early morning symptoms again bring SEPIA, NUX, PULSAT. and SULPHUR into intimate relationship.

Nux—Has less paretic stiffness, but more retching, with scanty, loose stools and much straining or ineffectual urging.

Sulphur—Very much like SEPIA, has evening sleepiness, restless or sleepless nights, and consequently tiredness and general aggravation of symptoms on awaking. But with SULPHUR the ebullitions are more marked ; the patient awakes often and is, at each such awaking, wide awake ; his night is passed in "cat-naps".

Puisatilla—Has not the evening sleepiness : sleep comes late, and as a result the patient is disinclined to rise early. But the majority of the symptoms are not, as with the other remedies, worse in the morning. At most, we may expect merely dry mouth, bitter taste or headache.

Chill, Eever and Sweat.

Chilliness prominent. Chill, with thirst, followed by night-sweat.

Chill worse in the evening or night; worse at every motion; worse from external warmth (chill, with headache).

Coldness, with dampness of the skin ; feet and hands icy-cold, as if from iced water. Hands cold and feet warm; when the latter become cold, the former grow warm.

Heat usually in flushes: worse afternoon and night, then anxious sweat.

Animated talking makes him hot.

Sweat more after than during excitement or exertion.

Offensive foot-sweat. Sweat about the genitals, offensive.

Night-sweat, cold on the breast and back ; more on the upper part of the body.

RELATED REMEDIES.

Sepia causes chilliness with want of animal heat, and hence closely resembles PULSATILLA.

Alternation of coldness and warmth of hands and feet is unique and very characteristic.

SEPIA & OTHER ALLIED REMEDIES.—(*contd.*).

Icy coldness, with moisture, reminds one of the lime salts. But though in SEPIA and in CALCAREA excitement and exercise induce profuse sweat, it appears, according to Bœnninghausen, during exercise with CALCAREA, and after exercise with SEPIA.

Heat in flushes, which is the only prominent febrile movement caused by SEPIA, has led to the use of this remedy during the climaxis, during pregnancy, and during uterine displacements. Symptomatically SULPHUR stands very near ; but other remedies, as LACHESIS, Kali Bich., AMYL NITRITE and GLONOINE are also similar.

Heat during animated conversation suggests, in addition to SEPIA, Amm. Mur.

Sweat in SEPIA cases is profuse and weakening. As in SILICA the foot-sweat is offensive, but soreness of the feet is more common under SILICA. Compare, in offensive sweat in the axillæ, PETROL., *Sulph.*, *Hepar*—on the chest LYCOP.—on the genitals Fluor. AC., Sulph., *Thuja*—on the feet SILICA, *Graph.*, THUJA, *Nitric Acid*, *Pulsat.*, *Baryta Carb.*

TARENTULA
&
OTHER ALLIED REMEDIES.

Poisons derived from the *Araneidea* act energetically, but less fatally than those from the Ophidians.

Prominent among the effects of spider-poisons are disturbances in the nervous system, anxiousness, trembling and choreic movements, Hysteric attacks and great restlessness are frequently produced. Oversensitiveness is observed, as from noises (Theridion, Tarentula). Nervous prostration ; periodicity.

Bitten parts become swollen, red, or even livid, with dark streaks along the course of the lymphatics. Bone-pains (Theridon, Tarentula, Diadema*). Fevers of an intermittent type. Hæmorrhages (Diadema, Tarentula, Tela). The system is profoundly affected by spider-poisons ; hence they may be used in serious and chronic ailments.

The bite of the LYCOSA TARENTULA causes swelling and discoloration of the part ; pain and itching ; and as systemic symptoms, coldness, præcordial anxiety and vertigo. Then follows a long and often incurable strain of nervous symptoms. These consist of a commingling of restlessness and convulsive tremblings, with, at the same time, prostration of strength, melancholia, and weak memory. Music and certain colors exert

* The 'Diadema' signifies 'Aranea Diadema'.

TARENTULA & OTHER ALLIED REMEDIES.—(*Contd.*).

a soothing effect ; and for a time quiet the agitated nerves and palliate the mental depression. The measure called the "Tarantula" seems especially effective. So soon as the sufferer hears its strains he becomes excited and begins to dance, and his melancholy vanishes. A profuse perspiration may follow, with relief to the whole system.

The characteristic nervous symptoms, with their accompaniments, are briefly as follows : Insane paroxysms—she pulls her hair, strikes her head with her hands ; general trembling ; restlessness of the legs, and often sexual excitement. She sings, dances and cries ; without fever.

HYSTERIA.—Feigned paroxysms. Laughter immoderate and in uncontrollable attacks. Sings until hoarse and exhausted. Attacks of suffocation, with crying and screaming. Præcordial anxiety ; tumultuous beating of the heart ; want of air. Beating of the heart ceasing suddenly, then the patient thinks she will die. Heart pains as if squeezed. Mood changeable ; quarrelsome, with weak memory, but with excited sexual passion ; lasciviousness, with indecent exposure ; contractions of the uterus.

Profound grief and anxiety.

Desire to cry ; general agitation.

Desire to joke, play and laugh. Fits of nervous laughter.

Contortions of the head and hands, with nervous agitation and rage. Must be constantly occupied or moving the hands and feet ; cannot keep quiet. Irregular movements of head and upper extremities. Music allays the choreic movements.

Spasms preceded by a dizzy feeling ; great præcordial anguish during the attacks.

Tendency to get angry and speak abruptly.

Melancholic mood very prominent.

Fear and trembling ; apprehensiveness.

Memory weak, with many of the symptoms.

Intense headache, compelling to move from place to place.

Must move the head or rub it against some object.

Headache worse on awaking ; pains as if head was knocked, with stiff neck.

Headache as if cold water was poured on the head ; better from pressure and fresh air.

Headaches are accompanied with trembling, oppression of the chest, palpitation of the heart, great nervousness and spinal tenderness, or with uterine symptoms. Constrictive headache, with uterine pains.

Dim vision. Luminous spots before the eyes.

Gastric symptoms, with sympathetic pains on the sides of the head, face, ears, teeth, malar bones etc.

Uterus feels as if it contained a foreign body.

TARENTULA & OTHER ALLIED REMEDIES—(*contd.*).

Contractions in the uterus.

Sensitiveness of the uterus, much borborygmus through the vagina. Pains in the uterus with expulsion of gas, preceded by hysteria.

Pain in the uterus with severe constrictive headache.

Swelling and induration of the uterus, with difficulty in walking.

Pain in hypogastrlum, hips and uterus, as if compressed ; unconquerable sleepiness.

Burning pain in the hypogastrium and the uterus, with sensation of great weight, interfering with walking as in prolapsus, and causing pruritus vulvæ.

Fibroid tumors, with loss of pale blood.

Menses profuse ; pruritus vulvæ follows.

Sleeplessness, with nervous restlessness.

Trembling of the limbs ; the crawling and itching at night compel constant motion.

Constant chill and coldness except when asleep at night ; feels bruised all over, particularly when moving ; pains in legs and head; bilious vomiting ; burning, scorching heat, alternating with intense coldness, causing trembling.

Burning heat, thirst ; longs for sleep, but so nervous, cannot.

RELATED REMEDIES.

Tarentula is evidently a remedy of great power ; but the uncertainty and lack of confirmation, which surround the symptoms published, render any exhaustive analysis impossible. All symptoms marked "16", Allen vol. ix, are decided to be invalid, because the prover was poisoned by a tarentula which "came through the mail, and decomposition had undoubtedly commenced,.........hence the symptoms were such as might come from the scalpel or any other kind of animal poisoning". (Allen, vol. x, p. 637.) Further, Dr. R. Hughes calls into question Baglivi's cases, of which Dr. Nunez himself states that some may have been from a scorpion, instead of from the tarentula. (Pharmacodynamics, 4th edition, p. 891.) The late Dr. Houard criticised Nunez's provings, claiming that all the symptoms were not attributable to the spider under consideration.* Still, there is a group of symptoms which we have endeavored to present as clearly as circumstances will permit, which most probably belongs to the LYCOSA TARENTULA.

In our limited experience, we have found **Tarentula** useful in several forms of disease, when the patient, male or female, is nervous, restless, and compelled to keep constantly on motion. The headaches are violent and sometimes relieved by rubbing the head against the pillow. Indeed, this hypersensitiveness of the peripheries of the nerves seems to be a

---

*We feel that we were too hasty in our defence of Dr, Nunez against the attack of Dr. S. A. Jones in the *North American Journal of Homœopathy*, several years ago. We take this occasion to modify our views, and to say to .Dr. Jones, "peccavimus".—E. A. F.

TARENTULA & OTHER ALLIED REMEDIES—*Contd.*).

general characteristic : for, the patient is comfortable only when busily moving the fingers, rubbing the hands together, moving the legs etc. The spine is often exquisitely sensitive, while trembling and ennui show the general exhausted condition. Choreic symptoms are well marked, as are also the indications pointing to paralysis agitans. Hysteria is clearly pictured, even to the deceptions which such persons are prone to practise. When the urine symptoms concur with the mental, we expect good results from the drug.

The **Tarentula Cubensis** is claimed as a rival of *Arsenic, Carbo Veg.* etc., in the treatment of carbuncle and kindred affections. It relieves the intense pains and hastens the eure. It should therefore be campared with *Arsenic,* and no less with LACHESIS, ANTHRACINUM and SILICA.

Of the remaining Araneideæ **Mygale** is the most similar in choreic symptoms, *Theridion* in vertigo and nervousness, and ARANEA DIADEAMA in intermittent fever.

Mygale Lasiodora has produced : Delirious talk about business, restlessness all night, fear of death; despondency, with anxious expression. Nausea, with strong palpitation of the heart, dimness of sight, general weakness. Tremulousness of the whole body, in the evening. Severe chill, thirty minutes, then fever, with trembling.

Clinically, however, the MYGALE has proved useful in chorea. We can recall one case in which the convulsive symptoms were speedily removed, and the patient, a little girl, remained well for several years. The following are derived from MSS. furnished us by the late Dr. G. Houard : "Muscles of the face twitch ; mouth and eyes open and close in rapid succession; cannot put the hand to the face, it is arrested midway and jerked down. Gait unsteady ; legs in motion while sitting, and dragged while attempting to walk. Constant motion of the whole body."

We have, so far as we know, no record of hysterical symptoms which can confuse the MYGALE and the TARENTULA.

The **Mygale** has also cured extreme chordee.

Aranea Diodema, so far as proved, does not develop the extreme excitation of the three mentioned above. Still there is evidence enough that it affects the nervous system : confusion of the head, and headache, after eating—relieved, though not cured, by smoking. Headache ceases in the open air. Flickering sensation in reading and writing, from which the headache grows worse. Sudden violent pains in the teeth of the whole upper and lower jaw at night, immediately after lying down. Restless sleep, with frequent waking, always with the sensation as if the hands and fore-arms were greatly swollen, as if they were as strong and large again as natural. (Confirmed).

The strongest effects of the DIADEMA, however, are exhibited in the intermittent symptoms. Here it rightly claims precedence over the other

TARENTULA & OTHER ALLIED REMEDIES.—(*Contd.*).

Araneideæ. Symptoms recur daily at the same hour—such as griping in the abdomen, chills etc. ; chilliness, as if the bones were made of ice ; bone-pains; heat and sweat may be absent; worse in wet places and during protracted damp weather; swelling of the spleen, in one case with blood-spitting.

Tarentula causes chills and shivering; constant chill and coldness, except at night when she sleeps; feels broken down, as if bruised all over, particularly when moving ; burning heat ; sweat. Used successfully in intermittents with the hysteric. Worse from dampness and in change of weather.

The provings of TARENTULA record the following : Rachitism due to syphilis ; diseases of the bones in general; general pains, particularly of the bones of the arms. Whether these are genuine it is not easy to determine. In osseous affections experience places *Aranea Diadema*, and particularly THERIDION, foremost of the Araneideæ.

The latter is often needed in scrofula, rachitis, caries and necrosis, "to reach the root of evil and destroy the cause," when well-chosen remedies fail. Bones pain as if they would fall assunder ; coldness, cannot get warm. We think that this drug may even cure ozæna with caries, since it attacks the bones, and has so often removed the following : discharge from the nose yellow, or yellowish-green, thick and offensive.

Diadema has violent, dull, burrowing bone-pains in the right os calcis, if the foot is moved from a quiet position ; on continued motion the pain generally disappears ; similar pains in the limbs.

A unique symptom of this remedy is a sensation in both the ring and the little fingers of both hands as if they had gone to sleep, and of formication.

Concerning other related remedies we may profitably study the following. Compare **Tarentula** with :

In choreic symptoms, ACTEA RAC., STRAMON., *Hyosc.*, *Crocus*, AGARICUS MUS., *Caust.* (Mygale is comparable with the same remedies.)

Hysterical symptoms ; IGNATIA, MOSCHUS, STRAM., *Plat.*, *Hyosc.*, Bellad., Nux Mosch., Nux Vom., Laches., Phos., Zinc., Origanum.

Of these, STRAM., IGNATIA, Hyosc, and Bellad. are most similar in the mental symptoms; MOSCHUS, IGNATIA, *Laches.*, in suffocation ; *Mosch.*, *Plat.*, *Zinc.*, *Hyosc.*, *Stram.*, Phosph., Origan., in sexual excitement,

In the constrictions of the uterus, heart, head etc., so prominent in TARENTULA, the following are nearest related: BELLAD., *Secale*, CHAM., IGNATIA, NUX VOM., PLAT., *Laches.*, *Sepia* (uterine) ; CACTUS, *Lil. Tig.*, *Agaric.*, LACHES., *Nat. Mur.*, Nux Mosch. (heart).

Hyperæthesia, general : BELLAD., *Hyosc.*, *Nux Vom.*, *Cinchon.*, Natr. Mur., Sepia ; AGARICUS, ACTEA RAC., *Stram.* (the last three of spine).

TARENTULA & OTHER ALLIED REMEDIES.—(*Contd.*).

Restlessness of the legs : *Ammon. Carb.*, *Actea Rac.*, *Caust.*, *Asafœt.*, Bellad., *Mosch.*, Natr. Mur., *Calc. Phos.*, Stram., ARSENIC, *Mephitis*, Sulph., Hyosc., *Zinc.*

Tremulousness : *Agaric.*, *Arg. Nit.*, *Bellad.*, *Actea Răc.*, *Cicuta*, *Ignatia*, *Stram.*, Caust., Zinc., Lach., *Plat.* etc.

Indurated uterus : *Plat.*, Alumen, Aurum, Sepia etc.

Theridion should be compared with :

In headache, worse from noise—Spig. ; from jarring the floor—*Bellad.*, *Sang.*

In vertigo, worse closing the eyes : LACHES., Apis, Piper Methys., Silica, Arsenic, Thuja, Petrol. etc.

In scrofula : Sulph., Calc. Ostr., Lycopod., Silica.

Pains in upper left chest : MYRTUS, PIX LIQUIDA, SULPH., *Anisium*, *Stell.*

As a promoter of reaction, compare with : Ambra Grisea, Valeriana, Castoreum, Sulphur (these especially when nervousness obtains with defective reaction), Opium, Lauroc. Psorinum etc.

Aranea Diadema should be compared with :

In periodical return of symptoms : CHIN. SULPH., Gelsem., *Cedron* ; the *snake-poisons*, Carbo Veg., Rhus V., Sulph. (annual return) ; Sabadilla (fever and sweat) ; *Cactus*, *Spigelia*, Helleb, *Bovista*, Lycopod ; Silica (fever and sweat),

Chill predominates, without heat : *Verat. Alb.*, *Lycopod.*, Capsic., Digit., Caust., Bryon. etc.

Worse on rainy days, or in damp places : *Nux Mosch.*, *Rhus Tox.*, Lycopod., *Calc. Ostr.*, Ceanothus, *Natr. Sulph.*

Swollen spleen, ague-cake : CEANOTHUS, Cinchona, Sul. Ac., (these and Aranea with hæmorrhages), Nux Mosch., Natr. Sulph., *Carbo Veg.*, Arsenic, Natr. *Mur.*

Ring and little fingers, as if asleep (ulnar nerve) : Conium, Natr. Mur. (ring), Lycopod., Sulph., Sabad. (ring), Thuja, Caust. (formication).

In choreic movements **Agaricus** is distinguished by the spasms of the eyes and eye-lids, spots here and there, which itch and burn. Redness of the inner canthi. This remedy is likewise of eminent use in irritation of the brain, with violent and rapid rolling of the head, increased bodily mobility, with twitchings of the muscles. Intellection diminished almost to

TARENTULA & OTHER ALLIED REMEDIES. –(*Contd.*).

imbecility. Here **Tarentula** agrees and may be compared when friction caused by the rolling of the head on the pillow seems to give relief.*

Stramonium is characterized by the following : Features continually changing ; now he laughs, now appears astonished ; tongue protruded rapidly ; head thrown backwards and forwards ; spasmodic twisting of the spine and whole body ; extremities in constant motion, though not always jerked—for sometimes their motion is rotatory, gyratory and even graceful. Muscles of the whole body in constant motion. Stammering. If the mind is affected, the patient is easily frightened ; awakes terrified ; assumes often an attitude of prayer, with fervent expression and clasped hands. Frequently lifts the head from the pillow.

Cinchon. and **Chin. Sulph.** are similar to DIADEMA in periodical return of symptoms : swollen spleen ; ague from living in damp places etc.

Cedron, which, it is asserted, will relieve the bite of the rattle-snake and modify hydrophobia, may be considered as probably an analogue of the spider poisons also. It is said to act best in nervous, excitable, and even voluptuous patients, especially females. The febrile and neuralgic symptoms return with clock-like regularity. It is used in ague, contracted in warm countries or in low marshy lands, in which latter respect it offers some similarity to the DIADEMA. But the former has won favor mainly in hot elimatcs, while the latter works well in chills contracted in cold and wet localities. The chill predominates, heat being slight or wanting. In CEDRON, on the contrary, there is congestion to the head, flying heat in the face alternating with the chill and dry heat, with full, quick pulse.

Sulph., **Calc. Ostr.** and **Lycopod.** are somewhat intimately associated with **Theridion**, since the latter operates when the formers, though apparently indicated, fail.

Lachesis is nearest related to THERIDION in vertigo, swooning etc., worse when the eyes are closed. Also in anthrax of sheep, which the Orange Spider is said to cure, if given before the tumefied parts turn blue. Very likely it will follow the THERIDION, and possibly save life even if the parts *do* become blue and threaten to become gangrenous.‡

---

* By a very ingenious selection of AGARICUS, by Dr. Korndœrfer, in the case of a two-year-old child, who had evident meningitis, and who was not relieved by Apis, Sulph. etc., the rolling of the head ceased, alarming fore-warnings of imbecility happily vanished, and the patient fully recovered, We used the drug in a case of typhoid, in which the child rolled her head and bit her night-gown. Some improvement followed. Tarentula was then given, with slight aggravation, followed by lasting improvement. The two should be remembered in impending imbecility.

‡ Thrombidium has been treated of as an analogue of Mercury.

THERAPEUTIC HINTS
FOR
BEDSIDE REFERENCE.

——[*]——

BLOOD, DEFICIENCY OF.

[ANÆMIA—CHLOROSIS.]

Alumina—Cold, chilly girls with inactive rectum and bladder; anæmic at puberty with pale, scanty menses and profuse leucorrhœa; marked debility. Sadness in the morning on awaking.

Argentum Met.—Shares with the *Nitricum* in chlorosis. Body shrivelled, complexion sallow, dyspnœa, palpitation, prolapsus, ulceration and induration of the uterus; foul leucorrhœa.

Arsenicum—A direct poison to red blood-corpuscles—useful in anæmias of malarial or toxic origin. Pernicious Anæmia; prostration with emaciation, œdema, anasarca, engrafted upon the well-known generalities of *Arsenicum.*

Calcarea Carb.—Anæmia of girls; diminished hæmoglobin and red blood-corpuscles, increased leucocytes—Chlorosis. Psoric, scrofulous, tuberculous diathesis and general symptoms of the drug. Sad and apprehensive. Rush of blood to the head and vertgo, on excitement, hearing bad news, sufferings of others. Cold feet, dry cough at night, partial sweat, soreness of chest beneath right clavicles. Menses too profuse, too soon.

Calcarea Ars.—Worthwhile a careful study in anæmia and chlorosis, with a mind upon *Calcarea* and *Arsenicum.* Fleshy women at climacterie, palpitation from sightest emotion, chilliness; hæmoglobin and red-corpuscles low.

Calcarea Phos.—Anæmic or chlorotic girls with symptoms of *Calcarea Carb.* and thin, spare, emaciated build of *Phosphorus*.

China—Anæmia from loss of vital fluids. Women who do not make blood after hæmorrhages and develop a gradually increasing anæmia, with feeble circulation and dropsy, directly following loss of blood. Pale, weak, sensitive to cold; ringing in the ears; faintings, poor digestion, bloated abdomen with intoleranee of fruit or milk and diarrhœa—after midnight, after eating,

Manganum—Chlorosis, even Pernicious Anæmia with no history of hæmorrhage but long period of seanty menses. Headache, irritability, sad and silent weeping mood; prefers to lie down and great relief therefrom.

———

BLOOD, DEFICIENCY OF—(*Contd.*)

Chininum Ars.—Constantly increasing Anæmia from prolonged suppuration and hæmorrhages ; Pernicious Anæmia.

Acetic Acid.—Anæmia from prolonged morning sickness; waxy skin, thirst.

Ferrum Met.—False plethora with abnormal paleness of all mucous membranes ; pale face flushing up red on emotion. Pulsating headache ; throbbing all over body ; palpitation. Anæmic murmur in the veins of the neck ; chilly with hectic flush in the evening and œdema ot the extremities ; though weak yet relieved by moving slowly about, but exhausted easily. Complementary to *Alumina* in Chlorosis and to *China* in Anæmia from loss of blood.

Ferrum Ars.—Sometimes serves better than *Ferrum* or *Arsenicum.*

Graphites.—Anæmic though odese ; cold, constipated ; rough, herpetic skin ; cracks and fissures ; late, scanty, pale, watery menses : low-spirited and chilly, indoors or outdoors. Complements *Ferrum*, having many symptoms in common.

Lactic Acid.—Anæmia with Diabetes ; nausea after eating ; canker sores in mouth ; salivation ; polyuria.

Natrum Mur.—Anæmias due to loss of animal fluids ; thin, worn face, general emaciation ; Menstrual irregularities ; copious or scanty, watery menses once in two or three months ; cut-finger bleeds only water ; the menstural flow, only a Leucorrhœa. Constipation, fluttering palpitation ; pulsation over whole body ; melancholic ; easily angered ; aggravated by motion, sudden noise, and consolation.

Natrum Ars.—Sometimes replaces *Nat. Mur.* and *Arsenicum.*

Kali Carb.—Anæmia with chilliness, cannot go out without becoming chilly and cold ; vertigo, humming in ears, weak heart, sweat, and backache, especially with female complaints and the well-known modality and characteristics of *Kali Carb.* Often complements *Nat. Mur.*

Phosphorus.—Anæmia in deep-seated chronic diseases in tall, slender, narrow-chested, Phthisical patients ; easily catching cold ; menses too early, too copious, bright red. Chronic loose stool ; great thirst for cold, refreshing drinks. Jaundice.

Ferrum Phos. and Cal. Phos. sometimes outclass their components.

Hydrastis.—Anæmia from deep-seated zymotic diseases, as Cancer, etc., with faintness, prostration, atony, emaciation ; yellowish-white skin,

Pulsatilla.—Chlorotic or Anæmic ; after Quinine or Iron tonics ; chilly, yet better in open air ; fleshy and pale with late, scanty, dark and painful protracted menstruation ; sad, crying easily, seeks consolation ;

BLOOD, DEFICIENCY OF—(*Contd.*).

short breath, anxiety, palpitation ; pain under clavicles of either or both sides ; absence of thirst, weak digestion, Diarrhœa.

Cyclamen.—Similar to *Pulsatilla* but more or less thirsty and dreads open air ; physical languor in the morning. Scarcely fit to go through the day's work, but goes on tolerably well.

Helonias.—Chlorosis or Anæmia from prolonged hæmorrhage in those enervated by luxury or worn out with hard work ; sleeplessness and Melancholia ; tired, weak, backachy females, better when attention is engaged or when doing something.

Picrid Acid.—Extreme prostration in Pernicious Anæmia ; burning pain along the spine, worse from excitement.

Sepia.—Similar to *Pulsatilla,* but differs in mental symptoms. Sepia is irritable, often vehement ; averse to household duties.

Secale.—Progressive General Anæmia with cachexia ; pale, bloodless, jaundiced ; body cool but worse from warmth.

Aletris.—Tired all the time like *Helonias* with anæmia and relaxation etc., of female organism. "The *China* of the uterine organs".

Sulphur.—Often to rouse up action of other remedies ; flushes of heat ; hot vertex ; cold feet ; burning of the soles ; oppression of the chest at night—must open the window ; weak, sinking feeling in the epigastrium at fore-noon.

Zincum.—Too anæmic to develop an exanthema or menses ; progressive general emaciation, burning along spine, twitching of muscles, general trembling ; jerking of body during sleep ; aggravated by wine or stimulants.

DROPSY

[ASCITES—ANASARCA.]

Acetic Acid.—Dropsy of the abdomen (Ascites) and lower limbs with pale, waxy, emaciated face ; great thirst for large quanity of water (*Apis* is thirstless) ; sour belching and Diarrhœa ; unable to sleep on the back (*Arsenic* sleeps better on the back).

Apis.—Enormous water in the abdomen with total absence of thirst (with thirst, *Acet. Acid*, *Arsenic*). Waxy, transparent, dry skin ; dark scanty urine, albuminuria ; body and abdomen sore ; swelling about the eye-lids (kidney involved) ; œdema of the feet (heart involved) ; cannot breathe except when sitting—even leaning back causes suffocation. Hydrothorax with inability to lie down ; great dyspnœa, suffocation and restlessness with a feeling that he is going to die, but there is not the fear of death of *Aconite* and *Arsenic*.

DROPSY—(*Contd.*)

Apocynum.—Especially in Dropsy from heart disease more than in Renal Dropsy, with bewilderment and heaviness of head, drowsiness and debility or disturbed sleep, constipation (Diarrhœa, *Acetic Acid*), no sweat (*Apis*). Chilly, > warmth < hot, (warmth <*Apis* > cold). Fluttering of heart ; pulse irregular, feeble, slow—now weak, now stronger. (*Digitalis*—pulse slow, but quickens on motion). Ascites with sinking feeling in stomach—cannot retain water or food (*Ars.*). Bloatedness of face after lying down, passing off when sitting up. Hydro-pericardium with bloated face, small, weak pulse, bluish finger-nails, inability to lie down.

Arsenic.—Advanced cases with swollen spleen and liver. Œdema more or less general, beginning with puffiness of the eyes and swelling of the feet, ending with general Anasarca. Great dyspnœa, and prostration, anxiety, restlessness and fear of death—all <after midnight, <lying down (*Helleborus* breathes better on lying down). Urine dark, scanty with renal casts ; face and whole skin pale and yellowish ; eating and drinking cause vomiting—great thirst for small quantity of water. Dropsy of lower limbs with small ulcers, oozing serum. (*Lycopodium*—with emaciation of the upper part of body, muscles of arm and chest shrunken, distended abdomen and œdema of the lower limbs, with little oozing ulcers.) Ascites from Cirrhosis of the liver and Alcoholic drinks.

Aurum.—Ascites from liver affections and Syphilis. Cirrhosis or fatty degeneration of the liver with grayish or ashy-white stool. Scanty greenish-white urine together with a longing for death.

China.—Ascites from loss of blood, hæmorrhage (*Apocynum*), and other debilitating discharges (Dropsy from uterine hæmorrhage, *Helonias* : from Amenorrhœa, *Helonias*, *Senecio*).

Digitalis.—Dropsies primarily from cardiac debility, later developing congestions of liver and kidneys with Cirrhosis and fatty degeneration. Local and general Dropsies with irregularly-acting, weakened heart and suffocative feelings ; Cyanosis ; doughy swelling, pitting upon pressure ; face pale and bluish ; finger-tips clubbed ; constant urging to urinate with scanty discharge or total suppression of urine. Dropsy of the scrotum and penis (*Apocynum*).

Helleborus.—General Dropsies—especially Ascites from Post-Scarlatinal Nephritis. Urine dark and scanty or smoky from admixture of blood, which on standing looks like coffee-grounds. (*Terebinthina* has Dropsy from congested kidneys, with smoky urine and a dull aching in the renal region ; breathes easier when lying down. (Easier when sitting up—*Ars.*, *Lachesis*.)

Kali Carb.—Ascites of cardiac and hepatic origin, especially in old people with, œdematous swelling between the eye-brows and the lids.

DROPSY—(*Contd.*)

Insufficiency of the mitral valves ; < 3 A. M. Also œdema of the left foot, extending to the right and upwards, becoming general. Nephritis.

Lachesis.—Dropsy or Ascities of drunkards or after Scarlatina, when the urine is dark, almost blackish and albuminous ; the skin over the œdematous parts is dark, blackish ; suffocative fits waking from sleep.

Merc. Sulph.—Dropsy, especially of the chest with dyspnœa, inability to lie down ; swollen extremities and profuse watery stools, with burning and soreness at anus, which greatly relieves.

Muriatic Acid.—Last stages of Dropsy from Cirrhosis of the liver, when a typhoid condition develops with drowsiness, emaciation, involuntary stool, dry mouth, aphthæ.

Phosphorus.—Ascites from Cirrhosis of the liver with varicose veins over the abdomen coursing upwards, with highly albuminous urine. Soreness of the hepatic region and Jaundice with grayish-white stool.

Plumbum.—When dropsical condition has lessened, but uræmia has developed with convulsions.

Spigelia.—Especially in Hydrothorax, when there is anxiety in the chest, palpitation and dyspnœa on least motion, even raising the arms ; can lie only on the right side with the back raised.

Sulphur.—Dropsy, especially Hydrothorax : after suppressed eruptions, with rough skin, morning sleep ; arrest of breathing at night, when turning to other side on bed, going off when sitting ; must have windows open. Morning Diarrhœa driving the patient out at 5 P. M.

EYES, AFFECTIONS OF

Aconite.—First stage of Catarrhal Conjunctivitis, from sharp, cold winds ; dryness, burning, heat, photophobia, anguish. Reduces inflammation caused by foreign bodies sticking in the eyes and thus helps their removal. Complemented by *Sulphur* and *Silicea*.

Arnica.—Retinal or sub-conjunctival hæmorrhage from trauma.

Ledum.—Complements *Arnica ;* black and blue spots from blows.

Symphytum.—Great pain in the eye-ball itself from blows.

Calendula.—Traumatic Conjunctivitis, Keratitis, Iritis.

Cantharis.—Inflammation caused by burns.

Hamamelis.—Inflammation, ulceration or hæmorrhage into anterior chamber caused by burn or blow.

Hypericum.—Effects of injury years before.

Apis.—Lids and cellular tissues œdematous ; chemosis ; burning, stinging pain, cannot bear warmth ; relieved by cold water ; sensation

EYES, AFFECTIONS OF—(*Contd.*)

of a foreign body; Ulceration, Retinitis, Keratitis, Blepharitis, Conjunctivitis.

Argentum Nit.—Most intense Chemosis; strangulated vessels; eye-balls feel big; carencula swollen; violent Purulent Opthalmia. Blepharitis; worse from warmth, heat of fire; better from open air, cold water. Ophthalmia Neonatorum.

Arsenic.—Parenchymatous Keratitis, Kerato-Iritis. Burning like fire, after mid-night; non-inflammatory œdema of lids, hot tears, violent pains, sandy feeling; corrosive, watery discharge, excessive photophobia—all like *Apis* without its stinging pains, and with great relief from warmth; restlessness more pronounced.

Asafœtida.—Severe boring pain in, over and around the eyes. Worse at night, ameliorated by rest and pressure. Irido-Choroiditis; Retinitis—Syphilitic or Mercurial.

Aurum.—Syphilitic affections with ulcerations, vascularity, photophobia, profuse lachrymation. Interstitial Keratitis, Iritis, Choroiditis; soreness around the eyes with sensitiveness to touch, relief from warmth.

Belladonna.—Conjunctivitis; Sclerotitis; sudden attack, severe pain; great intolerance of light; conjunctiva bright red; hot tears, dryness of the eyes; headache and other *Bell.* symptoms.

Calcarea Carb.—Scrofulous Blepharitis with aching, loss of eye-lashes; from working in the wet; profuse lachrymation, photophobia and other characteristics of the drug.

Calcarea Fluor.—Corneal Ulceration with hard edges. Cataract; has dissolved the capsule after operation. Pain in the eye-balls, better closing the eyes and pressing lightly.

Cal. Iod.—Scrofulous; ulcers on cornea, wrose getting fluent coryza; acrid tears on attempting to open eyes; worse cold.

Calcarea Phos.—Pain in the eyes; light hurts, especially artificial light; lachrymation, most with yawning; Cataract; ulcers on the cornea.

Calcarea Sulph.—Cataract. Chronic inflammation with ulceration of the cornea, thick yellow pus; dim, foggy vision, photophobia, flickering before the eyes; redness and fissures of the canthi.

Cantharis.—Inflammation with burning and smarting in the eyes, which look prominent and is accompanied with convulsive movements of the eyes, with a fiery sparkle in them; objects look yellow; eyes hot, tears scalding.

Capsicum.—Inflammation of the eyes with redness, burning and lachrymation; confusion of sight, better for an instant from rubbing.

EYES, AFFECTIONS OF—(*Contd.*)
Objects appear black when brought before the eyes ; sight entirely extinct, as if from Amaurosis.

Carbo Animalis.—Far-sighted, objects seem to him to be far off ; sensation as if the balls were detatched from the sockets ; dimness of sight on attempting to read, relieved by rubbing ; especially in old people.

Carbo Veg.—Pains in the eyes from over-use. Bleeding of the eyes with congestion of the head ; quivering and trembling of the lids and black, flying spots before the eyes. Myopia, near-sightedness, can see when objects are near to the eye, worse from exerting the eyes.

Carbolic Acid.—Very servere orbital neuralgia over the right eye i pupils dilated.

Carboneum Sulph.—Myopia, Diplopia, complete Achromatopsia ; Contraction of the field of vision for white and blue, red and green totally absent ; constant flashes, spots and spider's webs before eyes ; reading brings tears to the eyes ; atrophy of the optic papillæ ; optic disc pale, deeply cupped, less transparent than normal : congestion of the disc ; retina congested ; retinal arteries too small and tortuous ; retinal veins dilated and tortuous ; vision better in the twilight, after eating ; obliged to wink to see elearly.

Causticum.—Obscuration of the eyes, often sudden, as if eyes were covered or as if a gauge or mist before the eyes ; dark nets or swarms of insects seem to dance before the eyes. Ophthalmia with opacity of the cornea spreading over the pupil ; photophobia ; lachrymation ; ulceration. Paralysis of the optic nerve—vision gradually grows weaker until it is lost. Gradually increasing Paralysis of the eye-lids ; Cataract.

Cedron.—Severe pain in the eye-ball, radiating around the eye, shooting into nose ; Supra-Orbital Neuralgia, recurring at the same hour with clock-like regularity. Iritis, Choroiditis ; objects seem red at night, yellow by day (*Bell.* cured).

Cereus Bonplandii.—Pain through the globe of the eyes and the orbits with severe pain in the occiput.

Chamomilla.—Inflammation of the eyes ; shooting, burning, heat. Ecchymoses in and hæmorrhage of the eyes ; oozing of bloody water from the eyes of the new-born infant ; violent pressure in the orbit ; profuse, acrid, yellow, purulent discharges. Irritability of temper.

Chelidonium.—Orbital Neuralgia of the right eye with profuse lachrymation and stitching, tearing pains in and above the eye, better by pressure ; pupils contracted.

EYES, AFFECTIONS OF—(*Contd.*)

China.—Nocturnal blindness in anæmic retina ; sparkling, black, dancing spots and obscuration before the eyes ; intermittent Ciliary Neuralgia with pressure in the eyes ; photophobia ; pains worse from light, better in the dark ; on reading the characters appear pale and surrounded by a white edge.

Chininum Ars.—Intense photophobia and orbicular spasm ; gushing hot tears, with large ulcers on each eye ; worse from midnight to 3 A.M. Keratitis.

Cicuta Virosa.—Wavering of all objects before the sight—objects recede, approach and seem double ; luminous colored circle around all objects ; pupils get behind the upper lids as head inclines ; strabismus coming periodically, from cold, after a fall or a blow.

Cimicifuga.—Hyperæmia of iris, choroid and retina. Sharp neuralgic pains through the eye into the head ; Ciliary Neuralgia ; intense pains in the eye-balls, especially at night ; amel. by pressure, worse by slightest movement. Deep-seated throbbing and shooting pains in the eyes with photophobia from artificial light.

Cina.—Asthenopia from defective accomodation. Eyes ache with blurring of sight on reading, better by rubbing ; strabismus from worms or abdominal irritation ; pain in head and eyes from sewing, especially when presbyopia forms in middle-aged women.

Cinnabaris.—Pressive, shooting pains from lachrymal duct around the eye to the temple, from the inner canthus of the rt. eye ; severe shooting pains in bones of the orbit from inner to outer canthus ; redness of the whole eye with flow of tears and swelling of the face.

Cocculus.—Rheumatic Glaucoma. Pain in the eyes as if they were torn out of head. Dim-sightedness, after reading a short time : the print is all blurred ; confusion of sight, black spots and phantoms before the eyes ; photophobia ; no lachrymation.

Colocynth.—Violent neuralgic pains with severe burning, cutting, sticking in the eye, with profuse acrid lachrymation. Rheumatic Iritis ; sharp, cutting stabs, worse in evening and night, better from firm pressure ; as if eyes would fall out on stooping. Glaucoma.

Comocladia.—Pains in the right eye, feeling as if it were larger or were being pushed out of the head ; worse near a warm stove. Glaucoma.

Conium.—Intense photophobia and excessive lachrymation from slightest inflammation or even none at all. Cataract from contusion ; sees various colors before the eyes ; shooting, burning, cutting pains in the eyes when reading ; sick headache and visual disturbances on watching moving objects—defective accommodation. Hordeola ; Paralysis of the muscles of the eyes.

EYES, AFFECTIONS OF—(*Contd.*)

Clematis.—Follows *Merc. Cor.* in Iritis. Iritis from cold, with pressing pain, great photophobia, lachrymation and heat in the eyes with great sensitiveness to cold air, so that the patient covers the eyes.

Crocus Sativa.—Lachrymation in the room, not in the open air; tears rush from the eyes as soon as he begins to read; heat and lancinating pains in the eyes after surgical operations; constant necessity to wink or rub the eyes; visible quivering of the eye-lids.

Crotalus Horridus.—Keratitis, when there are cutting pains around the eyes; lids swollen in the morning; Ciliary Neuralgia with these cuttings, worse during menses. Intra-ocular hæmorrhage—blood exudes from the eyes; pressure in the eyes, as if would be pushed out from the head; very sensitive to light, especially artificial light.

Cyclamen.—Dimness of vision, diplopia, convergent strabismus; flickering of various colors before the eyes, sees countless stars.

Duboisia.—Hallucinations of vision: things seem elevated; drops a glass in mid-air instead of placing it on the table; imagined it was quite dark, when it was a bright summer after-noon; appearance of a red spot in the field of vision moving with the eye. Hyperæmia of the optic nerve; accommodation paralysed.

Euphrasia.—Most violent Acute Conjuntivitis: Rheumatic Iritis; great inflammation of all the tissues of the eyes, ulceration of the cornea. Cutting pain in the eyes, extending into the head; as if sands in the eyes. Much tumefaction of the mucous membrane, with redness, enlarged blood-vessels, smarting and itching, copious acrid lachrymation and marked photophobia—cannot bear sun-light or, even more especially, artificial light; must rub and wink.

Fluoric Acid.—Violent itching of inner canthus; fistula lachrymalis; sensation as of cold wind blowing through the eyes, even in a warm room.

Gelsemium.—Paralysis of the eye-lids and occular muscles; diplopia, double vision, ptosis; eye-balls oscillating laterally when using them; cannot tell which side of the street he is on; complete blindness coming on suddenly. Glaucoma; intra-occular inflammations with serous exudations, intense pain over the right eye, double vision and vertigo. Serous Iritis, Choroiditis, with gradual impairment of vision and heavy lids: detachment of the retina; strabismus from weakness of the muscles or following Diphtheria.

Glonoine.—Supra-Orbital Neuralgia—pulsating. Diseases of the eye from exposure to very hot, bright light, producing retinal congestion. Apoplexy of the retina; feeling as if eyes were pulled from within outward; protrution of the eyes; sparks and flushes before the eyes; letters appear smaller.

EYES, AFFECTIONS OF—(*Contd.*)

Graphites.—Scrofulous inflammation of the eyes ; cornea inflamed and covered with superficial uleers ; thickening of the eye-lids, along the edges with scurfs or scales. Blepharitis, worse in canthi, with cracking and bleeding of the edges ; ectropion or entropion ; wild eye-lashes turning towards the eye and irritating the conjunctiva. Hardened styes along the edges ; letters appear double or run together. Eczema about the eyes ; shooting and sandy feeling in the eyes ; photophobia especially by day.

Hepar Sulph.—Ulcers on cornea ; Iritis with pus in anterior chamber. Purulent Conjunctivitis with marked chemosis, profuse discharge , great sensitiveness to touch and air, with throbbing pain in and about the eyes ; eye-lids inflamed ; pain, as if balls were pulled back into the head ; bright circles before eyes. Speedily absorbs hypopyon ; valuable in Keratitis.

Ignatia.—Nictitation of the eye-lids with spasmodic action of the facial muscles. Neuralgic pains about the eyes which are exceedingly severe, often associated with globus hystericus. Phlyctenular Ophthalmia with intense photophobia and a feeling of sand in the eyes.

Jaborandi.—Eye-strain from whatever cause ; eyes easily tired ; heat, burning and smarting in globe on use ; vision becomes indistinct every few moments ; retinal images retained long ; pupils contracted, do not react to light. Staring eyes ; near-sighted ; white spots before eyes. Atrophic Choroiditis ; spasm of accommodation while reading.

Kali Bichrom.—Indolent ulcers and Conjunctivitis of scrofulous or syco-syphilitic origin. The eye-lids are swollen and agglutinated, especially in the morning, with thick yellow matter ; chemosis. Indolent Iritis, when there has been exudation posteriorly between the iris and lens, causing adhesions and with little or no photophobia even with severe ulceration or inflammation (opposite of *Conium*).

Kali Carb.—Tearing, stitching, shooting pains in eyes ; swelling of eyes and lids with difficulty in opening them ; excoriation and suppuration in corners of eyes. Spots dancing before sight on reading and looking into open air ; rainbow colors, spots (blue or green) and sparks before sight ; on shutting eyes painful sensation of light penetrating the brain ; photophobia, dazzling of eyes by day-light.

Kali Iod.—Syphilitic Iritis, after abuse of *Mercury* ; inflammation involving both choroid and iris. Syphilitic Pustular Keratitis, with chemosis, after abuse of *Mercury*.

Kali Sulph.—Purulent or yellow mucus in eye diseases ; yellow crusts ; yellow discharge ; Ophthalmia Neonatorum.

Kalmia.—Almost complete blindness when in erect position. Retinitis albuminurica ; pain in the back as if it would break. Sclero-choroiditis anterior, with glimmering before eyes. Severe pain in right eye extending over forehead—begins at sun-rise, increases till noon and leaves at sun-set.

EYES, AFFECTIONS OF—(*Contd.*)

Kreosote—Inflammation of eye-lids, in infant or adult, with continued heat and burning sensation in the eyes and frequent lachrymation of hot, scalding tears, early in the morning ; salty tears. Interstitial Keratitis, with pegged teeth.

Lachesis—Defective vision after Diphtheria ; dim vision, worse on awaking ; dark spots before eyes ; sight suddenly fades away ; dim sight from heart disease with faintness, palpitation and vertigo. Causes absorption of the blood in Retinal Apoplexy.

Lithium Carb.—Pain over eyes with half vision, right half invisible. Sun-light blinds him ; black motes before eyes which are sensitive after using them by candle-light.

Lycopodium—Ophthalmia Neonatorum, suppurative stage. Catarrhal Ophthalmia ; thick yellowish-green discharge ; night-blindness.

Mercurius—Scrofulous or Syphilitic Ophthalmia, markedly aggravated from the glare and heat of fire. Blepharitis from working in and about fires ; lids thickened at tarsal edges, with thin, acrid muco-pus discharge and little pimples over the cheeks. Superficial ulcers on the cornea with an opaque look as though pus were between corneal layers. Syphilitic Iritis when there is hypopyon.

Mercurius Biniod.—Similar to the above, but there is more glandular swelling.

Mercurius Cor.—Inflammatory symptoms of the eyes of the most violent character with burning, tearing, agonizing pains in the bones around eyes and most excessive photophobia and profuse excoriating lachrymation making the cheeks sore, almost taking the skin off. Perforating ulcers on the cornea with hypopyon. Syphilitic Iritis—almost a specific. Retinitis Albuminurica.

Mercurius Dulcis—Eye-troubles in scrofulous children with flabby bloatedness, pallor and swelling of cervical and other glands.

Mercurius Proto Iod.—Corneal ulcers, as if they have been clipped out with the finger-nail, usually accompanied with a thick yellow coating on base of the tongue and a tendency to a rapid extension of the ulceration.

Mezereum—Ciliary Neuralgia after operations ; the pains radiate and shoot downwards with a feeling as though a stream of cold air were blowing on the eye ; the bones are involved—a frequent sequence of *Mercury*.

Natrum Carb.—Keratitis and ulceration of cornea ; lancinations across eyes and stitches from within outwards with photophobia and swelling of lids ; abscess in lachrymal gland. Dim eyes—has to wipe them

EYES, AFFECTIONS OF—(*Contd.*)

constantly ; black dancing specks or bright sparkling before eyes ; inability to read small print, as in presbyopia.

Natrum Mur.—Weakness of the muscles of the eye, especially the internal recti, with stiffness of the lids when moving them ; marked asthenopia, letters blur and run together when reading. Scrofulous Ophthalmia with acrid tears and spasmodic closure of lids. Ulcers on the cornea with inflamed eyes, agglutinated in the morning. Stricture of the lachrymal duct ; fistula lachrymalis with escape of muco-pus on pressing on the sac ; tears stream down face on coughing. Scrofulous children with eruptions on border of hairy scalp. Incipient Cataract. Eye affections reflex from uterine diseases with drooping eye-lids ; cracks in the canthi and corners of mouth.

Natrum Sulph.—Itching on edges of lids and intense photophobia on waking in morning ; aching in eyes when reading ; burning in eyes, worse near fire, with great dryness or profuse lachrymation, morning and evening ; nocturnal agglutination of lids.

Nitric Acid.—Sometimes indispensable in Ophthalmia Neonatorum. Mainly useful for superficial ulcers of the cornea with sharp sticking, splinter-like pains. One of the best remedies for corneal opacities.

Nux Moschata.—Objects look larger, very distant or vanish ; sees two, instead of one ; dryness of eyes and sensation of dryness, which impedes movement of lids ; drooping eye-lids.

Nux Vomica—Scrofulous Ophthalmia and Blepharospasmus with agglutination of lids and photophobia in the morning ; can use eyes freely in the afternoon.

Onosmodium.—Vision blurred ; optic disc hyperæmic and retinal vessels enlarged ; muscular asthenopia ; occular muscles tense. Pain in eye-balls, between orbit and ball, extending to left temple. Useful in eye-strain, with dull, heavy, sore, aching eyes.

Paris Quadrifolia—Eye-balls feel too large, as though lids did not cover ; pains as if the eyes were drawn back by strings.

Petroleum.—Blepharitis Marginalis. Inflammation of the lachrymal canal, when suppuration has commenced and a fistula has formed ; the lids are red, raw, moist.

Phellandrium—Headache involving the nerves going to the eye, with a crushing feeling on the top of the head, burning of the eyes and lachrymation.

Phosphorus.—Diseases involving the deeper structures of the eye, as the retina, choroid and vitreous humour and affections of the nerves of the eye. Hyperæmia of the choroid and retina resulting in Choroditis

EYES, AFFECTIONS OF—(*Contd.*)

and Retinitis ; pains, as if in orbital bones and pressure as if eyes would be pressed out ; shooting, smarting, burning and heat in eyes, especially, in external canthi ; eyes feel full and sore to touch, vision greatly lessened ; sees better in morning, in twilight or by shading eyes with hands ; sees all sorts of abnormal colors, black spots in the air and gray veils over things ; as if looking through mist or fog ; objects look red ; letters appear red when reading. Retinitis with kidney affections.

Physostigma—Contraction of the pupil and of the ciliary muscles. short-sightedness, night blindness ; twitching of occular muscles. Glaucoma : paresis of accommodation, astigmatism. Spasm of ciliary muscles with irritability after using eyes. Increasing Myopia, Post-Diphtheritic Paralysis of eye and muscles of accommodation.

Platina—Objects look smaller than they are ; twitching of lids ; eyes feel cold ; cramp-like pain in orbits.

Piumbum—Optic nerve inflamed ; intra-ocular suppurative inflammation. Glaucoma, especially if secondary to spinal lesion.

Prunus Spinosa—Cilliary Neuralgia ; bursting pain in right eye, shooting like lightening through the brain to occiput ; sudden pain in the eye-balls, as if would burst ; better by lachrymation. Irido-Choroiditis.

Pulsatilla—Conjunctivitis with thick, yellow or yellowish-green, bland discharge, worse at night, with agglutination of lids in the morning. Ophthalmia after Measles. Purulent Ophthalmia and Ophthalmia Neonatorum—used before or after *Arg. Nit.* Fine granulations on the lids ; repeated, highly inflamed styes. Useful for the mild, passive, lymphatic temperament and locally profuse, thick, bland discharges and not much pain or photophobia.

Rhus Tox.—Scrofulous Ophthalmia with phlyctenules on or about the cornea and most intense photophobia, chemosis and tendency to the formation of pus ; spasmodic closure of the eye-lids and gushing forth of yellow pus on forcing the lids apart. Conjunctivitis on getting wet. Rheumatic or Traumatic Iritis with great intolerance to light ; inflammation extending to and involving the choroid with pains shooting through to the back of the head, worse at night, and profuse flow of hot scalding tears on opening the lids. Almost a specific in Orbital Cellulitis and much useful in Glaucoma. Ptosis, in rheumatic patients after exposure to dampness. Often beneficial after Cataract extraction, to control threatened Iritis and formation of pus.

Ruta—Eye-strain followed by headache ; eyes red, hot and painful from sewing or reading fine print ; disturbances of accommodation ; eyes burn, feel like balls of fire.

EYES, AFFECTIONS OF—(*Contd.*)

Santoninum—Sudden dimness of sight ; color-blindness ; strabismus due to worms.

Saponaria—Supra-orbital stitching pain, left side ; worse evening, motion ; violent eye-pains with hot stitches deep in eye-ball, photophobia. Exopthalmos, worse reading and writing ; increased intra-ocular pressure.

Sepia—Asthenopia attending uterine diseases. Conjunctivitis of a sluggish type, in scrofulous children, with muco-purulent discharge in the morning ; better morning and afternoon, worse in the evening. Cataract ; Trachoma, with or without Pannus ; scaly lids ; pustular lids with eruptions on face ; eyes irritable to light ; lids close in spite of him ; eye-lids droop ; aching, sticking pains, worse from rubbing.

Spigelia—Violent, sharp-cutting pains in the left eye, but lacks the congestion of *Belledonna* ; sensation that the eye-balls are too large. Shooting and stabbing pains accompanying Glaucoma, worse at night and on motion. Neuralgia of eyes especially the left, with great soreness, can scarcely bear a touch ; pain deeply seated in sockets. Ciliary Neuralgia coming and going with the Sun, worse at mid-day.

Silicea—Swelling of the lachrymal duct ; lachrymal fistula ; photophobia and dazzling in day-light. Sharp pain through the cyes which are tender to touch, worse when they are closed. Confusion of vision, letters run together on reading. Iritis, Irido-Choroiditis, with pus in the anterior chamber. Perforating or sloughing ulcer of the cornea ; abscess in cornea after traumatic injury ; styes. Cataract, in office workers ; after-effects of Keratitis, and ulcers corneæ, clearing the opacity. Encysted tumors of the lids.

Staphisagria—Recurrent styes which remain hardened, chalazæ. Affections of angles of eyes, particularly the inner. Lacerated or incised wounds of cornea.

Sulphur—Keratitis ; Conjunctivitis from a foreign body—as a grain of sand or cinder in the eye—with acrid discharge, hot tears flow out on opening the eyes, after *Aconite* fails. Scrofulous inflammation of the eyes with tendency to congestion ; the eyes are red and injected, with splinter-like pains, worse in hot weather or near a hot stove ; chronic cases.

Syphilinum—Chronic, recurrent, phlyctenular inflammation of cornea ; intense photophobia, profuse lachrymation ; pain intense at night. Diplopia, one image seen below the other ; feeling of cold air blowing on eye.

Tellurium Lids thickened, inflamed, itching ; Pterygium. Cataract following ocular lesions. Aids the absorption of infiltration in iris and choroid.

EYES, AFFECTIONS OF—(*Contd.*)

Terebinthina—Ciliary Neuralgia over right eye ; intense pain in eye and side of head. Amblyopia from *Alcohol.*

Thuja—Wart-like excrescence on iris ; vascular tumor on cornea. Ophthalmia Neonatorum ; Phlyctenular Conjunctivitis. Fungous tumor in orbit ; inflammatory swelling of lids with hardness ; granular lids with wart-like granulations ; red and painful nodosities on margin of lids ; dry and branny lids ; styes ; tarsal tumors ; chalazæ ; thick and hard knots. Lachrymation, especially in left eye, when walking in open air—the tears do not run off, but stand in the eye ; the eye must be warmly covered, pains when uncovered.

Zincum—Amblyopia, accompanied by severe headache, with severe pain at the root of the nose ; the pains are particularly worse at inner canthus of each eye ; pupils contracted ; opacities of the cornea following repeated long-lasting inflammations. Pterygium, with smarting, stinging pains at the inner canthus : granular lids. Prosopalgia with blurring of one-half of vision ; squinting ; worse, stimulants.

> **Zincum Sulph.**—In opacities of the cornea and granular lids, it is perferable to the *Metallicum.*

FEMALE GENITAL ORGANS

[AMENORRHŒA]

Aconite—Young, plethoric. Suppression from cold-bath, sudden and violent emotions as fear, anger etc., or from checked perspiration. Terrible pain in the lower abdomen ; dry-hot skin ; full, hard, bounding pulse ; great agitation, fear of death.

Apis—Congestion of the head due to suppression ; bearing down in the uterine region ; pain in right ovary ; no thirst ; pain in the back. Urine suppressed, or scanty and high-colored ; cannot tolerate heat applied or warm atmosphere ; occipital headache ; cardiac troubles ; waxen face ; swollen eye-lids ; nervous, hysterical, silly.

Belladonna—Amenorrhœa with rush of blood to the head ; terrible pain in head and lower abdomen ; worse by motion or jar ; wakefulness ; painful urination.

Cal. Carb.—Suppression due to working in water or from cold ; rush of blood to the head and chest ; vertigo, dyspnœa and palpitation on ascending. Fat, flabby, chilly, anæmic, with evening fever, sweat, dry cough at night and soreness of chest below the right clavicle.

FEMALE GENITAL ORGANS – *Contd.*

Cimicifuga—Suppression from emotion. Rheumatic or Neuralgic. Chorea, Hysteria, Mania. Heat and heavy pressure on top of the head ; crampy pains of abdomen.

Cocculus.—Leucorrhœa instead of menses. Similar to *Cimicifuga* in hysterical manifestations. Vertigo and nausea on riding ; pain in the back ; intense spasmodic pain in the pelvic region ; weak and nervous ; great weakness, cannot stand or talk.

Cuprum Met.—Amenorrhœa from suppressed foot-sweats. Violent cramps in the chest and abdomen ; nausea and frequent vomiting ; palpitation and spasm of heart ; cramps of fingers and toes,

Cyclamen —Amenorrhœa with headache and vertigo. Weeping mood, Melancholia; prefers loneliness ; drowsy ; swollen eye-lids ; chilly—prefers warmth ; worse, open air.

Gelsemium—Drowsy, dizzy and faint ; apathetic mood.

Glonoine—With violent rush of blood and throbbing, bursting pain in head ; worse from least motion ; better from firm pressure ; chest feels as if full of blood with great uncanny feeling in chest.

Helonias,—Suppression with congested kidneys ; urine scanty and turbid ; albuminuria ; backache and a constant feeling of tiredness.

Ignatia—Amenia from suppressed grief with much sighing.

Kali Carb.—Suppression with sour eructations and swelling of cheeks at every menstrual nisus, shooting pains over the abdomen, anæmic and weak heart ; swelling over eye-lids. Often brings on menses when *Nat. Mur.* fails.

Lilium Tigrinum—Amenia with heart effections, together with prolapse or retroversion. Burning, stinging pain in the ovaries ; partial, with occasional return of menses and absent again ; pain in the chest, from left nipple through to the back.

Lycopodium—From fright. Sad and weeping ; acid eructations and vomiting ; desires sweet things ; rumbling of the abdomen ; wind passes from vagina with a noise.

Mag. Carb.—Suppression with sore-throat and toothache at every menstrual nisus.

Mag. Mur.—With sleeplessness, constipation and hysterical, excited mood at every menstrual nisus.

Nat. Carb.—Suppression with pressing towards the genitals, as if the contents of pelvis would protrude ; a feeling as if menses would appear.

Nat. Mur. – Anxious and melancholy at the menstrual nisus ; nausea with flow of sweet saliva—spitting of blood ; long-lasting headache in

FEMALE GENITAL ORGANS – (*contd.*)

morning on waking ; constipation, fissures of the anus. Followed well by *Kali Carb.*

Nux Mosch.—From getting wet ; rheumatic, hysteric ; irresistible sleepiness and tendency to faint ; debility and exhaustion.

Opium—Suppression from fright, with great sopor and convulsions.

Phosphorus—Menses absent with tightness of chest, dry cough and spitting of blood. Similar to *Calc. Carb.*, but *Phos.* is tall. slender, Phthisical, with delicate, refined skin, sharp and handsome features, long silky eye-lashes, where as *Calc. Carb.* has slow development as a child, scrofulous, fat, flabby, with large features and thick upper lip.

Pulsatilla.—Amenia due to wet feet ; vicarious menses, epistaxis ; uterine colic ; morning sickness ; bad taste in mouth in the morning ; soreness of the apices of the lungs ; worse from warmth, must have fresh air.

Rhododendron—Always worse during rough, windy weather and before thunder-storm.

Sabina—Menses suddenly suppressed, followed by thick, fetid Leucorrhœa.

Senecio—Menstrual nisus, but no show ; gastric derangement, loss of appetite ; little or no urine pale and anæmic ; General Dropsy.

Sepia—Feeble women ; yellow saddle across the nose, dingy spots on the face ; *Pulsatilla* symptoms with frequent alternation of chilliness and heat ; constipation with a sense of weight at the anus ; foul Leucorrhœa.

Sulphur—Heat on the top of head, burning of palms and soles; hungry at noon, cannot wait ; weak and faint at about 11 A. M. ; piles, uterine pains. After failure of *Pulsatilla.*

Thuja—Suppression of menses with anxious restlessness, sleeplessness and constipation ; mental dullness and no desire for work ; embrace prevented by extreme sensitiveness of vagina (*Platina*) ; she has a fixed idea that she is pregnant ; she even declares that she feels the movement of the child.

Ustilago—Suppression of menses with vicarious menstruation from lungs and bowels and constant aching distress at the mouth of the womb ; pain in the left ovary ; general debility-and bearing down, as if everything would come through.

Veratrnm Alb.—Amenia with headache, vomiting, diarrhœa and cold sweat on forehead, at every menstrual nisus.

FEMALE GENITAL ORGANS—(*Contd.*)

[DYSMENORRHŒA—LEUCORRHŒA—MENORRHAGIA—METRORRHAGIA.]

Aconite—Plethoric, vigorous women coming down suddenly with a violent congestion and inflammation of the womb and the menses are suppressed or the flow may be profuse, simulating active hæmorrhage, with much excitability, restlessness, fear of death and violent labor-like pressing colic which forces her to bend double, but with no relief.

Belladonna—Most intensely painful Congestive Dysmenorrhœa with constant and violent drawing and bearing-down pain. Too early and too profuse menses of hot, bright red blood, with offensive clots. The violent dragging down is worse on lying down, and is relieved by standing (opposite of *Sepia*). Uterine hæmorrhage with bearing-down in the back, as if it would break, the violent pains that come suddenly and disappears suddenly and the general picture of *Bell.* decide.

Cactus Grandi.—Violent congestion of the uterus in young, vigorous women, with terrible spasms and cramping pains before the flow starts or just at the beginning, causing her to cry aloud. The menses are too early and scanty, and sometimes copious, with clots expelled with every paroxysm, extorting screams and with difficult urination. The menses are dark, black and thick, like pitch (*Cocc.*, *Mag. C.*) and the flow ceases on lying down (*Mag. C.* is opposite). The heart symptoms accompany.

Coccus Cacti.—Copious, frequent and prolonged flow of dark, thick blood, only in the evening and at night, while lying down, passing enormous black clots which make urination difficult till they have passed out and sharp pains in lower abdomen, first right, then left.

Chamomilla—Early and profuse discharge of offensive, black, clotted blood, with labor-like pains and cutting colic, tearing down the thighs, griping and pinching in uterus followed by discharge of large clots of blood, the flow occurring in fits and starts at irregular intervals. Membranous Dysmenorrhœa ; menstrual colic, amel. by heat. Emotion and anger will bring them on in *Chamomilla* patients.

Cocculus—Violent cramping and clutching pains with too early, too profuse, dark and clotted menses, gushing out in a stream on rising ; or irregular and scanty. Flatulence ; spasm of the chest with groaning and sighing and tendency to faint ; menses lessen during abdominal pains and become copious with their

FEMALE GENITAL ORGANS—(*Contd.*)

abatement (*Cimici.*—opposite). Very weak, can scarcely speak or is hardly able to stand. Purulent, gushing Leucorrhœa between or instead of menses.

Colocynth—Sharp, darting, paroxysmal pains several days before, with left ovarian pain, as if squeezed on a vise. Amel. by bending double, firm pressure and warmth ; yellow, thick, offensive Leucorrhœa between the menses.

Causticum.—Early or late and profuse menses mixed with large clots, offensive and acrid, causing itching of vulva ; too feeble and flowing only in the day-time, no discharge during night or when lying down. Menstrual colic of a griping, cutting character and relieved by bending double, appears previous to the menses with tearing in the back and limbs. Useful after *Colocynth* fails. Leucorrhœa profuse and flowing like menses but only at night or worse then, with itching and biting in vulva and between legs.

Bovista—Early and profuse menses occurring chiefly or only at night or early in the morning with Diarrhœa, before and during ; epistaxis, flow to blood between the periods from any little over-exertion. Leucorrhœa, thiek, viscid, yellowish-green, a few days before or after menses, dropping out in coagulated mass or clots, specially when walking. Tettery persons with puffy condition of the body.

Ambra Grisea—Atony of the uterus ; regular or too early but profuse menses with nose-bleed and increase of varicose veins on legs, if present, and discharge of blood between the periods at every little accident, excitement or extra effort. Leucorrhœa, only at night, of bluish-gray mucus.

Ammon. Carb. and **Mur.**—Too early and copious, acrid and blackish menses, often in clots, flows more profusely at night and when sitting and makes the thighs sore and burning, with Cholera-like symptoms at the commencement and is preceded by griping and colic, toothache, sleeplessness and fatigue, especially of thighs ; yawning and chilliness but smothers in a warm room. Discharge of blood from bowels during menses. The *Muriate* is preferable when there is a tensive pain in either groin which forces the patient to walk bent and stools crumbling at the anus. With the *Carbonate* the Leucorrhœa is profuse, watery, acrid, with sensation of excoriation and ulceration in vulva, while that with the *Muriate* is like the white of an egg, brown and slimy, preceded by pinching about the navel and violent pain in small of the back, especially at night.

FEMALE GENITAL ORGANS—(*Contd.*)

Calcarea Carb.—Excessively profuse and too long-lasting menses (atony of muscular coat of uterus and relaxation), coming too frequently, almost twice a month, from the least excitement or provocation (*Ambra*), light-colored or bright red, with copious, thick, yellow Leucorrhœa that is acrid and keeps up an itching, burning and smarting in the genitals (*Ammon. C.*, *Kreosote*). Colicky pains in back and hips, swelling and tenderness of the breasts (*Conium*, *Lac Can.*). The generals of the drug go to-gether to make up the *Calcarea Carb.* case.

Calc. Phos.—Too early and bright red or late and bright, then dark blood, with vlolent backache in young girls of the make up of the remedy, who complain of headache several days before and great sexual desire (*Murex*, *Platina*), followed by copious flow, griping, shooting pains from left to right, great weakness and sinking sensation (*Cocculus*). Leucorrhœa, like the white of an egg (*Ammon Mur.*, *Borax*) and the generals of the drug.

Trillium Pendulum--Pıofuse and premature menstrual flow or uterine hæmorrhages, during climaxis, with gushing of bright red blood on least movement with sensation as though the hips were falling to pieces, better by tight bandages ; hæmorrhage from fibroids. Copious, yellow, stringy Leucorrhœa ; the flow exhausts very much.

Erigeron—Alarmingly profuse flooding of bright red blood especially during climaxis, coming with a sudden gush and stopping again, and returning after least movement, with great irritation of rectum and bladder (*Cantharis*, *Lilium*, *Nux Vom.*) and prolapsus uteri.

Hamamelis – Passive hæmorrhage, with bearing down pain in back and soreness in abdomen, dark and profuse, occurring mid-way between menstrual periods, only during the day and none at night ; vicarious (*Bryo* , *Phos.*).

Helonias—Too frequent, too profuse, passive flow of dark coagulated .and offensive blood with a tired, dragging feeling in the back and constant—without any let up—soreness and weight in the womb. Dark, offensive and constant Leucorrhœa, which flows on every exertion. Tired, backachy females, with great languor and prostration, who are enervated by indolence, luxury or hard work, and have atony of the pelvic organs and tissues ; always better when attention is engaged.

Ipecac.—Profuse menstruation or uterine hæmorrhage with a constant nausea and discharge of bright-red blood with a gush ;

FEMALE GENITAL ORGANS—(*Contd.*)

constant oozing which every little while or with every effort to vomit, increases to a gush, with gasping for breath and faintness.

Phosphorus—Too early, too long-lasting and copious flow of bright red blood, with violent pain in ovaries, extending down the inner side of thighs, and pain in the back, as if it would break ; inflammation of the ovaries and uterus during menstruation accompanied with ice-cold feet and hands, nausea, blue rings around the eyes, loss of flesh and much fearfulness. Frequent and profuse hæmorrhages from uterus in Cancerous affections. Copious yellow Leucorrhœa, or white, watery, acrid and excoriating, causing blisters to form upon the genitals, burning and sashing in vagina and great weakness. Violent sexual excitement or complete aversion, with sterility. Vicarious menstruation.

Sabina—Menses too copious and last too long, sometimes not stopping before the next period begins ; liquid, bright red blood, intermingled with clots. The flow may be stopped for a while, when an enormous, partially decomposed clot is passed with labor-like pains and is followed by a bright red flow. There is a violent, dragging pain in the sacrum shooting and extending from sacrum to the pubis, and going around abdomen down the thighs. Bright-red blood, intermingled with clots coming in gushes, particularly profuse on motion with the characteristic pain.

Cimicifuga—Rheumatic Dysmenorrhœa, the menses being too soon, dark, copious and clotted, starting with severe spasms and cramps of the uterus, which continue all through and become more and more severe as the flow increases. "The more the flow, the greater the pain," with sensitiveness of the uterus and pain in the ovarian region, which shoots upwards and down the anterior surface of thighs and goes across the pelvis with bearing down and tightness around the hips. The mental gloom, nervousness, soreness of the eye-balls, pressing pain of the vertex, hysteric or epileptic spasms of the drug are all intensified during the flow. Also chilly, must be wrapped up (*Pulsatilla*). Leucorrhœa.

Caulophyllum—Neuralgic and Congestive Dysmenorrhœa with spasmodic, irregular and very violent and sharp cramps (*Viburnum Opulus*) especially the first two days of menses ; the pains are of an intermittent character and fly to other parts of the body. Profuse or scanty and light-colored flow with intermittent uterine pains (*Puls.*) and oozing from relaxed, flabby, displaced and passively congested uterus, especially after miscarriage or hasty labor. Profuse and weakening Leucorrhœa of little girls.

FEMALE GENITAL ORGANS—(*Contd.*)

Gelsemium—Neuralgic and Congestive Dysmenorrhœa with sharp, labor-like, bearing down pains extending to back and hips, even down the thighs, with a sensation as if the uterus were squeezed by hand and forced downward. These are associated with a frontal headache with a wild, confused feeling and dim vision and also loss of voice during the menses, which are usually scanty and delayed.

Viburnum Opulus—Spasmodic and Membranous Dysmenorrhœa, with most excruciating cramps and severe bearing down pains, together with drawing pains in anterior muscles of thighs (*Xanthox.*) and sharp shooting pains over ovaries, with great nervousness—cannot sit or lie still—coming on before the menses which are too late and scanty, lasting a few hours and offensive in odor. Thick, white, copious Leucorrhœa, excoriating, with redness, smarting and itching of genitals.

Borax—Membranous Dysmenorrhœa, too soon and too profuse flow with nausea and griping pain in stomach, extending into small of the back and lancinating pains in the groin and stitches in uterus. Profuse Leucorrhœa like white of an egg, perfectly bland but hot, with a sensation as if warm water was flowing, coming on between the menses.

Platinum—Too early and too profuse, long-lasting and often of short duration, dark-clotted or black, like tar, ropy and tenacious menses, with spasms and painful bearing down and sensitive ovaries, esp. the left, with burning pains. Albuminous Leucorrhœa flowing only in the day-time, often without pain or any sensation. The mental hauteur, extreme sensitivensss of the parts preventing coition or digital examination and Nymphomania are ever present.

Palladium—Menses during lactation. Pain and induration of the right ovary, worse from mental agitation from being in society. Transparent jelly-like Leucorrhæa, before and after menses, with shooting pain from navel into pelvis and bearing-down, relieved by rubbing ; cutting pain in uterus, relieved after stool. She likes to be flattered, and keeps up brightly when in company but much exhausted afterwards with aggravation of her pains.

Crocus—Too early, too profuse flow of dark, viscid, stringy blood or black clots, often hanging down in clots in long strings, and associated with a sensation as of something moving around in the abdomen. Foul-smelling, protracted and profuse flow, worse from least movement.

FEMALE GENITAL ORGANS—(*Contd.*)

Murex—Irregular menses, flowing in large clots, profuse and frequent, with intense pain, like something pressing on a sore spot in the pelvis, worse from sitting. Watery, greenish or thick bloody Leucorrhœa, only in day-time. Violent sexual excitement, augmented by least contact of the parts.

Magnesia Carb.—Menses too late and scanty, dark or black, almost like pitch, and washed out with difficulty. The flow is more profuse between the pains and at night or on first rising in the morning, is scanty during the day and even cease altogether in the afternoon and when walking; thin scanty Leucorrhœa, with pinching around umbilicus and itching of pudendum, coming on after the menses and flow more when walking about. The flow is preceded by coryza and sore-throat; neuralgic pains of the teeth and the face come on during the flow, with relief from walking about,

Magnesia Mur.—Painful cramps and spasms of the uterine region with black and pitch-like menses, accompanied by pain in the back when walking and in the thighs when sitting; flows more in the morning and after every stool, which are passed in hard lumps with great difficulty, often crumbling at the anus.

Pulsatilla—Tardy menses. Too late, scanty, thick, dark, clotted, changeable and intermittent, flows by fits and starts, with erratic pains, flying from one place to another and also uterine cramps, compelling her to bend double. Flow more in the day-time and while walking, very little at night. Milky, thin, white mucus or thin, burning, acrid Leucorrhœa with swelling of labia and soreness of pudendum, worse on lying down. Chilliness, nausea, downward pressure, painful, intermittent delayed, scanty and dark menses with pain in the back, and tired, faint feeling together with sad, melancholy, weeping mood, great difficulty of breathing in a warm room and relief from walking slowly about in the cool, open air are the decisive indications.

Cyclamen—Menses profuse, black, membranous, clotted, too frequent and anticipating, flowing less when moving about and more in the evenings, when sitting quiet, with migraine and blindness or fiery spots before the eyes; vertigo, worse walking in open air. A considerable thirst and general aggravation in cool, open air distinguishes *Cyclamen* from *Pulsatilla*.

Lilium Tig.—Menses early, scanty, dark, clotted, offensive; flow only when moving about, followed by abundant and excoriating,

FEMALE GENITAL ORGANS—(*Contd.*)

watery, yellowish or yellowish-brown Leucorrhœa, staining linen brown. Great relaxation of the pelvic organs and bearing down, as if all organs would escape, which forces her to press her hands upon the vulva. Pain in the ovaries, down the thighs and displacements of the uterus of all kinds, with constant urging for stool and urine, the latter with burning and smarting and a great need of some support to hold up the pelvic organs. Along with these, a nervous palpitation with suffocation, worse when lying on the rt. side ; also sadness and a sense of hurry with inability to do anything.

Sepia—The general symptoms are of utmost importance. Flushes of heat, over face and head, ascending from pelvic organs with anxiety, faintness and perspiration over the whole body ; great sadness, weeping and indifference ; headache, in terrific shocks, at every term with scanty flow, yellow saddle across the upper part of the cheeks and nose ; painful emptiness in the epigastrium, relieved by eating ; constipation ; fœtid, very offensive urine. When these are present *Sepia* is the remedy for irregular menses of every form—early, scanty, profuse, Amenorrhœa or Menorrhagia, associated with prolapsus of uterus and vagina ; pressure and bearing down, as if everything would protrude from pelvis, must cross limbs tightly to prevent ; violent stitches upward in the vagina from uterus to umbilicus. Profuse yellowish green or milky, offensive and excoriating Leucorrhœa, with darting pains in the cervix which is indurated, and the uterus also retroverted, prolapsed, enlarged and indurated. Sexual intercourse hardly endurable with a decided aversion there-to.

Natrum Mur.—Decided increase of sadness before menses which are too late, too short and scanty, or too early and profuse, flowing day and night ; dark ; fluttering palpitation and throbbing headache which persists even after the period ; pressure and pushing towards genitals from relaxation of ligaments and prolapsus uteri, particularly when she gets up in the morning —must sit down to prevent prolapsus. Profuse, thick, white, transparent and acrid Leucorrhœa with itching and smarting of vulva ; cutting in the neck of bladder or urethra after urinating ; backache relieved by lying flat on the back or by firm support. Pain in the small of the back as if broken ; paralysed feeling in lumbar region, worse morning after rising. In the generals it is almost similar to *Sepia*, which it complements.

FEMALE GENITAL ORGANS—(*Contd.*).

Secale—Passive hæmorrhage in feeble, cachectic women, with burning pains in uterus and a continuous oozing of thin, black, watery, fluid blood, continuing until next period. The flow comes in gushes and is always accompanied by strong bearing down pains, great prostration, pinched look, coldness—but cannot bear to be covered. The Leucorrhœa is green, brown and offensive. Thin, dark, sanious discharge from morbid growths in the uterus.

Carbo Animalis—Menses too early, not too profuse but last too long, causing great exhaustion, with stretching and yawning and a goneness of the stomach not relieved by eating. She is so weak even with a moderate flow, that she can hardly speak. Menorrhagia from chronic induration of the uterus ; also in cachectic women with glandular affections, carcinoma, etc. Blood black, clotted, putrid. Watery, burning, acrid, offensive Leucorrhœa when walking or standing, staining linen yellow.

Carbo Veg.—Great weakness and relaxation of the genitalia. The uterus drags down so that she cannot stand on her feet. There is a persistent hæmorrhage of a low type with slow, and continuous oozing of dark, even black and putrid blood, with small clots, due to uterine atony. Burning pains in chest and difficult breathing—wants to be fanned ; burning of the hands and soles of feet. Profuse, thin, foul and acrid Leucorrhœa or bloody mucus, excoriating the pudenda.

Kali Carb.—Too late and too scanty or too early, too copious, too long or too late, too profuse menses ; pale, acrid, fœtid, excoriating the parts it comes in contact and covering them with eruptions. Continued oozing after abortion, after curetting. At the menstrual period the flow is clotted and then after prolonged menstruation she settles back into a state of oozing until next month, and this goes on repeating. There is a troublesome backache, which makes walking difficult and is relieved by lying down. (*Natr. Mur.* is relieved by lying flat on back, with firm pressure).

Thuja—Inflammation, with pain in the left ovary, coming on at the time of menstruation and continuing during the flow and going down the thighs. Severe pain in the left ovary and left inguinal region increasing as the flow comes on, as if parts were being torn out, makes her cry aloud. Worse when walking, must sit or lie down. The menses are too early too scanty and too short and the Leucorrhœa is profuse, thick and greenish, running from one menstrual period to the other.

FEMALE GENITAL ORGANS—(*Contd.*)

Apis—Menses too scanty, irregular, lasting but one or two days, with sharp, burning, stinging pains and extreme soreness in the right ovarian region, before and during menstruation and worse from heat. When walking she is compelled to bend forward ; painful, dark, scanty urine. Menstruation delayed or suppressed ; sensation as if they were coming on ; sharp, stabbing pain in uterus at every period. Hæmorrhage from uterus coming on one week after menses, with profuse flow of blood. Acrid, profuse, green or yellowish Leucorrhœa.

Arg. Met.—Hard, indurated, cystic ovaries, especially the left. Prolapsus, with pain in the left ovary ; neck of the uterus very much swollen, spongy, deeply corroded with ulcers in different directions and congested, indurated and ulcerated cervix with burning, stinging pains, and copious, putrid, ichorous, yellowish-green bloody discharge and sometimes bloody water, with unbearable stench. Horribly offensive Leucorrhœa.

Arg. Nit.—Cutting pain in right ovarian region and back, radiating to thighs. Metrorrhagia, too soon and too copious, with thick coagulated blood. Violent palpitation, with faintish nausea. The nervous excitements and Hysterical manifestations of the drug are aggravated during the menstrual period, the patient being free from symptoms during the interim. Profuse Leucorrhœa of yellow corroding, bloody mucus with prolapsus and ulceration of os or cervix ; coition painful, followed by bleeding from vagina.

Aurum Met.—Menses too late and scanty ; uterus prolapsed and indurated ; Leucorrhœa thick, white. Menstrual and uterine affections with great Melancholia and suicidal tendency, worse at menstrual period.

Aurum Mur.—Enlargement and great hardness of uterus, cervix indurated. Chronic Metritis and prolapsus. Menses frequent, profuse, and excoriating ; copious, yellow, Leucorrhœa ; ulceration of the cervix ; heat, burning and itching of the vagina and labia. *Aurum Muriaticum Natronatum* is more preferable for the above conditions.

Graphites—Left ovary swollen, hard and indurated, with violent pains on touch, inspiration or hawking ; when most violent pains shoot in it. The uterus is displaced, with the os flung far back, pressing upon the posterior wall of the vagina. Menses too late, too scanty, of too short duration and too pale, The Leucorrhœa is quite profuse, watery and excoriating,

FEMALE GENITAL ORGANS—(*Contd.*).

Decided averion to coitus. Adapted to women who are anæmic, though obese, constantly cold, constipated, and are subject to rough herpetic condition of the skin.

Lachesis—Induration and enlargement of ovaries, especially the left. The uterine region is very senstive to the slightest touch ; pains in the ovaries and uterus, going from left to right. Menstrual pains increase violently until relieved by the flow. The flow intermits and during the intermission, violent pain in left ovary or headache. Delayed, scanty, acrid, highly offensive, and intermittent menses, with Leucorrhœa several days before, stiffening linen and leaving a greenish stain. Abrasion of os ; cervix very sensitive to touch and bleeds. Flushes of heat in day-time and chillls at night. All sufferings are worse before and after the flow, with amelioration during the flow.

Lycopodium—Sharp, shooting pains extending from right to left ovarian region (*Lachcs.* and *Lil. T.*—opposite direction). Menses too profuse, too long ; flow partly black, clotted or bright red or watery, with labor-like pain, and reappearing after 6 or 8 days. Dryness in vagina, with burning and painful coition. Bearing down pains, as if menses would appear. Itching and burning at vulva. Discharge of blood from genitals during every stool. Profuse, corroding Leucorrhœa and discharge of flatus from vagina.

Bromium—Constant dull pain with swelling, hardness and induration of the left ovary, worse before and during menses which are premature ; profuse flow of bright red blood or passive flow. Membranous Dysmenorrhœa with violent contractive pain and loud emission of large quantities of flatus from vagina.

Lac Caninum—Severe congestion and inflammation of the one or the other of the ovaries, especially the right, before menses, with extreme soreness and tenderness which makes every motion, even breath, painful. Parenchymatous Metritis ; flow of bright red and stringy blood, hot as fire, coming in gushes and clotting easily, with constant bearing down pain, as if everything would come out of vulva; and sharp, lancinating pains, like knives cutting upwards from os uteri, followed by a sensation of needles, darting upwards in uterus. Severe pain in the entire region, with profuse yellow, brown and bloody Leucorrhœa, two weeks after menses. Sharp pains in right ovary, completely ameliorated by a flow of bright red blood, which lasted an hour, and did not return.

FEMALE GENITAL ORGANS—(*Contd.*)

Escape of flatus from vagina. Leucorrhœa, very profuse during day, none at night, worse standing or walking. Breasts sore and sensitive to pressure during menses (*Conium, Calc. C.*).

Krerosote—Too early and profuse menses, lasting too long. Metrorrhagia, which inclines to be intermittent, at times almost ceasing and then commencing again. Large, dark, offensive clots and bloody ichor discharged, with sharp stitches darting from abdomen into vagina ; the flow is more profuse when lying down and ceases on sitting or walking about. Violent abdominal spasms, worse after too copious and long-lasting menses. Acrid, corrosive and offensive Leucorrhœa with itching, biting, smarting and burning in pudendum, between labia and thighs, and stitches from above downwards, causing her to start ; has the odor of green corn, stiffens like starch, stains the linen yellow. Strong desire for coition with bloody ichorous discharge after. All complaints worse after menses.

Ustilago—Vascular system of the ovaries is most powerfully affected, producing much congestion, enlargement and great irritation, with Ovaralgia, Dysmenorrhœa and especially Menorrhagia. Ovaries are inflamed, irritable, sensitive and swollen, with constant burning distress and pain from the left ovary to uterus ; often a sharp pain cutting like knives, shoots around the hip down the legs with great rapidity, and makes walking painful—has to limp. Uterus is hypertrophied, prolapsed ; cervix swollen, sensitive, spongy, bleeds when touched. Oozing of dark blood, highly coagulated, forming long, black, stringy clots with extreme pain during the period, which is rather too early. Menses profuse, too long-lasting, come in gushes of bright red blood, especially when rising from a seat, but more frequently dark, clotted, fetid and stringy blood. Discharge of blood on the slightest provocation. Excessive bearing down, as if everything would come through. Sometimes scanty menstruation with all the pains ; suppression of menses without apparent cause. Yellow, offensive, mild or excoriating, albuminous Leucorrhœa. Pale, thin, weak, very nervous subjects.

Xanthoxylum—Menses early, profuse and painful ; scanty or retarded ; grinding pain in pelvis, worse left side, extending down the thigh, along genito-crural nerves. Neuralgic Dysmenorrhœa with agonizing bearing down, as if everything would be pushed out. Backache as if broken, pain starting in iljac

FEMALE GENITAL ORGANS—(*Contd.*)

crest and shooting down into knees, with no relief in any position. Great increase of Leucorrhœa during the time when menses should appear. Neurasthenic patients who are thin, emaciated ; poor assimilation with insomnia and occipital headache.

Zincum—Inflammation and boring pain in left ovary, relieved by pressure and during menses, when all her complaints generally disappear. Too early and profuse menses especially at night, and when walking, when lumps and clots pass off ; also too late or suppressed menses. All complaints are associated with restlessness, depression, coldness, spinal tenderness and restless feet. As soon as flow appears there is relief of all symptoms like *Lachesis*, but in the latter the sufferings all return when the flow stops. *Cimicifuga* is opposite, having pain so long as there is flow, ceasing when the flow intermits and returnig when the flow appears again.

GASTRIC DISORDERS

[GASTRALGIA—GASTRITIS—ETC.]

Aconite—Beginning of inflammatory processes within the abdomen from exposure, sudden chilling of the stomach from drinking ice-water, with sharp, shooting pain and the high fever, anxiety and restlessness of the drug. Abdomen swollen, tender ; pressure in stomach ; repeated vomiting of bitter, bilious fluid or of blood ; forced to bend double but with no relief.

Alumina—Dyspepsia with deficiency of gastric juice ; dryness and constriction of œsophagus with difficulty in swallowing food, tingling of the tongue, heart-burn ; mouth dry ; potatoes disagree ; aversion to meat and craving for undigestible things. Sensitiveness of liver with stitching pains ; subborn constipation from inertia and dryness of rectum ; piles itch and burn.

Anacardium—"Great relief by eating" is characteristic. Its nervous sinking feeling or a dull pain in stomach extending to the spine or even violent Gastralgia, are all relieved by eating, but they all come again about 2 hours after eating. There is urging for stool which passes away when attempt is made, due to powerlessness of the rectum, hence

GASTRIC DISORDERS—(*Contd.*)

constipation. It has proved of great value in Duodenitis when prescribed on its modality.

Antim. Crud.—Gastric catarrh from cold or improper food, with white-coated tongue, nausea, vomiting as soon as he eats or drinks ; also vomiting from overloading the stomach with indigestible substances, fat food, acids, etc., or from excessive heat of summer ; vomiting of food or curdled milk ; loss of appetite, colic. Diarrhœa or Constipation.

Antim. Tart.—Continuous nausea, vomiting. Diarrhœa with foul eructations, yawning and drowsiness ; vomiting, green and watery, sometimes frothy and containing food ; violent straining to vomit with perspiration on forehead, coldness of the surface, hands and feet cold like ice, thirstless or drinking little and often.

Argentum Nitricum—Gnawing, ulcerative pain at the pit of the stomach, radiating in every direction, worse from food ; enormous distension with flatulence, relieved by belching up of flatus in enormous volume after long effort : nausea, retching, and vomiting of glairy mucus ; great longing for sugar but worse from sweets, producing Diarrhœa ; gastric ulcer, with gnawing pain, worse from pressure and immediately after eating ; these pains seem to increase and decrease gradually.

Arsenicum.--Inflammation, from slight irritation to the most destructive Gastritis and Enteritis. Burning pains in the stomach ; mouth dry, tongue white, as if white washed, or red with raised papillæ ; intense thirst, but drinks little, with vomiting as soon as taken ; distressing heart-burn and extreme tenderness of the pit, anxiety, restlessness, fear of death. Diarrhœa of undigested stool with violent tenesmus and burning of rectum, prostration, cold hippocratic face, cold extremities ; after abuse of ice, spoiled meat or sausages, Alcoholic excess, lobster, salads, etc.

Asafœtida—Enormous meteorism and violent Gastralgia with gurgling and rolling of wind which escapes upwards with great difficulty, none downwards ; burning of stomach and œsophagus and pulsation in the pit ; great disgust for food with difficult rancid eructations and spasmodic tightness of the chest ; sensation as if a ball started from stomach rose into the throat ; an empty, gone feeling in stomach at 11 A.M. Hysterical patients.

Belladonna—Spasmodic pain in the epigastrium, as if clutched by a hand, worse during a meal ; stitching pains, running towards the spine—must bend backwards and hold breath ; spasms of stomach, spasmodic hiccough ; abdomen tender, swollen, distended, hot—transverse colon protudes like a pad ; extreme sensitiveness to touch, to bed-clothes, to jar to pressure ; loss of appetite, aversion to water, dread of drinking, uncontrollable vomiting.

GASTRIC DISORDERS—(*Contd.*)

Bismuth—Gastralgia with burning, griping pains, going through to the spiue ; feeling of a load ; better from cold drinks, but water is vomited as soon as it reaches the stomach ; vomits all fiuids.

Bryonia—Pains, soon after taking food, which seems to lie like a stone in the stomach ; sharp, cutting pains extend to shoulders and back ; stomach sensitive to touch ; complexion yellow, mouth dry, taste bitter ; constipation and frontal headache, white-coated tongue ; stitching pains, extending to chest, worse from motion ; brought on by summer heat, on taking cold water after being heated or from vegetable food.

Cadmium Sulph.—Burning, cutting pains ; burning in stomach, extending up into œsophagus ; everything sour ; fluids burn all the way, up into the mouth and throat, and come up sour, mixed with blood or bile, with great prostration and tenderness over pit of the stomach ; distressing nausea and vomiting of yellowish-green mucus. Black vomit ; Carcinoma.

Calcarea Carb.—Cutting in the abdomen, which is hard and distended with incarcerated flatus ; pit of the stomach tender, cannot bear tight clothing around the waist ; milk disagrees ; sour eructations, sour vomiting ; loss of appetite, craving for indigestible things ; worse while eating. Hyperchlorhydria.

Cantharis—Violent burning in the stomach with severe colic ; vomiting of blood-streaked membrane, with violent retching ; burning thirst with aversion to all fluids ; drinking increases pain in bladder, and is vomited;

Carbo Veg.—Patient below par. Excessive flatulency with tendency to Diarrhœa. Violent spasmodic contraction in epigastric region, better by sour, rancid, putrid eructations and flatus per anus, which is offensive, moist and burning ; worse in warm sultry weather ; worse from fat, fish, oysters, ice-cream ; milk increases flatulence. Violent burning in the stomach, chest, abdomen, with crampy pain, forcing to bend double. Useful for effects of over-eating, eating tainted meats. etc., and where digestion is slow and food putrifies before it digests.

Chamomilla—Wind colic, abdomen distended like a drum ; tongue coated yellowish-white, bitter taste , irritable. Colic after anger.

Chelidonium—Aching, gnawing pain in stomach or constrictive pain, worse from pressure ; better by eating, by hot milk. Nausea, Constipation or Diarrhœa ; icterus and the characteristic pai*n* under lower border of rt. scapula.

China.—Dyspepsia from loss of animal fluids. Extreme slowness of digestion with pressure and cramps of stomach after eating ; constant

GASTRIC DISORDERS – (*contd.*).

satiety, yet can eat, but feels worse afterwards. Enormous flatulence, but belching does not relieve. Weak, sinking sensation at the pit of the stomach, relieved by eating, but gets an urging to stool after meals.

Colchicum—Appetite for different things, but as soon as sees or smells food, he shudders from nausea and is unable to take anything. Violent retching followed by copious forcible vomiting of food, and then of bile, renewed by every motion and kept at abeyance by lying quietly. Cold feeling in the stomach ; intolerance of clothing ; burning in the stomach ; vomiting, purging, offensive flatus, offensive Diarrhœa ; exhaustion.

Colocynth—Acute Gastritis. Violent, cutting, tearing pains, from different parts of chest and abdomen concentrate in pit of stomach with constant inclination to vomit ; better from hard pressure, bending double ; caused by vexation and indignation or after taking cold.

Dioscorea—Sharp pain in epigastrium, relieved by standing erect ; pain suddenly shifts and appears in remote parts, as fingers and toes; pain radiates from abdomen to back, chest, arms; worse bending forwards and while lying ; better walking about and bending backwards.

Ferrum Met.— Gastralgia with a heavy pressure in the stomach after every meal ; vomiting immediately after eating ; painless and involuntary Diarrhœa, immediately after eating ; food has no taste.

Graphites—Gartralgia with burning, crampy, colicky pain, relieved by eating, drinking especially hot milk, and lying down. Abdomen distended, with extreme tenderness to the pressure of clothing after eating ; sweet things nauseate and disgust the patient. Obstinate constipation ; piles ; fissures of anus.

Hepar Sulph.—Atonic Dyspepsia. Hunger—a gnawing, empty feeling in the forenoon, relieved by eating but cannot bear any pressure upon epigastrium after eating. Liability to derangement of stomach in spite of the most careful diet ; longing for strong tasting substances.

Hydrastis—Atonic Dyspepsia. Great lassitude, obstinate constipation , bitter taste ; gone feeling in stomach ; bread or vegetables disagree ; weakness of digestion with heavy, hard, thumping and fulness of chest and dyspnœa. Gastro-duodenal catarrh.

Hyoscyamus—Burning and inflammation of stomach with vomiting of blood ; incoherent speech, stupor, insensible to the state of his situation.

Ignatia—Dyspepsia from mental depression. Empty retching, relieved by eating ; all gone feeling and sinking in stomach, relieved by taking a deep breath ; paroxysms of cramps in stomach and stitching in the sides of abdomen.

GASTRIC DISORDERS—(*Contd.*).

Ipecac.—Gastric derangement from rich mixed food, fruits, ice-cream, etc. Clutching pains, going from left to right with constant deathly nausea, easy vomiting ; tongue clean or not coated.

Iris Versi.—Great burning distress in epigastrium ; shocks of colicky pains every few minutes in the umbilicus. Nausea, straining and belching of wind. Diarrhœa, burning at anus ; burning of œsophagus ; sick headache with blur before eyes.

Kali Bichrom.—Gastritis ; malignant disease of the stomach. Stomach swells up immediately after eating ; vomiting, sour or bitter, is renewed by every attempt at eating or drinking and is associated with a great deal of distress and burning rawness about stomach. Round, perforating ulcer of the stomach.

Kreosote—Deep and lasting disgust for food in convalescence from severe diseases ; food is thrown up undigested after several hours ; great and constant nausea, with tendency to vomit ; painful hard spots at or near the left of stomach ; water tastes bitter ; worse from cold, better from warm food.

Lachesis—Gnawing pain, relieved after eating, but soon a heavy pressure as from a weight in the stomach and other symptoms of indigestion show themselves. Abdomen bloated, sensitive to touch about waist ; constant tormenting urging in rectum, but not for stool.

Laurocerasus—Violent contractive and cutting pain in stomach ; burning or coldness in stomach and abdomen ; green, liquid, mucous stools ; suffocative spells.

Lycopodium.—Atonic Dyspepsia of weakly persons ; intestinal flatulent Dyspepsia. Hungry, but a few mouthfuls fill him up ; incarcerated flatus, causing bloating, distension and asthmatic symptoms with pains, shooting across from right to left ; worse from 4 to 8 P. M. Sensitiveness of gastric region only after a meal (*Lach.*—all the time).

Nux Vom.—Griping, clawing pains in stomach, relieved by hot drinks ; vomiting of food and of sour matter with violent retching. Gastralgia, radiating to the back, every morning, with vomiting and ineffectual urging to stool ; worse 2 hours after eating ; tongue coated posteriorly. Pyrosis, acid eructations, squeezing around waist ; headache in the morning ; sour taste.

Ornithogalum—Painful contraction of the pylorus with duodenal distension ; agonising feeling in chest and stomach, starting from pylorus, with flatus that rolls in balls from one side to the other ; loss of appetite, phlegmy retchings and loss of flesh. Pains increase when food passes pyloric outlet ; vomiting of cofee-ground-looking matter ; tongue coated.

GASTRIC DISORDERS—(*contd.*).

Petroleum—Severe pains in stomach radiating to chest with sweat and nausea ; always relieved by taking food ; tendency to Diarrhœa and vomiting. Diarrhœa during day-time, never at night, with colic before and hunger after stool.

Phosphorus—Cutting, burning pains and severe pressure in stomach after eating, with vomiting of food ; cramps in stomach ; unquenchable thirst. Hæmatemesis, better from drinking cold water. Regurgitation of food by mouthfuls, without nausea ; cold water is thrown up as soon as it gets warm in stomach.

Plumbum—Contraction in œsophagus and stomach ; excessive colic, radiating to all parts of body ; abdominal wall feels drawn by a string to the spine ; pain causes desire to stretch ; abdomen retracted. Obstructed flatus, with intense colic. Constipation —hard lumpy stools.

Ptelea—Griping in epigastric region with dryness of mouth ; constant sensation of corrosion, heat and burning in stomach ; stomach feels empty after eating. Retraction of abdomen ; tongue coated white or yellow, with red and prominent papillæ ; excess of saliva with bitter taste.

Pulsatilla—Pain, as from sub-cutaneous ulceration, an hour after eating ; great tightness in abdomen after a meal, must loosen clothing, and relieved by eating again. Sensation as of a lump in mid-sternum, as if food were lying there (*China* ; also *Abies*—hard-boiled-egg sensation). Bitter, sour, putrid eructations, or tasting of the ingesta ; regurgitation of the ingesta. Heart-burn, water-brush, accumulation of thick mucus in mouth ; diminished taste of and aversion to all food, especially warm ; aggravation after ice-cream, pastry, anything that is fatty and greasy. Erratic pains in chest with gastric symptoms. Colic, with chilliness, in the evening ; tongue coated with a thick, rough, white fur.

Sepia—Atonic Dyspepsia, in women suffering from portal stagnation or incidental to uterine diseases. Pain in stomach and abdomen after simple food ; tongue coated white ; taste sour, putrid ; all gone sensation in the pit of the stomach, not relieved by eating (similar to *Carbo Ani.* ; with *Anacardium, Nat. Carb.*, Nux and *Sulphur*, it is always better after meals). Nausea at smell or sight of food. Everything eaten tastes too salty. Sensitiveness of the pit of the stomach and a band of pain encircling hypochondria, with bloatedness of the abdomen ; tongue coated and often sore and covered with little blisters on edges and tip. Aversion to household duties. Worse forenoon and evening.

Stannum—Cardialgia with a cramp-like colic around the navel and a sinking gone feeling in the epigastrium. The pains increase and decrease

GASTRIC DISORDERS—(*Contd.*)

gradually and are better by hard pressure and walking about, which proves to be very fatiguing. Nausea and vomiting, in the morning, or excited by the odor of cooking (like *Colchi.*).

Staphisagria—Colic after anger. Severe pain following an abdominal operation ; sensation as if the stomach were hanging down relaxed, with a great desire for stimulants. Canine hunger, even when the stomach is full.

Uranium Nit.—Gastric and duodenal ulcers ; boring pain in pyloric region ; abdomen bloated ; excessive thirst, nausea, vomiting ; ravenous appetite.

GLANDS—DISEASES OF

Alumina—Inguinal glands : Bubo—Gonorrhœal, with yellowish discharge and burning and itching of the urethra.

Apis—Inflammation of glands ; with induration of cellular tissues ; the affected part pits on pressure.

Ars. Iod.—Axillary, inguinal or sub-maxillary glands—inflamed, with threatening suppuration.

Belladonna—Inflammation of glands and lymphatics. Heat, redness and swelling, with induration ; cervical, axillary or inguinal glands. When suppuration is inevitable it should give place to *Hepar* or *Merc. Sol.*

Badiaga—Mal-treated and indurated Buboes ; Syphilitic (also *Carbo Animalis* ; *Alumina*—Gonorrhœal).

Baryta Carb.—Inflammation of tonsils and formation of pus with enlargement of glands—in the neck, under the jaw and behind the ears, especially in the children who are backward mentally and physically ; every little exposure to damp or cold weather settles on the tonsils, with difficulty of deglutition, especially on empty swallowing.

Baryta Mur.—Painful swelling of glands, tonsils, the right parotid and the sub-maxillary glands, which are very hard and indurated. *Baryta Iod.* for chronic enlargements of tonsils with tumefaction of cervical glands and stunted growth.

Bromium—Scrofulous enlargement of the glands every where, with induration and great hardness and less tendency to suppurate, but if suppuration occurs, the hardness of the gland around the opening

GLANDS, DISEASES OF—(*Contd.*)

remains, with acrid discharge—Tuberculosis of the glands. (Comp. *Carbo. Animalis*).

Calc. Carb.—Scrofulous enlargement of lymphatic glands of the neck, axilla, etc., especially in *Calcarea*-children with Otorrhœa and hardness of hearing. Tuberculosis of the mesenteric glands.

Calc. Fluor.—Chronic induration of cervical glands with stony hardness ; also chronic hypertrophy of the tonsils.

Calc. Iod.—Enlarged tonsils, with little crypts or pockets ; also glands of the neck, in flabby children subject to colds.

Calc. Phos.—Like *Calc. Carb.* Tabes Mesenterica, with fetid Diarrhœa and Marasmus, in scrofulous and psoric constitutions.

Carbo Animalis—Buboes, Syphilitic or Gonorrhœal, hard as stone. Useful when they are opened too soon, leaving the surrounding tissue stony hard. Hard, indurated mammary glands (*Bromine*) studded with little nodes of stony hardness, with burning pains running from the breasts through to the axilla—with hard and indurated glands in the axilla ; Mammary Cancer (also *Carbo Veg.*).

Chamomilla—Induration of the mammæ of new-born babies ; also of children.

Cistus Canadensis—Malignant disease of the glands of neck and submaxillary glands, with caries of the jaw ; glands inflamed, indurated and ulcerated ; an impure breath is an indication.

Conium—Glands enlarged, stony hard, with little or no pain. Useful in the beginning of Carcinoma. Especially indicated after injuries to glands—mammary, axillary, testicles—when they become hard and indurated.

Graphites—Scrofulous swelling of cervical and lymphatic glands, with pain and sensitiveness, in patients who look fat, but are not healthy, with rough, harsh, dry skin and a tendency to Eczema and to take cold easily.

Heper Sulph.—Buboes and enlarged glands— at the stage of suppuration.

Silicea.—Inflamed suppurating glands with fistulous openings (*Calc. Fluor.*, *Fluoric Acid*) ; also scrofulous indurations and swelling of the glands.

Mercurius.—Inflmmation of the glands with emaciation in scrofulous and Syphilitic patients : sub-maxillary, axillary, and parotid glands.—Comes in after *Bell.* and *Rhus Tox.* Very efficacious in Syphilitic Buboes at the stage of suppuration. *Merc. Iod.*, when the Bubo has become indolent, with little or no pain—

GLANDS, DISEASES OF—(*Contd.*).

no tendency to suppuration or to heal. The action of *Iodium* seems to have been intensified in *Merc. Iod.*

Iodium—Large, hard and usually painless glands, about the neck or anywhere, which are torpid and sluggish, with indolent swellings. The mammary glands atrophy. Tabes Masenterica, with great emaciation, ravenous appetite and mental irritability. Better in the open air ; worse in warm room. Goitre.

Kali Bichrom.—Swelling of the parotid gland with sharp, shooting pain from the ear to the gland.

Kali Iod.—Glands swollen, ulcerated, atrophied ; Goitre. Bronchial and sub-maxillary glands. Buboes after the abuse of *Mercury*—or with Scrofula.

Lachesis—Swelling of the glands about the neck and of the lymphatics with a dark, purplish hue, threatening suppuration—in Diphtheria.

Lapis Albus—Chronic glandular swellings in scrofulous children with enlargement of mesenteric glands. The glands have a certain amount of elasticity and pliability rather than stony hardness. Enlarged and indurated cervical glands and Goitre, with Anæmia and increased appetite.

Mercurius—See under *Hepar Sulph.*

Nitric Acid—Mercuro Syphilitic inflammatory swelling and suppuration of inguinal and axillary glands.

Phosphorus—Fistulæ in the glands with thin, purulent, ichorous discharge (*Silicea, Fluor. Acid, Calc. Fluor.*).

Phytolacca—Excellent in its action on the mammary glands with a tendency to cake and threatening suppuration.

Rhus Tox.—Swollen, hot, painful glands. Erysipelatous swelling of glands and surrounding tissues, with a tendency to suppuration ; after strains and sprains.

Silicea—See under *Hepar Sulphur.*

Spongia—Goitre, hard and large with suffocative attacks. Hardness and swelling of testicles from checked Gonorrhœa and scrofulous induration and swelling of cervical glands with tension and pain on touch and motion.

Sulphur—Scrofulous glandular enlargement of the inguinal, axillary, sub-maxillary and sub-cutaneous glands in typical *Sulphur*-subjects.

Syphilinum—Glands in different parts of body, especially about the neck enlarged, indurated and painful. Hodgkin's disease : enormous swelling of glands of head and neck (Kent).

GONORRHŒA

Aconite—Inflammatory stage ; hot, burning, red and clear or bloody urine, passed with difficulty. The mental state of the remedy must be present.

Ferrum Phos.—Inflammatory stage, with heat in the urethra and scanty, watery or mucous discharge, also hæmorrhage ; troublesome nightly erections, chordee (*Acon.*).

Gelsemium—Inflammatory stage, with great urethral soreness and burning, slight whitish discharge and severe erections. Gonorrhœal Rheumatism and Orchitis.

Cannabis Indica—First stage, with chordee and increased sexual desire ; yellow discharge and frequent urination with burning, stinging in urethra before, during and after.

Cannabis Sativa—Comes in after *Aconite* when the disease has localised itself with thin, yellow, purulent discharge and smarting and burning on urination and chordee. Soreness of the urethra and prepuce, which is greatly swollen, to touch, so that the patient walks slowly with legs stretched apart.

Argentum Nit.—Follows *Cannabis Sat.* when the discharge becomes thick, purulent, more profuse, with cutting pains extending to the anus, when urinating.

Cantharis—When the inflammation has spread to the bladder with intense tenesmus ; urine scalds him and is passed drop by drop, with extreme pain and intolerable tenesmus ; the entire urethral canal scalds and burns before, during and after micturition ; urine is often mixed with blood and the discharge is yellow or bloody muco-pus. *Murcurius Sol.* and *Cor.*—follow *Cantharis*, when the discharge becomes worse at night and is green and purulent. *Merc. Cor.* causes more violent tenesmus, burning and swelling, and is very similar to *Cantharis*, while *Merc. Sol.* has more burning and smarting between the acts of micturition similar to *Cannabis Sativa* but differs from the latter in the character of the discharge. *Cantharis* gives place to *Cannabis Indica* when the chordee is well-marked.

Capsicum—White cream-like or thick, purulent, yellow discharge, with stitches and burning in the urethra between the acts of micturition ; excessive sensitiveness of the parts. Old cases, in those who have no endurance and are plump, flabby and sensitive to cold.

GONORRHŒA—(*Contd.*)

Chimaphilla—Urethritis, with purulent or bloody, ropy discharge and stricture, the stream being split or urine passing only in drops ; must strain before the flow comes.

Clematis—Formation of stricture ; urine flows by fits and starts ; has to wait a long time for the urine to come, then passes only a few drops with the most severe pain and burning along the urethra, which feels like a cord, painful on pressure, and at the glans penis, followed by a full, painless stream. Gonorrhœal Orchitis, with much painful swelling and stony hardness, and sensitiveness of the rt. cord. Often useful after the failure of *Puls.* to finish the cure.

Copaiva—Thin stream ; itching, biting, burning and great pain when urine reaches glans penis ; thin, milky discharge or large amount of viscid mucus or blood and mucus in the urine ; violet smell of urine.

Cubeba—See under *Pulsatilla*.

Digitalis—Strangury and frequent urging, especially when standing or sitting ; burning in the urethra with thick, bright yellow, purulent discharge : glans penis inflamed, with copious thick pus over its surface and the prepuce is puffed up and infiltrated with serum ; violent erections, chordee. It will do no good if the prepuce is indurated, but *Sulphnr* will.

Merc. Cor.—Has inflammation of the prepuce, dark purplish in color and less œdema than *Digi.* and the glans, hot and painful to touch, is dark red in appearance. Discharge is greenish, especially at night. Phimosis or Para-phimosis (also *Merc. Sol.*, *Canth.*, *Nit. Acid.*).

Pulsatilla—Ripe Gonorrhœa without much pain ; thick, bland, yellow, or more characteristically, yellowish-green discharge. Gonorrhœal Orchitis, from suppression, with sharp, dragging pains in the cord. *Puls.* restors the discharge and relieves the pain. But if the glands remain indurated and "hard as stone" in spite of *Puls.* then *Clematis* finishes it up.

Cubeba—Profuse, thick, yellowish-green discharge with burning and cutting still remaining after the first stage (*Puls.* is painless and bland.)

Hydrastis—Copious and persistently thick, yellow or green discharge without pain or soreness of urethra. The discharge is tenacious and here it is like *Kali Bich.*, which has a sensation after urinating, as if a drop remained far back in the urethra, which burns and worries him with fruitless effort to expel.

Argent. Met.—Old, stubborn cases with thick, yellow discharge without any pain or soreness; great hardness and inflammation of

GONORRHŒA—(*Contd.*)

the right testicle with crushing pain ; clothing increases pain on walking (same with *Arg. Nit.*).

Hamamelis—Orchitis, testicles swollen and extremely painful to touch, worse after mid-night.

Nat. Mur.—Is useful in Chronic Gonorrhœa with gleety discherge of clear or yellow pus and cutting in the urethra after urinating.

Nat. Sulph.—Cures obstinate cases ; loss of sensitiveness of penis and thick, yellowish or greenish discharge.

Kali. Sulph.—Advanced stage, with green or yellow, thick or thin and viscid discharge, with burning during urination, at the meatus.

Lithium Carb.—Thick and profuse greenish-yellow discharge alternating with Hæmaturia.

Petroleum—Useful in that "last drop". White or yellow discharge with great itching in the posterior half of the urethra and here it is similar to *Petroselinum*, which has, moreover, a sudden irresistible urge to urinate along with troublesome tickling and itching in urethra and pain at root of penis.

Medorrhinum—Often useful for chronic ailments due to suppressed Gonorrhœa and brings it back even after years in the form of Chronic Gleet and finally cures without treatment or by some other indicated remedy. Also used for profuse, yellow, purulent discharge, most copious in the morning, gumming up the orifice.

Sulphur.—Thick and purulent or thin, watery, gleety discharge with burning and smarting and bright-redness of the lips of the meatus. Phimosis, prepuce inflamed and indurated (**Digi.**—not indurated).

Sepia—Chronic mucous discharge without any pain and burning ; milky or yellowish discharge ; urine turbid and offensive.

Thuja—Lingering cases with prostatic complications. Gleet. Condylomata. Prostatic affections ; discharge thin and greenish ; red spots and erosions on the glans ; sudden stitches along the urethra from back to front or a sensation as if a drop of urine were passing along the urethra with cutting pains and forked stream of urine.

HEART, AFFECTIONS OF THE

Aconite—Cardiac congestion ; hyperæmia preceding Peri-carditis or Endo-carditis with fever, mental anxiety, oppression, palpitation, worse walking ; stitches, preventing erect posture or deep inspiration. Angina Pectoris, with intense pain down left arm, with numbness and tingling in fingers. Uncomplicated hypertrophy. Fears he will drop dead in the street.

> **Bromium**—In uncomplicated hypertrophy without valvular lesion, similar to *Aconite* but without its fear and anxiety. Also *Arnica* and *Rhus Tox.*—from over-exertion.

Anacardium.—Rheumatic Peri-carditis with double stitches, palpitation, weak memory ; coryza in the aged.

Apis—Cardiac inflammation and Dropsy, Hydro-thorax ; unable to lie down ; as if could not draw another breath ; feeling as though going to die, but no fear of death like *Aconite.* Peri-carditis, with sudden stinging pains, dyspnœa, and restlessness which is not of *Arsenic* type, but only a fidgety restlessness and anxiety.

Argentum Nitricum—Constant cardiac anxiety ; violent palpitation and throbbing through whole body from slightest emotion, worse in horizontal position ; better when walking fast.

Arsenic—Later stages ; Endo-carditis, Peri-carditis, Angina Pectoris ; after suppression of Measles, Scarlatina ; from sepsis, fatty degeneration of blood-vessels. Insufficiency of aortic valves—præcordial anxiety, oppression, palpitation, restlessness and œdema, puffiness of eyes, swelling of feet ; great thirst, drinks little at a time ; great dyspnœa, cannot lie on back ; worse after mid-night. Affects rather the left heart. Orthopnœa, Anasarca ; cannot go up-stairs.

Aurum Met.—Pure cardiac hypertrophy without dilatation. Increased force of heart-stroke and hyperæmia of lungs. Crushing weight under sternum, as if chest would burst ; worse from exertion; as if heart stopped beating, and then gave a tumultuous rebound. Fatty infiltration (*Ars.* ; *Phos.*—fatty degeneration). Atheroma of heart and blood-vessels ; great anguish and suicidal tendency.

Benzoic Acid—Gout and rheumatism affecting the heart with valvular deposits. Dark urine, of offensive odor is characteristic. Palpitation alternates with rheumatism.

Bromium—Cardiac Asthma from hypertrophy without valvular affections ; palpitation on beginning to move : from getting up from a sitting to a standing posture. Cardiac Asthma, better at sea than on land.

HEART, AFFECTIONS OF THE—(*Contd.*).

Bryonia—Peri-carditis with effusion, strong pulse, stitching pains preventing motion, even breathing ; persistent friction sound ; cramp in heart region, from slightest exertion, even raising the arm ; heart beats violently and rapidly.

Asclepias Tub.—Similar to *Bryonia* but not so acute ; pains relieved by bending forward.

Cactus Grandi.—Endo-carditis, Peri-carditis. Constriction, as if heart were squeezed by hand, or tightly bound around false ribs arresting breathing, with determination of blood to head and intense headache. Low-spiritedness, weeping. Cannot lie on left side. Pains increase gradually and subside gradually. Palpitation from emotion, fluttering like a bird's wings, worse at menses, on stooping, but a walk does not bring it on. Pains shooting into left arm, œdema and quick, tense, hard pulse, with the constrictive sensation. Angina Pectoris.

Calcarea Carb.—Anxious dread of heart disease. Nervous palpitation, dyspnœa and headache, worse on ascending, after eating, at night ; with anguish ; inclination to take deep breaths ; vertigo ; cold lower extremities. Copious menstruation.

Cimicifuga—Angina Pectoris ; pains radiate all over the chest ; numbness of left arm, feels as if bound to the body. Cerebral congestion and unconsciousness.

Colchicum—Heart disease following acute rheumatism. Peri-carditis ; violent cutting, stinging pains with great oppression and dyspnœa ; worse at night, when lying on Ieft side.

Convallaria—Heart symptoms associated with the uterine. Valvular diseases with scanty urine, dropsy and dyspnœa, out of proportion ; feeble heart, anæmic murmurs, pain and fluttering. Endo-carditis with extreme orthopnœa ; Angina Pectoris. Heart ceased, then started very suddenly.

Adonis Vernalis—Mitral and aortic regurgitation. Præcordial pain, palpitation, dyspnœa ; cardiac asthma ; fatty heart. Valuable in cardiac dropsy.

Lycopus—Præcordial pain, tumultuous action of heart ; rapid, irregular, tremulous pulse. Excessive hypertrophy after depressants or stimulants ; cardiac asthma.

Collinsonia—Palpitation, rapid but weak. Dropsy. After heart symptoms are relieved, piles or menses return ; heart symptoms and piles alternate.

Cratægus Oxyacantha—Fatty degeneration ; extreme dyspnœa on least exertion without increase of pulse. Heart dilated, first

HEART, AFFECTIONS OF THE–(*Contd.*)

sound weak ; failing compensation. Anæmia, œdema. Threatened heart failure during acute diseases.

Digitalis--Sub-acute inflammation of the heart. Weak, irregular, abnormally slow intermittent pulse ; weakness and dilatation of myocardium. Weakness, faintness, irregular respiration, coldness of skin, jaundice, hypertrophy of the liver. Hydro-pericardium, Hydro-thorax, Ascites; œdema of scrotum and penis ; Anasarca. Least movement causes violent palpitation ; sensation as if heart would stop beating on movement ; pulse very slow when at rest, accelerated on least exertion. Cardiac Dropsy with suppressed urine (*Apis*),

Gelsemium—Roused out of sleep feeling that heart would stop beating if he did not move about. Nervous chill, yet skin is warm ; wants to be held, that he may not shake so.

Apocynum—Mitral and tricuspid regurgitation. Fluttering of heart ; small, weak pulse ; heart-beat irregular, now weak, now stronger ; sinking at epigastrium ; hardly gets breath to speak, even after light meals ; swelling of feet and ankles. Anasarca, Cardiac Dropsy ; urine, suppressed or scanty.

Glonoine—Excessive throbbing of heart ; pulse rapid and forceful ; throbbing in vessels of neck, pulsating headache. Stooping causes pain in cardiac region ; laborious of action of heart ; blood rushes to heart and mounts to head ; stitches from heart to back ; worse lying on left side ; better on right side ; must have head high.

Kali Carb.—Deposits on valves ; late stage of Endo and Peri-carditis with sharp, stiching pains, worse on deep inspirations, coughing, but not on motion ; suffocation, inability to lie down. Insufficiency of mitral valves ; systolic murmurs. Pulse unequal, irregular, intermittent or rapid and weak. Follows *Spigelia*, when the sharp pains persist and there is 3 A. M. aggravation.

Kalmia—Gout or rheumatism shifts from joints to the heart after external applications ; sharp, servere pain, taking away breath, shooting down to stomach with numbness of the left arm. Tumultuous, rapid, visible beating of the heart. Hypertrophy with palpitation, shaking the whole frame ; worse lying on left side ; slow pulse.

Rhus Tox.—Rheumatic hypertrophy ; also from over-exertion ; uncomplicated hypertrophy without valvular lesions ; tingling numbness of left arm. Endo or Peri-carditis from wet, from sepsis. General symptoms of the remedy are decisive. Follows *Bryonia* well.

Phytolacca—Chronic rheumatic Endo-carditis ; shocks of pain in cardiac region, shooting into right arm.

HEART, AFFECTIONS OF THE—(*Contd.*)

Lachesis—Rheumatism of heart, late stage. As if heart were too large for the chest ; horrible smothering feeling about the heart awakens from sleep and compels him to leave the bed ; dread of going to sleep again ; cannot bear pressure on throat ; numbness of left arm. Hydro-pericardium and Hydro-thorax ; urine dark, almost black and offensive.

Kali Iod.—Repeated attacks of Endo- or Peri-carditis of rheumatic origin with sharp, darting pains, worse from walking. It also has a horrible smothering feeling about the heart, awakening from sleep and forcing him to go out—(like *Lachesis*).

Kali Bichrom.—Also has the symptom, as also *Graphites*. These have again a cold feeling about the heart. (*Petrol., Nat. Mur.*)

Naja.—Later than *Lachesis* in Endo-carditis with a dry, hard cough ; tumultuous action of heart with sharp sticking pain and a sense of oppression in chest, cannot lie a moment on left side, great relief on lying on right side (reverse of *Lilium Tig.*).

Ledum—Valvular deposits with Arthritis (also, *Lithium Carb., Kalmia, Benzoic Acid*, etc.)

Lilium Tigrinum—Cardiac disorders with uterine disease. Nervous palpitation ; heart as if grasped in a vise, awaking her suddenly ; much fluttering and faintness ; as if heart contained too much blood, which might be relieved by throwing it up. Violent palpitation and sharp pain from left nipple through chest to back, ameliorated by lying on left side and in open air.

Lithium Carb.—Rheumatic soreness, shocks and jerks, valvular deficiencies, fluttering of heart brought on by mental emotion (*Calc. Carb., Nat. Mur., Sepia*) ; cardiac pains on bending forward and relieved by urinating.

Nat. Mur.—Cold feeling about the heart during mental exertion. Hypertrophy, chronic valvular troubles ; strong pulsations, shaking the whole body ; fluttering palpitations with weak, faint feeling from motion or sudden noise. Sad tearful patients who are worse from consolation.

Nux Mosch.—Hysteria cordis ; violent action of heart ; palpitation and fainting followed by sleep ; disposition to faint from slight pains.

Nux Vomica—Hypertrophy from portal obstruction ; dilatation palpitation when lying down. Look for other *Nux Vomica* symptoms.

Phosphorus—Endo- or Myo-carditis during acute inflammatory Rheumatism or Pneumonia ; Peri-carditis. Palpitation from emotion, as when a visitor comes sundenly, from motion, particularly in the rapidly growing young. Fatty degeneration involving the right heart ; venous stagnation, puffiness of face. *Arsenic* affects right heart with greater oppression of breathing, more orthopnœa and more anasarca.

HEART, AFFECTIONS OF THE—(*Contd.*)

Pulsatilla—Rheumatic pains of heart ; pains shifting rapidly from place to place. Hypertrophy or dilatation of right ventricle, with numbness about elbow (see Amenorrhœa). *Sumbul* has heaviness and sharp shooting pains in the fingers with cardiac affections.

Spigelia—Front rank remedy in acute Rheumatic Carditis and Pericarditis. Sharp, shooting pains through heart to back and radiating down the arm, chest and spine ; great oppression and palpitation from any movement of arm or body ; great dyspnœa on change of position with tumultuous beating of heart. Systolic blowing ; pulse intermittent, not synchronous with heart-beat. Heart symptoms with Neuralgia. Can lie only on the right side with head high. Trembling of the carotids, of the chest ; purring, vibrating feeling over heart. The above conditions following closely or months after fever has subsided in a rheumatic attack makes *Spigelia* a front rank remedy in acute Rheumatic Carditis, Pericarditis, etc., along with *Aconite*, *Bryonia*, *Cactus*, *Colchicum*, *Kalmia*, *Kali Carb.*, *Rhus Tox.* and others. A careful consideration of their individual characteristics will amply repay. *Spigelia* antidotes the abuse of *Colchi.*, and precedes *Kali Carb.*

Spongia—Organic affections of heart, cannot lie flat on back ; aroused from sleep, as if smothering and sits up with an anxious look, flushed face and rapid, hard breathing. Rheumatic Peri-carditis, after effusion takes place (follows *Acon*.). Valvular insufficiency, bellow's murmur, loud blowing with each heart-beat ; stinging pain, violent gasping for breath ; as if breathing through dry sponge. Pulse frequent, hard, full or feeble. In treating heart cases it is always safer to begin with *Aconite*, *Bryonia*, *Spigelia*, *Spongia*, *Phosphorus*, etc. in the first stages, unless there be complete picture for *Arsenic*, *Lachesis* or other remedies which are usually indicated in later stages.

Sulphur—Palpitation, worse going up-stairs. Roused up at night with sudden rush of blood to heart, palpitation, gasping for breath, must have fresh air, must have doors and windows open.

Veratrum Viri.—Simple or rheumatic endo and peri-carditis ; cardio-pulmonary dyspnœa. Congestion to heart and lungs, with violent fever, fluttering of heart, throbbing carotids, rapid respiration etc.

Zincum—Sudden shocks and jerks in cardiac region. Swelling and great tenderness of cardiac region, severe palpitation, tearing pain and irregular spasmodic action of the heart ; occasionally one violent thump—(also *Conium* and *Aurum*).

LIVER, AFFECTIONS OF THE

Aconite—Great and violent inflammation, comes on suddenly, quickly following an exposure to dry cold of mid-winter, particularly in those with a strong heart and vigorous circulation. Violent tearing pains with aweful anxiety, restlessness, fear of death, great thirst. Jaundice from fear or anger, during pregnancy, in the new-born children.

Aurum Met.—Congestion of liver from cardiac disease. Liver large and hard, with burning cutting pains, gradually becomes cirrhosed or undergoes fatty degeneration, with ascites, constipation of grayish or ashy-white stools, foul breath, jaundice and suicidal melancholia (also *Aurum Mur.*)

Digitalis—Congestion, enlargement and soreness of the liver from organic disease of the heart ; hard and sensitive. Deathly nausea, vomiting of bile, awful sinking in the stomach, aversion to food, great thirst, bileless putty-like stools, jaundice, drowsiness, despondency and high-coloured, scanty and often suppressed urine. Dropsy and Ascites.

Myrica Cerifera—Almost similar to *Digitalis*, differing in this that with *Myrica* the heart is affected secondarily, thus producing slowness of the pulse. Also the jaundice of *Digitalis* is due to the condition of the heart, while with *Myrica* the bile is not properly formed and the elements remain in the blood. *Myrica* is more superficial in action than *Digitalis*.

Nux Vom.—Liver disorders of high livers and Alcoholic addicts. The liver is hard, sore and sensitive to pressure of clothing. Cirrhosis of high-livers and drunkards ; biliary or hæmorrhoidal colic, with severe pain in rt. side and stitches in the hepatic region, fitful urging for stool and urine. Irritability of temper. Jaundice evoked by anger (*Acon.*, *Bryo.*, *Chamo.*, *Nat. S.*) ; worse in the morning. Also see under *Sulphur*.

Magnesia Mur.—Enlarged and hard liver of puny, rachitic childern. Pain in liver, worse lying on right side (*Ptelea*, better). Feet are often œdematous, knotty stools like sheep dung or diarrhœa and large, coated, yellow tongue taking imprint of teeth.

Mercurius—Enlarged and indurated liver. The pains are worse lying on the right side but differ from *Mag. Mur.* in the characteristic stools. Other symptoms of *Mercurius* should be considered.

Lycopodium—Cirrhosis with Ascites, especially in drunkards. Dull, aching pain ; hunger, but a few mouthfuls fill him up,

LIVER, AFFECTIONS OF THE—(*Contd.*).

quickly followed by hunger again. Distress in stomach immediately after eating, tension in hypochondria after a meal. Flatulence, tending upwards, great fermentation in intestines with discharge of flatus and diarrhœa, yet usually constipated, with ineffectual urging to stool and an unfinished feeling (Comp. *Nux Vom.*). Nutmeg liver, atrophic form.

Lachesis—Enlarged liver of drunkards, going on to a low grade of symptoms with inflammation and abscess of liver, jaundice, tenderness to pressure all the time (*Lyco.* only after meal), intolerance of clothing ; constant urging in anus, but no stool follows or extremely offensive stools. Pain as if something had lodged in the right side, worse in spring. Gastric pains better during eating, but returns after one or two hours. Mental depression. Also liver complaints at climaxis, after Ague, from Syphilis. All symptoms worse after sleep.

Hepar Sulph.—During inflammatory process in Cirrhosis, tending towards the formation of an abscess. Soreness and stitches when walking ; depressed and irritable ; craving for sour and strong-tasting articles ; sensitiveness to dampness ; hyper-sensitiveness of the liver region to touch.

Silicea—Abscess of liver ; throbbing ulcerative pain, worse from touch, motion, lying on the right side. Constipation from inactivity of rectum (also *Kali Carb.*, *Calc. Carb.*, *Hydrastis*, *Merc.*, *Lyco.*).

Phosphorus—Waxy liver in long lasting bone disease : fatty degeneration of the liver from cardiac troubles ; acute yellow atrophy of the liver, hyperæmia. At first enlargement, fatty degeneration and finally atrophy with Jaundice and Dropsy. Suppurating Hepatitis with hectic fever, loss of appetite, unquenchable thirst, worse after eating and drinking ; chronic loose bowels. Hæmorrhages from different parts of the body. Malignant Jaundice from venous obstruction, often from Alcoholism ; worse during thunder-storms, windy weather, after mid-night.

Crotalus Hor.-Acute yellow atrophy of the liver. Malignant Jaundice, which comes on with astonishing quickness. Dark hæmorrhages from nose, mouth, etc. ; great prostration, skin mottled, rapidly increasing unconsciousness ; dark, scanty, bloody urine, containing albumen.

Plumbum—Cirrhosis ; first enlarged, then contracted. Sensation of heat and burning in liver ; persistent sticking, darting pain in the hepatic region ; constipation,

LIVER, AFFECTIONS OF THE—(*Contd.*)

Laurocerasus—Wasting away of liver, nutmeg liver. Sticking in liver, as if an abscess would burst ; constipation or diarrhœa ; rapid sinking of vital forces.

Nux Moschata.—Atrophic nutmeg liver ; enlargement of liver and spleen after intermittent fever.

Iodium—Hard, cirrhotic liver. Progressive emaciation, excessive weakness, Jaundice, loss of appetite, diarrhœa.

Natrum Phos.—Cirrhosis. Hepatic form of Diabetes; yellow creamy coating at the back part of tongue and roof of mouth ; intense pressure and heat on top of head ; acidity.

Hydrastis—Liver atrophied ; torpor of liver with pale, scanty stools. Marasmus, Jaundice. Bitter taste, obstinate constipation, lack of appetite, coated tongue, yellow urine.

Belladonna—Sudden congestion and inflammation. Bursting, pressing, throbbing pains ; extremely sensitive to touch, jar of the bed or motion, better by warmth. High fever, severe congestive headache, vomiting and thirst ; the pain suddenly comes and goes suddenly. A great remedy during an attack of Gall-stones Colic, relieving the pain instantanenusly.

Berberis Vul.—Gall-stones Colic. Sharp stitching, stinging pains, shooting in every direction, more particularly downwards to the umbilicus from the tenth rib, often with stitches in the kidneys, and frequent desire to urinate ; colic followed by jaundice.

Chelidonium—Relieves Gall-stones Colic in a few minutes when there are shooting, stabbing pains extending through to the back and marked jaundice. Also useful in various affections of the liver from simple congestion to a positive inflammation, characterized by simple soreness or sharp pains in the liver, shooting in every direction, going through thc chest like a rivet to the lower angle of the right scapula; bitter taste, yellow tongue, eyes, skin, urine ; even the perspiration is yellow. Intolerable itchlng of the skin. The stool is either clay colored, like putty, or yellowish diarrhœa.

Nat. Sulph.—Congestion of liver with soreness and sharp, sticking pains worse from touch or jar ; stool dark-green, bilious ; urine loaded with bile. Great flatulence. Worse lying left side, damp, wet weether. It has removed Gall-stones and has cured the condition permanently in many cases.

Calc. Carb.—Gall-stones Colic ; great chilliness during. Profuse sweat, abdominal spasms, bend double, clench hands, writhe

LIVER, AFFECTIONS OF THE—*(Contd.)*

with agony. Has often stopped the pain as by magic and has also cured permanently.

Carduus Mari.—Swelling of gall bladder with tenderness ; stools hard, difficult, knotty, alternates with bright yellow diarrhœa. Jaundice with intolerable itching, when lying down at night.

China—Is highly praised in Gall Stones colic both during the attack and to cure the condition permanently (also *Hydrastis, Ipec.*) Also see under *Sulphur*.

Podophyllum—Gall Stones with Jaundice. Pain from stomach towards gall bladder, with excessive nausea ; alternate constipation and diarrhœa. Also useful in Chronic Hepatitis with constipation and jaundice ; constantly rubs the liver region with hands.

Dioscorea—Gall Stones colic ; sharp pain from liver shooting upward to right nipple ; cutting pains, changing location and radiating to chest, back, arms ; worse bending forwards and while lying, better walking about and bending backwards ; much flatulence.

Chionanthus—Gall Stones colic; soft, pasty, yellow or clay-colored stool, jaundice and constipation. Pain in paroxysms, as if suddenly tied tightly with a cord and then gradually loosened.

Bryonia—Peri-hepatitis ; sharp stitches in right hypochondrium, worse from any motion, better lying on right side ; pain under rt. shoulder-blade ; swelling of the liver. Bitter taste, yellow-coated tongue, large, hard, dry and brown stool ; sensation of a stone or heavy weight in abdomen ; great thirst.

Ptelea—Has a sore, swollen liver, sensitive to pressure, greatly aggravated lying on the left side and better lying on the right. Its pains are of the nature of aching and heaviness in the liver region and not the sharp stitches of *Bryonia.*

Kali Carb.—Has sharp. shooting, stitching pains like *Bryo.*, but they are not necessarily worse on motion.

Chelidonium—Has pains like *Bryo*, but the pain under the right scapula going through the chest like a rivet is characteristic. They also differ in their stools.

Chenopodium—Has dull pain, lower than the angle of the rt. scapula, and nearer the spinal column, while *Ranunculus Bulb* has pain along the whole inner edge of the left scapula, at times below its inferior angle and through the left chest.

LIVER, AFFECTIONS OF THE—(*Contd.*)

Sulphur—Chronic affections. Passive congestion of the portal system from suppressed hæmorrhoidal or other habitual discharges. A sense of tightness or fulness in the abdomen and repletion after a small meal. The liver is congested, enlarged and sore on pressure. Goneness or faintness in the epigastrium—as if he must have food or sink, at 11 A. M. Cannot digest farinaceous food, cannot take milk. Constipation with ineffectual urging and Hæmorrhoids or alternating with Diarrhœa, and then he is subject to Gall Stones with tearing pain in the region of the duct, coming periodically. *Nux Vom.* has almost exactly the same symptoms and generally precedes in these affections. When *Nux* only partially relieves, *Sulphur* comes in to complete the cure.

Sepia—Venous congestion and portal stasis with heavy and sluggish liver. Constant aching pain in forehead and conjunctiva yellow, also around mouth and yellow red saddle over bridge of nose down cheeks ; imperfectly acting liver. Atonic Dyspepsia ; sluggish bowels, *Uric Acid* deposits in the urine and evidences of impaired digestion and assimilation ; a gone, faint feeling at forenoon, feels better by exercise.

Myrica Cerifera—Despondency ; dirty, dingy, yellowish hue of the eyes ; tongue coated dirty yellow ; weak, sinking feeling after eating ; ash colored stool and dark turbid urine ; also Jaundice and slow pulse—all resembling *Digitalis.* The Jaundice in either case is neither catarrhal or obstructive nor due to retention of bile. It is due to functional imperfection of the liver for which it cannot take from the blood the elements which go to form bile, and so they remain in the blood. The difference is that in *Digitalis* the liver condition follows the condition of the heart, which is the reverse in the case of *Myrica.*

China—Gastro-duodenal catarrh, dullness of head, yellow tongue, loss of appetite, bitter and sour taste and eructation, oppression of stomach and chest, worse after eating, flatulence ; swollen, sensitive liver. Jaundice (See under *Bell.*).

Nat. Mur.—A dull, heavy aching and distension about liver after eating, better as digestion advances ; tension in the liver, earthy skin, obstinate constipation, short breathing, palpitation and stitches in the spleen, worse from every motion. Malarial cachexia, enlargement and induration of both liver and spleen.

Arsenic—Abuse of *Mercury* and after Intermittents. Pressure and tension in the rt. hypochondrium : heat, restlessness, anxiety and irritability, alternating with low spirit ; vomiting of black masses, black stools.

LIVER, AFFECTIONS OF THE—(*Contd.*)

Nitric Acid.—Chronic derangement of the liver. Cadaverous smell from mouth (*Merc*) ; constipation ; great tearing pain in rectum, continuing a long time after stool, even more intense after a loose stool.

Taraxacum—A good liver remedy with indications, such as mapped tongue or tongue coated white which peels off in patches, leaving dark red, sensitive spots ; bitter taste, chilliness after eating or drinking, pain and soreness in hepatic region and Bilious Diarrhœa. Mapped tongue is also found under *Arsenic*, *Lachesis*, *Nat. Mur.* and *Nitric Acid.*

Leptandra—A prominant liver remedy with a dull aching in the right hypochondrium, in the gall-bladder region and the posterior portion of the liver with soreness and burning. Diarrhœa—stools horribly offensive and black, almost as black as pitch, with burning, distressing, colicky pain at the umbilicus. Vomiting of bile with burning distress and occasionally clay-colored stools ; tongue coated yellow or more frequently dark brown or black down the middle. *Mercurius* is distinguished from *Leptandra* in this that the latter lacks the tenesmus of *Mercurius* though the urging and griping continues after stool.

Aurum Muriaticum Natronatum—Useful in some obstinate cases of Jaundice with bilious vomiting and alternating white and black stools—as black as tar.

MALARIA

[BENIGN AND MALIGNANT.]

"Every case of intermittent Fever can, has, and must be cured with the potentized remedies, under the law of the Similars, Homœopathically." —Lippe.

"For the successful treatment of Intermittents the symptoms occurring BEFORE and DURING the CHILL, HEAT, SWEET and APYREXIA ; the TIME of OCCURRENCE of the paroxysm ; the PARTS of the BODY in which the chill first makes its appearance ; the REGULARITY of its STAGES ; the DEGREE or ABSENCE of THIRST, and the TIME of its APPEARANCE ; as well as THE CONSTITUTIONAL AILMENTS AROUSED BY THE FEVER, are all to be carefully noted."

"For the treatment of Intermittent Fever a more INTIMATE PERSONAL ACQUAINTANCE with our remedies is needed ; general knowledge will not suffice."—Allen.

MALARIA—(*contd.*)

Aconite—Chill comes usually in the evening, ascending from feet to the chest, aggravated on the slightest movement or by even lifting bed-clothes, followed by high fever with long lasting, dry, burning heat and burning thirst for large quantities of water—everything else tastes bitter, (Thirst at every stage, *Bryo.*, *Nat. Mur.* ; only during heat, *Ipecac.*) and restless tossing about with excessive anguish and oppression of chest. General, warm, streaming sweat, most profuse on covered parts and during sleep or on the side on which he lies. When the oppression of chest is great, with loud complaining and the characteristic fear of death, *Aconite* may be interpolated, without any hindrance to the action of the specific remedy for the case.

Antim. Crud.—Violent shaking chill, without thirst, at noon or afternoon, preceded by gastric disturbances with Melancholia, sadness and woeful mood. Chilly even in a warm room with great desire to sleep (*Apis*, chill worse in warm room but wants to sleep during hot stage). Great heat with sweat which breaks out simultaneously with or immediatly after chill and ceases suddenly, a dry heat remaining even for the whole night. The tongue is thickly coated—milky white, with want of appetite, nausea, vomiting and bitter taste (*Ipec.*, *Nux*, *Puls.*). It is one of the few remedies where sweat follows chill and is followed by heat.

Antim. Tart.—Yawning and stretching (*Eup. Perf.*), followed by chill at 3 or 6 P.M., without thirst, alternating with heat during the day, (*Ars.* chill and sweat or sweat and heat alternates—*Ant. Crud.*), with goose-flesh, back-ache, trembling and shaking. Short chill and long heat, with somnolency and profuse sweat on forehead or violent short heat after a long chill, worse by every motion (feels chilly if he moves, *Apis, Nux*) with intense thirst, marked during heat and sweat, which is often cold, clammy, sticky or else profuse all over, lasting all night, feeling worse during and better afterwards. Tongue, with red edges or red and white in alternate streaks and red and raised papillæ is characteristic. Gastric symptoms are pronounced with nausea, vomiting, weakness, exhaustion and great depression of spirits. Drowsiness following heat. Malignant Tertians with severe and long heat, much sweat, intense thirst, delirium.

Apis—Of great use in Malignant Malaria with the well-known cerebral symptoms of the drug fully depicted. Shuddering chill with thirst (*Alum.*, *Arn.*, *Carbo Veg.*, *Caps.*, *Igna.*) at 3 P.M. or between 3 and 4 P.M. or at 4 P.M. without chill (*Lyco.* without thirst). Chill and great oppression of chest, as though smothering, worse from heat, warmth or covering. Falls into a deep sleep as the severity of chill passes off (*Gels.*—sleepy as chill is leaving ; *Op.*—sleeps in all stages ; *Nux M*,—becomes drowsy as chill progresses, falls asleep at its close and continues through heat ;

MALARIA—(*Contd.*)

Podo.—Falls asleep at climax of heat and breaks with sweat). Heat with no thirst, deep sleep (*Op.*). Chilliness on moving or uncovering, (*Arn.*, *Nux*), but intolerant of heat of the room and itching, burning urticaria (*Urtica U.* ; before and during chill, *Hep*, ; during heat and sweat, *Rhus* ; during heat only, *Ignat.*) Sweat is generally absent or of a light grade ; often it breaks out, dries up, breaks out and dries up again, with no thirst but with weakness, trembling and sleep.

Arsenic—Of great use in Quotidian, Malignant, Tertian, and other types of Malarial Intermittents with marked periodieity, the chill returning at 1 to 2 P. M. 12 P. M. to 2 A. M., and irregular chills at any time, always anticipating by one hour every other day, preceded by yawning and stretching, malaise, debility and inclination to lie down, headache and vertigo. The chill is not clearly defined, and comes simultaneously or alternating with heat.with no thirst, or if thirsty, drinks frequently but little at a time, which increases the chilliness, and causes nausea and vomiting (drinking hastens and aggravates chill and causes nausea, *Eup*, *Perf.* ; causes headache, *Cimex* ; every drink causes shivering and chill, *Capsi.*). The chill is ameliorated by external warmth (*Ign.* ; worse by exterual heat, *Apis*, *Ipec.*) and may be attended with unconsciousness, cramps in chest and difficult breathing. The hot stage is intense, long-lasting, dry, burning, as if hot water were coursing through the blood-vessels (*Bryo*.. *Rhus*), with desire to uncover and insatiable thirst for cold water, drinking little and often, followed by vomiting, oppressed breathing (*Apis*), great restlessness and burning pain in spleen. During chill and heat, the previously existing symptoms are all aggravated and they are relieved when sweat breaks out (*Nat. M.* ; but headache is increased, *Eup. Perf.*), with great thirst for large quantities (*China*), and vomiting. The sweat is very often absent with dry heat all night. The tongue is furred, with red streak down the middle (*Ant. T.*) and red tip ; water tastes bitter. With or without sweat, every paroxysm is followed by great prostration during apyrexia, pale, sunken face, bloated abdomen, fetid watery debilitating Diarrhœa ; scanty, turbid urine ; anæmia ; constant chilliness, must be in a warm room.

Baptisia—A great remedy for Malignant and other types of Malaria prone to become low Typhoid. Every day chill at 11 A. M. or every afternoon, the temperature rising rapidly to 103°—106°, with a small, thready, weak, and variable pulse and early prostration. The full *Baptisia* low state is clearly pictured.

Belladonna—The typieal pieture of the drug irrespective of the paroxysm indicates the drug in Cerebral Malaria. Congestive chill, with red, hot face and icy-cold feet, which cannot be warmed, intense heat, burning within and without with great thirst, extreme distension of the

MALARIA—(*Contd.*)

superficial blood-vessels, violent bursting headache, throbbing carotids, dilated pupils, delirium, restlessness and sweat on covered parts only. The furious delirium or unconsciousness with convulsions are too characteristic of the drug to mention.

Bryonia—The general picture of the drug indicates it in Tertian or Quotidian Intermittents that are anticipating or postponing, with gastro-hepatic complications. Its fever comes at all periods, but preferably in the morning, with great thirst for large quantities of cold water during chill and violent dry, racking cough with stitching pains in ehest (cough before and during chill, without pain—*Rhus*) and a desire to lie down. All the sufferings are aggravated during hot stage, with dry, burning internal heat, as if blood in the veins were burning (*Ars.*, *Rhus*), with a desire to uncover and keep perfectly quiet and a bitter taste. This stage is followsd by profuse sweat, sour and oily, which relieves. The tongue is thick, yellow with dryness of the mouth and lips. Everything tastes bitter and the mouth is bitter when not eating. Constipation and scanty, high-colored urine. Full, hard, rapid and tense pulse. The symptoms during apyrexia are characteristic, the gastric symptoms predominating (*Ant. C.*, *Nux*, *Puls.*)

Cactus Grandi.—It is useful in Congestive Intermittents, with regular paroxysms of chills, at the same hour every day (*Aranea*, *Cedron*, *Gels.*, *Sabadilla*), characteristically at 11 A. M. or 11 P. M., without thirst but with gaeat congestions here and there, but particularly of the head. Chill not relieved by covering or external heat (*Aran.*) followed by great heat in the head, flushes in face, horrible anxiety, lancinating pain in heart, shortness of breath, suppressed urine, pains in bladder, stupefaction, insensibility, coma. Then comes profuse sweat with unquenchable thirst for largc quantities of cold water or violent vomiting when perspiration fails.

> **Aranea**—Useful for every type of Intermitents, even Pernicious, Malignant Malarias with great regularity of the paroxysms, the chill returning precisely at the same hour every day or every other day. The paroxysm is often unattended by either heat or sweat, consisting of long-lasting, bone-searching chill which is persistent and severe, with internal coldness, as if frozen, and not relieved by covering or external heat. Thirst is usually absent in all the stages. "Chill as soon as he touches the bed."
>
> **Cedron.**—Intermittent Fevers in low, marshy regions and the tropics. The paroxysm is characterized by a marked periodicity, occurring with clock-like regularity at 3 A. M. or P. M. Severe chill shaking the whole body, dry mouth, great thirst for cold water, icy-coldness of hands and of the tip of the nose. The

MALARIA—(*Contd.*)

heat comes with great desire and longing for warm drinks—"Cannot take anything but hot drinks during fever,"—emission of large quantities of pale urine and a desire to sleep as heat passes off (*Apis*). Sweat comes with profuse perspiration, with thirst. The chill or chilliness predominates, with chill, heat and sweat irregularly intermingled.

Sabadilla—Well-marked periodicity and great regularity, the chill returning at the same hour, generally in the afternoon and evening, with thirst and often without subsequent heat. Violent chilliness at 5 P. M., as if dashed with cold water, relieved by external warmth, with dry, spasmodic cough, pain in ribs, and tearing in all the limbs and bones (dry, teasing cough before and during chill, *Rhus*; racking cough during chill and heat with pleuritic stitches, *Bryo.*). The chill predominates and thirst begins, with desire for warm drinks, as chill leaves and before heat begins. The heat alternates with shivering; yawning, stretching, delirium and sweat often during or with the heat. The sweat is profuse over head and face, which are hot to touch, rest of body cold; sweat of soles of feet. The gastric symptoms predominate during apyrexia as in *Nux* and *Puls.*

Calcarea Carb.—Intermittents with epileptiform spasms; after abuse of *Quinine*. Chronic forms with Scrofula; cachectic constitution.

The constitutional symptoms existing or aroused by the fever are the guides and are generally found in the apyrexia. The chill begins in scorbiculous cordis, with spasms, or fixed, cold, agonizing weight, increasing with the chill and disappearing with it, at 2 P. M. or 11 A. M. one day, 4 P. M. the next, with thirst. But there is no thirst during the stage of heat or sweat which latter is hot, and comes on during the day from the least exertion (*Amm. M.*, *Bryo.*). The tongue is dry and coated white, with bitter, sour or foul taste. Chill, heat and sweat of single parts. The cause, such as working while standing in water, handling cold vegetables or fruits, or working in wet clay, is often indicative.

Calcarea Ars.—Renders excellent service in Chronic Malaria, especially in infants of *Calcarea*-constitutions, with Anæmia, enlarged liver and spleen and also in women, developing Pernicious Anæmia.

Camphora—Pernicious, sinking or congestive Intermittents with a perfect picture of collapse of Cholera. Long-lasting, terrible, shaking chills without thirst; with chattering of teeth, cold, blue extremities and death-like paleness of face, icy coldness of the whole body. Chill

MALARIA – (*Contd.*)

with anxiety, unconsciousness, spasms ; cold as marble, but cannot be covered (*Secale*), hot breath (cold, *Carbo Veg*). Chill is the predominant stage, followed by heat without thirst, with distension of veins, sometimes of single parts. Sweat is cold and profuse, over the whole body —most profuse during sleep (*China*) or on slightest motion (*Bryo.*) and is very weakening, debilitating and prostrating. The tongue is cold, trembling, flabby and covered with tough, yellowish mucus. Pulse is small, weak, slow, often imperceptible.

Capsicum—A valuable remedy in Intermittents of mid-summer. The paroxysm comes with thirst sometime before the chill which commences in the back, between the shoulders, worse after drinking and relieved by putting bags of hot water to the back—must have something hot to the back. Violent chill with general coldness of the body, painful swelling of the spleen, contraction of the limbs (*Cimex*), anxiety, giddiness, headache and intolerance of noise (*Bell.*). The chill is followed by sweat or by heat with copious and general sweat, without thirst. Great sleepiness after the fever.

Capsi., *China*, *Eup. Perf.*, *Nat. Mnr.*—all have thirst for sometime before the paroxysm beings—"Knows the chill is coming, because he wants to drink." Both *Capsi.* and *China* are wanting in the bone-pains and back-ache of the other two respectively.

Cocculus—Shaking chill at 8 A. M. without thirst, not relieved by external warmth and without subsequent heat (*Causti.*), with severe colic and lameness of the small of the back or at 11.A. M. with disgust for even the smell of food and ceasing when Diarrhœa and vomiting set in. Heat without thirst comes in flushes with burning cheeks, cold feet and intolerance of both cold and warm air. Sweat, of the body from evening till morning, is aggravated on slightest motion. When the fever threatens to assume a slow, sneaking, nervous form, attended with vertigo, dull pains in the head, general weakness, physical depression, and anorexia, with a comparatively clean tongue and a marked tendency to nausea, as if always nauseated, *Cocculus* should be thought of.

Colchicum—Is often useful for the Intermittents occurring late in autumn, when Epidemic Dysentery prevails. The gastric and abdominal symptoms are guiding. Desire for, or aversion to food, with loathing when merely looking at it and still more when smelling it. The smell of broth nauseates, and that of fish, eggs or fat meat almost makes him faint.

Carbo Veg.—Patients debilitated from protracted disease and abuse of *Quinine*. Annual return of paroxysms, at about 10 or 11 A. M.

MALARIA—(*Contd.*)

or in the evening, with violent chill and rigor with great thirst for cold water, one sided chill, generally of the left side, icy cold hands and feet, blue finger-nails, breath cold. Flushes of burning heat in the evening, with loquaciousness but without thirst, and a constant desire to be fanned. Marked picture of collapse with dyspnœa, coldness, copious sweat, exhaustion and weak, irregular, intermittent pulse, indicative of rapid sinking. MALIGNANT, PERNICIOUS or CONGESTIYE MALARIAL FEVERS.

China --Paroxysms every 7 or 14 days, with great thirst before the chill begins, which ceases as chill increases. General shaking chill over whole body, increased by drinking, with goose-flesh after every drink (every swallow increases the chill, *Eup. Perf.* ; drink causes vomiting, *Ars.* ; shuddering and chill after every drink, *Capis.* ; drinking makes headache and all symptoms unbearable, *Cimex*). Wants to be near the stove but it increases the chill (*Ipec.* ; relieved by heat of stove, *Ign.* ; relieved by external heat, *Ars.*). The chill is followed by long-lasting heat without thirst and a desire to uncover, fiery red face, and sometimes delirium. The sweat is profuse and debilitating, with intense thirst. SWEATING PROFUSELY DURING SLEEP. The tongue is white or yellow with bitter taste and indifference to all food, even when thinking of it. During apyrexia, face is sallow, dingy yellow, from bilious complications ; aching, sore and enlarged spleen, total loss of appetite or canine hunger. The feet become œdematous, and sleep is greatly disturbed, seeing figures as soon as closing eyes. Contra-indicated if there be mueh thirst in the cold and hot stages and the perspiration is not profuse and not debilitating.

Chininum Sulph.—Perfectly regular paroxysms at 10 or 11 A. M. and 8 or 10 P. M., anticipating two and a half hour every day. Violent shaking chills with blue lips and nails, paleness of the face and pain in the middle dorsal vertebræ, increased hunger and constipation ; followed by vioient heat with excessive thirst, redness of face and sometimes delirium and pain on spine on pressure. Sweat gradually breaks out, while perfectly quiet, with great thirst, which relieves all symptoms of head and chest (*Nat. Mur.* ; headache increased, *Eup. Perp.*) but pain in lumbar vertebræ on pressure continues. The apyrexia is short, with great thirst and the sweat hardly ceases before chill begins again ; the spinal pain continues. Spleen swollen and painful. It is contra-indicated where there is no thirst during all the stages and perspiration does not succeed the heat. The PAIN ALL DOWN THE SPINAL COLUMN ON PRESEURE, running through all the stages is also characteristic.

MALARIA—(*Contd.*)

Chininum Ars.—It proves of great utility in patients who are cold, pale and emaciated. Patients who have a tendency to take cold and crave warm food, drinks, and warm room. The periodicity is most marked in those who frequently suffer from Malarial Fevers and have developed a general increasing Anæmia, with fast, feeble, irregular pulse. They are weary of life, with anxious restlessness, driving to despair. The rigor comes in the forenoon, afternoon or evening, with a hard shaking chill, goose-flesh all over body, and pain in the back, at different parts or in the whole spine. The chill is worse by drinking and better in a warm room, or by external warmth. High fever follows the chill or sometimes fever and chill alternate, with a desire to uncover during heat. Cerebral congestion with great heat of the head and violent darting pains, most severe at night and during the chill and heat, but ameliorated with the sweat. The sweat is cold and profuse, DURING SLEEP GENERALLY but also after awaking, with great weakness and exhaustion. The tongue is sore, tastes bitter while eating, diminished or ravenous appetite aversion to meat, cannot digest eggs or fish. Chronic Diarrhœa, vomiting, epistaxis and great prostration with cold hands and feet, cold knees, cold legs, palpitation and dropsical swelling of the hands and feet. Studied with the mind on *Arsenicum*, *Chininum Sulph* and *China* a broader knowledge will be gained of this remedy.

Taraxacum—Useful when Intermittents develop into a slow fever, in dry, nervous, bilious subjects, without any marked periodicity. Feels chilly after eating and drinking, with icy coldness of the nose, hands and tips of fingers, followed by heat without thirst, with red and hot face. The tongue is mapped, covered with a white film, which feels raw and comes off in patches, leaving red sensitive spots with loss of appetite, bitter taste and eructations. The sweat is copious and debilitating and occurs invariably at night. Jaundice with pain, enlargement and induration of the liver, and stitches in the spleen. The ABUNDANT, DEBILITATING NIGHT-SWEAT IS THE GUIDING SYMPTOM and the tongue and the gastric symptoms serve to differentiate it from *China*, which also has abundant, debilitating sweats but occurring chiefly during sleep or when covered.

Cina—Is frequently indispensable for Continued Fevers and Intermittents of children, between two and ten years of age, the chill returning at the same hour every day, with ravenous hunger before

MALARIA—(*Contd.*)

and duriug chill, without thirst. Shivering ; creeping over the trunk, not relieved by external warmth, with pale, cold face and cold sweat on forehead and vomiting. The chill is followed by convulsions and high fever. Heat with thirst for cold drinks, face puffed, pale around mouth and nose with red cheeks, restless sleep—starts and screams as if frightened, short breath and dilated pupils. Violent fever, vomiting, Diarrhœa. Sweat is generally light and cold, especially on forehead, around nose and on hands, followed by vomiting of food and canine hunger. TONGUE IS ALWAYS CLEAN. Peevish, whinning, complaining children with general worm symptoms ; too serious or sensitive for joking ; crave sweets.

Chamomilla—Vies with *China* and *Arsenicum* in the treatment of Intermittents of children who are irritable and cross. Fever attacks in spring. Paroxysms at 11 A. M. or 4 P. M. lasting till 11 P. M. ; 9 A. M. or 9 P. M. Chill without thirst intermingled with heat, with one red and one pale cheek. Long-lasting heat with violent thirst and frequent startings in sleep. Sweat is hot and profuse on covered parts and at night. ON AWAKING THE SWEAT CEASES AND RETURNS ON FALLING ASLEEP (*Sabad.*).

Eupatorium Perf.—It vies with *Arsenicum*, *China* and *Nat. Mur*. as one of our shcet anchors in this disease. It cures all types, its symptoms are clear-cut and well-defined and its action is prompt and decisive. It cures without reference to time though chill at 7 to 9 A. M. is characteristic. In some cases there is a double periodicity, the chill coming in the morning of one day and in the evening of the next. In the prodrome there is insatiable thirst, but drinking causes nausea and vomiting and hastens the chill. Knows the chill is coming as he cannot drink enough. Yawning, stretching, backache and bone-pains in extremities as if broken. Chill, with intense thirst, begins in back with yawning, stretching, backache and bone-pains. Chill may leave and return with no heat in the interval (*Ars.* chill and heat alternates). Vomiting of bitter fluids and bile at close of chill (*Capsi.* sour vomiting at close of chill, *Lyco.*). Heat, with great weakness, cannot raise head while heat lasts ; rarely any thirst ; cheeks mahogony-red and intense throbbing headache ; body sore from head to foot. A swallow of water produces shivering. Sweat is scanty or absent ; or profuse, when it brings relief of all pains except headache, which is increased (relieves all pains *Nat. Mur.*). When chill is severe, sweat is light or wanting or *vice versa*. Tongue, coated white or yellow ; insipid, bitter taste for food. Bone-pains continue in every stages unless relieved by sweat.

MALARIA—(*Contd.*)

Arnica—The picture is the same as in all other diseases, viz.—bruised, sore, weary feeling ; great weakness, must lie down, yet bed feels too hard, so he must change position for a soft place. Before the chill, yawning, stretching and drawing pain, as if in the periosteum, aching twists and thirst for large quantities of cold water, which refreshes him. Chill is felt more severely in pit of stomach, with heat and redness of one cheek, thirst and pain in muscles of the back and extremities, as if bruised, and great soreness of whole body. Heat, with less thirst but increased soreness of flesh, restlessness as the bed feels too hard. The heat feels intolerable and wants to uncover (*Apis, Pnls.*), but feels chilly on uncovering or even moving in bed (*Apis, Nux, Rhus Tox.* in all stages). Sweat is absent in recent attacks ; in old cases, sour and offensive. The soreness of mucles continues through every stage and persist during apyrexia. In cases where *Arnica* is indicated, relapses are more frequent.

Gelsemium—Marked periodicity, with regularity of the paroxysms, at the same hour every day (*Aran., Ced., Sabad.*). The Remittents take on Intermittent types and *vice versa.* Fever without chill at 10 A. M. Afternoon-fever without chill in infants and children. Fever with chill is preceded by incontinence of urine. The chill is without thirst, running along the spine, up and down the back. During chill wants to be held that he may not shake so hard (*Lachesis*). Sleepy as chill is leaving (*Apis*). Heat is also without thirst, with intense burning in the face. Sleeps during the heat ; stupid, besotted, wants to lie still (*Bryon.*). Sensation of falling, child starts and grasps and screams out for fear of falling, cannot open eyes ; loquacity. Sweat comes on gradually and moderately with thirst, always with relief. Tongue is clean or nearly so, with bitter taste. The apyrexia is very short, with great prostration of whole muscular system. It is always to be thought of in recent uncomplicated cases, where chill begins in the extremities (in chronic cases, *Nat. Mur.*).

Ignatia – Irregularity of hour is characteristic, the chill coming at all periods, preceded by violent yawning and stretching. Great thirst for large quantities of water only during chill (*Bryo.* same in all stages ; *Capsi., Carbo Veg., Eup.*, before and during chill). Shaking chill with redness of face in the evening, relieved at once in a warm room or by a warm stove (*Caps.* by heat applied to the back ; *Ars., China, Kali C., Lach., Menyanthes, Sabadilla* are others relieved by external warmth). Chill proceeding from the abdomen (most sever in abdomen, *Meny.* ; from the stomach, *Cal.* ; running to and terminating in stomach,

MALARIA—(*Contd.*)

Arni.). Heat, of whole body in afternoon, without thirst, when external warmth is intolerable (*Puls.*), must be uncovered (*Acon.*, *Sec.*); one ear, one cheek and side of face red and burning (one cheek red and hot, the other pale and cold, *Chamo.*). Deep snoring sleep, during heat (*Apis*, *Opium*), with frequent sighing. Urticaria over whole body with violent itching, disappearing with sweat (*Apis*, urticaria as chill passes off and continues during heat and sweat; *Rhus*, during heat and sweat; before and during chill, *Hepar*; *Elaterium* when chill is suppressed). Sweat is light, warm, chiefly on extremities. Tongue is clean, saliva sour and food tasteless. The apyrexia is complete with pale face and eruption on the lips and the corners of the mouth. Great thirst during chill which is relieved by external warmth and heat aggravated by external covering is prominently marked only in *Ignatia*.

Ipecac—Intermittent Fever paroxysms returning at 9 or 11 A. M. or 4 P. M., from indiscretions in diet or consequent upon abuse of *Quinine*, with short and usually not-severe chill, preceded by violent retching, yawning, stretching, back-ache, profuse flow of saliva and persistent nausea. Chill, without thirst, worse in a warm room or from external heat (*Apis*; better by external heat, *Ars.*, *Ign.*) and lessened by drinking and in open air (*Causti.*; worse by drinking *Capsi.*, *China*, *Eup.*, *Nux*). Great oppression of chest and great lassitude and weariness during chill (prostration greatest after heat, *Ars.*); chill followed by nausea and vomiting, first of contents of stomach, hen of bile. The hot stage lasts long, even all night, with thirst, and great oppression of chest, can hardly breathe; nausea, vomiting and dry, hacking cough with stitches in chest (*Acon.*, *Bryo.*, *Rhus*). Sweat is light, partial and sour, but profuse after abuse of *Quinine*. Worse during sweat and better after it (better by sweat *Eup.*, *Gels.*, *Nat. M.*). The tongue is at first clean, then coated yellowish or white. Bitter taste of everything eaten (*Bryo.*; except water, *Acon.*), and nausea and vomiting even during apyrexia which is never clear, with loss of appetite and more or less gastric trouble.

Lachesis—The paroxysms come on every spring, after suppression by *Quinine* the previous autumn, with strongly marked periodicity from 12 A. M. to 2 P. M. Violent chill in the evening, with chattering of the teeth and longing for fire heat which makes him feel better (*Ign.*) and wants to be firmly held to relieve the chill and prevent shaking (*Gels.*); icy-cold feet, pleuritic stitches; in children, convulsions; violent pain in the small of back and limbs and violent headache and oppression of chest continues even in heat, with deep breathing or sleep or great loquacity and thirst, (loquacity during chill and heat, *Podo*).

MALARIA—(*Contd.*).

Heat in the evening with vermilion-red cheeks, must be uncovered (*Acon.*, *Sec.*), with shivering when lifting the bed-clothes (*Nux*) and great sensitiveness of throat at night. The Sweat is cold and profuse, with relief, smelling like garlic and stains yellow or it is bloody, staining red. The tongue trembles when protruded or catches behind the teeth, is mapped, or dry with red tip and brown centre. Every thing tastes sour (bitter, *Ipec.*).

Crotalus Horridus--Indicated in Pernicious, Malignant Intermittents coming on with an unusual rapidity and reaching a very low and grave condition in an unusually short time, with relaxation of the blood-vessels, bleeding from all the orifices of the body and rapidly increasing unconsciousness. Ushers in with a light chill, soon developing an intense burning heat with dry hot skin, red flushed face, very quick pulse, 130-150 or even more, temp. 104°-106° and often epistaxis. Delirium, with open mouth, cold skin, and vomiting of bile, or blood. Abdomen tympanitic, stool bloody and involuntary, urine scanty or suppressed. Hæmorrhage from ears, eyes, nose, lungs, of dark, fluid, offensive blood, which does not co-agulate, and even bloody sweat and oozing of blood from nails, gums, skin. Ecchymoses and Purpura Hæmorrhagica. The tongue is fiery red, smooth and polished (*Pyro.*), intensely swollen or dry and cracked, with a dark brown streak down the centre with deep red edges. Pulse feeble and rapid, or slow, small, trembling and scarcely perceptible. Sweat is cold and comes in sudden attacks ; dark-colored, of axillæ ; bloody (*Cur.*, *Lach.*, *Lyco.*).

Terebinthina—Low types of Malignant Malarias with copious hæmorrhage of black, fluid blood from nose, stomach, kidneys, lungs, bowels, with excessive tympanites and meteorismus. Chill with rigors, followed by heat with great thirst, hot and dry skin and red face and profuse cold, clammy sweat with great prostration and emaciation. Tongue is smooth, glossy, red, as if deprived of papillæ (*Crotal.*, *Pyro.*) or dry and red with elevated papillæ. The pulse is small, wiry, scarcely perceptible.

Curare—Pernicious Intermittents with continued chillness. Paroxysms at 2 or 3 P. M and continued well into night. Burning heat with partial or transient chills, incoherent speech, great prostration and paralysis of extremities. The sweat is cold and bloody, especially at night.

Lycopodium—Must not be rejected in Intermittents if the paroxysm does not occur at 4 P. M. and the red, sandy sediment be not present in the urine. The sediment rarely occurs in acute cases. The most

MALARIA—(*Contd.*)

severe and most frequent paroxysm is the evening one at 6 or 7 P. M. which lasts all night. The general symptoms as flatulence, sour eructations, taste and sweat and sour vomiting are much more reliable guides and if these be aggravated from 4 to 8 P. M., *Lyco.* is much more indicated. It is useful in Pernicious Intermittents with long-lasting chill coming on at 9 A. M. and finally passing off without heat or sweat. Also shaking chill at 7 P. M. commencing in the back, with numb, icy-cold hands and feet (*Ced.*, *Sep.*), as if lying on ice, cannot get warm even by external heat and drawing in all the limbs, back and whole body followed by sweat without intervening heat. The hot stage comes with great heat and redness of the face, frequent drinking of small quantities at a time (*Ars.*, *China.*) and irresistible sleepiness (*Apis*, *Ign.*) and nausea after cold drinks (nausea relieved by drinking, *Lobel.*), warm drinks being grateful (*Ced.*). Sour vomiting between chill and heat (bitter, bilious, *Eup.*, *Ipe.*). Must uncover (*Lach.*). Perspiration, sour and profuse, often immediately after the chill without intervening heat, with great thirst. Tongue is clean but dry, with vesicles on tip. The apyrexia is marked with a constant sense of fulness of stomach, rumbling in the bowels and obstinate constipation.

Menyanthes—A very efficient remedy in irregular Intermittents when chill is the predominant stage, with icy-coldness of the hands and feet as far up as the knees and warmth of the rest of the body ; chilliness most severe in the back, relieved by external heat. A disagreeable feeling of heat comes on, alternating or intermingled with chilliness. The whole paroxysm is characterized by absence of thirst during all stages, bitter-sweetish taste and ravenous hunger.

Sambucus—Hard, dry cough before the chill, the latter lasting a very short time, about half an hour, with dry heat on falling asleep, dread of uncovering and without thirst. Profuse non-debilitating sweat over entire body during waking hours ; on going to sleep, dry heat returns (sweat as soon as he closes his eyes to sleep, *China*, *Coni.* ; sweats when he sleeps, stops when awakens, *Thuja*). The whole paroxvsm is characterized by entire absence of thirst during all stages.

Natrum Muriaticum—Every type of fever belongs to it with the morning paroxysm predominating, especially at 11 A. M., though it makes little difference when the chill commences, if the rest of the symptoms indicate the remedy. It is almost the best friend a physician has in a malarious district. Caused by living in the vicinity of water, in damp regions or near freshly plowed fields and also after abuse of *Quinine*. Patient dreads the chill and knows it is coming because of languor, head-

MALARIA—(*Contd.*)
ache and thirst with vomiting of the recently drunk water. Then comes a long and severe chill from 10 to 11 A. M., beginning in the fingers and toes or small of back (*Gels.*), with blue lips and nails (*Nux*), chattering of the teeth, thirst, drinking often and much at a time (but produces vomiting, *Eup.* ; little and often, *Ars.*), and brusting headache, nausea, vomiting and sometimes complete unconsciousness. Then comes a long, severe heat with excessive weakness (during chill, *Lyco.* ; after the paroxysm, *Ars.*), intolerable hammering headache, increased thirst, drinks much and often which refreshes (*Bryo.* ; little and often, but with vomiting, *Ars.*) ; stupefaction and unconsciousness (*Bell.*, *Cact.*, *Op.*). Vomiting of bile between chill and fever (*Eup.*, *Lyco.*) or during heat, which latter is followed by a gradual appearance of sweat which relieves all pains, the headache decreasing gradually as the sweat increases and becomes profuse. The tongue is dry, with a thin, yellowish-white coating or there are blisters on a mapped tongue, looking like herpes on the sides (*Lach.*, *Tarax.*). Water tastes putrid (bitter, *Ars.*), longing for salt, aversion to bread and great loss of appetite during apyrexia. Lips covered with hydroa (*Ign.*, *Nux*, *Rhus*), ulceration of labial commissures.

Nux Vom.—Like *Nat. Mur.* it is also a remedy of every type of fever, the paroxysms coming at any hour of the day, but more frequently in the morning being irregular in its stages, the chill, heat and sweat coming in different successions. The onset is preceded by intolerable drawing pain through the thighs and legs and a sense of prostration. Often heat, and sometimes sweat comes before the chill. The chill is without thirst and is violent and shaking, with great coldness of the whole body, not relieved by external warmth or covering (*Ars.*, *Ign.*, *Ipe.*, *Apis*), bluish cold face and hands and pain in sacrum (in dorsal vertebræ, *Chin. S.*). Shivering and chillness after drinking (*Capsi.*, *Eup.*). Sleeps after chill (*Apis.*, *Ars*, *Camph.*, *Lyco.*, *Nux M.*, *Sab.* ; during heat— *Ant. T.*, *Apis*, *Caps.*, *Ced.*, *China.*, *Eup.*, *Gels.*, *Ign.*, *Lach.*, *Lyco.*, *Nat. M.*, *Nux M.*, *Op.*, Podo., *Rhus*, *Samb.*). Pernicious, congestive type of chills with vertigo, headache, anguish, delirium, terrible coldness of the body, blue face, nails and hands, vivid visions, distension of stomach, stitches in the sides and abdomen ; worse from slightest attempt to uncover or move in bed. The heat is long-lasting and violent, with great thirst, whole body burning hot, yet must be covered, cannot move or uncover in the least without feeling chilly (*Acon.*, *Bell.*, *Arni.*, *Capsi.*), with stitching headache, anguish, vertigo, delirium, pain in chest, sides, abdomen, cold feet and shivering. The sweating stage is light without thirst but with chillness from motion or allowing the air to strike him. The severest paroxysm of the congestive chill is followed

MALARIA—(*Contd.*)

by profuse perspiration (reverse of *Eup.*, which has light chill and profuse sweat and hard shaking chill with scanty sweat). Sweat relieves pains in limbs (*Eup.*, *Lyco.*, *Nat.*). The tongue is heavily coated white or yellow, with sour, putrid or bitter taste, must rinse the mouth. Gastric and bilious symptoms are always present during the apyrexia, with great weakness, chilliness and rupugnance to cold air.

Opium—Congestive and Epileptiform Intermittents with regular paroxysms and irregular stages, particularly in old persons and children. Shaking chill at 11 A. M. or afternoon, night or after midnight, without thirst ; with hot head, deep sleep, profuse sweat about the head and coldness of single parts. The heat rises very high, 105° or 106°, and whole body becomes covered with a scorching hot sweat and a rapid or slow, scarcely perceptible pulse ; deep, snoring sleep with open mouth, stertorous breathing, twitching of limbs, spasmodic contraction of the muscles of the face, sardonic smile and unconsciousness with besotted, bloated, purple face, glossy eyes and contracted pupils. Wants to be uncovered, wants the cool air and even gets into convulsions in a warm room with opisthotonos, head drawn back ; kicks the covers off (*Apis*). Sweat and heat intermingled, with aggravation of the existing symptoms. The apyrexia is marked by evidences of cerebral congestion with profound stupor, and complete indifference—makes no complaint what so ever.

Podophyllum—The morning paroxysm at 7 A. M. is characteristic and the chill is ushered in with severe backache in the lumbar region and is accompanied with aching in hypochondria, knees, ankles, elbows and wrists ; loquacity, and no thirst. The heat begins while he is yet chilly, with violent headache and excessive thirst. Great loquacity, constantly talking (*Carbo Veg.*, *Lach.*), which continues with delirium, until fever reaches its acme, when he falls asleep and perspires profusely ; when awakes he forgets all that had passed. The tongue shows imprint of teeth (*Merc.*) ; offensive breath which disgusts him (not perceptible to himself, *Puls.*). Falls asleep at climax of heat and sleeps during perspiration like *Apis*, but there is no urticaria and the perspiration is more profuse.

Pulsatilla—Intermittents of irregular type with irregular stages which are apt to run into each other (*Ars.*, *Nux*, *Podo.*), the 4 P. M. paroxysm predominating. Caused by dietetic irregularities and disorders of stomach (*Ant. T.*, *Ipe.*, *Nux*). Chill begins in the hands and feet with pain in limbs. Thirstless during chill even with dry mouth and lips ; licks the lips but does not want to drink. Often thirst appears before the chill, at about 2 or 3 P. M., and then comes chill without thirst, and with anxiety and

MALARIA—(*Contd.*)

oppression (from venous congestion) of the chest. Heat with thirst and uneasiness ; burning of the hands, seeks about cool places for them and desires to uncover (*Apis, Camph., Sec.*). The heat is generally of single parts or heat of one hand, coldness of the other or body hot, limbs cold. LONG CHILL, LITTLE HEAT, NO THIRST (short chill, long heat, no thirst *Ipe.*). At the end of the fever there may be general or partial sweat, which may last all night, with LOQUACITY during stupefied sleep (during heat, *Laches.* ; during chill and heat, *Podo.*). The pains continue during sweat (*Eup., Lach., Nat., Nux*). During apyrexia there is a constant chilliness and the spleen is enlarged and sensitive with prevalance of the gastric and bilious symptoms. With *Puls.* no two paroxysms are alike and the symptoms are ever-changing with increasing severity. Presence of thirst during heat is not a contra-indication.

Pyrogen.—Types of Intermittents which tend rapidly to malignancy. Chill is preceded by aching in the limbs great muscular soreness and bone-pains, the bed feels hard (*Arn., Bapti., Eup.*). Chill begins in the back between the scapulæ with chattering teeth, as soon as he touches the cold bed (*Aran.*), increased action of the heart and a sensation as if lungs were on fire, must have fresh air. Chilly when leaving the fire. Intense restlessness ; must move constantly to relieve aching and soreness of bones and muscles (*Arn., Bapti.*). Frequent urging to urinate as soon as chills come on, could tell when it was coming on that account. Heat comes with very high temperature, 103° to 106°, with circumscribed redness of the cheeks, great throbbing of temporal arteries and dry, burning skin ; pulse rapid, small, wiry 140 to 170. Sweat is profuse, horribly offensive and exhausting ; of single parts ; SWEATS DURING SLEEP, STOPS WHEN HE WAKES. (*Camph., China, Chamo., Sabad.*). Tongue clean and smooth, as if varnished ; fiery red and very dry and cracked with difficult articulation. Taste is bitter, fetid and breath horribly offensive. The symptoms of this remedy are very much like those of *Baptisia*, but the temperature is too intense for the latter. "When the temperature reaches 106° with great soreness and aching, *Pyrogen* will make a great change in a single day ; and if the pains are relieved by motion and heat, it will abort the fever."

Rhus Tox.—All types of Intermittents, the first two stages being often irregular, and the paroxysms coming at all periods except, perhaps, forenoon, the evening paroxysm being predominant—that at 7 P. M. lasting all night. Caused often by getting wet, cold bathing, living in damp rooms, sleeping in damp beds, damp wet weather. The chill is preceded by burning in eyes, stretching, severe pain in limbs and a dry, teasing, fatiguing cough (*Acon., Bryo., Ipe.*). The caugh continues during chill which is mixed and irregular. Severe chill, as if ice-water were

MALARIA.—(*Contd.*

dashed over him, or blood running cold through vessels. Coldness of left tibia, arm and left side of body. Shaking chill on going from open air into a warm room and great restlessness with relief (*Ars.* from mental anguish). Heat is excessive, as if dashed with hot water or as if blood was running hot through the vessels. The cough ceases with the heat but urticaria breaks out over entire body with violent itching, increased by rubbing, driving the patient frantic and pases off with the sweat which breaks out profusely over the whole body, except face (reverse of *Sili.*) or *Vice Versa*, but is not debilitating and also does not relieve the pains like *Nat. Mur.* SLEEPS DURING THE SWEAT (*Podo.*). Tongue takes imprint of teeth (*Merc.*, *Podo.*) ; tringular red tip and dry ; bitter or putrid taste after eating or drinking. Hydroa on upper lip.

Secale.—Proves of great service in PERNICIOUS or SINKING forms of Intermittents with violent, shaking chills, unquenchable thirst, intense icy- coldness of the skin, particularly of face and extremities (*Camph.*, *Meny.*, *Nux*, *Ver.*) ; pale, sunken face with bluish lips and diminished temperature of the body (*Camph.*, *Ver.*). The heat is severe, dry and long-lasting with great restless and violent thirst (*Ars.*, *Nat.*, *Rhus*) and is followed by profuse, cold, clammy sweat all over the body, except face (*Rhus* ; reverse of *Sili.*). The pulse is generally slow, contracted and at times intermittent and the tongue deathly pale. The whole picture resembles a Cholera-collapse with pale, drawn, collapsed, hippocratic face and intense icy-coldness of the whole body, characterized by a decided aversion to heat or being covered (*Camph.*).

Sulphur.—Frequently required in all forms of the disease to combat some latent malady aroused during the course of the fever. The chill comes at any time but is predominant in the evening. Frequent internal chilliness creeping from sacrum up the back, and shivering over whole body, without thirst. Hands and feet very cold, with livid, pale face and icy-coldness of genitals. Thirst comes with the heat which is intense, presistent and long continued ; skin dry, hot, burning ; temperature 103^{0}–105^{0}, little or no remission, day or night ; patient literally being consumed with fever ; great orgasm of the blood and violent burning heat of the palms and soles. Profuse, sour sweat breaks out all over the body at night with restless sleep or copious morning sweat, setting in after waking (*Samb.*). Bitter taste in the mouth in the morning, food tastes natural, longing for sweets. Great prostration after the paroxysm (*Ars.*). Burning heat on vertex.

Tuberculinum.—Stubborn cases that continue relapsing from a little cold or draft or fatigue or from mental exertion, over-eating and disordered stomach. Intermittents in Phthisical patients with ever-changing

MALARIA—(*Contd.*)

symptoms, often require the remedy. General excessive fatigue, even after a short walk, must lean on his companion ; great weakness from knees down, so that can scarcely walk. Drawing in the limbs in the evening, before and during the chill. Khows the chill is coming on because of the drawing in the limbs. Cough before and during chill and vomiting during fever with extreme heat, mixed up with chilliness extending into the fever and the sweat if there is any uncovering.

Thuja.— Persons of sycotic diathesis, who are always chilly from least change of weather often need the remedy. Paroxysms at 3 A. M. or 5 to 7 P. M. are characteristic. Shaking chill with thirst begining in the thighs, with much yawning and shivering through and through, from the slightest uncovering of the body in warm air and even the hot sun does not warm him (*Nux*, *Camph.*, *Canth.*), with blueness of nails, chattering of teeth, rapid and difficult respiration. Then thighs become hot, like a glowing coal, with cold hands and fcet and gradually face and cheeks become burning hot, lasting the whole day, with restlessness, severe headache and thirst ; drinking refreshes. Sweats profusely on his legs, where chill began or only on uncovered parts or even all over except the head (reverse of *Sili.*) ; profuse perspiration when he sleeps, which ceases when he awakes (reverse of *Samb.*) ; tongue clean, or red with vesiclcs or blisters on margin, tip painfully sore to touch. Bitter sour taste—has to rinse mouth (*Nux*). Feels perfectiy well as soon as paroxysm is over.

Veratrum Album.—Produces one of the best pictures of the "Sinking", "Congestive" or "Pernicious" types of Intermittents with a shadow of death overhanging. Severe, long-lasting, congestive chill not relieved by external warmth (*Aran.*, *Camph.*), and running from head to the toes of both feet, with thirst ; face cold, collapsed, extremities cold. The external coldness is predominant. Heat ascends from extremities to the head (chill descends), streaming up the back into the occiput with thirst and persistent cold sweat on the forehead, redness and burning heat in face and cheeks with contracted pupils and cold feet (*Op.* ; dilated pupils, *Bell.*). The sweat is without thirst ; profuse, cold and clammy (profuse, with thirst *Ars.*, *China*), offensive, bitter smelling, staining linen yellow. Tongue is coated white or yellowish-brown and is cold, with red tip and edges. The appetite remains voracious with craving for everything cold and aversion to warm things. There is an overwhelmingly rapid sinking and exhaustion with deathly pale and cold face, cold sweat on forehead, deep sighing with oppression of chest, persistently cold extremities and bluish, cold, in-elastic skin, vomiting, diarrhœa. The temperature is generally sub-normal or rarely elevated even in hot stage, from a general lack

MALARIA—(*Contd.*)

of vital heat, so much so that the patient rarely recovers from one paroxysm, ere another begins.

Elaterium.—Chilliness preceded by yawning and gaping with headache, soreness of the limbs and pain in the bowels which all run through the chill gradually increasing to violent tearing pains through-out the head, especially on the vertex in the heat with intense thirst and pains shooting to the very tips of fingers and toes and back again into the body and copious, liquid, frothy diarrhœa. When sweat comes, it is copious and gradually relieves all the symptoms. It thus compares with *Verat. Alb.* but the predominance of the characteristic cold stage of the latter is decisive. Urticarea all over the body after suppression of Intermittent Fever.

Verat. Viride.—Ranks equally with *Camph.* and *Verat. Alb.* in congestive, malignant types of Intermittents of sudden onset and rapid course with a slow, soft and weak pulse,—irregular and intermittent (*Digi.*), which suddenly increases and gradually decreases below normal and a white or yellow tongue with a red streak down the middle.

Congestive, Malignant, Pernicious Intermittents with extreme coldnese, thirst, cold collapsed face, great prostration, cold clammy skin, cold sweat on forehead and deathly pallor on face.

MALIGNANT INTERMITTENTS—Compare.—*Ars., Carb. Ac., Crot., Mur Ac., Psor., Pyr., Terb., Ver., V.*

PERNICIOUS—*Apis., Arn., Camph., Lyco., Nux., Op., Psor., Sul., Sul. Ac., Ver., Alb., Ver., V.*

RESPIRATORY ORGANS

APHONIA (LOSS OF VOICE)—HOARSENESS

Alumina.—Hoarseness ; paralytic weakness of the vocal cords, *Causticum, Gelsemium*) ; steadily increasing to loss of voice, worse in the morning (*Causticam*), with dryness and splinter-likc feeling in the throat when swallowing (*Arg. Nit., Hepar, Nit. Acid*). The voice is weak, can sing only for a little while.

Alumen.—Useful for chronic loss of voice from a low state of the economy, in patients who are always taking a fresh cold and scraping out all the time a little yellow mucus (*Arg. Met.* profuse).

RESPIRATORY ORGANS—(*Contd.*)

Argentum Met.—Loss of voice from inflammation or over-use and a sort of paretic weakness of vocal cords in singers and public speakers who suffer from an alternation of the timber of the voice. Tubercular states of the larynx (*Manganum*), cannot speak a loud word ; soreness, rawness and tickling in the larynx with a necessity to scrape out large quantity of gray mucus all the time (small quantity—*Alumen*) ; great weakness of the chest.

Arg. Nit.—Rawness, soreness and scraping with tenacious mucus in the throat, causing hacking and cough in singers and speakers with marked hoarseness and even total loss of voice. Sensation of a splinter in the throat (*Alumina, Hepar, Nit. Acid*).

Manganum.—Equal to *Arg. Met.* in singers and speakers, with chronic hoarseness and loss of voice in anæmic or Tubercular patients ; constant accumulation of mucus and hemming all the time.

Selenium.—Useful in Tubercular throat with hoarseness and large, hard glands of the neck (also see under *Arum Triphyllum*).

Spongia.—Sudden hoarseness in Tubercular patients (see also *Arum Triphyllum* and *Verbascum*).

Causticum.—Sudden hoarseness from paralytic weakness with morning aggravation. *Carbo Veg.* has evening aggravation,

Arum Triphyllum.—Hoarseness of singers or those who exert their voice a great deal. Voice uncertain and uncontrollable—suddenly goes up with a squeak if he attempts to raise it.

Graphites.—Singers cannot control their voice. They are hoarse and their voice cracks as soon as they begin to sing.

Rhus Tox.—Voice hoarse to begin with, but his voice improves on singing or talking a while.

Selenium.—Gets hoarse as soon as he begins to sing ; also after long use of voice. Much clear starchy mucus hawked out at the beginning of singing (see also *Senega*).

Spongia.—Voice gives out or gets cracked when singing or talking ; each cold settles on the throat with great dryness (*Alumina*). Hoareseness and hissing or croupy voice.

Carbo Veg.—Deep voice, which fails when tried to rase it. *Arnica* is also useful for hoarseness from over-use of voice, as shouting loudly (*Arg. Met., Arg. Nit.*). Generally painless aphonia, but sometimes with rawness and soreness ; worse in the evening and damp warm weather. Must frequently clear the throat in the evening.

RESPIRATORY ORGANS—(*Contd.*)

Causticum.—Rawness and soreness down the throat, with hoarseness, in the morning (*Alumina*), from dry cold or severe winter weather. Sudden loss of voice, cannot speak a loud word, caused by paresis of the vocal cords or by catarrhal states.

Ammonium Causticum.—A splendid remedy for aphonia with burning rawness in the throat (also *Ammon. Mur.*).

Eupatorium Perfoliatum.—Morning hoarseness in connection with great soreness rather than the burning and rawness of *Causticum.*

Phosphorus.—Evening hoarseness with extreme sensitivness of the box of the larynx, which hurts to touch, to talk or to cough. Tubercular diathesis.

Stannum.—Also *Arg. Met.* and *Phosphorus* have evening hoarsness, weak chest, hectic fever and copious sputum. But *Phosphorus* has more blood or blood streaks with the sputum, worse lying on left side, and thirst for cold water.

Gelsemium.—Paresis of the vocal cords in hysterical women especially after depressing emotions, so that they can scarcely utter any sound, can only whisper ; worse during menses and better after it. Nervous hoarseness—"Apprehension of some unusual ordeal, brings on symptoms." In paralytic weakness of the vocal cords *Gelsemium* should also be studied with *Causticum* and *Alumina.*

Senega.—Hoarseness with dry throat, copious tough mucus in the air-tubes and a tickling cough that ends with sneezing. Aphonia from severe cold or excessive use of voice.

Silicea.—Catarrhal hoarseness with dryness and roughness and cough, due to tickling at the supra-sternal fossa—very much like *Rumex.*

Spongia.—Also has a barking cough with hoarseness (also *Causticum* which is useful in chronic hoarseness with deep bass voice remaining after acute laryngitis).

Sulphur.—Sometimes needed in cases of hoarseness with deep hoarse cough—if the others fail.

Thuja.—Sometimes useful for hoarseness in the decidedly sycotic.

Trifolium Pratense.—Hoarseness and choking spells at night with cough.

Verbascum.—Hollow, hoarse, barking or trumpet-like cough, with hoarseness. The voice itself is deep and hard, basso-profundo, with hoarseness when reading aloud. *Drosera* has also a deep barking cough with hoarseness, but it has more laryngeal troubles.

RESPIRATORY ORGANS

(*Contd.*)

ASTHMA.

Antim. Tart.—Asthma with coarse rattling of mucus in chest, oppression of breathing, with pale cyanotic faee, prostration, coldness, cold sweat on forehead, must sit up to get air. The suffocative attacks come on at 3 A. M. like *Kali Bi.*, *Kali Carb.*, etc. There is grcat rattling with but very little expectoration and that too without any relief.

Argentum Nit.—Pure nervous asthma with spasms of the respiratory muscles and marked dyspnœa worse in crowded, stuffy or warm room. Wants doors and windows open, cold air, cold drinks, cold things,

Arsenicum—A prime remedy in asthma with aggravation after midnight and lying down and great anguish and restlessness. Asthma complicated with emphysema—expiration being much prolonged. Must sit up and incline the chest forward. Great dyspnœa with despair which abates as soon as raises frothy saliva or thick mucus, sometimes even streaked with blood. Worse from cold things, better from warmth, warm food, etc. It follows *Ipecac* well.

Apis.—Has a suffocative feeling and the patient does not see how he can take another breath.

Bromine.—Breathes very deeply as if could not get enough air into his lungs ; complicated with constriction of the glottis.

Cuprum Mct.—Useful in asthma when the spasmodic element predominates with constriction of the throat ; face gets blue and almost goes into convulsions. Violent attacks come suddenly and cease as suddenly. Worse at night, before and during menses, from mental emotions.

Ferrum Met.—Asthma worse after 12 o'clock at night, better from uncovering chest and slowly moving about.

Graphites.—Spasmodic Asthma. Suffocative spells arousing from sleep, must jump out of bed and eat something to ease the difficulty of breathing. Sensitive to cold in winter and to heat in summer. Fat. chilly, costive ; worse in a warm room and desires open air.

Lachesis.—Is aroused from sleep with asthmatic paroxysm, cannot bear the least pressure about the neck or chest and finally coughs up a quantity of watery phlegm with great relief.

Grindelia.—Stops breathing on falling asleep, wakes with a start and gasps for breath. Profuse, tough, whitish expectoration relieves.

RESPIRATORY ORGANS—(*Contd.*)

Ipecac.—Asthma in stout persons of lax fibre, adult or child, who are sensitive to warm, moist atmosphere. There is a constant feeling of constriction in chest with shortness of breath together with a violent, incessant, wheezing cough and rattling of mucus in chest, yet none is expectorated. Threatened suffocation with very difficult expiration, worse from least motion. Followed by *Arsenic.*

> **Lobelia.**—Great oppression and weak sensation in the chest which seems to come from the epigastrium, spreading into the chest with nausea, profuse salivation and a feeling of a lump in the stomach ; often preceded by prickling all over, even to fingers and toes. Worse from any exertion, slightest motion, cold, tobacco.

Kali Bichrom.—Asthma, worse from 3 to 4 A. M. (also *Kali Carb.*), liable to return in winter or in summer when chilly ; relieved from sitting up and bending forward and finally by the expectoration of stringy or ropy yellow mucus. It diflers from *Ars.* in this feature of tenacious sputum.

Nat. Sulph,—Useful in asthma excited or made worse by every spell of damp weather ; hydrogenoid constitution, sycotic basis. Dyspnœa with rattling in chest at 4 or 5 A., M ; cough with profuse, thick, glairy, greenish expectoration. Looseness of bowels after each attack. Must sit up and hold the chest with hands during the attack. Asthma of children.

Nux Vom.—Attacks brought on by gastric distrubance, in persons of irritable, billous temperament, with a feeling of fulness and oppression in stomach, particularly after a hearty meal. A constricted feeling at the lower part of chest, relieved by loosening clothing, belching and by recumbent position, raising the trunk and turning to the other side.

> **Zingiber.**—May also be used in servere paroxysms of asthma of gastric origin, coming at night towards morning, but with no anxiety.
>
> **Lycopodium.**—Asthma from abdominal irritation with marked flatulence. So also is *Carbo Veg.* The latter particularly in asthma of old people or who are much debilitated. They look as if they would die of the oppressed breathing and are relieved by belching and by hard fanning.

RESPIRATORY ORGANS

(*Contd.*)

BRONCHIAL CATARRH.

Aconite.—Vigorous persons, exposed to dry, cold winds or drafts or from checked perspiration, come down suddenly with violent congestions with severe fever, hot, dry skin, quick and hard pulse, intense restlessness, anxiety and fear of death, developing Bronchitis with short, dry, titillating cough. It ceases to be the remedy when exudation commences.

Ferrum Phos.—Is indicated in just such eases as indicate *Aconite,* but there is less of the extreme restlessness, anxiety and thirst.

Gelsemium.—Is characterized by lassitude, physical weakness, drowsiness, with a full flowing pulse and moderate congestion.

Ammon. Carb.—Chronic Bronchitis of the aged with atony of the bronchial tubes which favors bronchial dilatation and œdema pulmonum. Therc is copious mucus in lungs but can hardly cough lout loud and because of weakness cannot expel mucus like *Ant. Tart.* Slow, labored, stertorous breathing, bubbling sound. Winter catarrh. Worse, 3 to 4 A. M., cold weather.

Ammon. Mur.—Chronic Bronchitis with constant hacking and scraping, but only brings out small pieces of white mucus; burning in chest and coarse, rattling murmurs; icy-coldness between shoulders. Bronchiectasis, Emphysema.

Ammoniacum.—Chronic Bronchitis, with coarse rattling of chest in old people, worse cold weather.

Senega.—Chronic Bronchitis of the old. Cough with great accumulation of mucus, which seems to fill the chest, with much rattling, wheezing and difficult breathing. Fat pcople with lax fibre.

Pix Liquida.—Chronic bronchial catarrh with offensive purulent expectoration and a pain in the upper left chest going through to the back.

Antim. Tart.—At the beginning of Capillary Bronchitis of children, with sub-crepitant rales all through thc chest, wheezing breathing and loose cough but no expectoration. Often follows *Ipecac.* which is one of the best remedies for Broncho-Pneumonia or Capillary Bronchitis in infants. *Ipecac.* has great deal of mucus in chest with rales all through with diffio lt breathing and frequent spasmodic cough,

RESPIRATORY ORGANS—(*Coutd:*)

usually with gagging and vomiting of phlegm. If after *Ipecac.* there is great accumulation of mucus with coarse rattles or the chest is so filled with mucus that the child cannot cough, which grows less and less frequent and the child grows drowsy with hot head bathed in sweat, and symptoms of Cyanosis, indicating threatening Paralysis of the lungs *Antim. Tart.* often cures.

Terebinthina.—Is useful when the urine is apt to be scanty and dark from admixture of blood.

Hepar Sulph.—Is often useful in Capillary Bronchitis but differs from *Ant. Tart.* in this that the latter has loose rattling mucus and the former has a wheezing, purring sound, as if the exudate were more tenacious.

Kali Carb.—Also useful in Capillary Bronchitis of infants. The child has intense dyspnœa with great deal of mucus in chest raised with difficulty. Breathing is wheezing and whistling and the child has a choking cough.

Chelidonium.—Capillary Bronchitis especially after Measles or Whooping Cough, with difficult respiration, short fits of coughing and rattling of mucus in chest ; great oppression of chest with fan-like motion of alæ nasi, one hot and other cold foot. The well-known hepatic symptoms are decisive.

Lycopodium.—Also has fan-like motion of alæ nasi, and one hot and other cold foot. It is especially useful if there is stupor or drowsiness, tympanitis and opening of the mouth.

Phosphorus.—When the substance of the lungs becomes more and more involved with fan-like motion of alæ nasi, marked restlessness, intense thirst and burning all over the body.

Sulphur.—Bronchial catarrh with loud rales all through the chest, particularly the left lung and especially after the failure of *Ipecac., Ant. Tart,* or *Phos.*

Opium.—Capillary Bronchitis with severe aphonia. Difficult, intermittent or stertorous breathing, constant cough, sopor, face bluish, profuse sweat over whole body.

Baryta Carb.—In orthopnœa or threatened Paralysis of lungs in the aged, with loud rattling of phlegm but no expulsive power, it complements *Ant. Tart.* when the latter partially relieves.

Arsenicum.—Chronic Bronchitis of the aged, with dyspnœa from more or less extensive Emphysema and pulmonary congestions (See Asthma).

Calcarea Carb.—Chronic Bronchitis with Emphysema. Yellow, lumpy, sweetish or fetid expectoration which, when thrown into water,

RESPIRATORY ORGANS—(*contd.*).

is seen shooting to the bottom with a mucous trial behind, like a falling star. Teething children, with loose rattling cough and scrofulous individuals with the generalities of the drug.

Calc. Sulph.—Loose rattling cough in chronic catarrh, with copious expectoration of thick, lumpy, greenish or yellow or pus-like sputa in the morning. Here it compares with *Hepar* but unlike the latter it is better in cool air.

Pulsatilla.—Chronic loose cough after Measles or Broncho-Pneumonia after resolution, with copious expectoration of thick, yellowish-green mucus in the morning ; wants cold open air.

Kali Sulph.—Chronic catarrh of the air-passages with thick greenish-yellow mucus, rattling cough and breathing and dyspnœa. After Bronchitis or Pneumonia, rattling from every cold change in weather. It has all the modalities of *Pulsatilla* which it often complements.

Kali Bich.—Chronic Bronchitis where the tubes are filled with tough, tenacious exudation. Hard cough in the morning on waking up, with profuse yellow expectoration, coming out in long, stringy and very tenacious mass. The modalities are opposite of *Kali Sulph* or *Puls.*

Hydrastis.—Chronic cough in Bronchitis of the old, with cachectic state, loss of appetite and marked prostration. The sputa is thick, yellow, very tenacious, stringy and profuse.

Kali Iod.—Profuse, thick and heavy, greenish sputa, tasting salty (*Sepia*), which seems to come from deep in the chest with a pain through to between the shoulders. Exhausting night-sweats and general weakness. It also has a frothy or soap-suds-like sputa which is found in œdema of the lungs.

Stannum.—Profuse, purulent, greenish sputa, sweetish to taste, and a marked feeling of weakness in the chest ; can hardly talk.

Draconitum.—A violent attack of bronchial catarrh quickly and rapidly developing into yellowish, purulent discharge, with great burning and rawness in the trachea and bronchial tubes.

Balsam of Peru.—Loud rales and expectoration of thick, creamy and yellowish-white mucus, with night-sweats and hectic fever.

Pix Liquida.—Chronic bronchial catarrh with offensive, purulent expectoration and a pain in the upper left chest, going through to back (also *Guaiacum.*).

Sanguinaria.--Tough, rust-colored, offensive sputum, almost impossible to raise ; violent cough with pain in the trachea, as if torn

RESPIRATORY ORGANS—(*Contd.*)

asunder and after the cough, copious, loud, empty eructations. It is perhaps next in importance to *Capsicum* when there is a horribly offensive exhalation during coughing but not when quiet breathing.

Copaiva.—Chronic Bronchorrhœa with profuse expectoration of greenish, purulent, offensive mucus ; oppression of chest and labored breathing ; can only breathe easily when bolstered up in bed.

Carbo Animalis.--Hoarse cough, shaking the brain, as if it were loose in the head, and a cold feeling in chest (*Bromine, Camphor, Paris Quadri.*). Green, purulent and horribly offensive expectoration generally from the rt. lung, in which there may be a cavity.

Carbo Vegetabilis.—Spasmodic cough with deep, rough voice or aphonia and decided burning in the chest, particularly in Chronic Bronchitis of old people. The expectoration is profuse and is yellow and very fetid, more so than in *Carbo Animalis.* Great rattling in the chest and dyspnœa.

Silicea.—Brochial affections of rachitic children. Obstinate cough with copious, transparent or purulent expectoration. Laryngeal morning cough, immediately after rising, with tough, gelatinous and very tenacious sputum or expectoration of pus, which when thrown into water falls to the bottom and spreads like heavy sediment.

Sulphur.—Chronic catarrhs of long-standing, with secretion of large quantities of tenaeious mucus. Sensation of ice in chest, whenever chilled. Psoric diathesis, the general characteristics corresponding.

RESPIRATORY ORGANS

(*Contd.*)

PLEURISY.

Bryonia.—Has the closest picture of Pleurisy than any other remedy. It comes in when the stage of *Aconite* (See Bronchitis) is gone. The skin is not so hot though the fever continues, the face is not so red and the patient is not so restless as when *Aconite* was indicated and effusion has begun, as indicated by friction sounds. The patient is quiet, and full of pain, he lies on the affected side with the characteristic sharp, stitching pains which are worse on motion.

RESPIRATORY ORGANS—(*Contd.*)

Senga.—Violent attack of Pleurisy with *Bryonia* symptoms but worse from rest (*Rhus Tox.*) ; as if chest were too tight.

Arnica.—Aftcr injuries to chest-wall. Must often change position ; stitches in chest. Pneumo-thorax from external injuries. Is followed well by *Sulph. Acid.*

Belladonna.—Rt. side ; great soreness ; cannot lie on the affected side ; worse from jar of bed ; general picture of the drug.

Stannum.—Sharp knife-like stitches in the left axilla, going up to left clavicle.

Kali Carb.—Pleurisy with stitches in the left chest irrespective of motion ; palpitation and dry cough. Pain as if lower lobe of rt. lung were adhering to ribs. Puffiness of upper eye-lids. Worse at 3 A. M. and on inspiration.

Gaultheria.—Pleurodynia with pain in anterior mediastinum.

Guaiacum.—Rarely fails in Pleurodynia associated with Tuberculosis.

Borax.—Pleurodynia ; stitches in chest with inspiration and cough ; worse, upper part of rt. chest ; out of breath when going upstairs, with stitches in the rt. chest even when speaking.

Sulphur.—Comes in when despite *Bryonia* exudation goes on increasing, with sharp stitching pains going through to the left scapula, shortness of breath and oppression. Plastic exudation. It is one of the most valuable absorbents.

Apis.—One of the best remedies to .bring about absorption of the fluid. It comes in when the fever has abated and the pains are very little if prescnt, but there is great oppression, worse at night and from warmth ; feels as if he cauld not take another breath. Face pale and œdematous, feeble pulse, scanty urine. Great oppression and faintness from the quanitity of exudation. Chronic or latent cases,

Kali Iod.—Great difficulty in breathing with Hydro-thorax ; pleuritic effusion. Cannot lie in comfort at all on right side ; heart displaced ; absence of respiratory sounds in affected parts.

Cantharis.—Profuse sero-fibrinous exudations, excessive dyspnœa, displacement of heart, stitches in chest, dry hacking cough, profuse sweat, palpitation, tendency to faint. Scanty, albuminous urine.

Arsenicum.—Serous effusion. Painful asthmatic respiration ; dyspnœa increasing with the rapid accumulation of serous or bloody fluid in chest. Fear of death, **sweat, insomnia**, diarrhœa, great thirst, dropsical swellings. Pyothorax.

RESPIRATORY ORGANS—(*Contd.*)

Arsenicum Iod.—Pleuritic exudation, with great emaciation and prostration. **Tuberculous cases.**

Hepar Sulph.—Purulent, plastic or croupous exudation, often of long-standing, **with hectic fever and** emaciation. Chilliness; sensitiveness to **damp air, which brings** on eoughing.

Ranunculus Bulb.—Often very useful to absorb the effusion of serum. Acute **stabbing pains**; **dyspnœa**, anguish, distress. Also stitches about **chest at every** change of weather, often from pleuritic adhesions.

Abrotanum.—When a **pressing** sensation remains in the affected side, impeding breathing.

Asclepias.—Sharp stitches **through** the lower pact of left chest. worse from motion. Chronic Pleurisy in Tubercular patients.

RESPIRATORY ORGANS

(*Contd.*)

PNEUMONIA.

Aconite.—Frist stage, when the fever is high and is ushered in by a chill. Engorgement of the lungs, with hard, dry and rather painful cough. (See Bronchitis).

Veratum Viride.--Violent congestion marking the onset of Pneumonia, with great arterial excitement and violent action of the heart and full, hard, incompressible pulse. Difficult, slow, labored respiration and great cerebral congestion and a red streak through centre of the tongue; nausca on attempting to sit up; cold sweat. Orthopnœa, threatening Cardiac Paralysis from over-action of heart. Absence of the anxiety and alarm of *Aconite*. It ceases to be the remedy when hepatization takes place.

Ferrum Phos.—First stage, infantile or of adults, as long as no exudation has taken place, with full, round and soft pulse, very little thirst, less restlesness and anxiety, thus differing from *Aconite*. Also secondary Pneumonias in the aged and the debilitated.

Bryonia.—The remedy for Pneumonia and comes in after *Acon.*, *Ferr, Phos.* and *Verat. Viri.*, when croupous exudation has taken place and hepatization has commenced and owing to accompaying inflammation of the pleura there are the characteristic sharp pleuritic stitches, and a

RESPIRATORY ORGANS—(*Contd.*)

heavy pressure over the sternum. The rt. side is affected by preference and the patient lies perfectly quiet on the right or the painful side. The tongue is coated and dry, sputum scanty and rust-colored, thirst, constipation ; dark-red and scanty urine and the modalities of *Bryo.* are distinctive. It is the remedy PER EXCELLENCE in Croupous Pneumonia complicated by Pleurisy and is often complemented by *Phosphorus* and by *Sulphur.*

Iodium.—Right-sided Pneumonia with high temperature, especially when characteristic plastic exudation commences with cough and great difficulty of breathing, as though chest would not expand, blood-streaked sputum and a tendency to rapid extension of the hepatization. He has ravenous hunger, worse if he fasts, suffocates in the warm room, dreads heat, desires cold water applied to body and face. It has not the agonised tossing about of *Acon.* and the stiching pains of *Bryo.*

Kali Iod.—When hepatization has commenced and there is an absence of symptoms for either of *Bryo., Phos.* or *Sulphur.* Also when the hepatization is so extensive that there is cerebral congestion similar to *Belladonna*, as, red face, more or less dilated pupils which do not react to light, drowsiness and heavy breathing. Also in the stage of resolution, when instead of absorption and expectoration of the exudate, slow suppuration appears with hectic fever, emaciation and copious, purulent, green sputa whieh tastes salty ; also frothy sputa, like soap-suds, showing œdema pulmonum.

Sanguinaria.—Tough and rusty sputa during red hepatization, purulent and offensive in the third stage. Hectic fever, diarrhœa, night-sweat, prostration, burning of hands and feet. Failure of heart's action although the amount of hepatization cannot account for it ; weak and irregular pulse ; weak faint feeling about heart and covered with sweat ; nausea.

Sulphur.—Any stage of Pneumonia. In the beginning it will abort the whole process and when exudation sets in, as revealed by crepitations, it will greatly modify the course of the disease. In tropid cases, it will cause the imperfect and slow resolution to react, and prevent formation of tubercles. Also in Pneumonia with a typhoid tendency, and again at the later stage when the lungs refuse to return to their normal condition and a break-down of the lung tissue is apprehended. The indications are : hot palms and soles, hot vertex, weak spells especially in the forenoon. Diarrhœa, especially early in the morning ; suffocating spells, especially after midnight, wants doors and

RESPIRATORY ORGANS—(*Contd.*)

windows open ; restless and sleepless nights ; cutaneous eruptions ; lips are of a rich red color. *Sanguinaria* is preferable when the hepatized lung does not clear up properly and the sputum becomes purulent and the expectoration is very offensive even to the patient himself.

Carbo Veg.—In the third stage, when there is a threatening Paralysis on the lungs. The bronchial tubes are greatly dilated and there are loose rattling rales with cyanosis and symptoms of a perfect picture of a collapse, so characteristic of the drug.

Ammon.Carb.—Great debility and rattling of large bubbles with coldness, prostration and weakness of chest and difficulty to expel mucus. When the patient gets along nicely but suddenly develops symptoms of heart clot, it often prevents the failure of heart and saves life. Aggravation 3 to 4 A. M.

Antim. Tart.—Resolution sets in but fails ; pale, cyanotic face, coldness, prostration and cold sweat on forehead, oppression of breathing and great rattling of mucus but unable to bring it up ; dark, sooty, dilated nostrils, mouth open, parched, tongue dry and brown ; great thirst, vomiting, intense nausea, Diarrhœa ; great coma or sleepiness ; a picture of threatened Paralysis of the lungs ; worse at 3 A. M.

Arsenicum.—Double Penumonia with extreme prostration, hippocratic countenance, clammy perspiration, restlessness but can only move his head ; sudden œdema pulmonum from defect of right heart with danger of Paralysis of lungs. Here it will act as a stimulant and warm the patient up and is to be followed by *Sulphur or Phosph.* according to indications. Threatened gangrene with fetid or dingy green ichorous expectoration.

Chelidonium.—Infantile Pneumonia (*Ipecac.*, see Bronchitis) and Capillary Bronchitis with hepatic symptoms. Bilious Pneumonia ; deep red face, stitching pain under rt. scapula ; loose rattling cough, not easily raised. (Also see Bronchitis).

Mercurius.—Bilious Penumonia ; rt. lung is affected and icteroid symptoms are present ; yellow skin, sharp stitching pain through the lower portion of rt. lung to the back, blood-streaked sputum. Stool is slimy and there is tenesmus characteristic of the drug while that of *Chelidonium* is quite free.

Phosphorus.—Affection of the lower half of the right lung When hepatization is just coming on or just going off it breaks up the hepatization and promotes absorption or resolution. There is burning

RESPIRATORY ORGANS—(*Contd.*)

in the chest, hot cheeks, violent thirst for ice-cold water ; cough with pain under sternum. Pressure across upper part of the chest and constriction of the larynx ; mucous rales, laboured breathing with fan-like motion of the nose ; hard, dry, hacking cough with expectoration of blood or yellowish mucus with streaks of blood. Typhoid Pneumonia with threatened Paralysis of lungs. *Phosphorus* is a great tonic to the venous heart and lungs.

Hepar Sulph.—It comes in late in the disease when pus forms and there is suppuration instead of normal resolution ; also late stage of Croupous Pneumonia.

Lachesis.—Late stage, when it assumes a typhoid form and an abscess forms in the lungs with frothy, purulent sputa, mixed with blood, and profuse sweat. Brain symptoms such as low muttering and hallucinations appear. *Sulphur* is the better remedy to prevent suppuration when there are no typhoid symptoms but it should not be given after tubercles have formed. The proper remedy then is *Lachesis.*

Lycopodium.—Maltreated Pneumonia entering into a state of typhoid, particularly if suppuration of the lungs impends. Also when hepatization is so extensive that there is diaphragmatic breathing, great dyspnœa and fan-like motion of the alæ nasi. Right side, loose, full, and deep cough, circumscribed redness of face, coldness of one foot while the other is warm ; brings out a whole mouthful of light rust-colored mucus.

Cuprum Met.—Sudden suffocative attacks with coldness of the surface of the body, great prostration and dyspnœa, disproportionate to the amount of solidification. Beginning Paralysis of the lungs ; the body is covered with cold, viscid sweat.

Carbo Animalis.—Last stage, with suffocating, hoarse cough which shakes the brain, as if it were all loose in the head ; smothers on closing the eyes. (See also Bronchitis).

Elaps. – Both lungs affected, the right more than the left ; pain in the rt. side in the morning prevents sitting up ; cold feeling in chest after drinking ; cough with intense pains in the rt. apex, as if it were torn out ; sputum consists of black blood.

Kali Carb.—Later stages with great rattling in the chest during cough with little globules of pus in the sputa ; worse about 3 A. M. Hepatization of rt. lung, unable to breathe deeply or to lie on rt. side ; sweat on upper lip during sleep. Abscess of lung, with spitting of pus and blood.

RESPIRATORY ORGANS—(*Contd.*)

Kali Bich.—Croupous Pneumonia with loud rales and tough, stringy sputa with casts of elastic fibrinous nature.

Rhus Tox. – Typhoid Pneumonia often from re-absorption of pus; rales especially over the lower lobes; tearing cough, restlessness, stool and urine passed unconsciously; dry shooty tongue, red at tip; distension of abdomen; sputa bloody or blood-streaked, of the color of brick-dust, of putrid smell.

Hyoscyamus.—Has a high place in Pneumonia with cerebral symptoms and a typhoid condition characteristic of the drug.

Terebinthina.—Typhoid Pneumonia complicated with renal symptoms as burning and dull pain in the region of the kidneys, burning during micturition, strangury and albuminous urine which is dark, cloudy and smoky, containing decomposed blood, having the odor of violets (*Cantharis, Copiva*).

RESPIRATORY ORGANS

(*Contd.*)

COLD—CORYZA—CATARRH.

Aconite.—Sudden attack, quickly following exposure to dry, cold winds; dry, hot, burning and stopped up nose or fluent coryza with frequent sneezing and dropping of clear, hot water. Any of the two states with most violent throbbing frontal headache, fever, muscles sore and painful on sneezing; better in cold room and open air.

Allium Cepa. – From cold damp winds; acrid water drops constantly, burns like fire, excoriates the lips and wings of nose, sneezing with constantly increasing frequency with profuse lachrymation which is bland. Splitting laryngeal cough. Worse in a warm room and better in open air. *Arsenic* sneezes in open air and has not the laryngeal symptoms of *Allium.* Almost similar to *Mercurius* in its eye and nose symptoms but *Mercurius* has more distress in the frontal sinuses, has a tendency to perspire which gives no relief or even aggravates and the discharge though profuse is not almost as watery as with *Allium* and not as thick as with *Pulsatilla.*

Euphrasia—Similar to *Allium* in all respects with profuse bland nasal discharge and acrid, scalding tears which is reverse with *Allium.*

RESPIRATORY ORGANS—(*Contd.*)

Kali Iod.—Similar to both *Allium* and *Mercurius* in its profuse, watery, scalding coryza with more or less sore throat ; every little exposure to damp or even cool air starts the trouble with neuralgic pains in the cheeks involving the frontal sinuses and Antrum of Highmore.

Arsenicum.—Winter colds—thin, watery, excoriating discharge with dull throbbing frontal headache, sneezing which does not relieve and is worse going into open air. Burning in the nose which remains stopped up in spite of fluent discharge. Chilly patient worse from cold, except headache : relieved by warmth and wants to be near the fire all the time.

Sinapis Nigra.—Similar to *Ars.* in the heat, burning, rawness and dryness of the nose but there is no discharge.

Arsenicum Iod.—Preferable to *Ars.* when there is involment of the lymphatic glands, and when worse in a warm room which is contrary to *Arsenic* (See under Ripe Cold).

Natrum Ars.—Resembles *Ars.* almost entirely and is preferable when particularly worse in the forenoon and the patient breathes with mouth open at night.

Ammon. Carb.—Can only breath with mouth open. Useful in winter colds when with all the *Ars.* symptoms there is frequent sneezing with epistaxis when blowing the nose, and much rawness down the trachea and the bronchi, with aggravation towards morning, 3 A. M.. Sensitiveness to cold and relief in warm room.

Ammon. Mur.—One nose stopped up in the day and both at night. The throat is swollen, so that patient cannot open the mouth ; there is throbbing on the tonsils.

Sticta.—Incessant sneezing, burning in the eyes, excessive dryness of the nasal mucous membrane, constant need to blow but no discharge, stuffed feeling at the root of the nose with a dull frontal headache and a dry, hard, barking cough. Atrophic Rhinitis.

Chamomilla.—Coryza of children from cold, windy weather ; the nose is stopped up with dropping of hot watery mucus ; sneezing with dry, teasing cough which keep the child awake or may even occur during sleep.

Sumbucus.—Nose dry and obstructed ; sniffles of infants ; child starts up suddenly as if suffocating ; lets go of the nipple when nursing, cannot breath, cannot expire. (*Arum Triph.*)

Nux Vom.—Initial stage, caused by dry cold weather or by sitting on cold steps or in cold places. Sneezing, nose stuffed up at

RESPIRATORY ORGANS—(*Contd.*)

night and in open air but fluent in a warm room and during day, with scraping rawness in the throat, dullness or oppression in the frontal sinuses and watering of the eyes. Alternate freeness and obstruction of the nose ; worse in a warm room, better in open air (Opposite of *Arsenic.*)

Sanguinaria.—Copious, acrid, burning, watery discharge with stinging in nose ; rawness and burning in the nose and throat.

Sabadilla.—Spasmodic sneezing, with running nose, severe frontal pains, redness of eyes and lachrymation.

Saponaria.—Will often break up a cold. Coryza with stitching supra-orbital pain and hot stitches deep in eye-balls.

Lycopodium.—Complete stoppage of nose, breathes with open mouth and protrudes the tongue ; frontal sinuses involved.

Gelsemium.—Slowly developing acute coryza days after an exposure to warm moist, relaxing weather : colds of mild winter in contra-distinction to cold of violent winter of *Aconite* or *Belladonna*, which follows quickly and develops rapidly and violently after the exposure. Frequent sneezing with fluent excoriating coryza, sore throat, difficulty of swallowing from paretic state of muscles ; dry, tickling cough ; a feeling of hot water passing through the nostrils , relieved near the fire ; general prostration and often neuralgia of the face.

Rhus Tox.—Copious coryza with redness and œdema of the throat, severe aching of the body, sneezing, dry cough, worse from evening till mid-night and from uncovering body ; brought on from exposure to dampness, getting wet, etc. (Also *Dulcamara*)

Pulsatilla.—"Ripe cold" in which the discharges are green and bland, not in the least excoriating ; bad smell in the nose, as of old catarrh. If given in the beginning it usually spoils the case, for sneezing and excoriating discharges are not its characteristics. *Cyclamen* is similar to it in every respect but it has spasmodic sneezing and aversion to open air. *Bryonia* has great dryness of the nose with headache just over the frontal sinuses, with some stomach and bowel symptoms peculiar to it.

Hydrastis.—Similar to *Pulsatilla*. The nose is obstructed and there is rawness in both nares with constant urging to blow the nose and the discharges are stringy and more distinctly yellow and more profuse than *Kali Bich.* which is also useful in "ripe cold" with ropy and stringy yellow discharges with a hard pain at the root of the nose, shooting pains in the malar bones and loss of smell.

RESPIRATORY ORGANS—(*Contd.*)

Hepar Sulph.—Sneezes every time he goes into a cold, dry wind, with running from nose and then a thick, offensive discharge, smelling like old cheese. *Kali Sulph.* simulates *Hepar Sulph.* in its alternating watery flow and offensive discharge which is not so much stringy as with *Kali Bich.* and is more like the greenish-yellow discharge of *Puls.* which it follows well. *Hepar* comes in after partial relief by *Mercurius.*

Arsenic. Iod. & Kali Iod.—Are both worse in a warm room like *Pulsatilla* with thick yellowish discharge and much pains at the root of the nose. The *Ars. Iod.* discharge is excoriating and looks like thick, yellow honey and both differ from *Pulsatilla* in this that the latter has greenish-yellow and bland discharge.

Alumina.—Has weak or entire loss of smell with frequent hawking and difficult discharge of dry, yellowish-green mucus with pain at root of nose and a feeling as of a splinter when swallowing. This last symptom is also to be found in *Argent. Nit.*, *Hepar.*, *Nat. Mur.* and *Nitric Acid.*

Thuja.—Blows out much thick, green mucus mixed with blood and pus. It has also fluent coryza in the open air and dry in-doors. There is often a history of vaccination which did not take.

SKIN, AFFECTIONS OF

ABSCESSES—BOILS—CARBUNCLES—ETC.

Angustura.—Abscess of the ankle-joint.

Apis.—Pustules with stinging and burning pains, precursor of an abscess, diffuse erysipelatous inflammation or Cellulitis with a tendency to gangrene and destruction of tissue. Carbuncle.

Arnica.—Successive crops of small boils all over body. Soreness and suppuration ; pus does not discharge but shrivel up. Given internally and used externally it redevelops them.

Arsenicum.—Boils or Carbuncles : intense burning ; **worse after** mid-night ; better by heat—(*Secale* is better by cold but otherwise similar). Pus bloody, putrid ; prostration, sleeplessness **and restlessness** (*Carbo Veg.*, but without restlessness). When *Ars.* fails ***Anthracinum*** comes in. If prostration is accompanied with diarrhœa, evening fever and black core at the centre, *Tarentula Cubensis.* *Nitric Acid*

SKIN, AFFECTIONS OF—(*Contd.*)

has hæmorrhagic tendency on dressing or otherwise. *Kali Bich.* is sometimes useful to remove the slough. *Echinacea* is wonderfully good in Carbuncles with high sepsis and prostration.

Belladonna.—Abscesses (mammary or tonsillar). Sudden and violent in onset ; radiating redness, throbbing ; worse by jar ; useful before pus is matured ; if it fails and pus matures, *Hepar Sulph.* Also useful in gum-boils but if fails, *Merc. Sol.*

Bryonia.—Abscesses (mammary) ; pale red or less red than *Bell.* ; mamma stony hard and heavy ; stitching pain ; worse from motion. When suppuration threatens, it is followed by *Phytolacca, Phos., Sili.*

Calcarea Carb.—Abscesses with suppuration deep down in muscles. Mammary abscesses with enormous suppuration. When situated in a vital part, so that discharge may be dangerous, *Calcarea Carb.* will absorb the pus without any unfavorable after effect.

Calc. Picri.—Recurring small boils on parts thinly covered with muscles, as the shin-bones, coccyx, auditory canal, etc., (*Bell., Picric Acid, Sili.*).

Calc. Sulph.—Abscesses , pus has a vent, has ruptured but is slow to heal, with continuous discharge of yellow pus. Follows *Sili.*, when the latter has changed the thin ichorous to thick, laudable, yellow pus. Also deep abscesses like *Calc, Carb.* Painful abscesses about anus and gum-boils.

Carbo Veg.—Boils or Carbuncles ; bluish, burning, offensive pus ; gangrenous. Abscesses along with disease of the spine. It is like *Ars.* without restlessness.

Hepar Sulpb—Abscesses or Boils ; after *Bell.* when chills and sharp sticking pains denote beginning of suppuration. Given high it aborts the whole process but enhances suppuration if given low. *Mercurius* follows and brings on the discharge of pus and finish the process. If healing is still delayed, givc *Sili.* if pus is thin, or *Calc. Sulph.* if it is thick ; if takes on erysipelatous character, *Apis* ; if bluish, *Lachesis.*

Lachesis—Carbuncles ; surrounding area swollen and bluish, pus forms slowly ; thin, sanious, offensive pus ; cerebral symptoms ; prostration ; a darkish-red streak running along lymphatics.

Merc. Sol.—Suppurative processes slower than *Hepar*, (which see). Abscesses at roots of teeth, in the auditory canal. Suppurative Tonsillitis.

Nitric Acid—Carbuncles with a tendency to hæmorrhage on slightest touch or without any touch. Is often followed by *Kali Bich.*, which removes the slough and brightens up the sore. *Nitric Acid* is also

SKIN, AFFECTIONS OF—(*Contd.*)

useful in suppuration of inguinal and axillary glands ; Syphilitic (*Merc. Iod., Thuja, Carbo Ani., Badiaga*). Mastoid abscesses—inflammation beginning in the mastoid cells—*Capsicum* ; when pus forms, *Hepar, Sili* ; caries or necrosis—*Aurum, Nitric Acid, Silicea.* Also *Calc. Fluor.*, and *Fluoric Acid.*

Phosphorus.—Abscesses, mammary and above joints, with fistulous openings ; thin ichorous discharge ; complementary to *Silicea.* Red streaks radiate like *Bell.*

Silicea.—Obstinate abscesses ; dark, fetid, thin, watery pus ; promotes granulation after discharge. Is followed by *Fluoric Acid* in fistulous or ony abscesses. *Sili.* is better by warmth, while *Fluoric Acid* is better by cold. When *Sili.* has changed the thin, ichorous foetid pus to a thick, laudable one, but fails to cure, *Calc. Sulph.* follows well. *Sili.* is generally chilly but *Calc. Sulph.* is opposite.

Sulphur.—In chronic suppurative processes which refuse to be healed, it excites reaction and leads on to cure by itself or by another indicated remedy.

SKIN, AFFECTIONS OF

(*Contd.*)

ECZEMA

Anacardium.—Eczema with unberable itching, affecting chiefly the fingers, eye-lids, face, chest and around the neck and scrotum. They begin as itching vesicles that rapidly become pustular, large, flat and later confluent and discharge a yellowish fluid which hardens when they come in contact with air. Lichen. Neurotic Eczema.

Antim. Crud.—Eczema with thick, hard, honey-colored scales with oozing of green sanious pus which irritates the surrounding parts and burn and itch violently ; worse from bathing or working in water, and at night. Lichen Planus : Eczema Capitis.

Arsenic.—Chronic Eczema. Induration and hardening of the skin with vesicles which turn into pustules and form scabs : dry, scaly eruptions upon scalp, face, legs and genitals with acrid and sometimes fetid discharge with terrible burning and itching at night and in cold air ; amel. by external warmth.

SKIN, AFFECTIONS OF—(*Conid.*)

Asterias Rubens.—Itching vesicles break and form small ulcers which spread superficially on thighs, legs, ankles and instep, in scrofulous, sycotic constitutions.

Baryta Carb.—Eczema on dorsa of hands ; skin rough, dry and chapped. Moist vesicular eruptions with formation of thick moist crusts, with itching and burning, causing hair to fall off, in fat, dumpy children who take cold easily and have swollen glands on the neck and under the jaw and enlarged tonsils.

Bovista.—Eczema of back of hands, brought on by washing ; moist, vesicular formation of thick crusts and no relief from scratching. Eczema about mouth and nostrils.

Bromium.—Eczema covering entire scalp like a cap ; scalp tender ; dirty-looking offensive discharge.

Calcarea Carb.—Thick scales with yellow pus spreading from head to face ; slightly itching but scratches the head impatiently on awaking and makes it bleed ; teething children. Moist eruptions on legs, about naval and flexure of extremities. Eczema Scrofulosum.

Calcarea Phos.—Scurfy and scabby eruptions in anæmic, rachitic, scrofulous constitutions.

Calcarea Sulph.—Eczema with greenish-yellow scabs. Pimples on scalp.

Capcicum.—Burning vesicular rash on chest, forearm, and vulva, alternating with Asthma.

Cantharis.—Eczema on an inflamed, red surface with much burning and itching ; beginning in a small area spreads to involve a large surface. Scales form on scalp like an enormous dandruff ; worse from warmth ; urinary symptoms often present.

Causticum.—Pimples on tip of nose and excessively itching moist tetters on neck. Itching at various parts, especially on tip and wings of nose, face, scrotum, back, arms, palms and dorsum of feet.

Chelidonium.—Eczema of lower extremities from chronic affections of the liver. Red and painful pimples and pustules on various parts with itching of the skin.

Cicuta Virosa.—Eczema Capitis, no itching ; suppurating eruptions on scalp with burning pain and forming hard lemon-colored crusts covering the head as with a solid cap ; when suppressed, causes brain disease.

Condurango.—When rhagades are present, oozing out a fetid fluid ; cachectic or syphilitic.

SKIN, AFFECTIONS OF—(*Contd.*)

Conium.—Moist vesicles with gluey, sticky discharge forming hard crusts about face, arms and mons vernis ; worse from scratching. People suffering from vertigo, worse in bed.

Croton Tig.—Pure idiopathie Eczema, as is seen in children. Eczema of faee and genitals (also see Herpes).

Dulcamara.—Impetiginous Eczema of scrofulous children. Humid eruptions on cheeks with thick brown-yellow crusts on face, forehead and chin. Crusta Lactea ; thick crusts on scalp, causing hair to fall out. Ringworm of scalp ; glands about throat swollen.

Graphites.—Eczema Capitis of entire scalp, forming massive, dirty scales, which mat the hair ; scabs sore to touch ; itching. Eczema Impetiginoid, begins as moisture and eruptions behind the ears, spreading over cheeks and neck with fissures on and behind the ears. Eczema with profuse serous, sticky exudations. In blondes, inclined to obesity, dryness of the skin and absence of perspiration.

Hepar.—Humid eruptions on the head feeling sore ; of fetid odor ; itching violently on rising in the morning ; burning and feeling sore on scratching ; scabs easily torn off, leaving a raw, bleeding surface ; falling off of the hair with very sore, painful pimples and large bald spots on the scalp. Burning-itching on the body, with white vesicles after scratching. Humid soreness on the genitals, scrotum, and the folds between the scrotum and the thigh. Eczema, spreading by means of new pimples appearing just beyond the old parts.

Hydrastis.—Eczema on margin of hair in front of head, worse coming from the cold into a warm room ; oozes .after washing ; itching when warm ; scalp and face covered with thick crusts, which on removal expose red, and infiltrated patches.

Hydrocotyle.—Eczema with thick and scaby skin but less burning than *Arsenic.*

Juglans Cinera.—Eczema, especially on lower extremities, sacrum, hands and wrists, frequently recurring with intolerable itching and soreness.

Juglans Regia.—Tinea Favosa, especially on the scalp behind the ear, with intense itching at night. Crusta Lactea with soreness around ear ; scabs appear on arms and in axilla.

Kali Ars.—Dry Chronic Eczema. Skin of arms thicker and rougher than natural, covered with filimsy exfoliations, itching and tingling on getting warm, intensely fissured about joints ; occasional exacerbation with eruption of distinct vesicles.

SKIN, AFFECTIONS OF—(*Contd.*)

Kali Bichrom.—Dry, red and hot skin with burning and stinging ; dry eruptions like Measles ; violent itching of whole surface, then small pustules form mostly on arms and legs ; small pustules on the hands secrete a watery fluid when broken, which thickens into a yellow, tough mass. Eruptions begin in the hot and are better in cold weather.

Kali Brom.—Acne Simplex and Indurata on face and chest, especially in lymphatic constitutions. Moist Eczema of legs with Pityriasis of scalp ; rose-colored eruptions on lower extremities with pustules in centre of patches that become unbilicated, exuding a creamy moisture and forming thick yellow scabs.

Kali Carb.—Itching, burning, yellow or red scaly spots over abdomen and around nipples, sometimes with oozing after being scratched. Herpetic spots on face, burning and itching ; moist after scratching.

Kali Iod.—Eczema of thighs. Pityriasis of scalp. Small boils on face, head, neck, back and chest, suppurating and leaving scars ; itching herpes on the face.

Kali Mur.—Eczema and other eruptions on skin, with vesicles containing thick, white contents. Albuminoid Eczema or other skin diseases from bad Vaccination and also from suppressed or deranged uterine functions. Dry flour-like scales on skin. Obstinate Eczema, Crusta Lactea, scurfy eruptions on head and face of little children.

Kali Sulph.—Burning, itching, papular eruptions, exuding pus-like, yellowish-green moisture. (See also Psoriasis).

Lappa Major.—(*Arctium Lappa*)—Eczema of scalp with moist, offensive, greyish-white crusts ; eruptions spreading even to face, tearing and itching. Herpetic eruptions on rt. alæ nasi.

Ledum.—Eczema of face ; redness and tuberous, crusty eruptions on forehead, face and around nose and mouth, with itching, burning and smarting, in the open air.

Lycopodium.—Eruptions on the head, with abundant and fetid suppuration, sometimes with obstruction of the glands of the neck. Scurf over whole scalp, child scratches it raw at night and then it bleeds. Tetters, on legs and calves, yellowish brown, wrinkled or moist, purulent, full of deep cracks and thick scabs, itching violently. Worse after scratching, from 4 to 8 P. M., and from getting heated.

Manganum.—Chronic Eczema. Deep cracks in bends of elbows and joints with soreness, associated with amenorrhœa ; worse at menstrual period or at menopause.

Mercurius.—Humid fetid eruptions ; thick, yellow discharge or yellow crusts form on scalp, surrounded by an inflamed border ; itching worse

SKIN, AFFECTIONS OF—(*Contd*·)

at night in bed; violent and voluptuous itching over whole body, principally in evening or at night, worse by heat of bed and sometimes attended by burning after scratching.

Mezereum.—Head covered with a thick, leathery crust under which pus collects and mats the hair. Violent itching on scalp, scratching increases the itching; child continually scratches the face, and tears off the scab, so that the face becomes covered with blood and fat pustules form on the the raw spots. Eczema, itching intolerably, with copious serous cxudation, covering the whole leg with elevated white scabs, and roughness and scaling here and there, on back, chest, thighs and scalp; worse on parts devoid of fat, worse in warmth.

Natrum Carb.—Eczema on dorsum of hands.

Natrum Mur.—White scaly scabs on the head from ear to ear. Eruptions about mouth, bends of knees and folds of skin generally. Borders and corners of eye-lids raw and ulcerated. oozing a corroding gluey fluid.

Natrum Sulph.—Vesicular Eczema; thin watery discharge exuding from stiff, swollen fingers; palms raw and sore. Barbers's itch.

Nitric Acid.—Humid, stinging eruptions on vertex and temples, bleeding easily when scratched; also on auditory meatus, genitals, about arms and on hands.

Oleander.—Vesicular eruptions about head of children; scaly eruptions on back part of head behind ears, with biting and itching as from lice.

Petroleum.—Yellowish-green thick crusts on face and neck, occiput, scrotum, peræneum, and thighs. Itching, sore places or deep cracks on skin (*Graph., Lyco.*) chiefly on dorsa of hands (*Nat. Carb.*); eruptions between toes with foul sweat; worse in winter, better in summer.

Psorinum.—Dry or humid fetid eruptions; crusty eruptions with red areolæ; intolerable itching of the skin, worse in bed and from warmth; scratches until it bleeds; eruptions easily suppurate. Psoric constitution with an abnormal tendency to produce skin diseases (*Sulph.*); dry; inactive skin; rarely sweats; dirty look, as if never washed. Dry, scaly or moist and fetid suppurating eruptions on scalp, oozing a sticky offensive fluid. Eczema Rubrum. Heat of fire is tormenting to the face, must sit with the back to the fire; cold air ameliorates, bathing aggravates, must dry face with great care. Burning and intolerable itching; legs—from ankles to the crest of ilium—and arms from wrists to elbows, covered with dry scaly eruptions, itching violently at night with no relief from scratching until it bleeds.

SKIN, AFFECTIONS OF—(*Contd.*)

Rhus Tox.—Moist eruptions on head, forming thick crusts, with violent itching at night and extending to shoulders. Eczema Scroti on inside of thighs, discharging freely ; worse in wet and winter weather.

Rhus Ven.—Intense itching, worse by scratching, and relieved by hot water ; dry eruptions on back of hands in winter, disappearing in spring.

Sarsaparilla.—Itching eruptions on forehead and face like milk-crusts with burning, becoming humid on scratching ; base of eruption is much inflamed, child cries much ; crusts become detached in open air.

Sepia.—Eruptions during pregnancy and nursing. Itching on face, on arms, hands, back, lips, feet, abdomen and genitals, often changing to burning on scratching ; eruption is dry, or soon becomes moist and discharges copious offensive pus-like fluid, which becomes dry, cracks and exfoliates.

Silicea.—Itching, burning eruptions behind ears, ending in scabs discharging pus ; also on scrotum and hands ; spreading from back to head ; itching and sensitive pustules on scalp and neck, discharging copiously ; worse from scratching ; better covering warmly.

Staphisagria.—Burning, itching about head, face and ears of children. Yellow scaly eruptions on scalp, cheeks and behind ears, holding offensive pus, breeding lice ; scratching stops itching in one place, but it goes to another.

Sulphur.—Eczema Erythematosum ; eruptions of yellow crusts. Dryness and heat of scalp, with intense itching especially at night and scratching causes soreness, worse from wetting. The skin is rough, coarse, measly with much soreness in the folds of the skin and a tendency to pustulur eruptions. The great characteristic is the aggravation from washing,—does not like to be washed or to bathe, and the itching with intense burning after scratching.

Sulphuric Acid.—Crusta Lactea in children, with saffron-yellow, stringy, slimy stools ; moist eruptions with itching, changing locality on scratching.

Thuja.—Eczema worse after vaccination. Skin extremely sensitive to touch, burning violently after scratching. Dry scaly eruptions on head, extending to temples, eye-brows, ears and neck, with itching, tingling, biting. Eruptions only on covered parts ; worse from washing.

Ustillago.—Eczema Impetiginosum ; whole scalp one filthy mass of inflammation ; watery serum oozing from scalp. Scald-head.

Vinca Minor.—Eczema of head and face ; pustules itching, burning, and oozing badly-smelling moisture, matting the hair.

SKIN, AFFECTIONS OF—(*Contd.*)

Viola Tricolor.—Eruptions, particularly over face and head with intolerable itching and burning, worse at night. Crusta Lactea in children with swollen glands, forming thick incrustations and pouring out a large quantity of thick, yellow fluid, which mats the hair.

Zincum.—Eczema, in the anæmic and the neurotic. Dry eruptions all over body with formication of feet and legs as from bugs crawling over the skin, preventing sleep, better by gentle rubbing ; itching of thighs and bend of knees.

SKIN, DISEASES OF

(*Contd.*)

HERPES—ZONA OR SHINGLES.

Arsenic.—Herpes Zoster. Confluent eruptions, with intense burning and dry, parchment-like skin ; worse after mid-night and from cold ; better from warmth.

Cantharis.—Herpetic eruptions with great itching and violent burning, ulcerative pain on being touched.

Carbon. Oxygenisatum.—Herpes Zoster ; the vesications following the course of nerves, with great coldness of the surface and icy-cold hands.

Causticum.—Itching, burning, moist, vesicles especially on shoulders and neck, with tendency to ulceration ; worse at night.

Cistus Can.—Herpetic eruptions on various parts of body but especially on face, ears and back ; worse in cold air. Scrofulous subjects who are very sensitive to cold air.

Commocladia.—Herpes Zoster ; vesicular, pustular, ulcerative eruptions on legs with violent itching-burning and red stripes on skin. Tormenting itching and burning over whole body followed by vesication and desquamation of cuticle.

Croton Tig.—Redness and hide-bound feeling of the skin and formation of vesicles and pustules, which run into one another and speedily develop a sero-purulent exudation forming large brown scabs with desquamation and falling off of the pustules. Pustules with nearly a general inflammation. There is intolerable itching but cannot bear to scratch ; must rub it gently which is relieving. Herpetic eruptions on face and especially genitals with fearful itching followed by painful burning.

SKIN, DISEASES OF—(*Contd.*)

Dolichos.—Herpetic eruptions on axilla, spreading in rings forward to sternum and backward to spine, burning, smarting and neuralgic pains of the affected side following. Also dry, tettery eruptions on arms and legs with violent itching all over ; worse at night, warmth, scratching and cold water. A general intense itching without eruption worse by scratching, is nevertheless characteristic of *Dolichos*.

Dulcamara.—Herpes Zoster after taking cold, from cold, wet weather ; worse at night, better moving about, external warmth ; bleeding when scratched.

Graphites.—Herpes Zoster, especially on left side, particularly on left side of chest, abdomen and back. Itching blotches on various parts of body oozing a thick, watery, honey-like sticky fluid.

Iris Versi.—Herpes Zoster on the right side of the body, with gastric derangements and pain in liver. Eruptions with great itching at night, showing black points after scratching.

Kali Ars.—Herpes Zoster behind rt. ear and on rt. side of neck, shoulder, upper arm and chest and isolated vesicles on left side of neck with itching, stinging and burning ; worse at night, on undressing and by warmth.

Kalmia.—After the disappearance of herpes, violent tearing shooting neuralgic pains of the face or of those nerves that supply the part where the eruptions were ; the pains come suddenly with great violence, and after some time go as suddenly. The pains are worse in the day, coming and going with the Sun or else, worse at night with the lying down.

Kreosote.—Dry or moist, sero-purulent herpes in almost all parts of the body, especially on the back of hands and feet, on the palms, ears, popliteal region and on the knuckles of hands, itching violently towards evening and in open air ; better from warmth.

Lachesis.—Eruptions of every kind, appearing in every spring and fall ; at first vesicles of yellow color, then developing into dark pustules with coper-colored swelling of the parts affected and pains which drive to despair.

Mercurius.—Zona, like a girdle from the back around the abdomen, running together with suppurating pustules, forming dry scabs bordering the eruptions which itch violently and have a tendency to suppurate.

Mezereum.—Zona, following the course of the inter-costal or supra-orbital nerves, with severe neuralgic pains and violent itching, burning like fire. The inter-costal neuralgia continuing after the disappearance of the eruptions find a great remedy in *Mezereum*.

SKIN, DISEASES OF—(*Contd.*)

Nitric Acid.—Herpes on outer side of thighs and blackness of the pores of the skin.

Petroleum.—Herpes on nape of neck, chest, scrotum, inner side of thigh, peræneum, knees and ankles ; itching, followed by ulcers.

Psorinum.—Moist Herpes with intolerable itching and burning, after suppressed scabies ; worse before mid-night and in open air.

Ranunculus Bulb.—Herpes Zoster following the course of supra-orbital or inter-costal nerves with sharp neuralgic pains preceding.

Rhus Tox.—Herpes, especially on the right side, in the winter, (there being hardly any eruption in summer) with intolerable itching, burning and neuralgic pains alternating with pain in chest and dysenteric stools with fever and restlessness.

Rumex.—Vesicular eruptions from wearing flannel, worse when undressing and exposed to cold air.

Sarsaparilla.—Herpetic ulcers, extending in a circular form, forming no crusts ; red, granulated bases, white borders ; skin appears as after the application of a warm compress.

Sepia.—Herpes Circinatus (Ring-worm)—dry, especially on face of children at each evolution of fresh teeth. Tetters in general, moist, or dry. Scabious herpes with itching, stinging in different parts (face, arms, hands, back, hips, abdomen) which changes to burning when scratching ; worse during menses, pregnancy and lactation.

Sulphur.—Dry, scaly eruptions. Herpes of all types, with vesicles in groups, forming scabs ; re-appearance of repelled herpes ; burning after scratching : worse from wet poultices, washing and warmth in bed.

Tellurium.—Herpes Circinatus on whole body, more distinct on lower limbs ; vesicles, in intersecting rings, thickly covering the whole body or same on single parts.

Thuja.—Herpes Zoster ; eruptions all over the body, especially on abdomen, from suppressed gonorrhœa, with terrible itching, followed by burning after scratching.

Zincum.—Herpes Zoster, dry, over whole body or on back and on hands, with burning pains and tingling and formication between skin and flesh. Burning, jerking neuralgic pains following Zoster, worse in the evening and from slightest touch. Suppurating Herpes.

———

SKIN, DISEASES OF

(*Contd.*)

PSORIASIS.

Arsenicum.--Bran-colored scales on head coming down on forehead ; desquamation of the skin of the body. Small red pimples gradually increase and are covered with scarf-like fish-scales ; skin dry ; cold and bluish, with hot itching and violent burning.

Arsenic. Iod.—Marked exfoliation of skin in large scales, leaving a raw exuding surface beneath ; skin dry, scaly, itching, with watery oozing ; worse from washing.

Calc. Carb.—Skin of the body rough, dry, and as if covered with a kind of miliary eruptions, with burning, smarting and itching, forming scales.

Clematis.—Scaly tetters, discharging a sanious pus, with redness, heat and swelling of the skin, with insupportable itching in the heat of the bed and after washing ; worse on the face, hands and scalp around occiput ; looks inflamed during increasing and dry during decreasing moon.

Corallium Rubrum.—Psoriasis of palms and soles in persons who have in them a combination of Syphilis and Psora. Red spots on palms, at first of coral color, then darker and finally coppery.

Fluoric Acid.—Rough and hard skin and eruption of little red blotches on the body with persistent itching in small spots here and there over the body, with desquamation of scales ; itching worse from warmth, better from cold.

Graphites.—Obstinate dryness of the skin and absence of perspiration and scabious eruptions sometimes with secretion of corrosive serum or with itching in the evening and at night.

Hydrocotyle.—Dry eruptions and great thickening of the epidermoid of soles. Psoriasis Gyrata, on trunk and extremities, palms and soles.

Kali Ars.—Psoriasis in numerous patches with great itching, causing him to scratch till an ichorous fluid discharges, forming a hard cake ; the patches scale off and are replaced by smaller ones and leave behind them a red skin.

Kali Brom.—Rose-colored eruptions on lower extremities ; pustules in centre of patches become umbilicated, exuding a creamy moisture and forming thick, yellow scabs ; Syphilitic Psoriasis.

SKIN, DISEASES OF

(*Contd.*)

PEMPHIGUS.

Anacardium.—Blisters from the size of a pin's head to a pea, often scarlet red, spread over the whole body with burning and itching, worse evening in bed.

Arsenic.—With great burning ; amel, by warmth.

Belladonna.—Watery vesicles, especially on palms and tibia, so painful as to extort cries and groans ; vesicles discharging great deal of serum.

Cantharis.—Erysipelatous inflammation of the skin forming blisters which burn like fire when touched ever so lightly.

Carbonenm Oxygenisatum.—Large and small vesicles along the course of nerves with anæsthesia of the skin and icy-cold hands.

Causticum.—Large vesicles on chest and back with anguish and fever with violent itching at night.

Chininum Sulph.—Erythema, forming confluent vesicles and bullæ which ulcerate and dry into crusts.

Crotalus.—Pemphigus with low typhoid conditions and the fluid assumes a dark, sanguinous character or gangrene threatens.

Lachesis.—Large blisters of a yellow or bluish-black color, with swelling of parts affected, and pains which drive to despair ; gangrenous blisters.

Phosphorus.—Tense blisters, full to bursting, not painful,

Ranunculus Bulb.—Constantly-repeating eruptions of blisters, secreting an offensive gluey matter, forming crusts and healing from the centre ; discharge makes the parts sore. Pemphigus of new-born babies.

Ranunculus Scel.—Large isolated blisters, which burst and form an ulcer, discharging acrid-ichor.

Rhus Tox.—Vesicles upon red patch or with a spreading red, erysipelatous base ; the blisters contain a milky or watery fluid with a red areola around each bulla.

Thuja.—Pemphigus Foliaceus ; big-sized blisters with escape of serous fluid through small openings ; large, painful blisters.

SKIN, DISEASES OF—(*Contd.*)

Kali Sulph.—Dry, sensitive and burning skin, with painful, itching and stinging scaly eruptions with abundant desquamation.

Manganum.—Itching Tetters with eruptions on elbows, knees and calves ; skin thickened and fissured and finally white, shiny, hard and adherent scales are continually reproduced. Occasionally rheumatic pains. Itching, amel. by scratching. Often associated with Amenorrhœa, worse at menstrual period or at Menopause.

Mercurius.—Skin rough, and dry ; cracks and peels off constantly in white bran-like scales, especially of scalp, whiskers and eye-brows, without attacking face. Dry, itching and measly tetters with desquamation of skin ; worse at night and heat of bed.

Mezereum.—General desquamation of skin of body ; liver spots on chest and arms become dark and desquamate. Skin covered with elevated white scabs, with itching, especially at night (when in bed) more violent and painful (and changed to burning) after scratching.

Nitric Acid.—In Syphilitic persons.

Petroleum.—Skin dry, constricted, very sensitive, rough and cracked ; Psoriasis of hands. Thick, greenish crust, burning and itching ; worse in winter.

Phosphorus.—Dry, furfuraceous, tettery spots over whole body and desquamation of skin.

Phytolacca.—Squamous eruptions ; erythematous blotches, slightly raised, pinkish, slowly desquamating, ending in purple spots ; as old ones died away, others came.

Psorinum.—Skin as if never washed. Scaly condition of skin of whole body. Eruptions soon become a thick dirty looking mass of scabs and pus, painful and violently itching, preventing sleep, with constant desire to scratch ; pruritus worse at night, when undressing and by warmth of bed ; profuse desquamation of scales ; disappeared entirely in summer and reappeared when cold weather set in. Psoriasis Syphilitica.

Selenium.—Syphilitic Psoriasis of the palms with great itching.

Sepia.—Exanthema and Tetters in general with soreness of skin and humid places in bends of joints ; itching in different parts (See Herpes) ; anular desquamation.

Silicea.—Painful sensibility of skin, sometimes covered with pityriasis, with itching over whole body, worse at night.

Sulphur.—Psoriasis Inveterata, itching when warm ; scratching relieves the itching but is followed by burning ; itching and burning worse by washing.

SCIN, DISEASES OF—(*Contd.*)

Tellurium.—Psoriasis ; skin dry and hot ; itching worse in cool-air. (See Herpes).

Thuja. – Universal Psoriasis in persons of Sycotic diathesis ; eruption only on covered parts, burning violently after scratching.

SKIN, DISEASES OF

(*Contd.*)

URTICARIA.

Aconite.—Red, broad pimples like flea-bites and crawling sensation in the skin with agonising itching unchanged by scratching and dcsquamation.

Anacardium.—Urticaria Tuberosa ; eruption like that of Poison-oak ; burning, itching and intense redness of the skin.

Antim. Crud.—White lumps with red areolæ and fearful itching ; thick white-coated tongue ; gastric derangement.

Antim. Tart.—Red, 'tching rash over whole body ; eruption comes and goes ; makes him irritable, hot and thirsty.

Apis.—Heat, redness and extreme soreness of the skin with burning smarting and stinging pains and dyspnœa with Urticaria ; worse from heat and covering.

Arsenicum.—From eating shell-fish ; with burning, itching and restlessness ; alternating with croup and asthma.

Belladonna.— During profuse menstruation , after eating cabbage or sour-kraut.

Bovista.—Urticaria covering whole body on excitment, with rheumatic lameness, palpitation and diarrhœa. Urticaria on waking in the morning, worse from bathing ; itching on getting warm.

Calcarea Carb.—Nettle-rash which always disappears in cool, open air ; white nettlerash of children, itching intolerably ; chronic hives.

Causticum.—Chronic Urticaria, coming out more fully in fresh air ; worse from heat of bed.

Chloral.—Urticaria, in large wheals with intense itching and œdematous swelling of face, cheeks, eye-lids and ears, coming on from a chill ; better from warmth.

Cimicifuga.—Urticaria with menstrual disorders or rheumatism.

SKIN, DISEASES OF—(*Contd.*)

Conium.—Nettle-rash in consequence of violent bodily exercise with painful, pricking, itching of thc skin, worse from scratching.

Copaiva. —Nettle-rash, pale-red or bright red, large elevated blotches all over the body with violent itching, constipation, headache and some fever.

Dulcamara.—Miliary nettle-rash with dryness and heat of the skin and fever, from taking cold, associated with griping pain in bowels, nausea and diarrhœa ; with much itching ; after scratching it burns ; increases in warmth, better in cold.

Hepar.—Nettle-rash with violent itching and stinging, disappears as heat begins in Intermittents ; chronic cases.

Hydrastis.—Nettle-rash, raised nodular scarlet eruptions, excessively irritable, over whole body, preceded by feeling of illness, vomiting and general digestive disorder ; worse from scratching, at night.

Ignatia.— During the chilly stage of Intermittent Fevers.

Kali Brom.—Slightly elevated, smooth, red patches with hard base, itching at night in bed and in a high temparature ; appear in winter.

Kali Carb.—Miliary nettle-rash during menstruation.

Lycopodium.— Chronic cases with burning and itching in the day time, on getting heated or in evening before lying down.

Natrum Carb.—Red hard blotches with dryness of the skin and itching over whole body, as from fleas.

Natrum Mur.— Miliary eruption, with shooting pain and itching and pricking in skin ; rash over whole body and whitish hives on arms and hands. Nettle-rash after violent exereise. Complementary to *Apis*.

Petroleum.—Miliary urticaria with great sensibility of the surface of the skin ; chronic cases.

Psorinum.—Frequently repeated attacks of urticaria after suppressed Itch, with fine vesicles on top, which dry and peel off in fine scales ; appearing regularly after any exertion.

Pulsatilla.—Hives of gastric origin or during delayed or scanty menses. Chilly all the time, even in a warm room ; rheumatic tendency.

Rhus Tox.—Vesicular nettle-rash, itching and burning ; skin swollen red ; after getting wet ; worse in cold air ; fever ; thirst.

Sarsaparailla.—Miliary nettle-rash, on going into fresh air from a warm room.

Sepia.—Chronic nettle-rash ; breaks out during a walk in cold air and disappears in the warm room ; especially on the face, arms and

SKIN, DISEASES OF—(*Contd.*)

thorax. Eruptions in the form of wheals similar to those produced by a blow with a whip or a small rod.

Urtica Urens.—Raised, red blotches of urticaria ; burning heat with formication and violent itching. Consequences of suppressed nettle-rash. Rheumatism associattd or alternating with Urticaria Nodosa (*Bov.*). Ill-effects of eating shell-fish.

Ustilago.—Terrible itching at night, scratching produces large pale welts ; ovarian irritation with menstrual irregularities.

SYPHILIS

CHANCRES—CHANCROIDS

Arsenicum.--Phagedenic Chancres, livid, intense burning with sloughing; desperate cases with general constitutional symptoms of the drug.

Asafoetida.—Syphilis of shin-bones with nightly pains ; most sensitive ulcers, thin offensive pus. Caries and necrosis with extreme nocturnal pains ; after abuse of *Mercury*.

Aurum Met.—Secondary Syphilis, also infantile ; after abuse of *Mercury*. Ulcers in mouth, caries of the nasal bones and palate ; stinking discharge and passes on pieces of bones ; pain in facial bones around eyes. Melancholia and no desire to live. The *Muriate* is sometimes more useful, especially in Syphilitic Gonorrhœa.

Mezereum.—Relieves nightly shin-bone pains of syphilis ; slightest touch unbearable.

Stillingia.—Severe pains especially in long bones ; nodes on head and shin-bones ; worse at night, in damp weather ; excoriating coryza co-existing.

Phytolacca.—Syphilitic rheumatism affecting the middle of long bones or attachment of muscles ; worse at night and in damp weather.

Phosphoric Acid.—Ostitis of Mercurio-Syphilitic origin ; nocturnal pains, as if bones were scraped with a knife.

Carbo Animalis.—Constitutional or tertiary syphilis after abuse of *Mercury* ; coppery-red blotches on skin, especially on face. (See Bubo).

Carbo Veg.—Syphilitic ulcers with high edges ; thin, acrid, offensive discharge ; bleeds freely on touch.

SYPHILIS—(*Contd.*)

Cinnabaris.—Combination of Syphilis and Sycosis. Fan-shaped fiig-warts ; swelling of penis; violent itching of glands ; small ulcer on roof of mouth and tip of tongue, right side ; nasal catarrh. Stringy mucus in posterior nares. Red, swollen chancres discharging thin pus ; hard elevated edges, not sensitive.

Corallium.—Combination of Syphilis and Psora. Red, flat ulcers on glans and inner surface of prepuce, extremely sensitive. Smooth copper-colored spots on palms and fingers. Coral-red color of chancres.

Fluoric Acid.—Syphilitic ulcers of mouth and throat. Syphilitic caries and necrosis with burning, boring pains ; discharge thin, acrid ; pains in bones of arms and legs ; elevated red blotches on palms.

Hepar Sulph.—Mercurio-Syphilitic diseases of gums ; pains in bones. Chancres bleed readily ; margins elevated, spongy ; abuse of *Mercury* ; red borders, with sticking pains, sensitive, nightly pains.

Kali Bichromicum.—Perforated ulcers in nose, mouth, and throat ; copper-red color around ; indurated chancres ; deep ; pricking, itching in glans,

Kali Iod.—Gumma, involving the nerves. Rupia. Papular eruptions of scalp and down back ; bone-pains ; throbbing, burning in nasal and frontal bones ; greenish-yellow acrid coryza. Chancres with hard edges and curdy pus ; deep-eating ulcers.

Lachesis.—Chancres, gangrenous or phagedenic ; of the soft palate, fauces and throat. Ulcers with blue surrounding ; nightly bone-pains ; flat ulcers on legs ; caries of tibia ; sensitive and livid ; burning on touch ; abuse of *Mercury*.

Lycopodium.—Dark, grayish-yellow ulcers in throat, right side. Indolent chancres ; thick, rounded margins ; ulcers on legs refuse to heal ; burning tearing at night, poulticing or dressing ; golden-yellow pus.

Mercurius Bin-Iodide.—Hard, red swelling in front of prepuce, as thick and hard as lead pencil, with a hard chancre in its centre ; entirely painless.

Mercurius Cor.—Regular indurated Hunterian Chancre with lardaceous base ; excessive pain, swelling and inflammation. Destructive, serpiginous ulcers, eating out and destroying half of the penis in a few days.

Mercurius Proto-Iodide.—Painless chancres with great swelling of the inguinal glands, no tendency to suppurate.

SYPHILIS—(*Contd.*)

Mercurius Sol— Soft chancre or chancroid ; rather superficial than deep, dirty lardaceous base, fetid discharge.

Nitric Acid.—Ulcers spread more in circumference than in depth. Mercurio-Syphilitic cases. Phagedenic chancres with exuberant granulations, bleeding easily, raised and ragged edges, splinter pains. Buboes suppurating.

Thuja.—Splinter pains in chancres with moist excrescences on prepuce and glans.

Staphisagria.—Ulcers after abuse of *Mercury* ; discharge thin, acrid ; diseased bone beneath ; soft humid excrescences and dry figwarts about genital organs.

Sulphur.—Deep, suppurating ulcers on glans and prepuce ; burning, redness of prepuce ; phimosis ; glands indurated or suppurating.

WORMS

ASCARIDES—WORMS—HELMINTHIASIS

Aconite—Is lauded as of great value in relieving the nightly restlessness and intolerable itching of the anus caused by the Oxyuris (the thread, seat or pinworms) as they enter just within the sphincter and the folds of the anus. Each time this trouble comes the child is feverish, restless and sleepless at night.

Ratanhia & Teucrium.—Are also highly recommended in intolerable itching of the anus.

Ignatia.—When children become simply much excited from itching at anus at night. They also sometimes get convulsions with loss of consciousness and temporary inability to speak afterwards.

Ferrum.—Is indicated in itching at anus at night and involuntary micturition, in children of pale, wretched complexion, easily flushing.

Mercurius.—Is indicated for itching of the anus with continuous greediness for eating, all the while becoming steadily weaker, and have fetid breath ; in case of girls, inflammation of vulva from seat and round worms.

Sulphur.—For creeping in nose and biting in rectum and passage of lumbricoides, ascarides and tænia, with nausea before meals and faintness before dinner and restlessness at night.

Apocynum Andr. & Asclepias Syr.—Are useful for tickling sensation at the end of penis from ascarides.

WORMS—(*Contd.*)

Caladium.—Is the best remedy in little girls when the worms travel over the perinæum and get into the vagina producing great irritation. Also useful in women who suffer from pruritus vulvæ, from the same cause, which keep them awake at night and brings on nymphomania and induce masturbation.

(Symptoms like the following; Cachetic countenance, blue rings around the eyes, enlarged abdomen, fever, irritation of the brain, fits, convulsions etc., which have been ascribed to worms, are rather doubtful. In such cases a careful examination will, no doubt, lead to other exciting causes.)

For abdominal griping, increased secretion of mucus, diarrhœa, vomiting, irregular appetite or the reflex or sympathetic symptoms as itching of the nose, anus, genitals; enlargement of the pupils, squinting, increased flow of saliva, restless sleep with frequent starting and grating of teeth which are produced by round worms inhabiting in the small intestines and wander about and creep into remote cavities or organs a different group of medicines are required. Thus :—

Artemisia.—Convulsions from irritation of worms, passes stool and urine with the spasm. Strangury.

Baryta Mur.—Worm affections : fœtid breath, pain in region of navel, worse in the morning : great appetite, bloated abdomen, chronic painless diarrhœa, yellow slimy stools, vomiting, exhaustion and periodical attacks of convulsions.

Belladonna.—Drowsiness, starting in sleep, grating of teeth, involuntary micturition and defæcation ; squinting.

Cicuta Virosa.—Useful in convulsions from worms. The patient is suddenly rigid, with fixed staring eyes, bluish face, frothing at the mouth and unconscious. There are shocks and jerks through the body, frequent hiccough and crying, pain in the neck, dilated pupils, spasmodic drawing of the head backwards, tremor of hands, constriction of œsophagus. Trismus and alternate tonic and clonic spasms, opisthotonos. The convulsions are renewed from slightest touch, noise or jar. It seems to come in if *Cina* does not help.

Cina.—Most powerful for the elimination of round worms. The sickly appearance of the face, the blue rings about the eyes and the grinding of the teeth, rubbing of the nose, associated with canine hunger and itching of anus is the perfect picture of *Cina*. (For the oxyuris which appear about the anus and get into the rectum or vagina producing irritation *Cina* is of no avail). Restless sleep with rolling of eyes, squinting, face pale and cold or red and hot, loathing of food or

WORMS—(*Contd:*)

great hunger ; nausea, vomiting ; pain in the umbilical region : abdomen hard and distended ; constipation ; urine turbid when passed and turns milky after standing ; frequent sudden attacks of very high fever with convulsions and twitchings and contortions of limbs ; vomiting of lumbrici and ascarides.

Cuprum.—Is indicated in convulsions from worms with drawing in of the fingers, clenching of the thumbs and twitching of the muscles. There is spasmodic breathing and dyspnœa ; spasm of glottis, frothing at the mouth, grinding of the teeth, quick rotation of the eye-balls with the lids closed. The face becomes purple and there is spasm of the whole respiratory system of such a character that the child seems to be choking to death.

Indigo.—Convulsions from worms in melancholic children. Intense pain in the umbilical region, aggravated by pressure ; diarrhœa without injury to appetite or digestion.

Spigelia.—Used for worms when there are strabismus from abdominal irritation, jerking over eyes, paleness of face and blue rings around eyes. The patient feels faint and nauseated on awaking in the morning, relieved by eating breakfast. There is colic, worse about the navel, and the stood consists of mucus, fæces and worms.

Stannum.—According to Hahnemann, *Stannum* so stupefies the tape and round worms that they are easily dislodged by purgatives. It is also used for epileptiform convulsions from worms. The patient has a a pale face and dark rings around the eyes and colic which is relieved by hard pressure on the abdomen.

Terebinthina.—Worms have been removed by *Terebinthina.* Passes segments of tape worms. The child starts and screams out in sleep, pick at his nose, has a choking sensation and a dry, hacking cough. There is burning and tingling at the anus and rectum, lessened by applying cold water. Irritability and weakness of bowels, sharp appetite and thirst ; strange appetite after a square meal and foul breath. There are spasms and convulsions with staring look and clenching of fingers.

Besides those mentioned, recourse must be taken to the deep-acting, constitutional, anti-psoric remedies to eradicate the verminous diathesis. They must be prescribed on general constitutional basis—MUST BE PRESCRIBED FOR THE PATIENT, WITHOUT EVER THINKING OF PRESCRIBING FOR FOR THE WORMS. They will so correct the constitution that order will be established in the interior of the economy and the worms will no longer hatch out. Some amongst such remedies are : *Sulphur, Calcarea, Lycopodium, Silicea, Sabadilla, Merc. Sol and Chamomilla.*

INDEX